MW00583866

MOTOR CONTROL

Motor Control

Theories, Experiments, and Applications

Edited by

Frédéric Danion, PhD
Movement Sciences Institute
Centre National de la Recherche Scientifique
Theoretical Neuroscience Group
l'Université de la Méditerranée, Aix-Marseille II
Marseille, France

Mark L. Latash, PhD
Department of Kinesiology
The Pennsylvania State University
University Park, PA

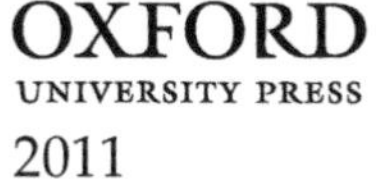

2011

OXFORD
UNIVERSITY PRESS

Oxford University Press, Inc., publishes works that further
Oxford University's objective of excellence
in research, scholarship, and education.

Oxford New York
Auckland Cape Town Dar es Salaam Hong Kong Karachi
Kuala Lumpur Madrid Melbourne Mexico City Nairobi
New Delhi Shanghai Taipei Toronto

With offices in
Argentina Austria Brazil Chile Czech Republic France Greece
Guatemala Hungary Italy Japan Poland Portugal Singapore
South Korea Switzerland Thailand Turkey Ukraine Vietnam

Published by Oxford University Press, Inc.
198 Madison Avenue, New York, New York 10016
www.oup.com

Library of Congress Cataloging-in-Publication Data

Motor control : theories, experiments, and applications/
edited by Frédéric Danion, Mark L. Latash.
p.; cm.
Includes bibliographical references and index.
ISBN 978-0-19-539527-3
1. Motor ability. 2. Human locomotion. I. Danion, Frédéric. II. Latash, Mark L., 1953-
[DNLM: 1. Movement—physiology. WE 103 M9175 2011]
QP301.M686 2011
612.7′6—dc22 2010014365

Preface

The brain is arguably the most fascinating object of scientific research. Voluntary movements are reflections of the brain activity and, as such, they provide a window into the functioning of this enigmatic organ. Movements have an advantage, as compared to such phenomena as memory, emotions, and cognition in general, in that they can be relatively easily quantified using the methods of classical mechanics. The goal of scientists in the field of motor control is to understand how the central nervous system interacts with the rest of the body and the environment so as to produce coordinated and purposeful movements. Under the word "understand," we mean to come up with a formal description operating with exactly defined variables that make physical and physiological sense. Researchers in motor control try to move toward achieving this goal using a variety of tools and approaches from different disciplines, such as neurophysiology, psychology, biomechanics, computational modeling, and, last but not least, physics. There are applied aspects to motor control that include, in particular, movement disorders, motor rehabilitation, and robotics. In contrast to many other valuable books that have focused on a specific aspect of movement studies, this book is an attempt to account for the diversity of the research performed in the field of motor control.

Over the past 20 years, motor control has become a recognized area of research. Over this time, many important developments have happened, including the emergence of an International Society of Motor Control, a journal "Motor Control," a series of biennial conferences "Progress in Motor Control," and the Annual Motor Control Summer School. The rapid development of this area also led to the publication of several books summarizing the recent progress and frequently emphasizing a particular direction of motor control research. This book, *Motor Control,* presents a comprehensive update on our current understanding. To achieve this goal, we invited leading scientists from various countries and with different backgrounds to present their current research and opinions on motor control. Last, but not least, another major goal of this project is to promote discussions and interactions across researchers from different subfields of motor control. We sincerely hope that this book will contribute to the integration of the fast expanding body of knowledge accumulated in the thriving field of motor control.

This book is designed primarily as a reference volume for researchers in the growing field of motor control. We hope that the book will be appreciated by our colleagues in a broad range of disciplines, from mechanics and engineering to psychology and neurophysiology. We also hope that the book will be useful for clinicians working in the areas of motor disorders and rehabilitation. The book can also be used as supplementary reading material for graduate students interested in the control of voluntary movements, movement disorders, robotics, and motor rehabilitation. Finally, although the book can be read one section after another, cross-referencing across chapters offers many alternative routes to navigate this exciting field.

Our thanks in producing this book go to all the contributing authors who managed to provide their chapters within the limited time frame and trusted in our ability to organize this project. We also wish to acknowledge the support of Oxford University Press in this project, especially of Craig Panner and David D'Addona for their work at different stages of this project. And last, we would like to thank the International Society of Motor Control for facilitating the exchange of ideas in the field of motor control.

Frédéric Danion
Mark Latash
Marseille, April 2010

Introduction

This volume is organized into six parts covering various aspects of motor control including theory, methodology, neurophysiology, biomechanics, motor learning, motor disorders, and robotics. The first part, Motor Control: Control of a Complex System, covers different theoretical and methodological approaches to motor control. The opening Chapter 1 by Latash reviews two influential hypotheses in the field, the referent configuration hypothesis (which represents a development of the equilibrium-point hypothesis) and a hypothesis on synergic control of movement that uses the computational apparatus developed within the uncontrolled manifold hypothesis. Latash suggests that a control hierarchy based on referent configurations at the whole-body, joint, and muscle levels may use synergic mechanisms stabilizing shifts of the task-related referent configuration expressed in salient for the motor task variables. He then describes a relatively novel phenomenon of anticipatory synergy adjustments and interprets it within the introduced framework.

The next chapter (Chapter 2), by Flanagan and Johansson, discusses how predictions influence not only our actions, but also our perceptual judgments. As an example, the authors focus on lifting tasks in which predictions about object mechanical properties, such as weight, play a critical role for both action and perception. Specifically, the chapter further addresses the relation between representations of objects employed by the action system and representations of the same objects used by the perceptual system to make judgments about object properties. Altogether, it is suggested that the brain maintains two distinct representations involved in predicting object properties: a slowly adapting one that supports perception and a rapidly adapting one that supports manipulatory actions.

Chapter 3, by Frank, Dotov, and Turvey, analyzes systems comprising agent, task, and environment as self-organizing open systems. They introduce an approach originating from physics that describes such systems as so-called canonical-dissipative oscillators. Such systems can be used to investigate the extent to which variables describing the agent, the task, and the environmental conditions affect control and coordination of movement. The authors apply the canonical-dissipative approach to study the emergence of oscillatory Parkinson's tremor, as well as to coordination in the context of paced and self-paced rhythmic limb movements.

Chapter 4, by Dodel et al. (a group headed by Jirsa), addresses issues of team performance as an extension of individual performance. The chapter examines the temporal nature of team behavior in a task in which four-member teams of various levels mimic an urban combat operation. The authors introduce a method based on the uncontrolled manifold approach that aims to identify crucial elements of team behavior in an observer-independent and time-resolved manner. Specifically, team behavior over time is represented as evolving manifolds in phase space. The authors suggest that expert team performance is distinguished by a larger degree of team coordination and team awareness.

The final chapter of the first part (Chapter 5), by Ting and Chvatal, examines methodological approaches to identification and quantification of multimuscle synergies. The chapter focuses on two methods that have been used recently, principal component analysis and non-negative matrix factorization. It addresses the implicit assumptions, practical issues, and caveats inherent to those methods. Using real data sets from human balance control and locomotion, the authors examine the robustness of these two methods across tasks and their implications for various muscle synergy hypotheses.

The second part, Cortical Mechanisms of Motor Control, presents two recent series of studies performed on monkeys. In Chapter 6, Riehle, Roux, Kilavik, and Grün describe a temporal coding hypothesis suggesting that not only changes in firing rate but also precise spike timing, especially synchrony, constitute an important part of the representational substrate for perception and action. In this framework, the concept of cell assemblies uses synchrony as an additional dimension to firing rate, as a candidate for information processing. Further, the chapter addresses possible mechanisms of performance optimization through practice achieved by boosting the computational contribution of spike synchrony while allowing an overall reduction in population activity.

Chapter 7, by Hatsopoulos, Olmedo, and Takahashi, presents a review of recently discovered spontaneous propagations of β frequency oscillations in the local field potential across the surface of the motor cortex along a rostral-to-caudal axis. These studies were performed on monkeys performing a variety of visuomotor tasks. The authors suggest a hypothesis that these propagating waves of local field potentials may promote proximal-to-distal recruitment of motor cortical neurons and therefore contribute to proximal-to-distal coordination as observed in multijoint movements such as throwing or jumping.

In the third part, three chapters reflect on Lessons from Biomechanics for motor control. In Chapter 8, Herzog analyzes the famous problem of motor redundancy at the level of multiple muscles crossing individual joints. He presents two of the classic ways in which biomechanics investigates movement control in redundant musculoskeletal systems. The first method is based on direct muscle force measurements in voluntary movements of animals, whereas the second method focuses on theoretical optimization approaches. The reviewed studies demonstrate that the mechanics of movements determine to a great extent muscle coordination strategies, and that muscle mechanical and physiological properties play a crucial role in movement control.

Chapter 9, by Prilutsky and Klishko, reviews the data on how quadrupedal animals operate their four extremities, select gaits, distribute loads between fore- and hindlimbs, divide labor among joints to generate the mechanical energy necessary for propulsion, and select specific muscles around individual joints to meet various task demands (slope, speed, required accuracy, and perturbations). The chapter provides new important perspectives on the interaction between central and afferent mechanisms in whole-body posture and locomotion control.

Duarte, Freitas, and Zatsiorsky, in Chapter 10, review a series of studies on the biomechanics of vertical posture. They present evidence suggesting that, during standing, humans maintain their posture not about a fixed point but about a position that in turn is also moving. Studies of unconstrained prolonged upright standing have shown that humans tend to oscillate about a moving reference position. Another example of this complex behavior is the postural sway of elderly adults. Commonly, older adults show an increase in postural sway, as compared to younger persons, when asked to stand as still as possible for a short period of time. However, during prolonged standing, elderly individuals adopt a "freezing" strategy reflecting their reduced ability to shift the body reference position in time.

The fourth part, Lessons from Motor Learning and Using Tools, includes four chapters. Chapter 11, by Imamizu, presents a review of functional magnetic resonance imaging (fMRI) studies of the human cerebellum. This chapter uses the language of internal models and describes the data in terms of the acquisition process of an internal model for a novel tool, modular organization of internal models for tools with different input-output properties, and switching mechanisms of internal models in the parietal-cerebellar network. The chapter also reviews studies of brain activity related to the imaginary use of common tools (e.g., scissors and a hammer). The author discusses how skills acquired in the cerebellum differ from those acquired in the frontal-parietal network, which have long been investigated in neuropsychological studies.

In Chapter 12, Sternad and Abe describe a technique to analyze motor variability by parsing it into three components termed *Tolerance*, *Noise*, and *Covariation*. This technique was used to analyze the results of three experiments focusing on the following questions: What aspects of variability decrease with practice? And, are actors sensitive to their intrinsic noise in selecting strategies? The authors show that changes with practice of the three components happen not simultaneously but in a ranked order. First, the subjects explore and find new ways of executing the task. This is followed by optimizing covariation, and finally the noise component experiences an improvement.

Frey, in Chapter 13, addressed a remarkable human ability to be able to forecast the demands of a wide variety of actions without performing movements. The chapter describes recent behavioral and fMRI work that focuses on identifying the brain mechanisms involved in prospectively selecting grasping actions based on use of the hands or recently mastered tool. Despite the complete absence of movements, the author find that the parietal and premotor regions implicated in the sensorimotor control of grasping also participate in these forecasts.

The last chapter in this part, by Avizzano, Ruffaldi, and Bergamasco, Chapter 14, addresses the use of virtual environment technology for training specific tasks. The chapter presents an integrated methodology to combine technological environments for training with specific pedagogical and training elements that are usually kept into account during traditional training.

The fifth part, which addresses Lessons from Studies of Aging and Motor Disorders, includes three chapters. Chapter 15, by Vaillancourt and Prodoehl, reviews models of basal ganglia function relevant to the pathophysiology of Parkinson disease that have emerged from studies in both nonhuman primates and rodents. It questions the relevance of those studies to early-stage Parkinson disease and to nonmotor signs of this disorder. Further, the chapter focuses on what is currently known regarding the motor and nonmotor features of early-stage patients with Parkinson disease who have not yet started any symptomatic treatment. A substantial focus of the chapter examines brain imaging studies of de novo Parkinson disease.

The chapter by Vasudevan, Torres-Oviedo, and Bastian (Chapter 16) reviews the adaptation of walking on a split-belt treadmill, a device that allows the researcher to control the speed of each leg independently. The authors have found that this learning is disrupted by cerebellar damage, but is undisturbed by cerebral damage following a stroke or hemispherectomy. This evidence suggests that the cerebellum, but not the cerebrum, is critical for predictive locomotor adjustments and offers the possibility of improving the locomotor patterns of people with cerebral damage through adaptive processes. The authors describe how, by using the split-belt treadmill to exaggerate a gait asymmetry, hemiparesis due to stroke or hemispherectomy can be corrected.

Swinnen, Heuninckx, Van Impe, Goble, Coxon, and Wenderoth, in Chapter 17, address the involvement of different brain regions into coordination of the ipsilateral hand and foot in elderly persons. The increased activation in brain regions involved in motor coordination, sensory processing/integration, visual imagery strategies, and cognitive monitoring points to a shift from automatic to controlled processing of movement in aging adults. Evidence suggests that the increased activation in some (but not all) brain areas is correlated with better performance. This suggests that altered brain function in the elderly can be "compensatory" in nature, possibly reflecting neuroplastic changes.

The last, sixth part of the volume reviews Lessons from Robotics and includes three chapters. Chapter 18 by Knuesel, Cabelguen, and Ijspeert reviews mathematical models and salamander-like robots that have been used to test hypotheses concerning the organization of the central pattern generators in the spinal cord and the mechanism of gait transition. These models and robots have been inspired by observations of the transitions between walking and swimming in salamanders. The findings reported in the chapter suggest that the ability of salamanders to switch between swimming and walking can be explained by a spinal cord circuit that is based on a primitive neural circuit for swimming.

Chapter 19, by Franceschini, Ruffier, and Serres, reviews studies on insects and insect-like flying robots. The authors present the concept of the optic flow regulator, a feedback control system based on optic flow sensors. They use both experiments and simulations to show that insect-like robots, a micro-helicopter and a micro-hovercraft, can behave very much like insects when placed in similar environments. The proposed simple and parsimonious control schemes function without any conventional devices, such as radio-altimeters, laser range-finders, radars, or GPS receivers. The simplicity of the proposed control puts little demand on neural resources and shows great potential for simplifying the design of aerial and space vehicles.

In the last chapter (Chapter 20), Guigon presents an overview of many problems inherent to the control of movements in humans and in robots. These problems include the problem of motor redundancy (Bernstein's problem), the interactions between posture and movement, the use of internal models, and issues of optimality and efficacy. Ways of solving such problems in humanoid robots are discussed.

We tried to make the book more readable by encouraging the authors to cross-reference other chapters and to present all the necessary background material in the introductory parts. Nevertheless, we appreciate that the breadth of this book will likely present a challenge to the readers. We hope, however, that the effort required to read the book will be rewarded by the many exciting ideas and perspectives that cover the spectrum of research activities united under the name "motor control."

Contents

Contributors

Masaki O. Abe, PhD
Departments of Biology, Electrical & Computer Engineering, and Physics
Northeastern University
Boston, MA

Carlo A. Avizzano, PhD
Perceptual Robotics Laboratory (PERCRO)
Scuola Superiore Sant'Anna
Pisa, Italy

Amy J. Bastian, PhD
Motion Analysis Lab
Kennedy Krieger Institute; and
Department of Neuroscience
The Johns Hopkins School of Medicine
Baltimore, MD

Massimo Bergamasco, PhD
Perceptual Robotics Laboratory (PERCRO)
Scuola Superiore Sant'Anna
Pisa, Italy

Jean-Marie Cabelguen, PhD
Neurocentre INSERM
F. Magendie Institute
Bordeaux University
Bordeaux, France

Stacie A. Chvatal, BS
The Wallace H. Coulter Department of Biomedical Engineering
Emory University and Georgia Institute of Technology
Atlanta, GA

Joseph V. Cohn, PhD
Defense Advanced Research Projects Agency
Arlington, VA

James P. Coxon, PhD
Motor Control Laboratory
Research Center for Movement Control and Neuroplasticity
Department for Biomedical Kinesiology
Katholieke Universiteit Leuven
Heverlee, Belgium

Silke M. Dodel, PhD
Center for Complex Systems and Brain Sciences
Florida Atlantic University
Boca Raton, FL

Dobromir G. Dotov, PhD
Department of Psychology
Center for the Ecological Study of Perception and Action
University of Connecticut
Storrs, CT

Marcos Duarte, PhD
Escola de Educação Física e Esporte
Universidade de São Paulo
São Paulo, Brazil

Philip W. Fink, PhD
Center for Complex Systems and Brain Sciences
Florida Atlantic University
Boca Raton, FL

J. Randall Flanagan, PhD
Department of Psychology
Centre for Neuroscience Studies
Queen's University
Kingston, Ontario
Canada

Nicolas Franceschini, PhD
Biorobotics Lab, Institute of Movement Science
Centre National de la Recherche Scientifique
l'Université de la Méditerranée, Aix-Marseille II
Marseille, France

Till D. Frank, PhD
Department of Psychology
Center for the Ecological Study of Perception and Action
University of Connecticut
Storrs, CT

Sandra M.S.F. Freitas, PhD
Escola de Educação Física e Esporte
Universidade de São Paulo City
São Paulo, Brazil

Scott H. Frey, PhD
Department of Psychology
Lewis Center for Neuroimaging
University of Oregon
Eugene, OR

Daniel J. Goble, PhD
Motor Control Laboratory
Research Center for Movement Control and Neuroplasticity
Department for Biomedical Kinesiology
Katholieke Universiteit Leuven
Heverlee, Belgium

Sonja Grün, PhD
RIKEN Brain Science Institute
Wako-Shi, Japan

Emmanuel Guigon, PhD
Institut des Systèmes Intelligents et de Robotique
UPMC University of Paris; and CNRS
Paris, France

Nicholas G. Hatsopoulos, PhD
Department of Organismal Biology and Anatomy
Committee on Computational Neuroscience
University of Chicago
Chicago, IL

Sofie Heuninckx, PhD
Motor Control Laboratory
Research Center for Movement Control
and Neuroplasticity
Department for Biomedical Kinesiology
Katholieke Universiteit Leuven
Heverlee, Belgium

Walter Herzog, PhD
Human Performance Laboratory
Faculties of Kinesiology, Engineering, and Medicine
University of Calgary
Calgary, Alberta
Canada

Auke Ijspeert, PhD
School of Engineering, Institute of Bioengineering
EPFL, Ecole Polytechnique Fédérale de Lausanne
Lausanne, Switzerland

Hiroshi Imamizu, PhD
National Institute of Information and
Communications Technology (NICT)
Advanced Telecommunications Research (ATR)
Institute International
Seika-cho, Soraku-gun, Kyoto
Japan

Viktor K. Jirsa, PhD
Center for Complex Systems and Brain Sciences
Florida Atlantic University
Boca Raton, FL; and
Movement Sciences Institute
Centre National de la Recherche Scientifique
Theoretical Neuroscience Group
l'Université de la Méditerranée, Aix-Marseille II
Marseille, France

Roland S. Johansson, MD, PhD
Physiology Section
Department of Integrative Medical Biology
Umeå University
Umeå, Sweden

Bjørg Elisabeth Kilavik, PhD
Mediterranean Institute of Cognitive Neuroscience (INCM)
Centre National de la Recherche Scientifique
l'Université de la Méditerranée, Aix-Marseille II
Marseille, France; and
RIKEN Brain Science Institute
Wako-Shi, Japan

Alexander N. Klishko, PhD
School of Applied Physiology
Georgia Institute of Technology
Atlanta, GA

Jeremie Knuesel, PhD
School of Engineering, Institute of Bioengineering
EPFL, Ecole Polytechnique Fédérale de Lausanne
Lausanne, Switzerland

Mark L. Latash, PhD
Department of Kinesiology
The Pennsylvania State University
University Park, PA

Eric R. Muth, PhD
Department of Psychology
Clemson University
Clemson, SC

Leonel Olmedo
Department of Organismal Biology and Anatomy
Committee on Computational Neuroscience
University of Chicago
Chicago, IL

Ajay S. Pillai, PhD
Center for Complex Systems and Brain Sciences
Florida Atlantic University
Boca Raton, FL

Boris I. Prilutsky, PhD
School of Applied Physiology
Georgia Institute of Technology
Atlanta, GA

Janey Prodoehl, PT, PhD
Department of Kinesiology and Nutrition
University of Illinois at Chicago
Chicago, IL

Alexa Riehle, PhD
Mediterranean Institute of Cognitive Neuroscience (INCM)
Centre National de la Recherche Scientifique
l'Université de la Méditerranée, Aix-Marseille II
Marseille, France; and
RIKEN Brain Science Institute
Wako-Shi, Japan

Sébastien Roux, PhD
Mediterranean Institute of Cognitive Neuroscience (INCM)
Centre National de la Recherche Scientifique
l'Université de la Méditerranée, Aix-Marseille II
Marseille, France; and
Bernstein Center for Computational Neuroscience (BCCN)
Neurobiology and Biophysics
Institute of Biology III
Albert Ludwig University
Freiburg, Germany

Emanuele Ruffaldi, PhD
Perceptual Robotics Laboratory (PERCRO)
Scuola Superiore Sant'Anna
Pisa, Italy

Frank Ruffier, PhD
Biorobotics Lab, Institute of Movement Science
Centre National de la Recherche Scientifique
l'Université de la Méditerranée, Aix-Marseille II
Marseille, France

Dylan D. Schmorrow, PhD
Office of the Secretary of Defense
Vienna, VA

Julien Serres, PhD
Biorobotics Lab, Institute of Movement Science
Centre National de la Recherche Scientifique
l'Université de la Méditerranée, Aix-Marseille II
Marseille, France

Dagmar Sternad, PhD
Departments of Biology, Electrical & Computer Engineering, and Physics
Northeastern University
Boston, MA

Roy Stripling
Human Performance Training and Education
Office of Naval Research
Arlington, VA

Stephen P. Swinnen, PhD
Motor Control Laboratory
Research Center for Movement Control and Neuroplasticity
Department for Biomedical Kinesiology
Katholieke Universiteit Leuven
Heverlee, Belgium

Kazutaka Takahashi, PhD
Department of Organismal Biology and Anatomy
Committee on Computational Neuroscience
University of Chicago
Chicago, IL

Lena H. Ting, PhD
The Wallace H. Coulter Department of Biomedical Engineering
Emory University and Georgia Institute of Technology
Atlanta, GA

Gelsy Torres-Oviedo, PhD
Motion Analysis Lab
Kennedy Krieger Institute
Baltimore, MD; and
Department of Neuroscience
The Johns Hopkins School of Medicine
Baltimore, MD

Michael T. Turvey, PhD
Department of Psychology
Center for the Ecological Study of Perception and Action
University of Connecticut
Storrs, CT

David E. Vaillancourt, PhD
Departments of Kinesiology and Nutrition
Bioengineering and Neurology and Rehabilitation
University of Illinois at Chicago
Chicago, IL

Annouchka Van Impe
Motor Control Laboratory
Research Center for Movement Control and Neuroplasticity
Department for Biomedical Kinesiology
Katholieke Universiteit Leuven
Heverlee, Belgium

Erin V. L. Vasudevan, PhD
Moss Rehabilitation Research Institute
Albert Einstein Healthcare Network
Elkins Park, PA

Nicole Wenderoth, PhD
Motor Control Laboratory
Research Center for Movement Control and Neuroplasticity
Department for Biomedical Kinesiology
Katholieke Universiteit Leuven
Heverlee, Belgium

Vladimir Zatsiorsky, PhD
Department of Kinesiology
The Pennsylvania State University
University Park, PA

Part 1

Motor Control

Control of a Complex System

1

Anticipatory Control of Voluntary Action

Merging the Ideas of Equilibrium-point Control and Synergic Control

Mark L. Latash

There is little argument that animals can behave in a predictive manner: A predator chasing a prey does not run, fly, or swim toward the prey's current location but tries to intercept it at a future point along the likely (anticipated) trajectory. Many human actions involve similar behaviors. Obvious examples include catching a ball, swinging a tennis racket, and pressing a brake pedal to stop at the approaching red light or releasing it when you expect the light to turn green. However, anticipatory actions are not limited to situations involving a moving, changing external target or signal.

One of the first examples of anticipatory actions studied in the field of motor control was anticipatory postural adjustments (APAs, reviewed in Massion 1992). APAs represent changes in the activation of postural muscles that are seen in a standing person prior to an action that produces (directly or indirectly) a mechanical postural perturbation. Starting from the pioneering paper by Belen'kii and co-authors (1967), APAs have been discussed as the means of producing muscle forces and moments of forces counteracting the expected perturbation (Bouisset and Zattara 1987, 1990; Friedli et al. 1988; Ramos and Stark 1990). I will revisit the notion of APAs at the end of this chapter and try to offer an alternative hypothesis on their origin and function.

The central nervous system (CNS) has to act in an anticipatory manner not only when engaged in tasks of intercepting a moving target, as in the predator–prey example, or in producing movements with an explicit postural component, as in studies of APAs, but also when it produces virtually any natural human voluntary action. The necessity to act in an anticipatory fashion is typically discussed in relation to the design of the human body, which makes it look inferior to human-built artificial moving systems such as robots. Indeed, the speed of information transmission along neural fibers is much lower than along electric wires, and muscles look sluggish when compared to powerful torque motors.

Many researchers of the past contemplated the apparent problems posed to the CNS by such factors as the relatively long time delays in the transmission of both sensory (afferent) and motor (efferent) action potentials, the relatively slow muscles with their nonlinear viscoelastic properties, and the complex mechanical interactions both within the body (due to the mechanical coupling of body segments) and between the moving body and the environment (Bernstein 1935, 1967; van Ingen Schenau et al. 1995; van Soest and van Ingen Schenau 1998). Indeed, if one starts with classical mechanics, to produce a movement of a material object from one point in space to another, requisite forces have to be applied to the object to induce its required movement. All the mentioned features of the human body design look like sources for a host of computational problems for the neural controller if it has to precompute and produce such requisite force time profiles. How can the CNS make sure that proper forces act at an effector at a certain time, when it has to send signals to the motoneuronal pools that innervate muscles moving the effector in advance, based on outdated sensory information? When the efferent signals reach the motoneurons and—ultimately—the muscles, the muscle state will change, and the muscle forces will differ from those that could have been expected based on the sensory signals available to the controller when it issued the efferent command.

Apparently, to make sure that muscles produce required forces at proper times, the controller has to predict many things. First, it has to predict what efferent signals will be required to ensure the desired movement of the effector in future. This is presumably accomplished with the help of inverse models. Second, the controller has to predict what will happen with the effectors when the efferent signals reach them (accomplished with direct models). Both model types have to be used simultaneously to ensure accurate motor action, because forces and effector states (such as, for example, muscle length and velocity) are tightly coupled. In fact, several papers presented arguments in favor of cascades of internal models, both inverse and direct, as the basis for accurate voluntary actions (Kawato 1999; Wolpert et al. 1998).

This field of study, commonly called *internal models* research, has been developed to deal with such problems and address the regularities of such predictive actions (reviewed in Kawato 1990; Shadmehr and Wise 2005; see also Flanagan and Johansson, this volume). Unfortunately, from the subjective view of the author, this field has been tightly linked to force-control schemes (i.e., the assumption that the CNS in some fashion precomputes efferent signals that make sure that "requisite forces are generated" [cf. Hinder and Milner 2003]). The idea of force-control (or muscle activation control, which is similar to force-control; Gottlieb et al. 1989; Gottlieb 1996; Feldman et al. 1998) has been critically reviewed in both classical and recent papers (Bernstein 1936; Ostry and Feldman 2003; Feldman and Latash 2005;

Latash 2008), so it makes little sense to repeat all the arguments against this position here.

It is rather interesting that, in personal conversations, quite a few champions of the internal model approach try to distance themselves from force-control views and claim that "it does not matter what the internal models precompute." First, this view seems to make the idea of internal models very fuzzy and imprecise. Using such terms does not help to bring clarity and exactness into the field of motor control; hinting at approaches to discuss complex scientific issues produces a very suboptimal route to understanding the nature of these issues. Second, in virtually all publications that make comparisons with experimental data, it is either explicitly or implicitly assumed that internal models do deal with forces and torques (for example, see Shadmehr and Mussa-Ivaldi 1994; Hinder and Milner 2003).

The purpose of this chapter is to put predictive (anticipatory) actions into the perspective of a physiologically based motor control theory and a theory of synergic actions. I accept the equilibrium-point hypothesis, or to be more exact, its recent development in the form of the referent configuration hypothesis (Feldman et al. 2007; Feldman and Levin 2009) as *the* motor control theory. I also accept the principle of abundance (Gelfand and Latash 1998) and the recently developed view on the problem of motor redundancy that uses the computational approach of the uncontrolled manifold (UCM) hypothesis (Scholz and Schöner 1999; for review see Latash et al. 2002b, 2007). These hypotheses can be united naturally into a single coherent scheme on the control and coordination of voluntary movements. In particular, they offer a fresh view on the neural organization of anticipatory actions.

A GENERAL SCHEME OF MOVEMENT CONTROL

The equilibrium-point hypothesis (Feldman 1966, 1986; Feldman and Levin 1995) is, to my knowledge, the only theory in the field of motor control that specifies a physiological variable that is used by the CNS as a control variable. The equilibrium-point hypothesis posits that the threshold properties of neurons are used to modify input signal ranges, to which the neuron responds with action potentials. This mode of control can only be used in the presence of feedback signals to the neurons related to variables that the neurons produce (for example, in the presence of length- and force-related feedback to α-motoneurons). A deafferented neuron cannot in principle be controlled using this method, and the controller has to invent alternative methods of control, such as directly setting the total input to the neuron and, hence, its output (cf. the α-model, Bizzi et al. 1982).

The idea of threshold control is illustrated in Figure 1.1 (see Latash 2010). A group of neurons, N1, project to a target (this may be another group of neurons, a muscle, or a group of muscles) with an efferent signal (EFF), ultimately resulting in salient changes for the motor task mechanical variables.

I will address these variables collectively as the actual configuration (AC) of the body. The input into N1 is produced by a hierarchically higher element that uses changes in subthreshold depolarization (D, see Fig. 1.1B) of N1, thus defining a minimal excitatory afferent input (AFF) that leads to N1 response. Command D may also be viewed as defining a referent configuration (RC) of the body—a value of AC at which the neurons N1 are exactly at the threshold for activation. The difference between RC and current AC is sensed by another neuron ("sensor" in Fig. 1.1A), which generates a signal AFF projecting back on N1.

Panel B of Figure 1.1 illustrates the physiological meaning of control signal D. Note that N1 activity is zero when the AFF signal is under a certain threshold magnitude, and it increases with an increase in AFF above this threshold. The graph in Figure 1.1C illustrates the output level of N1 (EFF) as a function of the afferent signals (AFF) sent by the sensor neuron for two values of the subthreshold depolarization (D_1 and D_2). Note that setting a value for the control signal D does not define the output of N1. Note also that, for a fixed AFF input (e.g., A_1), the output may differ (cf. E_1 and E_2) depending on the value of D (cf. D_1 and D_2).

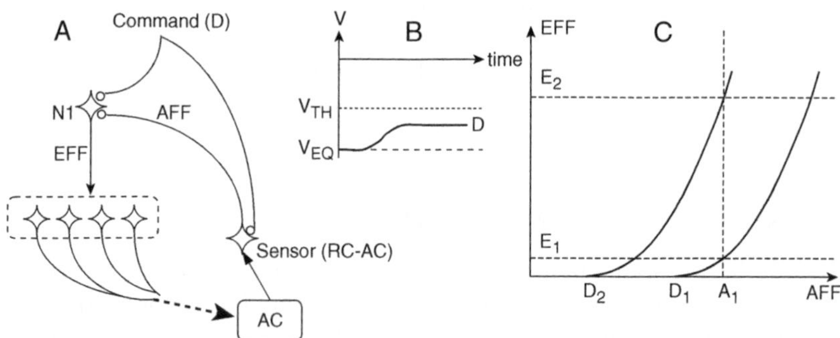

Figure 1.1 **A**: The idea of threshold control. A group of neurons, N1 project on a target that responds to the efferent signal (EFF) with changes in a set of mechanical variables addressed as actual configuration of the body (AC). The difference between the centrally set referent configuration (RC) and AC is sensed by another neuron (sensor), which projects back on N1. This feedback system is controlled by setting subthreshold depolarization (D) of N1 to define a minimal excitatory input from the sensor neuron (AFF) that leads to N1 response. **B**: An illustration of the physiological meaning of the control signal D. **C**: The output of N1 (EFF) as a function of the afferent signals (AFF) for two values of the subthreshold depolarization (D_1 and D_2). Note that setting a value of the control signal D does not define the output of N1. Note also that for a fixed afferent input (A_1), the output may differ (cf. E_1 and E_2) depending on D (cf. D_1 and D_2). Modified by permission from Latash, M.L. (2010) Stages in learning motor synergies: A view based on the equilibrium-point hypothesis. *Human Movement Science* (in press), with permission of the publisher.

The drawing in Figure 1.1A illustrates a feedback system controlled in a feedforward way. The control variable D, however, may be produced by a similar system using another neuronal pool with a feedback loop. In general, the scheme in the upper drawing may be viewed as representing an element of a control hierarchy.

For a single muscle, the illustration in Figure 1.1 is analogous to manipulating the threshold of the tonic stretch reflex (λ, see Feldman 1966, 1986), whereas the reflex mechanism (together with peripheral muscle properties) defines a relationship between active muscle force and length. Within the classical equilibrium-point hypothesis, the tonic stretch reflex is viewed as a built-in universal feedback system common to all skeletal muscles. As a result, all motor control processes move through this lowest level of the neuromotor hierarchy.

Within this scheme, control of any motor act may be viewed as consisting of two processes. First, a salient output variable has to be coupled to a salient sensory variable. Second, the output of this loop has to project onto appropriate hierarchically lower loops, ultimately ending up with tonic stretch reflex loops for all participating muscles. Setting the threshold for activation of the hierarchically highest neuronal group will trigger a chain of events at all levels of the hierarchy, ultimately leading to a state at which all elements (including the muscles) show the lowest levels of activation compatible with the set RC value (note that RC may involve variables related to muscle coactivation) and environmental and anatomical constraints. This has been addressed as the *principle of minimal final action* (Latash 2008).

Consider, for example, the task of moving the endpoint of a multijoint effector into a specific point in space in the presence of an external force field. The salient mechanical variables for this task are the force vector (F) at the endpoint and its coordinate vector (X). Imagine that there is a neuronal pool with the output that ultimately defines the force vector (certainly, after a chain of transformations similar to the elementary transformation in Fig. 1.1) and the afferent input corresponding to the coordinate vector. Setting a threshold for activation of the pool expressed in coordinate units (X_{TH}) may be described with an equation linking the force and coordinate vectors: $F = f(X - X_{TH})$, where f is a monotonically increasing function. To reach an equilibrium at the required location, $F = -F_{EXT}$, where F_{EXT} is the external force vector. Then, the problem is reduced to finding X_{TH} that would satisfy the equation: $F_{EXT} + f(X_{FIN} - X_{TH}) = 0$, where X_{FIN} is the desired final coordinate vector.

In fact, during voluntary movements, a person can define not only a point in space where the endpoint comes to an equilibrium, but also by how much the endpoint would deviate from X_{FIN} under small changes in F_{EXT}. This property is commonly addressed as *endpoint stability* (cf. impedance control, Hogan 1984) and quantified using an ellipsoid of apparent stiffness (Flash 1987). For a single joint with one kinematic degree of freedom, apparent stiffness may be described with only one parameter. For the limb endpoint in three-dimensional space, the ellipsoid of stiffness, in general, requires six parameters to be defined (the directions and magnitudes of the three main axes). However, humans cannot arbitrarily modulate all six parameters; these seem to be linked in such a way that the three axes of the ellipsoid of stiffness scale their magnitudes in parallel (Flash and Mussa-Ivaldi 1990).

So, in the most general case, two complex (vector) variables may be used to describe control of an arbitrary point on the human body, {R;C}, where $R = X_{TH}$, and C is related to setting stability features of X; C can be expressed as a range of X within which muscles with opposing mechanical action are activated simultaneously. Note that C does not have to be directly related to physically defined links between variables, such as stiffness or apparent stiffness. Setting feedback loops between an arbitrary efferent variable and an arbitrary afferent variable may produce neural links between variables that are not linked by laws of mechanics. Imagine, for example, a loop between a neuronal pool that defines mechanical output of an arm and a sensory variable related to the state of the foot. Such a loop may be used to stabilize the body at a minimal time delay when a person is standing and grasping a pole in a bus, and the bus starts to move unexpectedly.

The next step is to ensure that an {R;C} pair projects onto appropriate, hierarchically lower neural structures (Fig. 1.2). For the earlier example of placing the endpoint of a limb into a point in space, the next step may be viewed as defining signals to neuronal pools controlling individual joints {r;c} (cf. Feldman 1980, 1986). And, finally, the signals have to be converted into those for individual muscles, λs, using the "final common path" (to borrow the famous term introduced by Sherrington 1906) of the tonic stretch reflex.

As illustrated in Figures 1.1 and 1.2, each of these steps is likely to involve a few-to-many mapping (i.e., a problem of redundancy), which is considered in the next section.

THE PRINCIPLE OF ABUNDANCE AND MOTOR SYNERGIES

All neuromotor processes within the human body associated with performing natural voluntary movements involve several few-to-many mappings that are commonly addressed as problems of redundancy. In other words, constraints defined by an input (for example, by a task and external forces) do not define unambiguously the patterns of an output (for example, patterns of joint rotations, muscle forces, activation of motoneurons, etc.), such that numerous (commonly, an infinite number of) solutions exist. This problem has been emphasized by Bernstein (1935, 1967), who viewed it as the central problem of motor control: How does the CNS select, in each given action, a particular solution from the numerous seemingly equivalent alternatives? The formulation of this question implies that the CNS

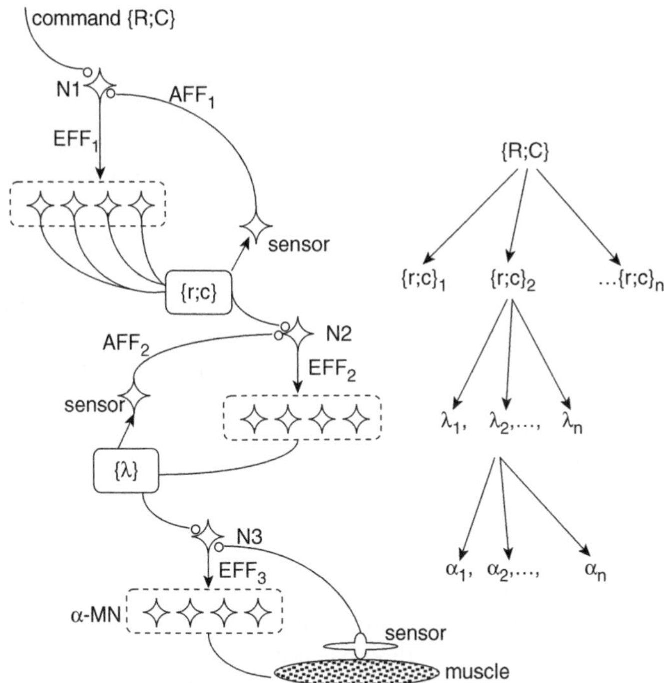

Figure 1.2 Left: An example of a control hierarchy from a referent body configuration {R,C} to signals to individual joints {r,c}, to signals to individual muscles (λ). Tonic stretch reflex is a crucial component of the last stage. At each step, a few-to-many mapping takes place. Right: A schematic illustration of the same idea.

does select a single, optimal solution when it is faced with a problem of motor redundancy, possibly based on an optimization principle (reviewed in Prilutsky 2000; Rosenbaum et al. 1993, Latash 1993; see also Herzog, this volume). This view has been supported by experimental studies claiming processes of freezing and releasing of degrees of freedom in the course of motor learning (Newell and van Emmerik 1989; Vereijken et al. 1992).

An alternative view is that the numerous degrees of freedom do not pose computational problems to the CNS but rather represent a rich (and even luxurious!) apparatus that allows the CNS to ensure stable behavior in conditions of unpredictable external forces and when it has to perform several tasks simultaneously (Zhang et al. 2008; Gera et al. 2010). This approach has been termed the *principle of abundance* (Gelfand and Latash 1998). It formed the foundation of a particular view on the organization of apparently redundant sets of elements into motor synergies.

According to this view, synergy is a neural organization that ensures a few-to-many mapping that stabilizes certain characteristics of behavior.

Operationally, this definition means that, if a person performs a task several times, deviations of elemental variables from their average patterns covary, such that variance of an important performance variable is low. The definition implies that synergies always "do something" (they provide stability of salient performance variables), they can be modified in a task-specific way (the same set of elemental variables may be used to stabilize different performance variables), and a large set of elemental variables may be used to create several synergies at the same time, thus stabilizing different features of performance. For example, the expression "a hand synergy" carries little meaning, but it is possible to say "a synergy among individual finger forces stabilizing the total force" or "a synergy among moments of force produced by individual digits stabilizing the total moment of force applied to the hand-held object." A number of recent studies have suggested that sometimes covariation among elemental variables does not stabilize a performance variable but rather contributes to its change (Olafsdottir et al. 2005; Kim et al. 2006); in such cases, one may say that a synergy acts to destabilize the performance variable in order to facilitate its quick change.

The introduced definition of synergy requires a computational method that would be able to distinguish a synergy from a nonsynergy and to quantify synergies. Such a method has been developed within the framework of the UCM hypothesis (Scholz and Schöner 1999; reviewed in Latash et al. 2002b, 2007). The UCM hypothesis assumes that a neural controller acts in a space of elemental variables and selects in that space a subspace (a UCM) corresponding to a desired value for a performance variable. Further, the controller organizes interactions among the elements in such a way that the variance in the space of elemental variables is mostly confined to the UCM. Commonly, analysis within the UCM hypothesis is done in a linear approximation, and the UCM is approximated with the null-space of the Jacobian matrix linking small changes in the elemental variables to those in the performance variable.

Consider the simplest case of a mechanically redundant system: two effectors that have to produce a certain magnitude of their summed output (Figure 1.3). The space of elemental variables is two-dimensional (a plane), whereas the desired magnitude of the summed output may be represented as a one-dimensional subspace (the solid line). This line is the UCM that corresponds to this performance variable ($PV = E_1 + E_2$). As long as the system stays on that line, the task is performed perfectly, and the controller does not need to interfere. According to the UCM hypothesis, the controller is expected to organize covariation of E_1 and E_2 over a set of trials in such a way that the cloud of data points recorded in the trials is oriented parallel to the UCM. Formally, this may be expressed as an inequality $V_{UCM} > V_{ORT}$, where V_{UCM} stands for variance along the UCM and V_{ORT} stands for variance along the orthogonal subspace (shown as the dashed slanted line in Figure 1.3). Another, more intuitive pair of terms have been used to describe

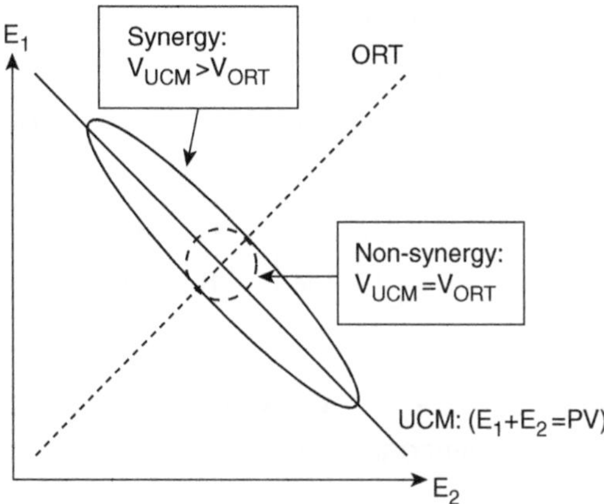

Figure 1.3 An illustration of two possible data distributions for a system that uses two elemental variables (E_1 and E_2) to produce a value of their combined output (performance variable – PV). Two components of variance are illustrated, "good" (V_{UCM}) and "bad" (V_{ORT}). The same performance variance may be achieved with (*solid ellipse*, $V_{UCM} > V_{ORT}$) and without (*dashed circle*, $V_{UCM} = V_{ORT}$) a synergy.

the two variance components: "good" and "bad" variance (V_{GOOD} and V_{BAD}). V_{BAD} hurts accuracy of performance, whereas V_{GOOD} does not, while it allows the system to be flexible and deal with external perturbations and/or secondary tasks (Gorniak et al. 2008; Shapkova et al. 2008). For example, having large V_{GOOD} may help a person to open a door with his elbow while carrying a cup of hot coffee in his hand.

HIERARCHIES OF SYNERGIES

According to the seminal paper by Gelfand and Tsetlin (1966), an input into a synergy (they used the term "structural unit") is provided by a hierarchically higher synergy, while its output serves as an input into a hierarchically lower synergy. A typical example of a control hierarchy is the control of the human hand during prehensile tasks. Commonly, such actions are viewed as controlled by a two-level hierarchy (Arbib et al. 1985; MacKenzie and Iberall 1994) (Fig. 1.4). At the upper level, the task is shared between the thumb and a virtual finger (an imaginary digit with a mechanical action equal to the summed actions of all actual fingers). At the lower level, the virtual finger action is shared among the actual fingers. Note that, at each level, a problem of motor redundancy emerges with respect to the resultant force and moment of force vectors (reviewed in Zatsiorsky and Latash 2008; Latash and Zatsiorsky 2009).

Several studies have demonstrated the existence of two-digit synergies at the upper level, typically stabilizing the total force and total moment of

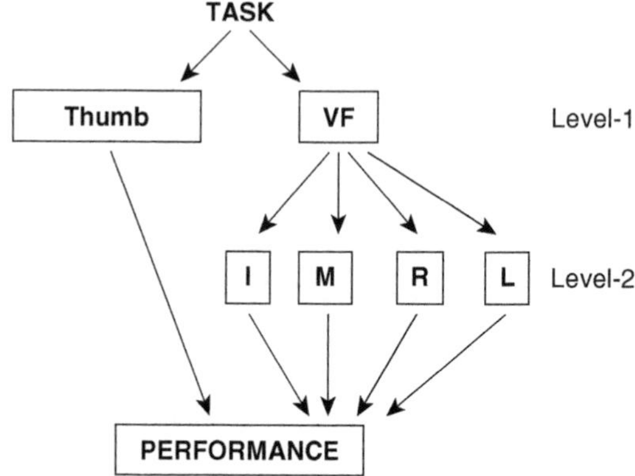

Figure 1.4 An illustration of a two-level hierarchy controlling the human hand. At the upper level (*Level-1*), the task is shared between the thumb and the virtual finger. At the lower level (*Level-2*), action of the virtual finger is shared among the actual fingers (I, index; M, middle; R, ring; and L, little).

force acting on the hand-held object (Shim et al. 2003, 2005; Gorniak et al. 2009), and four-digit synergies at the lower level, typically stabilizing the total pressing force by the virtual finger, its moment of force, and force direction (Shim et al. 2004; Gao et al. 2005). However, a few recent studies have shown that trade-offs may occur between synergies at different levels of a control hierarchy (Gorniak et al. 2007a,b; 2009). Indeed, imagine the task of constant total force production by two pairs of fingers, two per hand. At the upper level, the task is shared between the hands. Figure 1.3 suggests that a force-stabilizing synergy should correspond to $V_{GOOD} > V_{BAD}$. Note, however, that each hand's force variance gets contributions from both V_{GOOD} and V_{BAD}. So, large V_{GOOD} favors a strong synergy at the two-hand level, but it produces large V_{BAD} at the within-a-hand level (by definition, hand force variability is V_{BAD} when considered at the lower level).

Note that the hierarchy in Figure 1.4 resembles that illustrated earlier in Figure 1.2. It suggests that the problems of redundancy within the hierarchy of control variables in Figure 1.2 may be resolved by arranging synergies at each level that stabilize the variables assigned at the hierarchically higher level. In other words, there may be {r;c} synergies stabilizing {R;C} and {λ} synergies stabilizing {r;c}. There are reasons to expect such synergies: In particular, several studies have demonstrated multijoint kinematic synergies stabilizing the trajectory of a limb's endpoint during tasks that required accurate positioning of the endpoint in a given external force field (Domkin et al. 2002, 2005; Yang et al. 2007). Relatively high variability at the joint level, together with relatively low variability at the endpoint level (see also the classical study of Bernstein 1930), strongly suggest the existence of {R;C}-stabilizing {r;c} synergies. In addition, one of the very few studies that tried to reconstruct control variables during a multijoint action within the framework of the equilibrium-point hypothesis (under an assumed simplified model!) showed similarly timed profiles of the equilibrium trajectories for the two joints (Latash et al. 1999). In that study, the subjects performed quick flexion and extension movements of one of the two joints in the wrist–elbow system. A quick movement of one of the joints was associated with moments of force acting on the other joint. As a result, to prevent flapping of the apparently "static" joint required precise control of the muscles acting at that joint (Koshland et al. 1991; Latash et al. 1995). The similar time patterns and scaling of the peak-to-peak equilibrium trajectories at the two joints are signatures of a two-joint synergy at a control level, a synergy between $\{r;c\}_{ELBOW}$ and $\{r;c\}_{WRIST}$ that stabilized {R;C} for the arm endpoint.

Another important link exists between the ideas of equilibrium-point control and those of motor synergies: The control with referent configurations may, by itself, lead to synergies at the level of elemental variables. This issue is discussed in the next section.

SYNERGIES PRODUCED BY CONTROL WITH REFERENT CONFIGURATIONS

Consider grasping an object with two opposing digits, the thumb and another digit that may be either a finger or a virtual finger representing the action of all the fingers that act in opposition to the thumb (Fig. 1.5). In a recent paper (Pilon et al. 2007), it has been suggested that this action is associated with setting a referent aperture (AP_{REF}) between the digits. The rigid walls of the object do not allow the digits to move to AP_{REF}. As a result, there is always a difference between the actual aperture (AP_{ACT}) and AP_{REF} that leads to active grip force production.

Typically, three mechanical constraints act on static prehensile tasks (for simplicity, analysis is limited to a planar, two-dimensional case). First, the object should not move along the horizontal axis (X-axis in Fig. 1.5). To achieve this result, the forces produced by the opposing effectors have to be equal in magnitude: $F_{X1} + F_{X2} = 0$. (They also have to be large enough to allow application of sufficient shear forces, given friction; this issue is not crucial for the current analysis). Second, the object should not move vertically; this requires $L + F_{Z1} + F_{Z2} = 0$, where L is external load (weight of the object). Finally, to avoid object rotation, the moments of force (M) produced by each digit have to balance the external moment of force (M_{EXT}): $M_{EXT} + M_1 + M_2 = 0$.

Each of these equations contains two unknowns; hence, each one poses a typical problem of motor redundancy. Consider the first one: $F_{X1} + F_{X2} = 0$. According to the principle of abundance, it may be expected to involve a two-digit synergy stabilizing the resultant force at a close to zero level (documented by Shim et al. 2003; Zhang et al. 2009; Gorniak et al. 2009a,b). Note, however, that setting AP_{REF} by itself leads naturally to such a synergy.

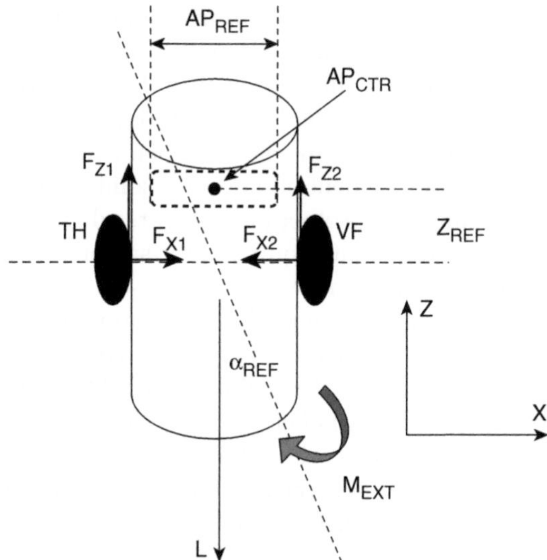

Figure 1.5 An illustration of four salient components of the referent configuration in the task of holding an object with two digits. Three components are the size, and two coordinates of the referent aperture (AP_{REF}). The fourth component is the referent angle with respect to the vertical (α_{REF}).

Setting a smaller or larger AP_{REF} (certainly, within limits), centered closer to one digit or the other, is always expected to result in $F_{X1} + F_{X2} = 0$. The forces produced by each of the digits and the spatial location of the handle where the forces are balanced may differ across trials. This mode of control is possible only if the two opposing digits belong to the same person. If they belong to two persons, the two participants have to set referent coordinates for each of the effectors separately, rather than a referent aperture value. This may be expected to lead to significantly lower indices of synergies stabilizing the resultant force in the X direction (confirmed by Gorniak et al. 2009b).

Similarly, setting a common referent coordinate for the two digits may be expected to result in a synergy between F_{Z1} and F_{Z2} that stabilizes the load-resisting force, and setting a referent object tilt value may result in a synergy between M_1 and M_2 that stabilizes the rotational action on the object counterbalancing the external moment of force. This simple example illustrates how the principle of control with referent values for important points on the body, {R;C}, in combination with the principle of minimal final action may lead to synergic relations among elemental variables without any additional smart controlling action. To realize this principle, sensory feedback on the salient variable (for example, AP_{ACT}) has to be used as an input into a neuron whose threshold is set at AP_{REF} by the controller (see Fig. 1.1A). If $AP_{ACT} > AP_{REF}$, the neuron generates action potentials that ultimately lead to shifts of λ for muscles producing closure of the opposing digits (possibly using the hierarchical scheme illustrated in Fig. 1.2). The digits move toward each other until $AP_{ACT} = AP_{REF}$ or, if the digits are prevented from moving, active grip force production occurs.

Are there synergies that are *not* organized in such a way? In other words, can any synergy be associated with setting the referent value of a variable and then allowing the principle of minimal final action to lead the system to a solution? A recent study (Zhang et al. 2008) has shown that, when subjects were required to produce a constant force level through four fingers pressing in parallel, they showed force-stabilizing synergies (in a sense that most finger force variance was confined to the UCM, i.e., it was V_{GOOD}) but different subjects preferred different solutions within the UCM compatible with $V_{GOOD} > V_{BAD}$.

Why would the subjects care about specific data distributions within the UCM, a space which, by definition, has no effect on their performance? Are there self-imposed additional constraints that individual subjects could select differently? This is possible and, if the subjects use referent values for different variables to impose such additional constraints, data point distributions within the task-related UCM may be expected to differ.

On the other hand, imagine holding an object with a prismatic grasp (the four fingers opposing the thumb). Setting a referent aperture leads to covariation between the normal force of the thumb and the resultant normal force produced by the four fingers. How will referent positions of the individual fingers covary, given a fixed referent aperture? This question has no simple answer. The four fingers may be characterized by four referent positions, $X_{R,i}$ (i = index, middle, ring, and little fingers). There is an infinite number of $X_{R,i}$ combinations that satisfy a given AP_{REF}. Even if the subject self-imposes another constraint (for example, related to a required total rotational hand action), this still results in only two equations with four unknowns. Note that setting the values of the referent aperture and referent hand orientation with certain variability imposes constraints on V_{BAD} in the space of finger referent positions, but the person is free to combine this V_{BAD} with any amount of V_{GOOD}, thus leading or not leading to multifinger synergies stabilizing the overall hand action. There seems to be no obvious way to describe such synergies with referent magnitudes of performance variables. The existence of such synergies is corroborated by their presence or absence in different subpopulations and after different amounts of practice (Latash et al. 2002a; Kang et al. 2004; Olafsdottir et al. 2007, 2008).

FEEDBACK AND FEEDFORWARD MODELS OF SYNERGIES

Several models have been offered to account for the observed synergies, based on a variety of ideas including optimal feedback control (Todorov and Jordan 2002), neural networks with central back-coupling (Latash et al. 2005), feedforward control (Goodman and Latash 2006), and a model that combines ideas of feedback control, back-coupling, and equilibrium-point control (Martin et al. 2009). Most models with feedback control allow for modulation of the gains of feedback loops. In particular, the back-coupling model explicitly suggests the existence of two groups of control variables related to characteristics of the desired action (trajectory) and stability properties of different performance variables.

Figure 1.6A illustrates the main idea of the model. The controller specifies a desired time profile for a performance variable (for example, the total force produced by several fingers) and also a matrix of gains (G) for the back-coupling loops that look similar to the well-known system of Renshaw cells. Changing G was shown to lead to stabilization of total force, with and without simultaneous stabilization of the total moment of force produced by the fingers (Latash et al. 2005). Figure 1.6B emphasizes the existence of two groups of control variables, CV1 and CV2, related to trajectory and its

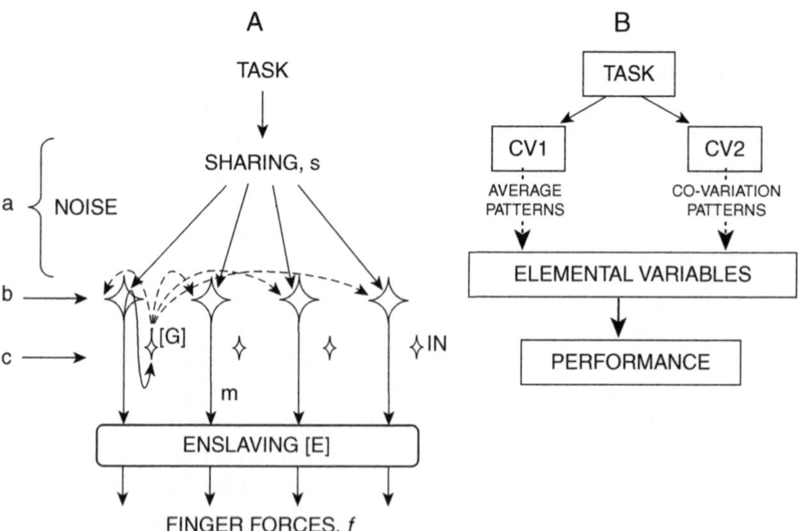

Figure 1.6 **A**: An illustration of a scheme with back-coupling loops for the task of four finger accurate force production. The task is shared among four signals (*level a*) that are projected onto neurons (*level b*) that generate finger mode signals (*m*). The output of these neurons is also projected onto neurons (*level c*) that project back to the neurons at level b. These projections can be described with a gain matrix G. **B**: The scheme assumes two groups of control variables, those that define average contributions of the elements (elemental variables) to the output performance variable and those related to covariation among the elemental variables. Modified by permission from Latash, M.L., Shim, J.K., Smilga, A.V., and Zatsiorsky, V. (2005). A central back-coupling hypothesis on the organization of motor synergies: a physical metaphor and a neural model. *Biological Cybernetics* 92: 186–191, with permission of the publisher.

stability, respectively. This simple scheme suggests, in particular, that a person can produce different actions without changing synergies that stabilize salient performance variables (CV1 varies; CV2 stays unchanged). It also suggests that one can change synergies without an overt action (CV2 varied; CV1 unchanged). Both possibilities have been confirmed experimentally (reviewed in Zatsiorsky and Latash 2008; Latash and Zatsiorsky 2009).

In particular, if a person is asked to maintain a constant force level by pressing with a set of fingers, and then to produce a quick change in the force level, the index of a force-stabilizing synergy (the normalized difference between V_{GOOD} and V_{BAD}) shows a drop 100–150 ms prior to the first visible changes in the total force (Olafsdottir et al. 2005). Similar changes in synergy indices computed for different variables have been reported in experiments in which the subjects perturbed one finger within a redundant set (Kim et al. 2006) or the whole set of digits (Shim et al. 2006) by a self-initiated action. These changes in synergy adjustments prior to an action have been termed anticipatory synergy adjustments (ASAs).

ANTICIPATORY SYNERGY ADJUSTMENTS

Anticipatory synergy adjustments have been viewed as the means of turning off synergies that stabilize those performance variables that have to be changed quickly. Indeed, if a synergy tries to bring down deviations of a performance variable from its steady-state value, it will also counteract a voluntary quick change in this variable (cf. the posture-movement paradox, von Holst and Mittelstaedt 1973; Feldman 2009). It is unproductive to fight one's own synergies, and turning them off in preparation to a quick action (or a quick reaction to a perturbation) sounds like a good idea. Note that, during ASAs, synergy indices show a slow drift toward lower values (corresponding to weaker synergies) and, close to the time of action initiation, there is a dramatic drop in these indices corresponding to complete dismantling of the corresponding synergies.

Figure 1.7 illustrates an example of ASAs (Shim et al. 2006). In this experiment, the subjects were required to hold a handle instrumented with six-component force/torque sensors for each of the digits. The four fingers opposed the thumb. The handle had an inverted T-shaped attachment that was used to suspend loads at three sites to create different external torques. A perturbation was produced by a quick action of lifting the load, which could be performed by the experimenter (Fig. 1.7A) or by the subject's other hand (Fig. 1.7B). The plots show time profiles of the index (ΔV) of a force-stabilizing synergy among individual finger forces. The index was computed in such a way that its positive values corresponded to a force-stabilizing synergy (higher ΔV mean stronger synergy). Note an early drop in ΔV (shown as $t\Delta_V$) when the load was lifted by the subject; this ASA is absent when the same perturbation was triggered by the experimenter.

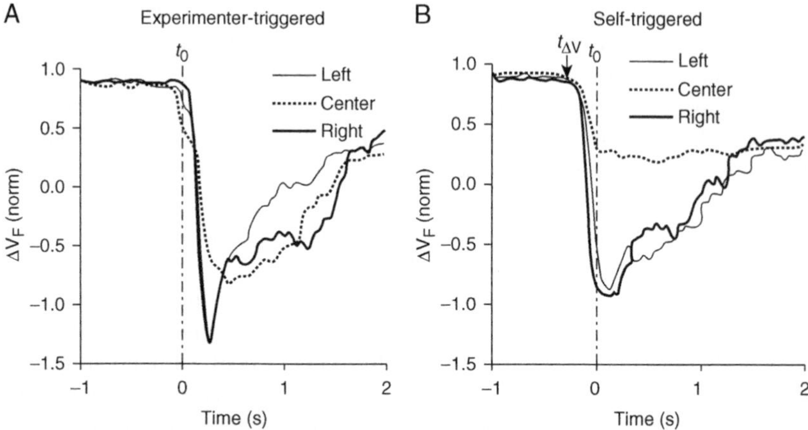

Figure 1.7 The subject was required to hold a handle with a set of loads. Then, one of the loads (attached under the handle [center], to the left, or to the right of the handle) was lifted at time t_0 by the experimenter (*A*) or by the subject himself (*B*). Changes in an index of force stabilizing multidigit synergy (ΔV_F) are illustrated. Note the anticipatory synergy adjustments ($t_{\Delta V}<t_0$) in (*B*) but not in (*A*). Modified by permission from Shim, J.K., Park, J., Zatsiorsky, V.M., and Latash, M.L. (2006) Adjustments of prehension synergies in response to self-triggered and experimenter-triggered load and torque perturbations. *Experimental Brain Research* 175: 641–653, with permission of the publisher.

The existence of ASAs suggests that synergy adjustments may be at least partly independent of changes in the control variables such as {R;C}. Indeed, the lack of an overt action suggests that {R;C} values have not changed. The existence of ASAs most naturally fits the scheme in Figure 1.6, within which "trajectory control" (with {R;C} changes) is clearly separate from the control of synergy producing back-coupling loops (with the G matrix). This scheme does not mean, of course, that during all natural actions synergies are created independently of {R;C} control variables, but it suggests that, in addition to {R;C}-created synergies, there may be synergies of a different origin that can be adjusted independently of {R;C}.

Several features of ASAs make them similar to APAs:

- First, both APAs and ASAs are seen about 100 ms prior to the initiation of a voluntary action.
- Second, APAs and ASAs are not seen when a similar perturbation is unexpectedly triggered by the experimenter for the subject.
- Third, both APAs and ASAs are delayed and emerge nearly simultaneously with the action initiation when a similar task is performed under a typical simple reaction time instruction (Lee et al. 1987; De Wolf et al. 1998; Olafsdottir et al. 2005).

- Fourth, elderly people show a decrease in the amplitude and delayed initiation of both APAs and ASAs (Woollacott et al. 1988; Olafsdottir et al. 2007).

These occurrences are too many to be viewed as simply coincidences. Therefore, I would like to suggest a hypothesis that ASAs and APAs are intimately related to each other.

A DUAL-FUNCTION HYPOTHESIS ON THE NATURE OF ANTICIPATORY POSTURAL ADJUSTMENTS

As mentioned earlier, APAs are traditionally viewed as the means of generating forces and moments of force that act against the anticipated perturbation (Bouisset and Zattara 1987; Friedli et al. 1984; Ramos and Stark 1990). There are, however, observations that cast doubt on this established view.

First, typical magnitudes of changes in mechanical variables acting on the body during APAs are very small. For example, typical shifts of the center of pressure (COP) coordinate in the anterior-posterior direction, within the APA time interval, observed prior to quick arm movements or load manipulations are of the order on 1 mm (Cordo and Nashner 1982; Massion 1992; Aruin and Latash 1995). On the other hand, typical spontaneous COP shifts during quiet standing (postural sway) are on the order of 10 mm (Winter et al. 1996; Zatsiorsky and Duarte 1999). Why would the CNS care about producing these precisely timed microscopic COP shifts on the background of spontaneous COP shifts that are larger by an order of magnitude?

Second, several studies explored changes in APA characteristics with changes in a variety of task variables, such as the magnitude of perturbation, type of action associated with the perturbation, and postural stability (Aruin and Latash 1995, 1996; Aruin et al. 1998; Shiratori and Latash 2000). Typically, these studies report significant changes in indices of muscle activation (such as integrals of rectified electromyograms [EMGs] over the typical time intervals), whereas changes in the shifts of the mechanical variables are small and, frequently, under the level of statistical significance. Overall, it seems that the CNS facilitates reproducible changes in muscle activation indices that have little net mechanical effect. What could be the reason for these adjustments?

I would like to offer a dual-function hypothesis on APAs. According to this hypothesis, APAs represent a superposition of two processes, only one of which has substantial net mechanical effects, while the other reflects reorganization of patterns of covariation among muscle activations or among higher-order variables such as muscle modes (groups of muscles with proportional scaling of activation levels, Krishnamoorthy et al. 2003a,b).

The first changes in muscle activation patterns reflect ASAs with the purpose of attenuating those synergies that are used to stabilize mechanical variables during quiet stance (or another steady-state task).

These variables must change quickly to ensure balance under the expected perturbation. As described in previous sections, turning off a synergy prior to a quick change in the performance variable is a reasonable strategy (cf. Olafsdottir et al. 2005).

The second process is the generation of net changes in relevant mechanical variables, such as COP coordinate and shear force vector, that will help stabilize posture when the perturbation comes. After a synergy stabilizing a relevant performance variable has been attenuated, the variable may be changed quickly. These changes may spread over a large time interval, including the typical APA interval, as well as later feedback-triggered postural adjustments (Nashner 1976; Nashner and Cordo 1981). Naturally, the second process is expected to start after the first one. However, under time pressure, these two processes may be expected to start simultaneously as, for example, in experiments under the simple reaction time instruction (cf. Lee et al. 1987; De Wolf et al. 1998; Olafsdottir et al. 2005).

Currently, no published evidence directly supports this hypothesis. Partly, this is due to the inherently noisy EMG signals that lead to the necessity to integrate EMG signals over relatively large time intervals in the analysis of muscle mode synergies (see also Danna-Dos-Santos et al. 2007; Robert and Latash 2008). However, to be fair, only a couple of studies have even tried to apply this method of analysis to APAs (Krishnamoorthy et al. 2003b, 2004). So, I believe that it is only a matter of time before ASAs will be demonstrated and studied as a component of APAs.

POSTURAL SYNERGIES AND THE EQUILIBRIUM POSITION CONTROL

Several attempts have been made to link the control of vertical posture to ideas of control with referent body configurations. These relate to such different actions performed by standing persons as quiet stance (postural sway), voluntary sway, and jumping after a counter-movement.

Spontaneous movements of the body during postural sway have commonly been viewed as oscillations of an inverted pendulum about the ankle joint (Winter et al. 1998; Morasso and Schieppati 1999). In most such models, the control of the body has been viewed as involving a modulation of the apparent stiffness of muscles crossing the ankle joint (Winter et al. 1996, 1998; Kiemel et al. 2006). There have been heated discussions on whether ankle joint apparent stiffness is sufficient to ensure balance (Winter et al. 1996, 1998; Morasso and Schieppati 1999; Loram et al. 2005). A recent study has also shown that a single-joint or even a double-joint (hip plus ankle) model of the body may be inadequate because it fails to account for important compensatory joint actions in other joints during quiet stance (Hsu et al. 2007).

Ankle stiffness control models implicitly accept the α-model of the equilibrium-point hypothesis (see Bizzi et al. 1982): they consider centrally produced changes in the slope of the torque–angle relationship of the ankle joint but not in its zero point. In contrast, the equilibrium-point hypothesis (its λ version, Feldman 1966) suggests that the CNS controls joints through changes in the threshold values of joint angle for activation of the opposing muscles, whereas joint apparent stiffness is one of the emerging performance variables. According to this view, at any moment of time, torque at the ankle joint is defined by the joint instantaneous equilibrium position (which is a time function) and the deviations of the joint's actual position from the equilibrium position. In other words, postural equilibrium is maintained with respect to a moving, rather than stationary, referent point. Moving the referent joint position allows the generation of much higher torques than could be expected if this position were kept constant.

This general view was implemented in a series of studies that decomposed whole-body postural sway into two components termed *rambling* and *trembling* (Zatsiorsky and Duarte 1999, 2000). Rambling represents migration of the referent point, with respect to which the equilibrium is instantly maintained. Points of instantaneous equilibrium were found at the instances when the horizontal ground reaction force was zero (Zatsiorsky and King 1998). The center of pressure (COP, coordinate of the vertical resultant force acting on the body) coordinates at these points were measured, and the rambling trajectory was then obtained by approximating the consecutive instant equilibrium points with cubic splines. Trembling represents the COP oscillation about the rambling trajectory. According to the rambling-trembling hypothesis of Zatsiorsky and Duarte, rambling reflects mostly supraspinal control processes, whereas trembling is defined primarily by the peripheral mechanical properties of the postural system and proprioceptive spinal reflexes.

Recent studies of multimuscle synergies in postural tasks have assumed a hierarchical control system, with muscles being united into groups (muscle modes or M-modes) at the lower level of the hierarchy, and gains of M-mode involvement are manipulated at the higher level (Krishnamoorthy et al. 2003a,b; Danna-Dos-Santos et al. 2007; Robert et al. 2008). The idea that muscles are united into groups during a whole-body task is not new. It was suggested by Hughlings Jackson (1889) and Bernstein (1967), and developed in a number of recent studies of postural and locomotor tasks (Ivanenko et al. 2004; Ting and Macpherson 2005; Torres-Oviedo and Ting 2007; see also Ting, this volume). The novelty of our approach is in considering the next hierarchical level that allows multimuscle (multi-M-mode) synergies to link to potentially important physical variables such as COP shifts, changes in trunk orientation, shear forces, and the like.

Some of the recent studies on the composition of M-modes suggest rather direct links to the referent configuration hypothesis. For example, it is reasonable to expect that, when a controller faces a challenging postural task, it tries to unite muscles into groups such that each group produces a change in the referent body configuration that does not endanger the postural equilibrium. Figure 1.8A illustrates possible kinematic effects of changes in muscle activation patterns corresponding to two groups of M-modes observed in a recent study (Robert et al. 2008) that required the subjects to perform a rather unusual action: the generation of a quick pulse of shear force in the anterior-posterior direction without moving the COP. The solid lines show new referent configurations that the body tries to reach. Note that both referent configurations correspond to a change in the body posture that is compatible with only a minor change in the location of the center of mass (COM) in the anterior-posterior direction. In other words, both referent configurations are compatible with vertical posture.

In several earlier studies, patterns of changes in the muscle activation patterns corresponding to the most reproducible M-modes involved combined activation of the ventral muscles (the "push-forward" mode) or combined activation of the dorsal muscles (the "push-back" mode) (Krishnamoorthy et al. 2003a,b; Danna-Dos-Santos et al. 2007). These patterns correspond to changes in the referent body configuration illustrated in Figure 1.8B. Note that these referent configurations are associated with substantial changes in the COM location. As such, the M-modes within this set always have to covary to avoid losing balance.

A trade-off seems to exist between mechanical efficacy and safety (Latash and Anson 1996, 2006). In relatively common tasks, such as stepping, quick

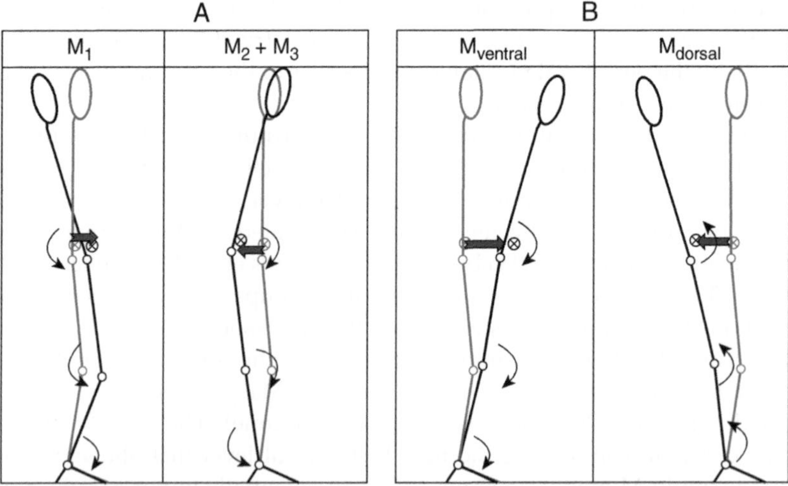

Figure 1.8 Illustrations of the referent configurations corresponding to sets of muscle modes (M-modes) observed in an experiment with an unusual task (*A*) and a typical voluntary body sway experiment (*B*). The referent configurations are shown with respect to a typical vertical posture (*gray lines*). The associated shifts of the center of mass are shown with the arrows. Modified by permission from Robert, T., Zatsiorsky, V.M., and Latash, M.L. (2008) Multi-muscle synergies in an unusual postural task: Quick shear force production. *Experimental Brain Research* 187: 237–253, with permission of the publisher.

arm motion, or load manipulation, the CNS organizes muscles into M-modes that are most effective in producing the required mechanical effects. In contrast, when the task is novel (as in the cited study by Robert et al. 2008), the controller organizes muscles into M-modes corresponding to shifts in the referent body configuration that are safe, although not necessarily mechanically optimal.

Different "atypical" M-modes were observed in studies when the subjects performed relatively natural tasks while standing on a board with a decreased support area (Krishnamoorthy et al. 2004; Asaka et al. 2008). Those M-modes involved co-contraction of the agonist–antagonist muscle pairs acting about the major leg joints that could be interpreted as a change in the range of joint angle values within which the muscle pairs could be active simultaneously without a change in the body referent configuration. This is another example of using a set of M-modes that, even when recruited individually, are not expected to lead to major COM deviations and loss of balance.

CONCLUSION

Getting back to the issue of anticipatory control of voluntary actions, a few conclusions may be drawn. There is no argument that anticipatory actions exist. However, their existence does not mean that the controller is each time solving complex problems related to the neural and mechanical aspects of voluntary movement production. More likely, the controller manipulates referent body configurations based on experience, which allows elaborating relatively simple rules. For example, if a person knows that an expected perturbation will produce body deviation from the vertical forward by about 10 degrees, the referent configuration may be shifted by 10 degrees backward, slightly in anticipation of the perturbation. An expected perturbation of a different magnitude may be associated with an appropriately scaled anticipatory shift of the referent configuration.

There is, however, another, more subtle component of anticipatory actions related not to production of net mechanical effects but to facilitation of future quick changes in the referent configuration. This is achieved by the attenuation of synergies stabilizing that particular aspect. This component is exemplified by the phenomena of anticipatory synergy adjustments. At present, these phenomena have been documented only for multidigit pressing and prehensile tasks. However, the existing tools for quantification of multimuscle synergies allow us to expect that demonstration of anticipatory synergy adjustments during standing is only a matter of time.

I would like to finish on an optimistic note. The field of motor control has been developing rapidly over the past 10 years, with important progress achieved in the areas of both control and coordination of voluntary actions. The development of the referent configuration hypothesis for multielement actions and the development of the notion of motor synergies give hope for a unified theory of motor control, based on a solid physiological and physical foundation. Such a theory will not require assuming that the CNS performs complex computations and then somehow converts the symbolic results of such computations into mechanical actions. It will offer a fruitful framework to analyze anticipatory motor actions.

ACKNOWLEDGMENTS

Preparation of this chapter was partly supported by NIH grants NS-035032 and AG-018751.

REFERENCES

Arbib, M.A., T. Iberall, and D. Lyons. 1985. Coordinated control programs for movements of the hand. In, *Hand function and the neocortex*, ed. A.W. Goodwin and I. Darian-Smith, 111–129. Springer-Verlag: Berlin.

Aruin, A.S., W.R. Forrest, and M.L. Latash. 1998. Anticipatory postural adjustments in conditions of postural instability. *Electroencephalography Clinical Neurophysiology* 109: 350–59.

Aruin, A.S., and M.L. Latash. 1995. Directional specificity of postural muscles in feed-forward postural reactions during fast voluntary arm movements. *Experimental Brain Research* 103: 323–32.

Aruin, A.S., and M.L. Latash. 1996. Anticipatory postural adjustments during self-initiated perturbations of different magnitude triggered by a standard motor action. *Electroencephalography Clinical Neurophysiology* 101: 497–503.

Asaka, T., Y. Wang, J. Fukushima, and M.L. Latash. 2008. Learning effects on muscle modes and multi-mode synergies. *Experimental Brain Research* 184: 323–38.

Belen'kii, V.Y., V.S. Gurfinkel, and Y.I. Pal'tsev. 1967. Elements of control of voluntary movements. *Biofizika* 10: 135–41.

Bernstein, N.A. 1930. A new method of mirror cyclographie and its application towards the study of labor movements during work on a workbench [in Russian]. *Hygiene, Safety and Pathology of Labor*, 5: 3–9, and 6: 3–11.

Bernstein, N.A. 1935. The problem of interrelation between coordination and localization [in Russian]. *Archives of Biological Science* 38: 1–35.

Bernstein, N.A. 1967. *The co-ordination and regulation of movements*. Oxford UK: Pergamon Press.

Bizzi, E., N. Accornero, W. Chapple, and N. Hogan. 1982. Arm trajectory formation in monkeys. *Experimental Brain Research* 46: 139–43.

Bouisset, S., and M. Zattara. 1987. Biomechanical study of the programming of anticipatory postural adjustments associated with voluntary movement. *Journal of Biomechanics* 20: 735–42.

Cordo, P.J., and L.M. Nashner. 1982. Properties of postural adjustments associated with rapid arm movements. *Journal of Neurophysiology* 47: 1888–1905.

Danna-Dos-Santos, A., K. Slomka, V.M. Zatsiorsky, and M.L. Latash. 2007. Muscle modes and synergies during voluntary body sway. *Experimental Brain Research* 179: 533–50.

De Wolf, S., H. Slijper, and M.L. Latash. 1998. Anticipatory postural adjustments during self-paced and reaction-time movements. *Experimental Brain Research* 121: 7–19.

Domkin, D., J. Laczko, M. Djupsjöbacka, S. Jaric, and M.L. Latash. 2005. Joint angle variability in 3D bimanual pointing: uncontrolled manifold analysis. *Experimental Brain Research* 163: 44–57.

Domkin, D., J. Laczko, S. Jaric, H. Johansson, and M.L. Latash. 2002. Structure of joint variability in bimanual pointing tasks. *Experimental Brain Research* 143: 11–23.

Feldman, A.G. 1966. Functional tuning of the nervous system with control of movement or maintenance of a steady posture. II. Controllable parameters of the muscle. *Biophysics* 11: 565–78.

Feldman, A.G. 1986. Once more on the equilibrium-point hypothesis (λ-model) for motor control. *Journal of Motor Behavior* 18: 17–54.

Feldman, A.G. 1980. Superposition of motor programs. I. Rhythmic forearm movements in man. *Neuroscience* 5: 81–90.

Feldman, A.G. 2009. New insights into action-perception coupling. *Experimental Brain Research* 194: 39–58.

Feldman, A.G., V. Goussev, A. Sangole, and M.F. Levin. 2007. Threshold position control and the principle of minimal interaction in motor actions. *Progress in Brain Research* 165: 267–81.

Feldman, A.G., and M.L. Latash. 2005. Testing hypotheses and the advancement of science: Recent attempts to falsify the equilibrium-point hypothesis. *Experimental Brain Research* 161: 91–103.

Feldman, A.G., and M.F. Levin. 1995. Positional frames of reference in motor control: their origin and use. *Behavioral and Brain Sciences* 18: 723–806.

Feldman, A.G., and M.F. Levin. 2009. The equilibrium-point hypothesis–past, present and future. *Advances in Experimental Medicine and Biology*, 629: 699–726.

Feldman, A.G., D.J. Ostry, M.F. Levin, P.L. Gribble, and A.B. Mitnitski. 1998. Recent tests of the equilibrium-point hypothesis (λ model). *Motor Control* 2: 189–205.

Flash, T. 1987. The control of hand equilibrium trajectories in multi-joint arm movements. *Biological Cybernetics* 57: 257–74.

Flash, T., and F. Mussa-Ivaldi. 1990. Human arm stiffness characteristics during the maintenance of posture. *Experimental Brain Research* 82: 315–26.

Friedli, W.G., M. Hallett, and S.R. Simon. 1984. Postural adjustments associated with rapid voluntary arm movements. I. Electromyographic data. *Journal of Neurology, Neurosurgery, and Psychiatry* 47: 611–22.

Gao, F., M.L. Latash, and V.M. Zatsiorsky. 2005. Control of finger force direction in the flexion-extension plane. *Experimental Brain Research* 161: 307–15.

Gelfand, I.M., and M.L. Latash. 1998. On the problem of adequate language in movement science. *Motor Control* 2: 306–13.

Gelfand, I.M., and M.L. Tsetlin. 1966. On mathematical modeling of the mechanisms of the central nervous system [in Russian]. In *Models of the structural-functional organization of certain biological systems*, ed. I.M. Gelfand, V.S. Gurfinkel, S.V. Fomin, and M.L. Tsetlin, 9–26, Nauka: Moscow. (A 1971 translation edition is from MIT Press, Cambridge, Massachusetts.)

Gera, G., S.M.S.F. Freitas, M.L. Latash, K. Monahan, G. Schöner, and J.P. Scholz. 2010. Motor abundance contributes to resolving multiple kinematic task constraints. *Motor Control* 14: 83–115.

Goodman, S.R., and M.L. Latash. 2006. Feedforward control of a redundant motor system. *Biological Cybernetics* 95: 271–80.

Gorniak, S.L., M. Duarte, and M.L. Latash. 2008. Do synergies improve accuracy? A study of speed-accuracy trade-offs during finger force production. *Motor Control*, 12: 151–172.

Gorniak, S.L., V.M. Zatsiorsky, and M.L. Latash. 2007a. Hierarchies of synergies: An example of the two-hand, multi-finger tasks. *Experimental Brain Research* 179: 167–80.

Gorniak, S.L., V.M. Zatsiorsky, and M.L. Latash. 2007b. Emerging and disappearing synergies in a hierarchically controlled system. *Experimental Brain Research* 183: 259–70.

Gorniak, S.L., V.M. Zatsiorsky, and M.L. Latash. 2009a. Hierarchical control of static prehension: I. Biomechanics. *Experimental Brain Research* 193: 615–31.

Gorniak, S.L., V.M. Zatsiorsky, M.L. Latash. 2009b. Hierarchical control of static prehension: II. Multi-digit synergies. *Experimental Brain Research* 194: 1–15.

Gottlieb, G.L. 1996. On the voluntary movement of compliant (inertial-viscoelastic) loads by parcellated control mechanisms. *Journal of Neurophysiology* 76: 3207–29.

Gottlieb, G.L., D.M. Corcos, and G.C. Agarwal. 1989. Strategies for the control of voluntary movements with one mechanical degree of freedom. *Behavioral and Brain Science* 12: 189–250.

Hinder, M.R., and T.E. Milner. 2003. The case for an internal dynamics model versus equilibrium point control in human movement. *Journal of Physiology* 549: 953–63.

Hogan, N. 1984. An organizational principle for a class of voluntary movements. *Journal of Neuroscience* 4: 2745–2754.

Hogan, N. 1985. The mechanics of multi-joint posture and movement control. *Biological Cybernetics* 52: 315–31.

Hsu, W.L., J.P. Scholz, G. Schöner, J.J. Jeka, and T. Kiemel. 2007. Control and estimation of posture during quiet stance depends on multijoint coordination. *Journal of Neurophysiology* 97: 3024–35.

Hughlings Jackson, J. 1889. On the comparative study of disease of the nervous system. *British Medical Journal* 355–62, Aug. 17, 1889.

Ivanenko, Y.P., R.E. Poppele, and F. Lacquaniti. 2004. Five basic muscle activation patterns account for muscle activity during human locomotion. *Journal of Physiology* 556: 267–82.

Kang, N., M. Shinohara, V.M. Zatsiorsky, and M.L. Latash. 2004. Learning multi-finger synergies: An uncontrolled manifold analysis. *Experimental Brain Research* 157: 336–50.

Kawato, M. 1999. Internal models for motor control and trajectory planning. *Current Opinions in Neurobiology* 9: 718–27.

Kawato, M. 1990. Computational schemes and neural network models for formation and control of multijoint arm trajectory. In *Neural networks for control*, ed. T. Miller, R. Sutton, and P. Werbos, 197–228. Cambridge MA: MIT Press.

Kiemel, T., K.S. Oie, and J.J. Jeka. 2006. Slow dynamics of postural sway are in the feedback loop. *Journal of Neurophysiology* 95: 1410–18.

Kim, S.W., J.K. Shim, V.M. Zatsiorsky, and M.L. Latash. 2006. Anticipatory adjustments of multi-finger synergies in preparation for self-triggered perturbations. *Experimental Brain Research* 174: 604–12.

Koshland, G.F., L. Gerilovsky, and Z. Hasan. 1991. Activity of wrist muscles elicited during imposed or voluntary movements about the elbow joint. *Journal of Motor Behavior* 23: 91–100.

Krishnamoorthy, V., S.R. Goodman, M.L. Latash, and V.M. Zatsiorsky. 2003a. Muscle synergies during shifts of the center of pressure by standing persons: Identification of muscle modes. *Biological Cybernetics* 89: 152–61.

Krishnamoorthy, V., M.L. Latash, J.P. Scholz, and V.M. Zatsiorsky. 2003b. Muscle synergies during shifts of the center of pressure by standing persons. *Experimental Brain Research* 152: 281–92.

Krishnamoorthy, V., M.L. Latash, J.P. Scholz, and V.M. Zatsiorsky. 2004. Muscle modes during shifts of the center of pressure by standing persons: Effects of instability and additional support. *Experimental Brain Research* 157: 18–31.

Latash, M.L. 1993. *Control of human movement*. Urbana IL: Human Kinetics.

Latash, M.L. 2008. *Synergy*. New York: Oxford University Press.

Latash, M.L. 2010. Stages in learning motor synergies: A view based on the equilibrium-point hypothesis. *Human Movement Science* (in press).

Latash, M.L. and J.G. Anson. 1996. What are normal movements in atypical populations? *Behavioral and Brain Sciences* 19: 55–106.

Latash, M.L., and J.G. Anson. 2006. Synergies in health and disease: Relations to adaptive changes in motor coordination. *Physical Therapy* 86: 1151–1160.

Latash, M.L., A.S. Aruin, and M.B. Shapiro. 1995. The relation between posture and movement: A study of a simple synergy in a two-joint task. *Human Movement Science* 14: 79–107.

Latash, M.L., A.S. Aruin, and V.M. Zatsiorsky. 1999. The basis of a simple synergy: Reconstruction of joint equilibrium trajectories during unrestrained arm movements. *Human Movement Science* 18: 3–30.

Latash, M.L., N. Kang, and D. Patterson. 2002a. Finger coordination in persons with Down syndrome: Atypical patterns of coordination and the effects of practice. *Experimental Brain Research,* 146: 345–55.

Latash, M.L., J.P. Scholz, and G. Schöner. 2002b. Motor control strategies revealed in the structure of motor variability. *Exercise and Sport Science Reviews* 30: 26–31.

Latash, M.L., J.P. Scholz, and G. Schöner. 2007. Toward a new theory of motor synergies. *Motor Control* 11: 275–307.

Latash, M.L., J.K. Shim, A.V. Smilga, and V. Zatsiorsky. 2005. A central back-coupling hypothesis on the organization of motor synergies: A physical metaphor and a neural model. *Biological Cybernetics* 92: 186–91.

Latash, M.L., and V.M. Zatsiorsky. 2009. Multi-finger prehension: Control of a redundant motor system. *Advances in Experimental Medicine and Biology* 629: 597–618.

Lee, W.A., T.S. Buchanan, and M.W. Rogers. 1987. Effects of arm acceleration and behavioral conditions on the organization of postural adjustments during arm flexion. *Experimental Brain Research* 66: 257–70.

Loram, I.D., C.N. Maganaris, and M. Lakie. 2005. Active, non-spring-like muscle movements in human postural sway: How might paradoxical changes in muscle length be produced? *Journal of Physiology* 564: 281–93.

MacKenzie, C.L., and T. Iberall. 1994. *The grasping hand*. Amsterdam: North-Holland.

Martin, V., J.P. Scholz, and G. Schöner. 2009. Redundancy, self-motion, and motor control. *Neural Computing* 21: 1371–1414.

Massion, J. 1992. Movement, posture and equilibrium – interaction and coordination. *Progress in Neurobiology* 38: 35–56.

Morasso, P.G., and M. Schieppati. 1999. Can muscle stiffness alone stabilize upright standing? *Journal of Neurophysiology* 82: 1622–26.

Nashner, L.M. 1976. Adapting reflexes controlling human posture. *Experimental Brain Research* 26: 59–72.

Nashner, L.M., and P.J. Cordo. 1981. Relation of automatic postural responses and reaction-time voluntary movements of human leg muscles. *Experimental Brain Research* 43: 395–405.

Newell, K.M., and R.E.A. van Emmerik. 1989. The acquisition of coordination: Preliminary analysis of learning to write. *Human Movement Science* 8: 17–32.

Olafsdottir, H., N. Yoshida, V.M. Zatsiorsky, and M.L. Latash. 2005. Anticipatory covariation of finger forces during self-paced and reaction time force production. *Neuroscience Letters* 381: 92–96.

Olafsdottir, H., N. Yoshida, V.M. Zatsiorsky, and M.L. Latash. 2007. Elderly show decreased adjustments of motor synergies in preparation to action. *Clinical Biomechanics* 22: 44–51.

Olafsdottir, H.B., V.M. Zatsiorsky, and M.L. Latash. 2008. The effects of strength training on finger strength and hand dexterity in healthy elderly individuals. *Journal of Applied Physiology* 105: 1166–78.

Ostry, D.J., and A.G. Feldman. 2003. A critical evaluation of the force control hypothesis in motor control. *Experimental Brain Research* 153: 275–288.

Pilon, J.-F., S.J. De Serres, and A.G. Feldman. 2007. Threshold position control of arm movement with anticipatory increase in grip force. *Experimental Brain Research* 181: 49–67.

Prilutsky, B.I. 2000. Coordination of two- and one-joint muscles: Functional consequences and implications for motor control. *Motor Control* 4: 1–44.

Ramos, C.F., and L.W. Stark. 1990. Postural maintenance during movement: Simulations of a two joint model. *Biological Cybernetics* 63: 363–75.

Robert, T., and M.L. Latash. 2008. Time evolution of the organization of multi-muscle postural responses to sudden changes in the external force applied at the trunk level. *Neuroscience Letters* 438: 238–41.

Robert, T., V.M. Zatsiorsky, and M.L. Latash. 2008. Multi-muscle synergies in an unusual postural task: Quick shear force production. *Experimental Brain Research* 187: 237–253.

Rosenbaum, D.A., S.E. Engelbrecht, M.M. Busje, and L.D. Loukopoulos. 1993. Knowledge model for selecting and producing reaching movements. *Journal of Motor Behavior* 25: 217–27.

Scholz, J.P., and G. Schöner. 1999. The uncontrolled manifold concept: Identifying control variables for a functional task. *Experimental Brain Research* 126: 289–306.

Shadmehr, R., and F.A. Mussa-Ivaldi. 1994. Adaptive representation of dynamics during learning of a motor task. *Journal of Neuroscience* 14: 3208–3224.

Shadmehr, R., and S.P. Wise. 2005. *The computational neurobiology of reaching and pointing*. Cambridge, MA: MIT Press.

Shapkova, E.Yu, A.L. Shapkova, S.R. Goodman, V.M. Zatsiorsky, and M.L. Latash. 2008. Do synergies decrease force variability? A study of single-finger and multi-finger force production. *Experimental Brain Research,* 188: 411–425.

Sherrington, C.S. 1906. *The integrative action of the nervous system*. London: Yale University Press.

Shim, J.K., M.L. Latash, and V.M. Zatsiorsky. 2003. Prehension synergies: Trial-to-trial variability and hierarchical organization of stable performance. *Experimental Brain Research* 152: 173–84.

Shim, J.K., H. Olafsdottir, V.M. Zatsiorsky, and M.L. Latash. 2005. The emergence and disappearance of multi-digit synergies during force production tasks. *Experimental Brain Research* 164: 260–70.

Shim, J.K., J. Park, V.M. Zatsiorsky, and M.L. Latash. 2006. Adjustments of prehension synergies in response to self-triggered and experimenter-triggered load and torque perturbations. *Experimental Brain Research* 175: 641–53.

Shim, J.K., B. Lay, V.M. Zatsiorsky, and M.L. Latash. 2004. Age-related changes in finger coordination in static prehension tasks. *Journal of Applied Physiology* 97: 213–24.

Shiratori, T., and M.L. Latash. 2000. The roles of proximal and distal muscles in anticipatory postural adjustments under asymmetrical perturbations and during standing on rollerskates. *Clinical Neurophysiology* 111: 613–23.

Ting, L.H., and J.M. Macpherson. 2005. A limited set of muscle synergies for force control during a postural task. *Journal of Neurophysiology* 93: 609–13.

Todorov, E., and M.I. Jordan. 2002. Optimal feedback control as a theory of motor coordination. *Nature Neuroscience* 5: 1226–35.

Torres-Oviedo, G., and L. Ting. 2007. Muscle synergies characterizing human postural responses. *Journal of Neurophysiology* 98: 2144–56.

Van Ingen Schenau, G.J., A.J. van Soest, F.J.M. Gabreels, and M.W.I.M. Horstink. 1995. The control of multi-joint movements relies on detailed internal representations. *Human Movement Science* 14: 511–38.

Van Soest, A.J., and G.J. van Ingen Schenau. 1998. How are explosive movements controlled? In *Progress in motor control,* v. 1, *Bernstein's traditions in movement studies,* ed. M.L. Latash ML, 361–87. Urbana IL: Human Kinetics.

Vereijken, B., R.E.A. van Emmerick, H.T.A. Whiting, and K.M. Newell. 1992. Free(z) ing degrees of freedom in skill acquisition. *Journal of Motor Behavior* 24: 133–42.

Von Holst, E., and H. Mittelstaedt. 1950/1973. The reafference principle. In *The behavioral physiology of animals and man. The collected papers of Erich von Holst*, ed. R. Martin (trans.), 139–173. Coral Gables FL: University of Miami Press.

Winter, D.A., A.E. Patla, F. Prince, M. Ishac, and K. Gielo-Perczak. 1998. Stiffness control of balance in quiet standing. *Journal of Neurophysiology* 80: 1211–21.

Winter, D.A., F. Prince, J.S. Frank, C. Powell, and K.F. Zabjek. 1996. Unified theory regarding A/P and M/L balance in quiet stance. *Journal of Neurophysiology* 75: 2334–43.

Wolpert, D.M., R.C. Miall, and M. Kawato. 1998. Internal models in the cerebellum. *Trends in Cognitive Science* 2: 338–47.

Woollacott, M., B. Inglin, and D. Manchester. 1988. Response preparation and posture control. Neuromuscular changes in the older adult. *Annals of the New York Academy of Sciences* 515: 42–53.

Yang, J.-F., J.P. Scholz, and M.L. Latash. 2007. The role of kinematic redundancy in adaptation of reaching. *Experimental Brain Research* 176: 54–69.

Zatsiorsky, V.M., and M. Duarte. 1999. Instant equilibrium point and its migration in standing tasks: Rambling and trembling components of the stabilogram. *Motor Control* 3: 28–38.

Zatsiorsky, V.M., and M. Duarte. 2000. Rambling and trembling in quiet standing. *Motor Control* 4: 185–200.

Zatsiorsky, V.M., and D.L. King. 1998. An algorithm for deter mining gravity line location from posturographic recordings. *Journal of Biomechanics* 31: 161–64.

Zatsiorsky, V.M., and M.L. Latash. 2008. Multi-finger prehension: An overview. *Journal of Motor Behavior* 40: 446–76.

Zhang, W., J.P. Scholz, V.M. Zatsiorsky, and M.L. Latash. 2008. What do synergies do? Effects of secondary constraints on multi-digit synergies in accurate force-production tasks. *Journal of Neurophysiology* 99: 500–13.

Zhang, W., H.B. Olafsdottir, V.M. Zatsiorsky, and M.L. Latash. 2009. Mechanical analysis and hierarchies of multi-digit synergies during accurate object rotation. *Motor Control* 13: 251–279.

2

Object Representations Used in Action and Perception

J. Randall Flanagan and Roland S. Johansson

The remarkable skill of the human hand in object manipulation tasks is not the result of rapid sensorimotor processes or powerful effector mechanisms. Rather, the secret lies in the way that the nervous system organizes and controls manipulation tasks. Skilled and dexterous object manipulation requires the ability to tailor motor commands, predictively, to the goals of the task and the physical properties of manipulated objects (Johansson and Flanagan 2009; see also Frey, this volume). Thus, the ability to estimate these properties, based on sensory cues and memory, is essential for dexterous performance. Skilled manipulation also requires the ability to predict the sensory outcomes of motor commands. By comparing predicted and actual sensory feedback, the sensorimotor system can monitor task progress and take appropriate goal-directed corrective actions if a mismatch occurs. In addition, the sensorimotor system can update information about the physical properties of objects, as well as the mechanical interaction between objects and the body, so as to reduce future mismatches. The first part of this chapter focuses on predictive control mechanisms in object manipulation tasks and the way the sensorimotor system represents the physical properties of objects.

In addition to manipulating objects, we use our hands to perceive object properties, including weight. Judgments about weight are comparative in nature rather than absolute (Ross 1969; Ellis and Lederman 1998; Flanagan et al. 2008). That is, weight judgments are biased by expectations about weight. Various weight illusions reveal this bias, including the size–weight and material–weight illusions (Ross 1969; Ellis and Lederman 1999; Flanagan et al. 2008). Thus, a small cube is judged heavier than an equally weighted large cube, and a cube covered in foam is judged heavier than a cube covered in metal, because the small and foam-covered cubes are heavier than expected based on size and surface material, respectively. Hence, expectations about object weight are essential in perceiving object weight, just as they are in controlling fingertip forces when lifting objects. The second part of this chapter examines representations of object weight used when making judgments about weight and considers the relation between these representations and those employed by the sensorimotor system when lifting objects.

PREDICTIVE AND REACTIVE CONTROL MECHANISMS IN PRECISION GRIP LIFTING

Object manipulation tasks are composed of a series of actions or phases that are often bounded by mechanical events that represent subgoals of the task (Flanagan et al. 2006; Johansson and Flanagan 2009). These events involve either the making or breaking of contact between the fingertips and an object, or between a grasped object and another object or surface. Consider, for example, the task of lifting a block using a precision grip with the tips of the index finger and thumb on either side (Fig. 2.1). In this task, contact between the digits and object marks the end of the initial reach phase, and the breaking of contact between the object and tabletop marks the end of the subsequent load phase during which the vertical load force, applied by the digits, is increased. Tactile signals associated with such mechanical contact events play an essential role in the control of object manipulation tasks. Not only do these signals confirm completion of the current action phase, they provide critical information for controlling subsequent phases (Johansson and Westling 1984; Westling and Johansson 1987; Jenmalm and Johansson 1997). For example, when the fingertip contacts an object, ensembles of tactile afferents provide rich information about the magnitude, direction, and spatial distribution of forces, the shape of the contact site, and the friction between the skin and the object (Goodwin et al. 1998; Jenmalm et al. 1998; Jenmalm et al. 2000; Birznieks et al. 2001; Johansson and Birznieks 2004; see Johansson and Flanagan, 2009 for a detailed review).

The precision grip lifting task has been used extensively to investigate both predictive and reactive sensorimotor control mechanisms in object manipulation. Using this task, Johansson and Westling (1988a) examined the control of fingertip forces when lifting objects whose weight could be accurately predicted based on previous lifts (see Fig. 2.1A). When lifting such an object just off a surface, during the load phase, people smoothly increase the vertical load force to a target level that slightly exceeds the weight of the object. Moreover, the rate at which load force is increased is proportional to weight. Thus, the load force rate function typically features a single peak that scales with weight. To ensure grasp stability, the grip force (normal to the grasp surfaces) is modulated in phase with the

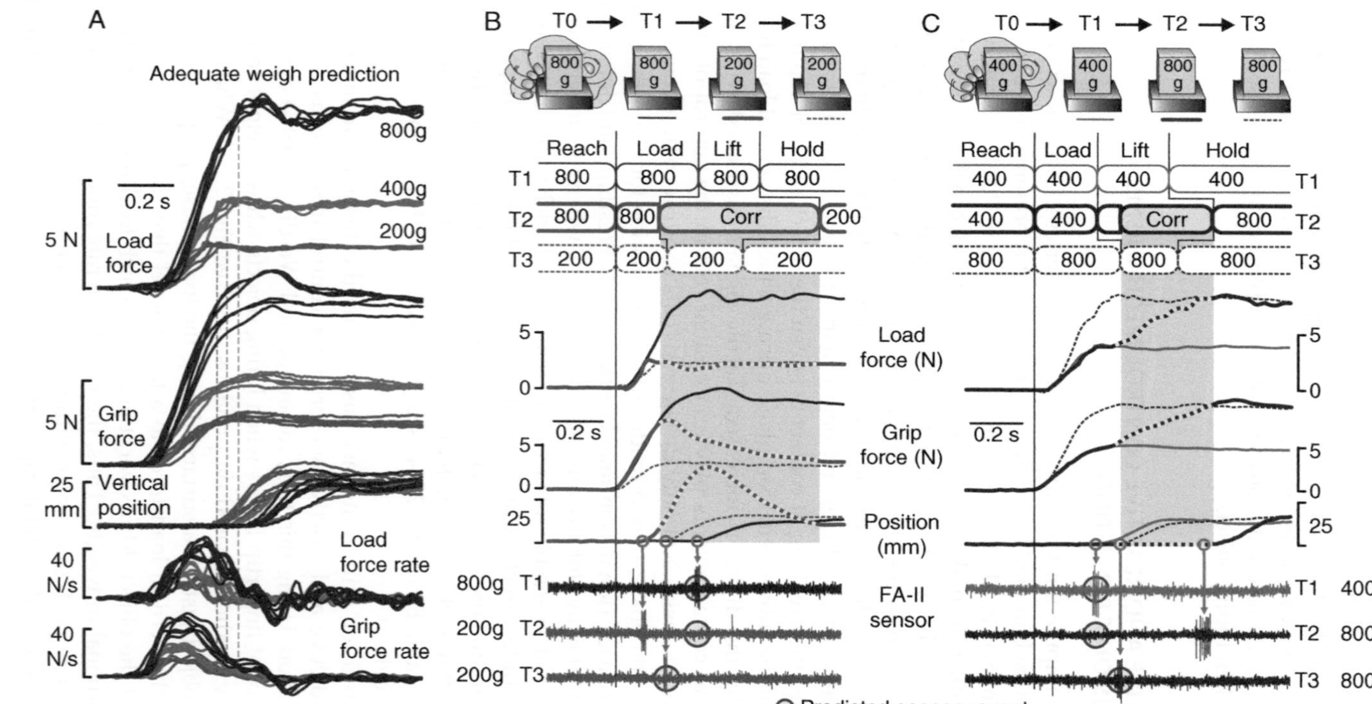

Figure 2.1 Adaptation of motor output to object weight. **A**: Fingertip forces and object position during the initial part of adequately programmed lifts with three objects of different weights (data from 24 single trials from a single participant superimposed).

load force, with a gain that depends on the friction between the digits and surface. Importantly, the increase in load force during the load phase is controlled predictively based on the expected weight of the object.

In the task used by Johansson and Westling (1988a), expectations about object weight were based on knowledge gained from previous lifts of the same object, and such knowledge has been referred to as *sensorimotor memory*. However, reasonable predictions about object weight can often be obtained, prior to the first lift, from other sources of information. Thus, Gordon and colleagues (1993) have shown that people can identify families of objects (e.g., candlestick holders, books, and loafs of bread) based on visual or haptic information and then use learned size–weight associations linked to these families to retrieve weight estimates (Gordon et al. 1991b; Gordon et al. 1991a; Gordon et al. 1991c; Mon-Williams and Murray 2000). In a recent study by Cole (2008), participants first lifted an opaque brown bottle 20 times. After a delay of 15 minutes, the participants then lifted a slightly smaller bottle that was similar in appearance. Although the participants were not aware of the change in bottle size, they nevertheless scaled their lifting forces appropriately for the smaller bottle. Based on

Figure 2.1 (*Continued*) **B** and **C**: Force adjustments and single unit tactile afferent responses to unexpected changes in object weight. Gray circles and vertical lines indicate the instance of lift-off for each trial and the arrowheads point at the signals generated by the lift-off in a FA-II (Pacinian) afferent. The circles behind the nerve traces indicate the corresponding predicted sensory events. **B**: Three successive trials (T1–3) in which the subject lifted an 800 (*blue curves*), a 200 (*red solid curves*), and then the 200 g object again (*red dashed curves*). The forces in T1 were adequately programmed for the prevailing weight because the participant had previously lifted the 800 g object (T0). The forces in T2 were erroneously programmed for the previously lifted 800 g object. In T2, sensory information indicating lift-off occurred earlier than expected, which triggered a corrective action (*yellow-dashed red curves*) terminating the strong force drive and bringing the object back to the intended position. **C**: Three successive trials (T1–3) in which the subject lifted a 400 (*green curves*), an 800 (*blue solid curves*), and then an 800 g object again (*blue dashed curves*). The forces in T2 were erroneously programmed for a 400 g object and the absence of sensory information at the expected lift-off time elicited a corrective action (*yellow-dashed blue curves*) that involved additional force increases until terminated by sensory input signaling lift-off. **B** and **C**: The top diagrams represent sequential action-phase controllers parameterized for different weights. Corrective actions ("Corr") were triggered about 100 ms after a mismatch between predicted and actual sensory information related to lift-off and were linked to an updating of weight parameterization in the remainder of the trial and the next trial. Modified from Johansson, R.S., and J.R. Flanagan. 2009. Coding and use of tactile signals from the fingertips in object manipulation tasks. *Nature Reviews Neuroscience* 10: 345–59, with permission of the publisher. (See color plate.)

these results, Cole (2008) concluded that people automatically make use of visual size cues in addition to memory of object density to scale lift forces when lifting. However, because not all families of objects have constant density, a more general conclusion would be that people learn size–weight maps for families of objects. It has been argued that predictions about the load force (and grip force) required to lift an object are based on an internal model that captures the mechanical properties (e.g., weight) of the object (Johansson and Westling 1988a; Kawato 1999; Imamizu et al. 2000; Wolpert and Ghahramani 2000; Wolpert and Flanagan 2001; Flanagan et al. 2006; see also Imamizu, this volume). However, these results suggest that people do not typically store the weights of individual objects in memory but instead store a more general representation (i.e., a size–weight map) associated with a family of objects. As noted, people appear to learn different size–weight maps for different families of objects such as books, loafs of bread, and candlestick holders (Gordon et al. 1993). Presumably, people can also use object material to estimate size–weight maps and learn associations between material and size–weight maps through experience (Wetenkamp 1933; Ross 1969). Thus, we learn that objects made of Styrofoam and objects made of stainless steel have very different densities or size–weight maps.

Although we rely on weight predictions for smooth and dexterous lifting, there are inevitably instances where our predictions go awry, and this can often result in pronounced performance errors. These errors are signaled by mismatches between actual sensory events and expected events that form part of the sensory plan of the task; that is, the sequence of sensory events expected as the phases of the task unfold (Johansson and Flanagan 2009). Moreover, these mismatches give rise to intelligent, phase-dependent corrective responses. These mechanisms have been well documented for erroneous weight predictions (Johansson and Westling 1988a) and are illustrated in Figures 2.1B and C. Figure 2.1B shows load and grip forces, the vertical position of the object, and predicted and actual sensory events from a fast-adapting type II (FA-II) tactile afferent for three successive trials (T1–T3) where the weight of the object changes, unexpectedly, from 800 to 200 grams in the second trial (T2). The figure also depicts the different phases of the lift for each trial and the expected weight in each phase. When the object being lifted is lighter than predicted and the load phase of the lift is programmed for a heavier weight (T2 in Figure 2.1B), the object lifts off earlier than expected and is lifted higher than intended. The sensory events elicited by the lift-off occur before the predicted sensory events of the sensory plan (Johansson and Flanagan 2009). This mismatch automatically triggers a learned corrective action, or smart reflex, that involves termination of the load phase force followed by corrective motor commands that bring the object back to the intended position. Due to the substantial delays in sensorimotor control loops, this corrective action, which takes ~100 ms to initiate, cannot prevent an overshoot in the lifting movement. Figure 2.1C is similar to Figure 2.1B, and shows three successive trials in which the weight of the object changes, unexpectedly, from 200 to 800 grams in the second trial (T2). When the object is heavier than expected (T2 in Figure 2.1C), the object does not lift off at the expected time because the load force increase is targeted for a lighter weight. In this case, the sensory events elicited by lift-off neither occur before nor at the point predicted by the sensory plan. This mismatch, resulting from the absence of an expected sensory event, triggers a different learned corrective action that involves slow, probing increases in fingertip forces until terminated, reactively, by sensory events signaling lift-off.

The results shown in Figures 2.1B and C demonstrate that the sensorimotor system reacts to both the presence of an unpredicted sensory event and the absence of a predicted sensory event. Moreover, the nature of the corrective actions triggered by these mismatches depends on the phase of the action and is built into the controller for that phase (see "action phase controllers" in Figure 2.1). This phase-dependent use of sensory feedback provides a nice example of optimal, or at least intelligent, feedback control that is central to recent computational models of sensorimotor control (Todorov and Jordan 2002; Scott 2004; Todorov 2004). In addition to triggering corrective actions, these sensory mismatches lead to an updating of memory representations related to object weight, which in turn improves predictive control in subsequent action phases and tasks involving the same object. Thus, for example, in the third trials (T3) shown in Figures 2.1B and C, increases in load force and grip force are tailored for the 200 and 800 g objects, respectively. In the absence of strong visual or haptic cues about object weight, this updating generally occurs in a single trial (as shown in Figures 2.1B and C). However, in the presence of misleading size cues about weight, repeated lifts may be required for complete updating (Gordon et al. 1991b; Flanagan and Beltzner 2000; Flanagan et al. 2008).

Although sensory feedback is continuously predicted and monitored throughout all action phases involved in a manipulation task, tactile signals associated with mechanical contact events play an especially important role in the control of object manipulation tasks. The example shown in Figure 2.1 focuses on tactile signals related to object lift off. However, distinct tactile signals also encode other mechanical events. For example, whereas FA-II afferents quickly and reliably signal the transient mechanical events that occur when an object is lifted off or placed on a surface, slow-adapting type I (SA-I) and especially fast-adapting type I (FA-I) afferents signal making and breaking of contact between the digits and the object (Westling and Johansson 1987; see Johnasson and Flanagan, 2009 for a review). We have argued that these mechanical events, which mark the completion of task phases, serve as critical sensorimotor control points in object manipulation tasks (Johansson et al. 2001; Flanagan et al. 2006). By comparing predicted and actual tactile signals linked to mechanical events, the central nervous system can evaluate whether task subgoals (such as object grasp and lift-off) have been successfully completed and can launch appropriate corrective actions as needed. Moreover, information about object properties provided by tactile signals, including texture, shape, and weight, can be used to parameterize subsequent action phases (e.g., Johansson and Westling 1984; Johansson and Westling 1988a; Jenmalm and Johansson 1997; Jenmalm et al. 1998). Thus, when lifting an object aloft, information about the friction between the skin and object surface obtained as the digits contact the object at the end of the grasp phase can be used to determine the appropriate ratio of grip force to load force during the subsequent load, lift, and hold phases (Johansson and Westling 1984). Importantly, mechanical events related to task subgoals also give rise to distinct signals in other sensory modalities including vision, audition, and proprioception. Thus, the comparison of predicted and actual sensory signals related to mechanical events and task subgoals can occur in multiple sensory modalities. Furthermore, that fact that the same events give rise to discrete sensory signals in multiple modalities means that these events provide an opportunity for multisensory alignment.

When lifting objects, grip force is increased in synchrony with and in proportion to load force (Figure 2.1A), and the rate of change of grip force, relative to the rate of change of load force, is tailored to the expected frictional conditions between the skin and the contact surface (Johansson and Westling 1984). Recently, it has been suggested that the modulation of grip force with changes in load force, seen in precision grip lifting and many other manipulation tasks, arises mechanically from the compression of finger pads rather than neural control mechanisms (Pilon et al. 2007). However, we know with certainty that this conjecture (for which the authors provide no evidence) is simply incorrect. There is clear and very strong evidence that neural mechanisms drive the coupling between grip force and load force and that the contribution of mechanical factors is minimal. Because we have recently discussed this issue in detail (Flanagan et al. 2009), we will only briefly deal with it here, taking advantage of the data shown in Figure 2.1B. As noted earlier, when a participant expects to lift an 800 g object but actually lifts a 200 g weight (cf. T2 in the figure), the object lifts off earlier than expected. Due to biomechanical factors, including muscle shortening, there is a rapid cessation of load force increase at the moment of lift-off. However, grip force continues to increases for some 100 ms after lift-off (before it decreases due to a reflex-mediated mechanism triggered by the earlier than expected lift-off). For the first 100 ms or so after lift-off, the grip force profile is indistinguishable from the profile observed when the participant both expects and receives the 800 g object (compare T1 and T2 in Figure 2.1B). Thus, for a critical 100 ms window there is a clear dissociation between changes in grip force and changes in load force, and grip force is unaffected by dramatic changes in load force. Similar dissociations between changes in grip force and changes in load force have been demonstrated in a number of different tasks in which load forces are unpredictably decreased or increased (Cole and Abbs 1988; Johansson and Westling 1988b; Johansson et al. 1992; Flanagan and Wing 1993; Häger-Ross et al. 1996; Blakemore et al. 1998; Turrell et al. 1999; Witney et al. 1999; Delevoye-Turrell et al. 2003; Hermsdorfer and Blankenfeld 2008). These results clearly demonstrate that load force and grip force are not mechanically coupled, and show that both anticipatory and reactive changes in grip force are achieved through neural control mechanisms.

Prediction, Control, and Internal Models

In numerous studies, we and others have examined the coupling of grip force and load force while moving objects held in a precision grip, where the direction of movement is orthogonal to the grip axis (e.g., Flanagan et al. 1993b; Flanagan and Wing 1993; Flanagan and Wing 1995; Flanagan and Wing 1997; Blakemore et al. 1998; Danion 2004; Descoins et al. 2006; Danion and Sarlegna 2007). This work has shown that grip force is modulated in phase with changes in acceleration-dependent loads that arise when moving inertial loads. Furthermore, grip force is modulated in phase with load force when moving objects with different dynamics specifying the relation between forces applied to the object and its motion (Flanagan and Wing 1997). Figure 2.2A shows single-trial kinematic and force records obtained in a task in which the participant moved a grasped object, instrumented with force sensors, in a horizontal direction between two positions. The object was attached to a linear motor that could be servo-controlled to create inertial, viscous, and elastic loads that depended on acceleration, velocity, and position of the object, respectively. After experiencing each of these loads for a few trials, participants were able to generate smooth movements that were roughly similar, in terms of kinematics, for the three loads. Of course, by design, the load force profiles produced during these movements were very different. The key finding was that the grip force was modulated in phase with load force for all loads.

The result shown in Figure 2.2A indicates that the sensorimotor system knows about, and cares about, object dynamics. When moving a hand-held object, the mapping between arm motor commands and load forces depends on the dynamics of the object. Therefore, to predict accurately the load forces that arise during movement, the sensorimotor system needs to take the dynamics of the object in account. In other words, the sensorimotor system must have stored knowledge, or an internal model, that captures the mechanical behavior of the object while interacting with the hand. Moreover, the sensorimotor must also take into account (i.e., have an internal model of) the dynamics of the arm. The ability of the sensorimotor system to account for arm dynamics is illustrated in Figure 2.2B, which shows fingertip forces recorded in a task in which participants slid an object, instrumented with a force sensor, across a near-frictionless horizontal surface

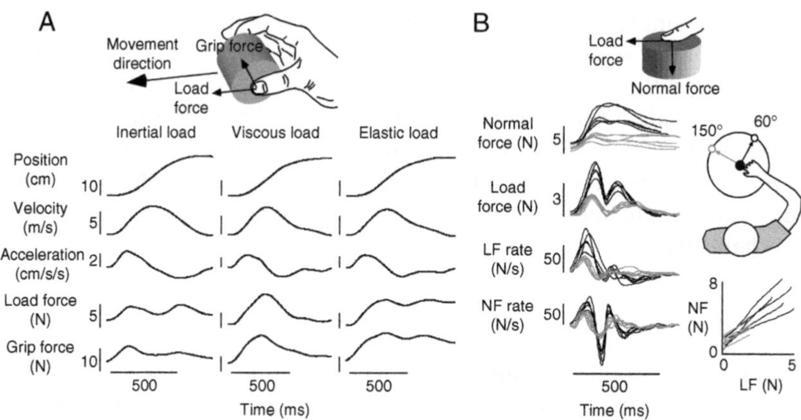

Figure 2.2 Anticipatory adjustments in grip force for movement-related changes in load force. **A**: Single kinematic and force records from one subject moving a hand-held object with three different loads. For all three loads, grip force changes in parallel with fluctuations in load force measured as the resultant load tangential to the grasp surface. All calibration bars start at zero. **B**: Normal and load forces records (data superimposed from ten single trials from a single participant) when sliding an object across a frictionless horizontal surface to one of two targets located at 60 degrees (*red traces*) or 150 degrees (*blue traces*). Subjects held the object, instrumented with a force sensor, beneath the index finger. The lower right panel shows normal force plotted as a function of tangential force from movement onset to the initial peak load force (same ten trials). Modified from Flanagan, J.R., and A.M. Wing. 1997. The role of internal models in motion planning and control: evidence from grip force adjustments during movements of hand-held loads. *Journal of Neuroscience* 17: 1519–28; and Flanagan, J.R., and S. Lolley. 2001. The inertial anisotropy of the arm is accurately predicted during movement planning. *Journal of Neuroscience* 21: 1361–69, with permission of the publisher.

from a central target position to targets located in different directions (Flanagan and Lolley 2001). Movements to the 60-degree target (*black traces*) primarily involve rotation of the forearm about the elbow, and therefore encounter relatively low inertia; whereas movements to the 150-degree (*gray traces*) target involve rotation of the entire arm about the shoulder, and therefore encounter relatively high inertia. Because of this difference in inertia, the acceleration of the hand (and object) is greater for the 60-degree target, in comparison to the 150-degree target, and greater load forces and load force rates are observed. Importantly, the differences in load force and load force rate across the two movement directions is matched by similar differences in normal force and normal force rate. Once again, we see that grip force (i.e., the normal force) is modulated in phase with, and thus anticipates, changes in load force. The bottom right panel of Figure 2.2B further illustrates the coupling between the grip and load forces by showing normal force plotted as a function of load force from movement onset to the initial peak of the load force. These results clearly show that the sensorimotor system takes the inertial properties of the arm into account when predicting and generating required grip forces. Such prediction could be achieved by using a copy of the arm motor command (i.e., efference copy) together with internal models of the object and arm, and information about the configuration of the arm and object (Kawato 1999; Wolpert and Ghahramani 2000; Wolpert and Flanagan 2001; Flanagan et al. 2006).

The term *forward model* refers to an internal model (i.e., a neural process) that can be used to predict the consequences of motor commands. Thus, a forward model pertaining to object dynamics could be used to predict load forces that arise when moving grasped objects. However, internal models pertaining to object dynamics can also be used to estimate the motor commands required to achieve desired sensory consequences. Such models are referred to as *inverse models*. Work examining adaptation of reaching movements to hand-held objects with novel dynamics (i.e., force fields) has clearly established that the sensorimotor system can learn, and store in memory, knowledge of object dynamics that can be used to generate motor commands under appropriate conditions (e.g., Shadmehr and Mussa-Ivaldi 1994; Brashers-Krug et al. 1996; Gandolfo et al. 1996; Conditt et al. 1997; Shadmehr and Brashers-Krug 1997; Thoroughman and Shadmehr 2000; Lackner and DiZio 2005; Cothros et al. 2006).

It is important to point out that internal models of objects, as defined by most researchers in the field, are not necessarily complete or veridical representations of the dynamics of the object. Indeed, most studies examining how people adapt to novel loads have shown that learning is action and context specific (e.g., Thoroughman and Shadmehr 2000; Wang and Sainburg 2004; Nozaki et al. 2006). For example, studies examining reach adaptation to loads applied to the hand have shown limited transfer of learning when the object—or force field linked to the object—is rotated relative to the arm (Shadmehr and Mussa-Ivaldi 1994; Malfait et al. 2002). These results suggest that people do not learn the full dynamics of objects with novel loads but instead learn a mapping between object motion and context- and action-specific motor commands (Shadmehr and Moussavi 2000; Mah and Mussa-Ivaldi 2003). It is an open question whether, with sufficient practice in manipulating an object with novel dynamics, people form a single internal model that approximates the true dynamics of the object or a set of internal models tailored to specific contexts and actions (Ahmed et al. 2008).

Some researchers consider the concept of an internal model to be so general that it is unhelpful or even vacuous. However, it is important to understand the context in which this concept first gained momentum in the field of motor control. In the 1980s, researchers at the Massachusetts Institute of Technology (MIT) and elsewhere began to use concepts from robots in an effort to understand human motion planning and control. One of the important insights obtained from work in robotics is that motor learning and control are improved if the controller has knowledge about the dynamics of the system it controls (Atkeson 1989). At the same time, proponents of the equilibrium-point hypothesis, including the first author of this chapter, argued that the sensorimotor control system did not need to know about the detailed dynamics of the arm (Flash 1987; Feldman et al. 1990; Flanagan et al. 1993a; see also Latash, this volume). According to the latter view, smooth movements arise as a natural consequence of simple shifts in the equilibrium position of a limb, and there is no need to plan a movement trajectory or consider dynamics in order to convert the planned trajectory into motor commands. As noted earlier, subsequent work on trajectory adaptation and anticipatory grip force control when moving hand-held loads has shown that the sensorimotor system does learn and make use of detailed knowledge of arm and object dynamics. However, the question of whether the system plans desired trajectories remains contentious (Kawato 1999; Todorov and Jordan 2002; Scott 2004; Todorov 2004) and it is possible that equilibrium-point control could be combined with knowledge about dynamics (i.e., an internal model) to generate movement (Flanagan et al. 1995). Over the last few decades, the idea that the sensorimotor system makes use of internal models has served as an important starting point for a great deal of innovative research aimed at understanding how such models are learned and represented, and how they might be implemented in the brain (for reviews see Wolpert and Ghahramani 2000; Shadmehr et al. 2010; see also Imamizu, this volume).

Distinct Object Representations in Action and Perception

As discussed earlier, the ability to predict accurately the weights of objects we interact with is essential for skilled manipulation. However, weight predictions are not just used in the control of action; they also influence our perception of weight. There is strong evidence that weight judgments are biased by expected weight, such that an object will be judged to be relatively heavy or light if it is heavier or lighter than expected, respectively (Ross 1969; Ellis and Lederman 1998; Flanagan et al. 2008). This bias is revealed by weight illusions, including the size–weight illusion (Charpentier 1891), in which the smaller of two equally weighted and otherwise similar objects is judged to be heavier; and the material–weight illusion (Wolfe 1898; Seashore 1899), in which an object that appears to be a dense material is judged to be lighter than an equally weighted and otherwise similar object that appears made of a less dense material. The fact that expectations about weight that bias weight judgments can be acquired through experience is well illustrated by the "golf ball" illusion (Ellis and Lederman 1998), in which experienced golfers (but not nongolfers) judge a golf ball to be lighter than a practice golf ball doctored to be equal in weight to a real golf ball.

The size–weight illusion is the most powerful and robust of the weight illusions, and this is presumably because, for a given family of objects, size is generally a very strong predictor of weight. This illusion, first described well over 100 years ago (Charpentier 1891; Murray et al. 1999), is experienced by almost all healthy people (Ross 1969; Davis and Roberts 1976), including children as young as 2 years of age (Robinson 1964; Pick and Pick 1967), and is not weakened when participants are verbally informed that the objects are equally weighted (Flourney 1894; Nyssen and Bourdon 1955; Flanagan and Beltzner 2000). The size–weight illusion is present when only visual cues about size are available, as when lifting viewed objects by strings, but is most powerful when haptic cues about object size are available, as when the hand grasps the objects directly (Ellis and Lederman 1993).

Experiments in which participants lift objects of varying size and weight have shown that predictions about weight, used in action, are independent of predictions about weight used when judging weight (Flanagan and Beltzner 2000; Flanagan et al. 2001; Grandy and Westwood 2006; Chang et al. 2007). In our first study (Flanagan and Beltzner 2000), we asked participants to repeatedly lift a small cube and an equally weighted large cube in alternation for a total of 40 lifts. Although participants initially scaled lifting force to object size, they quickly adapted the lifting force to the true weights of the cubes after about ten lifts. After 40 lifts, we assessed the strength of the illusion and found that the illusion did not differ from that observed in a control group who had not performed the repeated lifts. Thus, despite the fact that the sensorimotor system learned the true weights of the two cubes, at the perceptual level, participants still expected the large cube to be heavier than the small cube and therefore judged the large cube to be lighter than the small cube. This result also ruled out the hypothesis that the size–weight illusion arises from a mismatch between actual and expected sensory feedback related to lifting (Ross 1969; Granit 1972; Davis and Roberts 1976).

More recently we have shown that, in fact, the size–weight illusion can be altered by experience (Flanagan et al. 2008). We constructed a set of 12 blocks, consisting of four shapes and three sizes (Fig. 2.3A), whose weights varied inversely with volume (see circular cylinders in Figure 2.3B; the other shapes had the same sizes and weights). All blocks had the same color and texture. Participants gained experience with these size–weight inverted objects by repeatedly lifting and replacing them (in a random order), moving them from the tabletop to one of four force sensors or vice versa (Fig. 2.3A). Thus, in one-half of the lifts, we could measure the vertical load force participants applied to the object prior to lift-off. Three groups of participants performed lifts. Participants in Group 1 performed 1,050 lifts in a single session. Participants in Group 2 performed 1,200 lifts a day for 3 successive days and 120 lifts on day 4 and participants in Group 3 performed 240 lifts a day for 11 days. In all three groups, the size–weight illusion was tested once all lifts had been completed. We also tested the illusion in a control group of participants who never lifted the inverted size–weight objects.

Figure 2.3C shows load force and load force rate records from two trials in which one of the small, heavy objects was lifted. In initial trials, participants typically underestimated the weight of the small objects, and several increases in load force, associated with distinct peaks in load force rate, were required to achieve lift-off (*gray vertical lines*). However, in later trials in the same session, participants accurately predicted the weight of the small objects such that lift-off occurred after a single, rapid increase in load force. To quantify lift performance, we determined the load force at the time of the first peak in load force rate (LF_1; see gray circles in Figure 2.3C), focusing on trials with the small and mid-sized objects for which we could accurately measure the initial peak in load force rate. For each participant and object size, we computed the median value of LF_1 for each successive block of five lifts from a force sensor (collapsing across object shape). Figure 2.3D shows LF_1 as a function of trial block for Group 2; the first eight blocks and last four blocks on day 1 and the first four blocks on day 2 are shown. The horizontal gray lines are included as visual references, and the dashed line shows an exponential fit to the day 1 data. For the small, heavy objects, LF_1 increased substantially over the first eight blocks (i.e., 40 lifts of a small object from a force sensor and ~240 lifts in total) and had almost fully adapted by the 15th block. Moreover, participants retained this adaptation on day 2. When initially lifting the mid-sized, mid-weighted objects, participants' estimates of object weight were quite accurate, and modest changes in LF_1 occurred across trial blocks. Similar learning of the applied load force was seen in all three experimental groups. That is, all groups of participants fully adapted their lifting forces to the true weights of the objects on day 1 and retained this adaptation if lifting on subsequent days.

To test the size–weight illusion, we used a small and a large cube equal in volume to the small and large inverted objects, respectively, and both equal in weight to the mid-sized inverted objects (Fig. 2.3B). These cubes had the same color and texture as the size–weight inverted objects. Based on the absolute magnitude estimation procedure, in which participants lifted each cube and assigned numbers corresponding to their weights, we quantified the strength and direction of the illusion. A positive score of 100 indicates that the small object was judged 100% heavier than the large objects; a negative score of 50 indicates that the large object was judged 50% heavier than the small object. Figure 2.3E shows the strength of the illusion measured for the Groups 1–3 and the controls. On average, the control participants judged the small cube to be 141% heavier than the large cube. Participants in Group 1 also judged the small object to be heavier than the large objects, but the strength of the illusion was attenuated relative to the controls. Participants in Group 2 did not judge the cubes to be

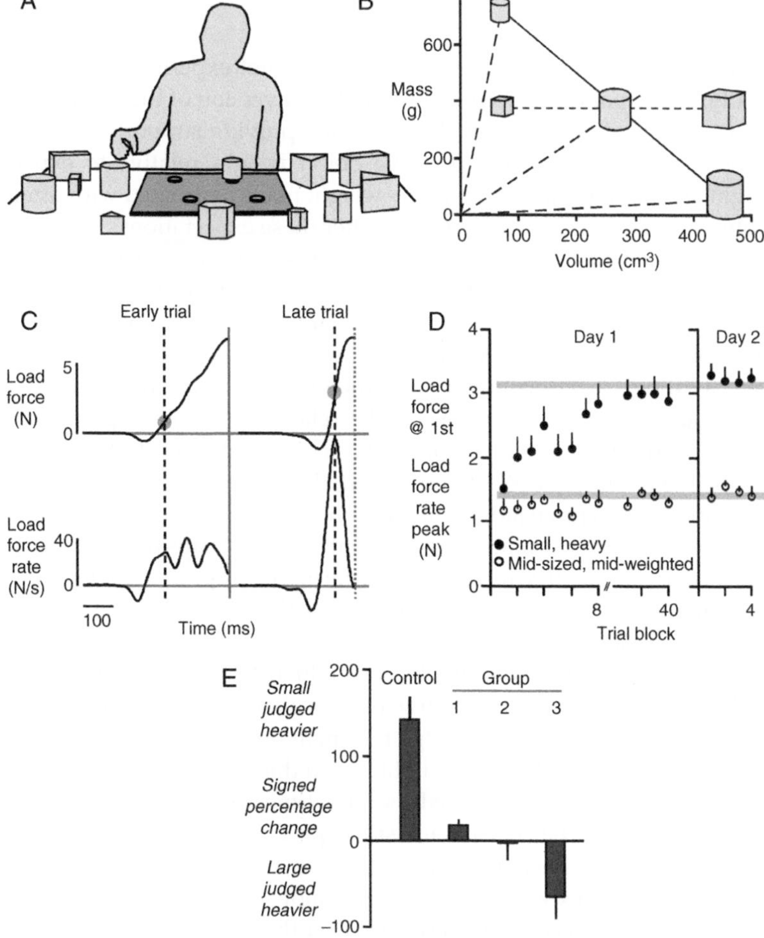

Figure 2.3 Adaptation of lifting forces and weight judgments to size-weight inverted objects. **A**: While seated, participants lifted the objects from the tabletop and placed them on to one of four force sensors or vice versa. All objects were covered with a thin sheet of balsa wood and painted green. A data projector, located above the participant, provided instructions about which object to place on a given force sensor and which object to remove from a given force sensor. **B**: Relation between volume and size for the size-weight inverted objects (circular cylinders given as the example) and for the small and large equally weighted cubes. **C**: Individual load force and load force rate records from an early and a late trial in which a small, heavy object was lifted. The black dashed vertical lines mark the time of the initial peak in load force rate and the gray dotted vertical lines mark the time of lift-off. **D**: Load force at the time of the initial peak in load force rate for the small and mid-sized objects as a function of trial block and day. Each point represents the average across participants and the height of each vertical bar represents 1 SE. **E**: The height of each bar represents the strength and direction of the size–weight illusion, measured as the signed percentage change score, across participants and the height of each error bar represents 1 SE. Modified from Flanagan, J.R., J.P. Bittner, and R.S. Johansson. 2008. Experience can change distinct size-weight priors engaged in lifting objects and judging their weights. *Current Biology* 18: 1742–47, with permission of the publisher.

significantly different in weight and thus did not experience the illusion. Finally, participants in Group 3 exhibited an inversion of the illusion when tested after 11 days of lifting. These results provide support for the dual proposition that (1) people perceive object weight relative to expected weight, generated from learned size–weight maps associated with families of objects, and that (2) experience can alter these expectations.

The fact that participants in all three groups fully adapted their lift forces to the inverted size–weight objects and yet exhibited striking differences in the strength and direction of the size–weight illusion supports the claim (Flanagan and Beltzner 2000) that sensorimotor predictions about weight used in lifting are independent of predictions about weight that influence weight judgments. This finding can be related to the idea, proposed by Goodale and Milner and their colleagues (e.g., Goodale et al. 1991; Culham et al. 2003; Goodale and Westwood 2004), that the control of action and the formation of perceptual judgments rely on neural mechanisms that use and represent sensory information in different ways. Perhaps the even broader point is that the way in which sensory information is processed depends on the demands of the task, rather than on whether the task is perceptual or motor per se (Smeets and Brenner 2006).

Note that expectations about object weight, used when judging weights, are distinct from verbal or cognitive reports about weight. In the standard size–weight illusion, subjects judge the small object to be heavier because they expect the small object to be lighter, and this expectation biases weight perception. If the illusion is tested a second time, the subject will still judge the smaller object to be heavier (and still expect it to be lighter) even though they just said it was heavier. Thus, it is clear that the previous judgment does not alter the expectation of weight underlying the size–weight illusion. Indeed, if expectations were based on the previous report, then the illusion would flip every time it was tested!

The different adaptation rates observed for lifting forces and the size–weight illusion suggest that distinct, adaptive size–weight maps (or priors) underlie the weight predictions used when lifting objects and predictions about weight used when judging their weights. We have suggested that size–weight priors used when judging the weights of familiar objects are resistant to change because they are based on well-established and stable correlations between size and weight that apply to families of objects (Flanagan et al. 2008). For weight perception, this resistance is important. If size–weight priors engaged when judging weight were modified quickly, people would effectively lose their ability to recognize and tag objects as being relatively heavy or light and to communicate this information to others. Conversely, because the sensorimotor system must deal with specific objects, the weights of which may, or may not, be well predicted from visual cues, it is critical that size–weight priors used when lifting objects adapt quickly.

We have argued that, with extensive experience lifting the size–weight inverted objects, people adapt their size–weight priors for these objects such that they learn a single inverted size–weight map for these objects (Flanagan et al. 2008). However, it is also possible that participants in our study learned separate size–weight maps for the small, mid-sized, and large objects. We are currently carrying out experiments to test this alternative account. Regardless of how these experiments pan out, the main conclusion still stands. That is, our results indicate that the brain maintains two distinct representations involved in predicting the weights of objects: a slowly adapting representation that supports weight perception, and a rapidly adapting one that supports manipulatory actions. Importantly, these representations are associated with families of objects, rather than individual objects, and allow generalization across objects within these families (Cole 2008; Flanagan et al. 2008). Similar representations likely encode the dynamics of objects with more complex dynamics in addition to simple inertial loads (Ingram et al. 2010).

REFERENCES

Ahmed, A.A., D.M. Wolpert, and J.R. Flanagan. 2008. Flexible representations of dynamics are used in object manipulation. *Current Biology* 18: 763–68.

Atkeson, C.G. 1989. Learning arm kinematics and dynamics. *Annual Review of Neuroscience* 12: 157–83.

Birznieks, I., P. Jenmalm, A.W. Goodwin, and R.S. Johansson. 2001. Encoding of direction of fingertip forces by human tactile afferents. *Journal of Neuroscience* 21: 8222–37.

Blakemore, S.J., S.J. Goodbody, and D.M. Wolpert. 1998. Predicting the consequences of our own actions: The role of sensorimotor context estimation. *Journal of Neuroscience* 18: 7511–18.

Brashers-Krug, T., R. Shadmehr, and E. Bizzi. 1996. Consolidation in human motor memory. *Nature* 382: 252–55.

Chang, E.C., J.R. Flanagan, and M.A. Goodale. 2007. The intermanual transfer of anticipatory force control in precision grip lifting is not influenced by the perception of weight. *Experimental Brain Research.* Epub ahead of print.

Charpentier, A. 1891. Analyse experimentale quelques elements de la sensation de poids [Experimental study of some aspects of weight perception]. *Archives de Physiologie Normales et Pathologiques* 3: 122–35.

Cole, K.J. 2008. Lifting a familiar object: visual size analysis, not memory for object weight, scales lift force. *Experimental Brain Research.* Epub ahead of print.

Cole, K.J., and J.H. Abbs. 1988. Grip force adjustments evoked by load force perturbations of a grasped object. *Journal of Neurophysiology* 60: 1513–22.

Conditt, M.A., F. Gandolfo, and F.A. Mussa-Ivaldi. 1997. The motor system does not learn the dynamics of the arm by rote memorization of past experience. *Journal of Neurophysiology* 78: 554–60.

Cothros, N., J.D. Wong, and P.L. Gribble. 2006. Are there distinct neural representations of object and limb dynamics? *Experimental Brain Research* 173: 689–97.

Culham, J.C., S.L. Danckert, J.F. DeSouza, J.S. Gati, R.S. Menon, and M.A. Goodale. 2003. Visually guided grasping produces fMRI activation in dorsal but not ventral stream brain areas. *Experimental Brain Research* 153: 180–89.

Danion, F. 2004. How dependent are grip force and arm actions during holding an object? *Experimental Brain Research* 158: 109–19.

Danion, F., and F.R. Sarlegna. 2007. Can the human brain predict the consequences of arm movement corrections when transporting an object? Hints from grip force adjustments. *Journal of Neuroscience* 27: 12839–43.

Davis, C.M., and W. Roberts. 1976. Lifting movements in the size-weight illusion. *Perception and Psychophysics* 20: 33–36.

Delevoye-Turrell, Y.N., F.X. Li, and A.M. Wing. 2003. Efficiency of grip force adjustments for impulsive loading during imposed and actively produced collisions. *Quarterly Journal of Experimental Psychology A* 56: 1113–28.

Descoins, M., F. Danion, and R.J. Bootsma. 2006. Predictive control of grip force when moving object with an elastic load applied on the arm. *Experimental Brain Research* 172: 331–42.

Ellis, R.R., and S.J. Lederman. 1993. The role of haptic versus visual volume cues in the size-weight illusion. *Perception and Psychophysics* 53: 315–24.

Ellis, R.R., and S.J. Lederman. 1998. The golf-ball illusion: Evidence for top-down processing in weight perception. *Perception* 27: 193–201.

Ellis, R.R., and S.J. Lederman. 1999. The material-weight illusion revisited. *Perception and Psychophysics* 61: 1564–76.

Feldman, A.G., S.V. Adamovich, D.J. Ostry, and J.R. Flanagan. 1990. The origins of electromyograms – explanations based on the equilibrium point hypothesis. In *Multiple muscle systems: biomechanics and movement organization*, eds. Winters J, Woo S., 195–213. London: Springer-Verlag.

Flanagan, J.R., and M.A. Beltzner. 2000. Independence of perceptual and sensorimotor predictions in the size-weight illusion. *Nature Neuroscience* 3: 737–41.

Flanagan, J.R., J.P. Bittner, and R.S. Johansson. 2008. Experience can change distinct size-weight priors engaged in lifting objects and judging their weights. *Current Biology* 18: 1742–47.

Flanagan, J.R., M.C. Bowman, and R.S. Johansson. 2006. Control strategies in object manipulation tasks. *Current Opinions in Neurobiology* 16: 650–59.

Flanagan, J.R., S. King, D.M. Wolpert, and R.S. Johansson. 2001. Sensorimotor prediction and memory in object manipulation. *Canadian Journal of Experimental Psychology/Revue Canadienne De Psychologie Experimentale* 55: 87–95.

Flanagan, J.R., and S. Lolley. 2001. The inertial anisotropy of the arm is accurately predicted during movement planning. *Journal of Neuroscience* 21: 1361–69.

Flanagan, J.R., K. Merritt, and R.S. Johannson. 2009. Predictive mechanisms and object representations used in object manipulation. In *Sensorimotor control of grasping: physiology and pathophysiology*, eds. Hermsdörfer J, Nowak DA, 141–60. Cambridge: Cambridge University Press.

Flanagan, J.R., D.J. Ostry, and A.G. Feldman. 1993a. Control of trajectory modifications in target-directed reaching. *Journal of Motor Behavior* 25: 140–52.

Flanagan, J.R., J. Tresilian, and A.M. Wing. 1993b. Coupling of grip force and load force during arm movements with grasped objects. *Neuroscience Letters* 152: 53–56.

Flanagan, J.R., J.R. Tresilian, and A.M. Wing. 1995. Grip force adjustments during rapid movements suggest that detailed movement kinematics are predicted. *Behavioral and Brain Sciences* 18: 753–54.

Flanagan, J.R., and A.M. Wing. 1993. Modulation of grip force with load force during point-to-point arm movements. *Experimental Brain Research* 95: 131–43.

Flanagan, J.R., and A.M.Wing. 1995. The stability of precision grip forces during cyclic arm movements with a hand-held load. *Experimental Brain Research* 105: 455–64.

Flanagan, J.R., and A.M.Wing. 1997. The role of internal models in motion planning and control: evidence from grip force adjustments during movements of hand-held loads. *Journal of Neuroscience* 17: 1519–28.

Flash, T. 1987. The control of hand equilibrium trajectories in multi-joint arm movements. *Biological Cybernetics* 57: 257–74.

Flourney, T. 1894. De l'influence de la perception visuelle des corps sur leur poids apparrent [The influence of visual perception on the apparent weight of objects]. *L'Année Psychologique* 1: 198–208.

Gandolfo, F., F.A. Mussa-Ivaldi, and E. Bizzi. 1996. Motor learning by field approximation. *Proceedings of the National Academy of Science USA* 93: 3843–46.

Goodale, M.A., A.D. Milner, L.S. Jakobson, and D.P. Carey DP. 1991. A neurological dissociation between perceiving objects and grasping them. *Nature* 349: 154–56.

Goodale, M.A., and D.A. Westwood. 2004. An evolving view of duplex vision: separate but interacting cortical pathways for perception and action. *Current Opinions in Neurobiology* 14: 203–11.

Goodwin, A.W., P. Jenmalm, and R.S. Johansson. 1998. Control of grip force when tilting objects: effect of curvature of grasped surfaces and applied tangential torque. *Journal of Neuroscience* 18: 10724–34.

Gordon, A.M., H. Forssberg, R.S. Johansson, and G. Westling. 1991a. The integration of haptically acquired size information in the programming of precision grip. *Experimental Brain Research* 83: 483–88.

Gordon, A.M., H. Forssberg, R.S. Johansson, and G. Westling. 1991b. Integration of sensory information during the programming of precision grip: Comments on the contributions of size cues. *Experimental Brain Research* 85: 226–29.

Gordon, A.M., H. Forssberg, R.S. Johansson, and G. Westling. 1991c. Visual size cues in the programming of manipulative forces during precision grip. *Experimental Brain Research* 83: 477–82.

Gordon, A.M., G. Westling, K.J. Cole, and R.S. Johansson. 1993. Memory representations underlying motor commands used during manipulation of common and novel objects. *Journal of Neurophysiology* 69: 1789–96.

Grandy, M.S.E.C., and D.A. Westwood. 2006. Opposite perceptual and sensorimotor responses to a size-weight illusion. *Journal of Neurophysiology* 95: 3887–92.

Granit, R. 1972. Constant errors in the execution and appreciation of movement. *Brain* 95: 451–60.

Häger-Ross, C., K.J. Cole, and R.S. Johansson. 1996. Grip-force responses to unanticipated object loading - load direction reveals body-referenced and gravity-referenced intrinsic task variables. *Experimental Brain Research* 110: 142–50.

Hermsdorfer, J., and H. Blankenfeld. 2008. Grip force control of predictable external loads. *Experimental Brain Research* 185: 719–28.

Imamizu, H., S. Miyauchi, T. Tamada, Y. Sasaki, R. Takino, B. Putz, et al. 2000. Human cerebellar activity reflecting an acquired internal model of a new tool. *Nature* 403: 192–95.

Ingram, J.N., I.S. Howard, J.R. Flanagan, and D.M. Wolpert. 2010. Multiple grasp-specific representations of tool dynamics mediate skilful manipulation. *Current Biology*, in press.

Jenmalm, P., S. Dahlstedt, and R.S. Johansson. 2000. Visual and tactile information about object-curvature control fingertip forces and grasp kinematics in human dexterous manipulation. *Journal of Neurophysiology* 84: 2984–97.

Jenmalm, P., A.W. Goodwin, and R.S. Johansson. 1998. Control of grasp stability when humans lift objects with different surface curvatures. *Journal of Neurophysiology* 79: 1643–52.

Jenmalm, P., and R.S. Johansson. 1997. Visual and somatosensory information about object shape control manipulative fingertip forces. *Journal of Neuroscience* 17: 4486–99.

Johansson, R.S., and I. Birznieks. 2004. First spikes in ensembles of human tactile afferents code complex spatial fingertip events. *Nature Neuroscience* 7: 170–77.

Johansson, R.S., and J.R. Flanagan. 2009. Coding and use of tactile signals from the fingertips in object manipulation tasks. *Nature Reviews Neuroscience* 10: 345–59.

Johansson, R.S., C. Hager, and R. Riso. 1992. Somatosensory control of precision grip during unpredictable pulling loads. {II}. Changes in load force rate. *Experimental Brain Research* 89: 192–203.

Johansson, R.S., and G. Westling. 1984. Roles of glabrous skin receptors and sensorimotor memory in automatic-control of precision grip when lifting rougher or more slippery objects. *Experimental Brain Research* 56: 550–64.

Johansson, R.S., and G. Westling. 1988a. Coordinated isometric muscle commands adequately and erroneously programmed for the weight during lifting task with precision grip. *Experimental Brain Research* 71: 59–71.

Johansson, R.S., and G. Westling. 1988b. Programmed and triggered actions to rapid load changes during precision grip. *Experimental Brain Research* 71: 72–86.

Johansson, R.S., G. Westling, A. Backstrom, and J.R. Flanagan. 2001. Eye-hand coordination in object manipulation. *Journal of Neuroscience* 21: 6917–32.

Kawato, M. 1999. Internal models for motor control and trajectory planning. *Current Opinions in Neurobiology* 9: 718–27.

Lackner, J.R., and P. DiZio. 2005. Motor control and learning in altered dynamic environments. *Current Opinions in Neurobiology* 15: 653–59.

Mah, C.D., and F.A. Mussa-Ivaldi. 2003. Generalization of object manipulation skills learned without limb motion. *Journal of Neuroscience* 23: 4821–25.

Malfait, N., D.M. Shiller, and D.J. Ostry. 2002. Transfer of motor learning across arm configurations. *Journal of Neuroscience* 22: 9656–60.

Mon-Williams, M., and A.H. Murray. 2000. The size of the visual size cue used for programming manipulative forces during precision grip. *Experimental Brain Research* 135: 405–10.

Murray, D.J., R.R. Ellis, C.A. Bandomir, and H.E. Ross. 1999. Charpentier (1891) on the size-weight illusion. *Perception and Psychophysics* 61: 1681–85.

Nozaki, D., I. Kurtzer, and S.H. Scott. 2006. Limited transfer of learning between unimanual and bimanual skills within the same limb. *Nature Neuroscience* 9: 1364–66.

Nyssen, R., and J. Bourdon. 1955. [Study of the incidence and degree of size-weight illusion in dementia and oligophrenia in adults.]. *Acta Neurological et Psychiatrica Belgica* 55: 391–98.

Pick, H.L., and A.D. Pick. 1967. A developmental and analytic study of the size-weight illusion. *Journal of Experimental Child Psychology* 5: 363–71.

Pilon, J.F., S.J. De Serres, and A.G. Feldman. 2007. Threshold position control of arm movement with anticipatory increase in grip force. *Experimental Brain Research* 181: 49–67.

Robinson, H.B. 1964. An experimental examination of the size-weight illusion in young children. *Child Development* 35: 91–107.

Ross, H.E. 1969. When is a weight not illusory? *Quarterly Journal of Experimental Psychology* 21: 346–55.

Scott, S.H. 2004. Optimal feedback control and the neural basis of volitional motor control. *Nature Reviews Neuroscience* 5: 534–46.

Seashore, C.E. 1899. Some psychological statistics. 2. The material-weight illusion. University of Iowa Studies in Psychology 2.

Shadmehr, R., and T. Brashers-Krug. 1997. Functional stages in the formation of human long-term motor memory. *Journal of Neuroscience* 17: 409–19.

Shadmehr, R., and Z.M. Moussavi. 2000. Spatial generalization from learning dynamics of reaching movements. *Journal of Neuroscience* 20: 7807–15.

Shadmehr, R., and F. Mussa-Ivaldi. 1994. Adaptive representation of dynamics during learning of a motor task. *Journal of Neuroscience* 14:5: 3208–24.

Shadmehr, R., M.A. Smith, and J.W. Krakauer. 2010. Error correction, sensory prediction, and adaptation in motor control. *Annual Reviews of Neuroscience*, in press.

Smeets, J.B., and E. Brenner. 2006. 10 years of illusions. *Journal of Experimental Psychology. Human Perception and Performance* 32: 1501–04.

Thoroughman, K.A., and R. Shadmehr. 2000. Learning of action through adaptive combination of motor primitives. *Nature* 407: 742–47.

Todorov, E. 2004. Optimality principles in sensorimotor control. *Nature Neuroscience* 7: 907–15.

Todorov, E., and M.I. Jordan. 2002. Optimal feedback control as a theory of motor coordination. *Nature Neuroscience* 5: 1226–35.

Turrell, Y.N., F.X. Li, and A.M. Wing. 1999. Grip force dynamics in the approach to a collision. *Experimental Brain Research* 128: 86–91.

Wang, J., and R.L. Sainburg. 2004. Interlimb transfer of novel inertial dynamics is asymmetrical. *Journal of Neurophysiology* 92: 349–60.

Westling, G., and R.S. Johansson. 1987. Responses in glabrous skin mechanoreceptors during precision grip in humans. *Experimental Brain Research* 66: 128–40.

Wetenkamp, L. 1933. Über die materialtäuschung. Ein beitrag zur lehre von der objektion. *Zeitschrift für Psychologie* 130: 172–234.

Witney, A.G., S.J. Goodbody, and D.M. Wolpert. 1999. Predictive motor learning of temporal delays. *Journal of Neurophysiology* 82: 2039–2048.

Wolfe, H.K. 1898. Some effects of size on judgments of weight. *Psychological Review* 5: 25–54.

Wolpert, D.M., and J.R. Flanagan. 2001. Motor prediction. *Current Biology* 11: R729-R32.

Wolpert, D.M., and Z. Ghahramani. 2000. Computational principles of movement neuroscience. *Nature Neuroscience* 3 Suppl: 1212–17.

3

A Canonical-Dissipative Approach to Control and Coordination in the Complex System Agent-Task-Environment

TILL D. FRANK, DOBROMIR G. DOTOV, AND
MICHAEL T. TURVEY

Rhythmic repetitive motor activities such as walking and stair climbing contribute significantly to the spectrum of everyday activities of humans. Rhythmic motor tasks seem to confront human actors with two fundamental challenges. First, a permanently changing action must be produced. Second, the produced action must be stabilized against perturbations. One may argue, however, that these challenges actually do not exist when considering motor control systems from the closely related perspectives of self-organization (Kelso 1995; Haken 2004) and dynamic systems theory (Bernstein 1967; Beek, Peper, et al. 1995). On this consideration, oscillatory repetitive activity is a generic property of open systems supplied by energy sources. It is often sufficient just to excite such a system with a sufficiently large stimulus for a permanently changing activity pattern to emerge. The stimulus itself does not need to contain any specification of the emerging oscillatory pattern. The pattern emerges due to self-organization.

Stability can also be considered as an in-built part of self-organizing systems because such systems in general are nonlinear and nonlinearity, in turn, invites systems to produce stable patterns. In line with this reasoning, it does not come as a surprise that in various disciplines such as chemistry, biology, and physics, a plenitude of systems can be found that exhibit stable oscillatory activity patterns. In other words, a decision to admit agent-task-environment (ATE) systems to the class of nonlinear, self-organizing systems means that we expect to see those systems exhibit repetitive motor activities that are stable against perturbations and emergent from the impact of unspecific stimuli. The ability to perform rhythmic repetitive motor tasks may be regarded as a "natural" property of nonlinear self-organizing systems.

If this perspective on oscillatory motor control holds, then the question arises how to proceed from qualitative considerations to more explicit and quantitative issues. How can we link observation with dynamic systems modeling and the theory of self-organization? A fair amount of research has been directed at this question. In Kay et al. (1987), hand oscillatory movements about the wrist in the horizontal plane were mapped to a class of limit cycle oscillators. The limit cycle oscillators were a mixture of van der Pol oscillators and Rayleigh oscillators. Both oscillators feature different nonlinearities. Kay et al. determined coefficients of these nonlinear terms from experimental data. In particular, the decay of perturbations, related to the relaxation toward the limit cycle, was used as a measure of the strength of the limit cycle attractor (Kay et al. 1991).

A related study on single-limb forearm oscillations in the horizontal plane aimed to generalize the Rayleigh model by means of a frequency-dependent coefficient that rendered the impact of the Rayleigh nonlinearity frequency-dependent (Beek et al. 1996). In addition, oscillations of a handheld pendulum in the sagittal plane concurrent with an isometric force production task have been studied in terms of van der Pol and Rayleigh oscillators that exhibit nonlinear stiffness in addition to (ordinary) linear stiffness (Silva et al. 2007). The coefficients of the stiffness terms were found to vary with the self-selected oscillation frequencies (manipulated via differences in pendulum length) and the magnitude of the required isometric force.

Although the aforementioned studies and others like them (Eisenhammer et al. 1991; Beek, Schmidt et al. 1995; Daffertshofer et al. 1999; Delignieres et al. 1999; Mottet and Bootsma 1999; van den Berg et al. 2000) have provided substantial insights, they have not as yet provided a pragmatic approach permitting researchers to identify model parameters of excitation and stability on the basis of experimental data. In physics, such a pragmatic approach has been developed, the so-called *canonical-dissipative approach* (Haken 1973; Graham 1981; Feistel and Ebeling 1989; Ebeling and Sokolov 2004; Frank 2005b). It has been particularly successful in the domains of self-propagating agents, "active" particles, and mutually-coupled many-particle systems (Erdmann et al. 2000; Frank and Daffertshofer 2001; Schweitzer et al. 2001; Frank 2003, 2005a; Schweitzer 2003; Erdmann et al. 2005; Frank and Mongkolsakulvong 2008). Our goal in this chapter is twofold: to present the canonical-dissipative approach, and to exemplify how it can be applied to rhythmic activity emerging in ATE systems viewed from a self-organizational perspective.

CANONICAL-DISSIPATIVE APPROACH TO OSCILLATORY ACTIVITY

Canonical-dissipative systems manifest properties of conservative systems as described by classical Hamiltonian mechanics and dissipative systems as described by dynamic systems theory. As shown in Table 3.1, conservative systems of Hamiltonian mechanics exhibit, on a phenomenological level, the conservation law of energy and exhibit, on a descriptive level,

Table 3.1 Characteristics of conservative, canonical-dissipative, and dissipative nonequilibrium systems

Conservative systems	Canonical dissipative systems	Dissipative nonequilibrium systems
Exhibit energy conservation and the dynamics satisfies Hamiltonian evolution equations	After a transient period we have (i) energy conservation and (ii) the dynamics satisfies Hamiltonian evolution equations	In general, energy is not conserved and the dynamics does not satisfy Hamiltonian evolution equations
Cannot account for damping (friction), pumping (excitation), fluctuations (variability)	Address damping, pumping, and fluctuations	Address damping, pumping, and fluctuations

Hamiltonian evolution equations. Phenomena such as damping (friction), pumping (excitation), and fluctuation (variability) are not considered. In contrast, dissipative systems typically feature damping, pumping, and fluctuations. No conservation of energy occurs, as there is typically a flow of energy, matter, and/or information through these systems. Such fully developed dissipative systems in general do not satisfy Hamiltonian evolution equations. Canonical-dissipative systems can account for damping, pumping, and fluctuations just as dissipative systems do. Energy is not an invariant, and Hamiltonian equations do not hold if we observe these kind of systems in their transient regimes. However, after a transient period, energy becomes an invariant and Hamiltonian mechanics becomes an accurate description (Haken 1973; Graham 1981; Ebeling and Sokolov 2004). That is, a canonical-dissipative system exhibits a transient and a nontransient time domain. The latter time domain is also referred to as *long-term* or *asymptotic behavior*. In the transient time domain, a canonical-dissipative system looks more like a truly dissipative system, whereas in the long-term domain a canonical-dissipative system exhibits a variety of properties similar to those of a truly canonical system. We may rephrase this property using the notion of fixed points, limit cycles, and other types of attractors (Strogatz 1994; Haken 2004). Accordingly, the dynamics of canonical-dissipative systems converges during transient periods to attractor spaces that define the long-term behavior of the system and, in turn, can be described in terms of Hamiltonian equations. In particular, energy is an invariant for canonical-dissipative oscillators along their limit cycles.

In what follows, we restrict our considerations to the oscillatory case. From a mathematical point of view, the evolution equation of an oscillatory canonical-dissipative system can be split into two parts. One part determines the behavior on the limit cycle. This part is described by the

Hamiltonian function H. The other part expresses the attraction toward the limit cycle and involves a function g that depends on H.

On the Limit Cycle

On the limit cycle, the Hamiltonian function H has the same interpretation as the ordinary Hamiltonian function of conservative systems. H reflects the total energy. That is, H is the sum of kinetic and potential energy terms and may even involve mixed energy terms. Energy measures are considered as generalized energies. That is, we do not necessarily measure energy in units of Joule, kg m^2/s^2, or calories. Recall that the dynamic models of interest are low-dimensional descriptions of high-dimensional perception-action processes. Accordingly, energy measures reflect types of energies that exist on the level of postulated underlying low-dimensional coordinate spaces. For example, the kinetic energy of a low-dimensional dynamic does not necessarily reflect the kinetic energy of the limb whose oscillatory behavior is described by that dynamic.

The state variable of interest is the time-dependent state variable $q(t)$ of the underlying low-dimensional dynamic that is known to emerge in high-dimensional self-organizing systems (Haken 2004). Typically, however, we do not have direct access to this variable. One of the observables at hand is the position $x(t)$ of a limb with respect to an appropriately defined reference (or zero) position. If other pieces of information $y_1(t),\ldots,y_n(t)$ about the ATE system are available (muscle activity, electroencephalograph [EEG], magnetoencephalograph [MEG], electrocardiogram [ECG], breathing, skin resistance, gaze, sensory stimulation, environmental changes, etc.) then we say we have information about a time-dependent state vector $M = (x,y_1,\ldots,y_n)$ available. The state vector can be used to make inferences about the variable $q(t)$. For example, we may introduce a set of orthogonal vectors $W_0,\ldots,W_n$ and expand $M(t)$ into a series of this set like $M(t) = q(t)W_0 + R(t)$, where W_0 denotes the most dominant component and R contains all other components. The vector W_0 and the amplitude $q(t)$ in this example can be determined by means of principal components analysis (see Ting and Chvatal and Dodel et al., this volume). In experimental designs focusing solely on the behavioral activity, and in which only information about a limb coordinate $x(t)$ is collected, we take $x(t)$ instead of $q(t)$. In what follows, we will consider this latter case, in which only information about the position x is available.

Let x denote the position. Let E_{pot} denote a suitable defined measure of potential energy. Then, E_{pot} is a function of x. Let Δt denote the sampling interval. The generalized velocity v can then be defined by $v(t) = (x(t + \Delta t) - x(t))/\Delta t$. Likewise, the kinetic energy E_{kin} can be computed from $E_{kin} = v^2/2$ at every time step t. Note that, in line with the comment on units made above, we have put here the mass equal to 1. Finally, let E_{mix} describe mixed energy terms that depend both on the coordinate x and the velocity v.

Having introduced these different types of energy terms, the Hamiltonian function at time t can be defined by

$$H(t) = E_{kin}(v(t)) + E_{pot}(x(t)) + E_{mix}(x(t), v(t)) \qquad \text{(Eq. 1)}$$

The shape of the oscillator limit cycle is determined by the function H. For example, the standard canonical-dissipative oscillator involves a harmonic potential function $E_{pot} = \omega^2 x^2/2$ and there is no mixed energy term. In this case, limit cycles correspond to closed elliptic trajectories in the phase space spanned by x and v. For an example, see Figure 3.1 (panels A and B). The canonical-dissipative approach can account for limit cycles that exhibit all kinds of trajectories. For example, when adding a mixed term $E_{mix} = \alpha x^2 v^2/2$, where α is a positive parameter, a more square-like limit cycle can be observed (see Fig. 3.1 C).

Approach to the Limit Cycle

The approach to the limit cycle is determined by a function, g, that depends on H. The function g describes a restoring mechanism in the energy space. That is, just like a spring force that pushes a mass attached to the spring back to a stationary position that is defined by the spring's rest length, the function g describes processes that increase or decrease the Hamiltonian energy $H(t)$ such that it eventually approaches a stationary value. If fluctuations are neglected, then this stationary value corresponds to a parameter of the canonical-dissipative oscillator. Let b denote this parameter. We will refer to the stationary total energy as *fixed-point energy*. The function g can depend in linear or nonlinear fashion on H. The standard canonical-dissipative oscillator involves a linear restoring function g (Haken 1973; Graham 1981; Ebeling and Sokolov 2004) as defined by

$$g(H) = -\gamma\,(H - b) \qquad \text{(Eq. 2)}$$

with $\gamma \geq 0$. As we will discuss next, γ and b, the two parameters involved in g, are crucial for our understanding of motor control systems as self-organizing systems.

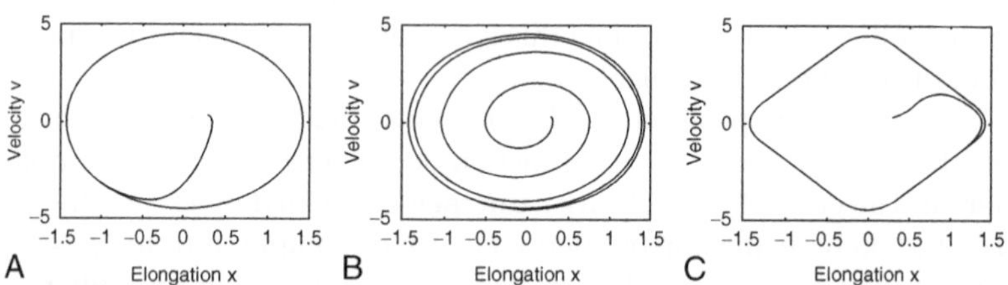

Figure 3.1 Limit cycle and approach to the limit cycle. Parameters: $\omega = \pi$, $\gamma = 1$, $b = 10$ (*A*), $\omega = \pi$, $\gamma = 0.1$, $b = 10$ (*B*), and $\omega = \pi$, $\gamma = 1$, $b = 10$, $\alpha = 2$ (C).

Roughly speaking, the parameter b quantifies the amount of excitation of the system under consideration. More precisely, b should be interpreted as the excess excitation or net pumping of the oscillator. That is, if we would be able to quantify the amount of raw pumping, on the one hand, and the amount of energy losses (e.g., due to friction), on the other hand, then b would be a measure for the difference between these two quantities. Therefore, b should be interpreted as a net pumping parameter. Assuming that the energy scale for the Hamiltonian H has a lower boundary at $H = 0$ (i.e., H cannot assume values smaller than zero), then parameter values $b > 0$ indicate that the excitation is stronger than the losses due to friction, whereas parameter values $b < 0$ indicate that the losses dominate the excitation. For $b < 0$ the nonoscillatory state (exhibiting $H = 0$) is stable. In contrast, for $b > 0$ the nonoscillatory state is linearly unstable, and the system dynamics bifurcates to an oscillatory state with $H > 0$. In that case, nonlinear terms ensure that the oscillation amplitude does not increase beyond any boundary (i.e., the nonlinear terms ensure that the dynamics approaches a limit cycle). Consequently, $b = 0$ is a critical parameter value (see also section "Conclusion" and Fig. 3.7 panels A and B). The parameter b has a qualitative property (as reflected by its sign) and a quantitative property (as reflected by its magnitude). The quantitative property of the parameter b can be used to compare the net excitation level of an oscillatory behavior under different conditions. The larger b is, the stronger is the degree of excitation. Therefore, b can be used to study to what extent experimental manipulations of an ATE system affect the net excitation level of a rhythmic behavior exhibited by that system. How do variables of agent, task, and environment affect the unspecific stimulus, postulated earlier, that results in the observed rhythmic activity?

The parameter $\gamma \geq 0$ describes how strongly the oscillatory behavior is attracted by the limit cycle when studying the oscillator behavior in its appropriate energy space. For example, for the standard canonical-dissipative oscillator involving the function g as defined by Eq. (2), it can be shown that the Hamiltonian energy H satisfies the following differential equation

$$\frac{d}{dt}H = -\gamma\,(H - b)v^2 \qquad \text{(Eq. 3)}$$

Since the squared velocity is positive in any case, we see that if H is larger than the fixed-point energy b, then the Hamiltonian energy will decay as a function of time until H approaches the value of b. In contrast, if H is smaller than b, then H will increase as a function of time and, again, $H(t)$ will converge to b. The approach toward the fixed-point energy b goes along with the approach of the trajectory in phase space toward the oscillator limit cycle. The faster H converges to its fixed-point energy, the faster trajectories reach the limit cycle. This implies that perturbations decay on the characteristic time scale that is defined by the energy dynamics. This time scale is primarily determined by the parameter γ. The larger the parameter γ, the stronger the restoring processes, the faster the relaxation of H to the fixed-point value b, and the faster the approach of trajectories in phase space toward the oscillator limit cycle. Panel A in Figure 3.1 illustrates the approach to the limit cycle for a canonical-dissipative system with relatively large parameter γ (here $\gamma = 1.0$). Panel B depicts a trajectory for the same system when the parameter γ is reduced (from $\gamma = 1.0$ to $\gamma = 0.1$), that is, when the system exhibits a relatively small parameter γ. Since the decay of perturbations is associated with the notion of stability, we conclude that γ is a parameter that describes the stability of the canonical-dissipative oscillator. With the parameters γ and b at hand, we have identified the two parameters that inform us about the excitation and stability of repetitive rhythmic activities emerging in ATE systems under various natural conditions and experimental manipulations.

STANDARD CANONICAL-DISSIPATIVE OSCILLATOR

The stochastic evolution equation of the standard canonical-dissipative oscillator corresponds to a Langevin equation involving the random variables $x(t)$ and $v(t)$. For the sake of convenience, we will write down this equation as a second-order stochastic differential equation involving only the generalized coordinate x:

$$\frac{d^2}{dt^2}x = -\omega^2 x - \gamma \frac{d}{dt}x\,(H - b) + \sqrt{Q}\,\Gamma(t)$$

(Eq. 4)

$$H = \frac{1}{2}\left(\frac{d}{dt}x\right)^2 + \frac{\omega^2 x^2}{2}$$

The function $\Gamma(t)$ is a Langevin force (Risken 1989). If we observe the dynamics defined by Equation 4 at finite sampling times, then this Langevin force yields a sequence of independent, Gaussian-distributed random numbers with mean equal to zero and variance of 1. The parameter $Q \geq 0$ amplifies the impact of the Langevin force $\Gamma(t)$. Q and Γ taken together describe a fluctuating force that persistently perturbs the rhythmic behavior of the ATE system. We say that there is a source of perturbation, a so-called noise source, which results in fluctuations of the oscillatory behavior. In this context, Q is also referred to as *noise amplitude* or *strength of the fluctuating force*. Equation 4 determines both the approach of the oscillator dynamics to the limit cycle, as well as the behavior of the oscillator on the limit cycle. Figure 3.2 illustrates these issues. In the deterministic case (i.e., for $Q = 0$) from Equation 4, we obtain the energy equation (Equation 3). If the approach to the limit cycle requires several oscillation periods, as in the case shown in Figure 3.1 (panel B), then we can average the energy H across one cycle to obtain H_a like $H_a = \langle H \rangle_{\text{cycle}}$. In this case, the virial theorem

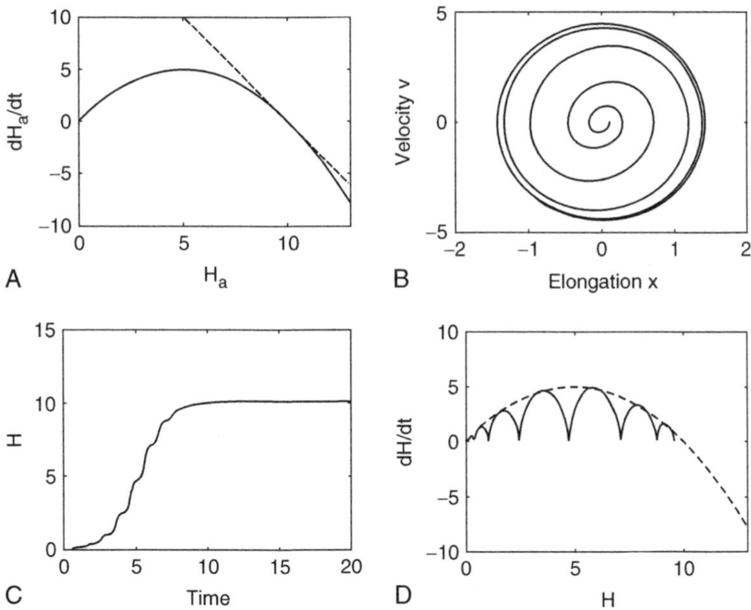

Figure 3.2 **A**: Stability plot dH_a/dt versus H_a (*solid line*) with a linearization (*dashed line*) of the graph at the stable fixed point $H_a = b$ (here $b = 10$). **B**: Trajectory in phase space computed from Equation 4. **C**: Instantaneous Hamiltonian $H(t)$ computed by means of Equation 4b for the trajectory shown in B. **D**: Stability plot dH/dt versus H for the energy function $H(t)$ shown in C. Parameters for all panels: $\omega = \pi$, $\gamma = 0.1$, $b = 10$, $Q=0$.

(Bartlett 1975) gives us the relation $H_a = 2<v^2>_{\text{cycle}}$ such that Equation 3 becomes $dH_a/dt = -2\gamma H_a (H_a-b)$. Figure 3.2 (panel A) shows dH_a/dt on the vertical axis versus H_a on the horizontal axis (for $b = 10$). There is an unstable fixed point at $H_a = 0$ and a stable fixed point at $H_a = b$. The dashed line is the linearization at the stable fixed point. The slope of the dashed line is determined by the parameter γ. The larger γ is, the steeper the graph. Panel B shows the trajectory in phase space of a simulation of model Equation 4 for $Q = 0$ (and $b = 10$). The variable H approaches the stationary value $H = b$ as shown in panel C. Recall that H is the instantaneous energy at every time point t (and not the cycle averaged energy H_a). If we plot dH/dt versus H then we obtain the graph shown in panel D, which has as an envelope the graph obtained previously from our theoretical considerations on H_a. In short, Figure 3.2 illustrates that H shares the same stability properties as the cycle-averaged energy H_a. However, as mentioned in the previous section when discussing Equation 3, in general (i.e., irrespective of whether it takes several or only a few cycles for the dynamics to approach the limit cycle), from Equation 3 it follows that the energy H approaches a stable fixed point value.

From our previous discussion, it follows that the two key parameters of interest are the net pumping parameter b and the stability parameter γ. How can we link these parameters with experimentally accessible observables? Several studies have been concerned with parameter estimation techniques for oscillator models of human rhythmic movements. The techniques discussed in these studies primarily exploit the observation of the oscillator position. However, as shown earlier, the properties of canonical-dissipative systems rely on the Hamiltonian function H and on how the energy H is attracted toward a fixed-point level. Therefore, in the context of the canonical-dissipative approach toward an understanding of rhythmic movements in ATE systems, it is promising to study how the parameters γ and b are mapped to $<H>$ (mean H) and SDH (standard deviation of H) of a given Hamiltonian function H.

Figure 3.3 summarizes the results that can be derived for the standard canonical-dissipative oscillator defined by Equation 4. The results presented in Figure 3.3 can be obtained by exploiting both analytical considerations and numerical solution methods (see Appendix). According to Figure 3, the oscillator frequency ω affects neither $<H>$ nor SDH. The parameter b affects $<H>$. For large enough parameter values of b we have $<H> = b$. The stability parameter has an effect on $<H>$ in the case of weak attractors (i.e., when γ is small). For large enough stability parameters (e.g., $\gamma \geq 2$ in the example shown in Figure 3.3), $<H>$ does not change significantly with γ. Rather, it is the case that when γ becomes sufficiently large, then $<H>$ converges to a saturation value. This saturation value depends exclusively on the net pumping parameter b. For weakly excited oscillators, there is an effect of the net pumping parameter b on SDH. However, if the net pumping parameter b is sufficiently large (e.g., $b \geq 2$ in the example shown in Figure 3.3), then SDH does not change with b (i.e., SDH is not affected significantly by b). With respect to γ, SDH decays monotonically, decaying to zero when γ tends to infinity (meaning that energy fluctuations disappear in the case of an infinitely strong attractor).

In sum, if the ATE system under consideration exhibits relatively strong attractors and relatively strong net excitement stimuli, then the model parameters b and γ simply map to the observables $<H>$ and SDH. First, $<H>$ is equivalent to the net pumping parameter b. Second, there is a reciprocal relationship between energy variability and stability: SDH increases when γ decreases, and vice versa. This reciprocal relation is not affected by the amount of net pumping. Therefore, observation of $<H>$ and SDH can be used to make inferences about the magnitude of the model parameters γ and b.

When oscillator attractors are weak or when the net pumping of the standard canonical-dissipative oscillator is relatively small, then the dependent variables $<H>$ and SDH are both affected by the stability parameter γ and the net pumping parameter b. Consequently, it becomes more technically involved to make inferences about b and γ on the basis of the observation of $<H>$ and SDH.

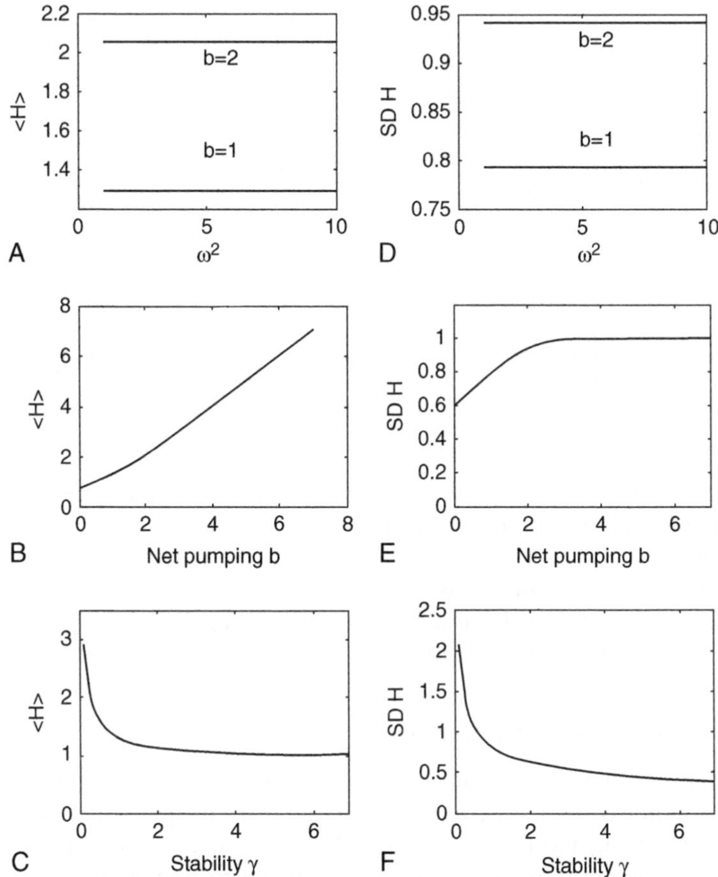

Figure 3.3 Properties of the standard canonical-dissipative oscillator. **Left column (A–C)**: mean Hamiltonian energy <*H*> as a function of squared frequency ω^2, net pumping b, and stability γ (from top to bottom). **Right column (D–F)**: energy standard deviation SD*H* as a function of ω^2, b, and γ (from top to bottom). For details, see also Appendix.

As already noted, ω affects neither <*H*> nor SD*H*. The reason for this is that, in the case of the standard canonical-dissipative oscillator, the distribution of H depends only on the parameters γ, Q, and b but does not depend on ω (see Appendix). In view of the Hamiltonian function $H = v^2/2 + \omega^2 x^2/2$ (see Equation 4) this property does not appeal to our intuition. Therefore, the question arises: What happens when ω is increased but all other parameters are held constant? The result of a numerical simulation for the deterministic case is shown in Figure 3.4. The oscillators in both simulations have the same energy on the limit cycle (in the example, we have $H_{stationary} = b = 10$). The oscillator shown in the panel B oscillates

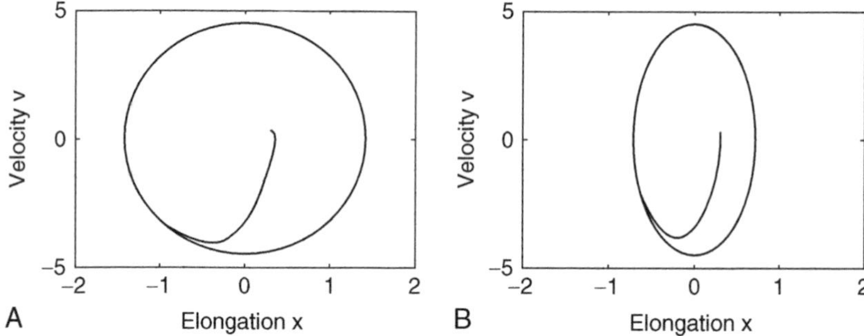

Figure 3.4 Illustration of the effect of frequency ω on the oscillation amplitude. **From left to right**: Frequency increase results in a decrease of amplitude. Parameter: $\omega = \pi$ (*panel A*) and $\omega = 2\pi$ (*panel B*). Other parameters: $b = 10$, $\gamma = 1$.

with twice the frequency of the oscillator shown in the panel A. Since both oscillators exhibit the same total (Hamiltonian) energy, the amplitude of the faster oscillator is smaller. Note that, in the deterministic case, we have $H_{stationary} = \omega^2 \text{AMP}^2/2$, where AMP is the oscillator amplitude. This equation tells us again, that if we increase ω but keep the fixed-point energy $b = H_{stationary}$ constant, then the oscillator amplitude AMP will decrease.

Parkinsonian Oscillatory Tremor

Oscillatory tremor of parkinsonian patients is believed to originate from neural motor control systems that operate far from equilibrium (Lee and Stein 1981; Lang and Lozana 1998a,b; Deuschl et al. 2000). We applied the standard canonical-dissipative oscillator model to tremor oscillations in order to see whether regularities involving the variables $\langle H \rangle$ and SD*H* can be found. In particular, in respect to the ATE system formulation, do these regularities depend on subject-dependent variables such as whether the patients are under treatment or not? We examined two publicly available data sets that include data from five patients under treatment (set 1) and six patients off treatment (set 2). Patients of both data sets were diagnosed with high-amplitude parkinsonian tremor. (For detailed descriptions of the participants, see Beuter et al. 2001.) Tremor data were recorded for about 60 seconds with a sampling rate of 100 Hz. Peripheral tremor was measured at the index finger. Note that finger velocities were recorded rather than finger positions. We determined ω using spectral analysis. Subsequently, we computed the instantaneous Hamiltonian energy values at every recorded time point using Equation 4. From the instantaneous values of *H*, we calculated the mean value $\langle H \rangle$ and SD*H* for every patient in the two data sets. In addition, we computed the average amplitude $\langle AMP \rangle$, where amplitude was defined with respect to the limit cycle trajectories in phase space. That is, instantaneous amplitude values were defined as the coordinates on the horizontal axis when limit cycle trajectories passed through the horizontal axis. In the case of the tremor data, the horizontal axis was spanned by the finger velocity, whereas the vertical axis was spanned by finger acceleration. Figure 3.5 shows <*H*>, SD*H*, and <*AMP*> for set 1 data (first row) and set 2 data (second row). That is, the first row (A–C) depicts the results for patients under treatment, whereas the second row (D–F) provides the respective figures for patients off treatment. The Hamiltonian energy values for patients under treatment were found to be of 3 orders in magnitude lower than the energy values for patients off treatment. Likewise, the amplitudes typical for the patients under treatment were several magnitudes lower than the typical amplitudes produced by off-treatment patients. As summarized in Table 3.2, we examined to what extent the measures <*H*>, SD*H*, and <*AMP*>, were correlated with tremor oscillation frequency. Linear regression analysis did not yield significant results for patients under treatment. For off-treatment patients, there were statistically significant positive correlations between <*H*> and ω^2 ($r = 0.93$, $F(1, 4) = 26.1$, $p < 0.01$) and between the amplitude <*AMP*> and ω^2 ($r = 0.97$, $F(1, 4) = 70.8$, $p < 0.001$).

Single-joint Rhythmic Movement

Dotov et al. (2009) reported an experiment in which six participants maintained a steady and continuous oscillation of a hand-held pendulum about the wrist joint (with forearm supported by an arm-rest) at a self-paced frequency and at three metronome-paced frequencies (4.21, 5.22, and 8.36 rad/s). The forward extremity of the pendulum motion was synchronized with the discrete pacing signal. Figure 3.6 shows <*H*>, SD*H*, and <AMP> for each participant in the three paced conditions (first row) and the self-paced condition (second row). The measures <*H*> and SD*H* increased across the three paced-frequency conditions. Repeated-measure ANOVA showed a significant effect of frequency on <*H*>, $F(2, 10) = 8.0$, $p < 0.01$, partial $\eta^2 = 0.61$, and SD*H*, $F(2, 10) = 8.7$, $p < 0.01$, partial $\eta^2 = 0.64$. There was no significant effect for <*AMP*>. The linear trend was significant for both <*H*> and SD*H*, $F(1, 5) = 9.6$, $p < 0.05$, partial $\eta^2 = 0.66$, and $F(1, 5) = 9.4$, $p < 0.05$, partial $\eta^2 = 0.65$, respectively (see Table 3.2).

The self-paced condition, with one ω per participant, exhibited a single effect: <*H*> and ω were positively correlated ($r = 0.94$) such that <*H*> increased with ω^2, $F(1, 4) = 31.9$, $p < 0.01$.

CONCLUSION

The Parkinson tremor data sets discussed in the previous section were previously used by Beuter et al. (2001) to show that the characteristic high-amplitude finger tremor essentially disappears under treatment conditions. Our approach using a canonical-dissipative oscillator model supports this

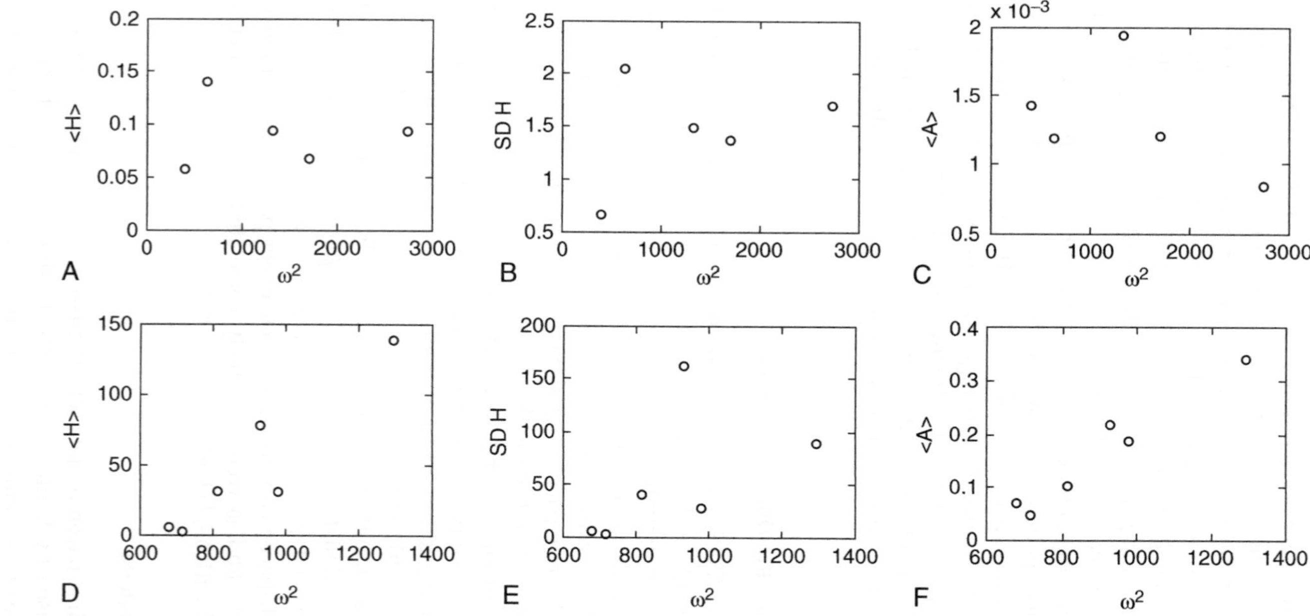

Figure 3.5 Relationship between measures <*H*>, SD*H*, and AMP and ω^2. **First row (A–C)**: Parkinson data for patients on treatment. **Second row (D–F)**: Parkinson data for off-treatment patients.

Table 3.2 Summary of results

Subject-variable	Task	Environment	<*H*>	SD*H*	AMP
Treatment on	Posture		n.s.	n.s.	n.s.
Treatment off	Posture		Positive correlation	n.s.	Positive correlation
	Pendulum Swinging	Paced	Increase	Increase	n.s.
	Pendulum Swinging	Self-paced	Positive correlation	n.s.	n.s.

Statistically significant effects were found in terms of positive correlations between squared frequency and the measures <*H*>, SD*H*, AMP or in terms of linear trends reflecting an increase of the measures <*H*>, SD*H*, AMP with squared frequency.

finding. We found that <*H*> and <*AMP*> of the finger oscillations were reduced by a factor of about 100 due to treatment. Moreover, we found that, for off-treatment patients, <*H*> scaled with ω^2 but SD*H* did not. This observation is consistent with the notion that the amount of excitement or net pumping scales with ω^2. More precisely, we speculate that the net pumping parameter b depends linearly on ω^2 and, in addition, reflects a relatively strong excitement. In this case, SD*H* is in the saturation regime of the net pumping parameter (see Fig. 3.3, panel E) and does not vary with b, whereas <*H*> scales linearly with b (see Fig 3.3, panel B).

It has been suggested that the progressions of Parkinson disease involves a Hopf bifurcation (Friedrich et al. 2000; Titcombe et al. 2001). Likewise, treatment in terms of medication and deep-brain stimulation results in an inverse Hopf bifurcation. The Hopf bifurcation and the inverse Hopf bifurcation occur in the standard canonical-dissipative oscillator when the net pumping parameter b exceeds or falls below the critical value $b = 0$. Consequently, we assume that the parameter b depends on the subject-dependent variable "treatment." Our hypotheses are summarized in Figure 3.7. Figure 3.7 also suggests that the hypothesized correlation between net pumping b and tremor ω^2 is probably affected by the medical treatment.

Our analysis of hand-pendulum oscillations showed that both <*H*> and SD*H* scaled with ω^2 in the paced condition. Higher trends were not statistically significant. The increase of <*H*> and SD*H* could be explained by assuming that the net pumping b increases with ω^2 and that the underlying oscillator dynamics is only weakly excited (see panels B and E in Figure 3.3 for small values of b). However, the increase in SD*H* due to b is limited by the existence of the saturation domain. Therefore, if b affects SD*H*, then one should observe a nonlinear increase exhibiting a curvature. In short, we would expect to see a higher-order trend to be significant. Alternatively, it is plausible to assume that the increase of <*H*> and SD*H* is due to a loss of the attractor stability (see panels C and F of Figure 3.3,

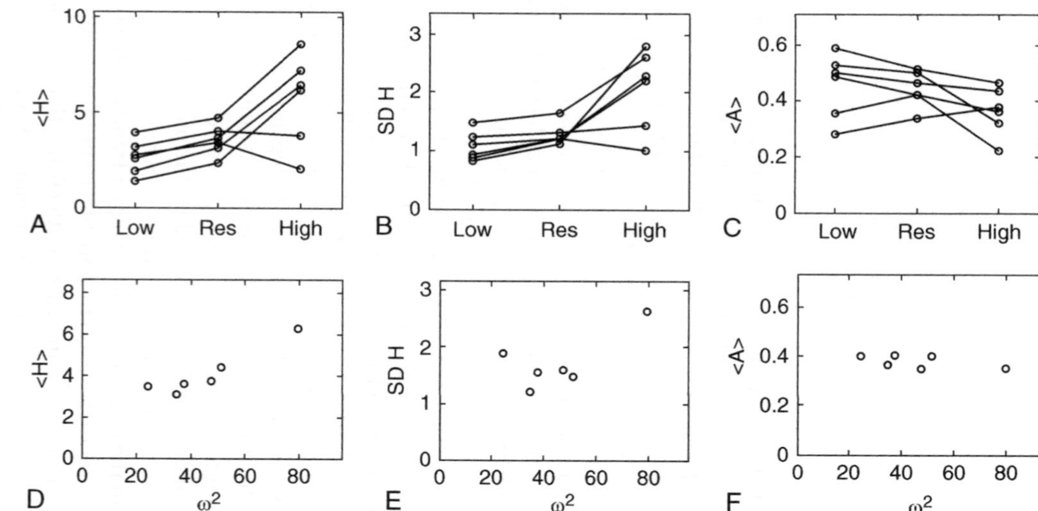

Figure 3.6 Relationship between measures *<H>*, SD*H*, and AMP and ω^2. **First row (A–C)**: Hand-pendulum oscillation data for metronom-paced condition. **Second row (D–F)**: Hand-pendulum oscillation data for self-paced conditions.

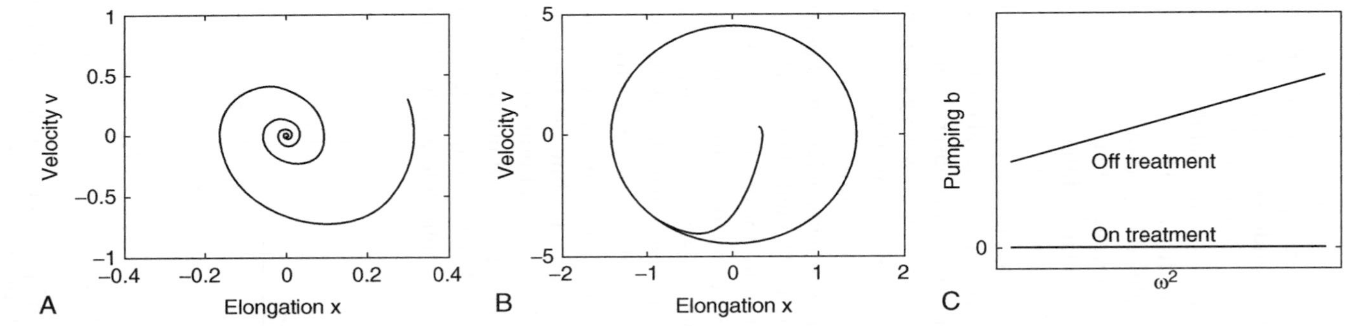

Figure 3.7 **A** and **B**: Hopf bifurcation of the standard canonical-dissipative oscillator induced by the net pumping b. Parameters $b = -1$ (*panel A*) and $b = 10$ (*panel B*). **C**: Results of the Parkinson tremor data sets interpreted in terms of correlations between b and ω^2.

when γ approaches zero). In fact, this speculation finds partial support from a previous study by Goodman et al. (2000), in which it was found that stability is affected by required pacing frequency. Although in Goodman et al. (2000) a U-shaped relationship was found, the linear increase in SD suggests that the stability, as indexed by the parameter γ, decays monotonically. In this context, one should realize, however, that the stability parameter γ primarily relates to the stability of the energy dynamics, whereas the stability measure discussed in Goodman et al. (2000) addressed stability in appropriately defined high-dimensional coordinate spaces that are assumed to contain the relevant system dynamics. To what extent these stability measures capture similar or different aspects of dynamic stability has not been yet explored. In the case of self-selected oscillation frequencies, we found a statistically significant positive correlation between $\langle H \rangle$ and ω^2, a correlation possibly due to a causal relationship between $\langle H \rangle$ and ω^2, and no similar effect for SD*H*. This observation is again consistent with the assumption that there is a relatively strong excitement, such that variations in the degree of excitement do not affect energy variability but affect the mean of the oscillator energy. Figure 3.8 summarizes our hypothesis on controlling the rhythmic movements of handheld pendulums.

Comparing Figure 3.7 (panel C) with Figure 3.8 (panel A), we speculate that maintaining finger posture for off-treatment Parkinson patients and self-paced pendulum oscillations for young healthy adults have a certain pattern in common. In both cases, we speculate that there is a positive correlation between the pumping parameter b and the squared oscillation frequency. Moreover, it is plausible to assume that self-paced oscillatory activities of human agents emerge due to Hopf bifurcations—one of the most fundamental bifurcations leading to oscillatory behavior. Both Parkinson tremor and self-paced pendulum oscillations may be induced, therefore, by increasing an unspecific stimulus (here, modeled in terms of the net pumping parameter b) beyond a critical threshold. Parkinson tremor has been modeled on the neurophysiological level in terms of interacting

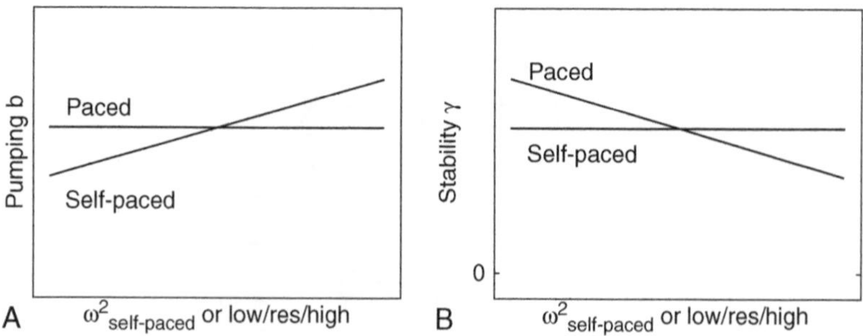

Figure 3.8 Results of the hand-pendulum oscillation data interpreted in terms of correlations and trends between b and ω^2 (*panel A*) and γ and ω^2 (*panel B*). (Refer to Figure 3.6 for labels).

neuron populations exhibiting pathological synchronization (see, e.g., Tass et al. 1998; Tass 2002). Just as in the canonical-dissipative oscillator model, in the neuronal network model the pathological state emerges via a bifurcation. The control parameter is the coupling strength between the neurons of the network. The canonical-dissipative oscillator model with the bifurcation parameter *b* may be used as a departure point to link neurodynamic modeling with behavioral modeling.

We reported a positive correlation between $<H>$ and ω^2 for paced and self-paced pendulum oscillations (Fig. 3.6 panels A and D) and high-amplitude finger tremor of off-treatment Parkinson patients (Fig. 3.5 panel D). This is consistent to a certain extent with the data on single-limb oscillations reported in Kay et al. (1987). In this study, mean oscillation amplitudes for required oscillation frequencies are reported (see their Table 1) for both hands. We computed for each required frequency and hand condition an estimate of $<H>$ according to: $<H> = <AMP>^2\ \omega^2/2$ (see above). The $<H>$ values thus obtained are shown in Figure 3.9A. The scatter plot suggests that there is a positive correlation between $<H>$ and ω^2. However, when applying the same procedure to the data published in Beek et al. (1996) (see their Table 1), we obtain a scatter plot as shown in Figure 3.9B that suggests the opposite relationship between $<H>$ and ω^2. In terms of the net pumping parameter *b*, we would be inclined to say that, for the Beek et al. (1996) data, the net pumping *b* is constant or decays with ω^2, which would explain the reduction of $<H>$ when ω^2 is scaled up.

As mentioned at the beginning of this chapter, the studies by Beek et al. (1996) and Silva et al. (2007) support the hypothesis that the coefficients of

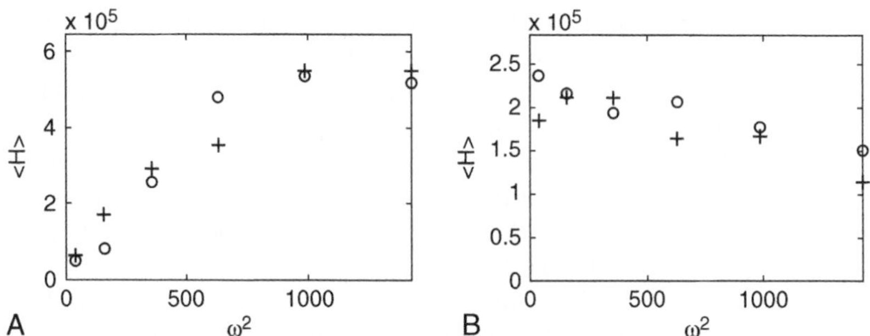

Figure 3.9 Estimated mean Hamiltonian energies as function of required squared frequencies as obtained from a re-analysis of published data (*circles*, left hand; *plus signs*, right hand). **A**: Data from Kay, B.A., J.A.S. Kelso, E.L. Saltzman, and G. Schöner. 1987. Space-time behavior of single and bimanual rhythmic movements: Data and limit cycle model. *Journal of Experimental Psychology: Human Perception and Performance* 13: 178–92. **B**: Data from Beek, P.J., Rikkert, W.E.I., and P.C.W van Wieringen. 1996. Limit cycle properties of rhythmic forearm movements. *Journal of Experimental Psychology: Human Perception and Performance* 22: 1077–93.

nonlinear oscillator terms that describe the relative importance of these terms depend in general on ω. Taking the canonical-dissipative perspective, this argument does not come as a surprise. Canonical-dissipative systems exhibit nonlinearities that involve energy expressions, such as the Hamiltonian energy function. The Hamiltonian energy in turn depends in general on the oscillation frequency. As a result, the oscillator nonlinearities will depend explicitly on frequency parameters. For example, in the case of the standard canonical-dissipative oscillator, we may substitute explicitly the Hamiltonian function defined in Equation 4 into the stochastic second-order equation defined by Equation 4. In doing so, the two parts of Equation 4 become

$$\frac{d^2}{dt^2}x = -\omega^2 x + \gamma\, b\frac{d}{dt}x - \frac{\gamma}{2}\left(\frac{d}{dt}x\right)^3 - \frac{\gamma\omega^2 x^2}{2}\frac{d}{dt}x + \sqrt{Q}\Gamma(t) \qquad \text{(Eq. 5)}$$

Equation 5 involves a nonlinear term proportional to $\omega^2 v x^2$.

Postscript

The perception, action, and cognition of an agent are, in general, context-dependent. That is, perception, action, and cognition depend on agent-specific, task-specific, and environment-specific constraints (Newell 1986; Davids et al. 2008). The canonical-dissipative approach provides a tool to examine how these constraints probably affect the overall excitation and the stability of the relevant underlying processes. The measure of excess excitation or net pumping (reflected above by the parameter *b*) describes how far the ATE system is pushed away from its bifurcation point, where the bifurcation point is defined as the condition under which damping and pumping are in exact balance. This implies that, by means of the canonical-dissipative approach, the distance of a process to its bifurcation point at which the perceptual, behavioral, or cognitive process under consideration emerges at all can be measured. Agent-specific constraints related to development and aging may affect this distance. In the context of disease progression, this idea has led to the notion of dynamic diseases (Mackey and Glass 1977; Glass and Mackey 1988).

An objective of the present study was to make some of the basic concepts of the canonical-dissipative approach available for inquiry into control and coordination in ATE systems. In particular, the standard canonical-dissipative oscillator described in detail here should be considered as one of the most parsimonious canonical-dissipative systems. However, more sophisticated canonical-dissipative models have been developed, primarily in the physics literature. For example, systems involving interacting agents have been studied from the perspective of interacting canonical-dissipative particle systems (Erdmann et al. 2005). Future research on ATE systems may take advantage of such cross-disciplinary efforts.

APPENDIX

From Equation 4, an analytical expression for the joint probability density that describes the distribution of x and v can be derived. This probability density in turn can be transformed into a probability density $P(H)$ that describes the distribution of the Hamiltonian energy values H. The probability density reads

$$P = \frac{1}{Z}\exp\left(-\frac{\gamma}{Q}[H-b]^2\right) \qquad \text{(Eq. A1)}$$

The normalization factor Z can be computed from the integral

$$Z = \int \exp\left(-\frac{\gamma}{Q}[H-b]^2\right) dH \qquad \text{(Eq. A2)}$$

This integral can be determined numerically for every parameter b and every ratio γ/Q. Having determined Z, the first and second moments of H can be computed by solving numerically the following integrals

$$\langle H\rangle = \frac{1}{Z}\int H \exp\left(-\frac{\gamma}{Q}[H-b]^2\right) dH \qquad \text{(Eq. A3)}$$

and

$$\langle H^2\rangle = \frac{1}{Z}\int H^2 \exp\left(-\frac{\gamma}{Q}[H-b]^2\right) dH \qquad \text{(Eq. A4)}$$

The first moment corresponds to the mean value of H. Having determined numerically the values of the first and second moments, the standard deviation σ can be calculated from

$$\sigma = \sqrt{\langle H^2\rangle - \langle H\rangle^2} \qquad \text{(Eq. A5)}$$

Figure 3.3 was computed using the aformentioned relations. Parameters for panels A and D: $\gamma/Q = 1.0$, $b = 1$, and $b = 2$. The integral (A2) was computed as Rieman integral $Z = \Sigma\ exp(-\gamma(H_k-b)^2/Q)\ \Delta H$ with $H_k = k\ \Delta H$ and $k = 1,2,3,\ldots$ Likewise (A3) and (A4) were computed numerically as $\langle H\rangle = Z^{-1}\ \Sigma\ H_k\ exp(-\gamma(H_k-b)^2/Q)\ \Delta H$ and $\langle H^2\rangle = Z^{-1}\ \Sigma\ (H_k)^2 exp(-\gamma(H_k-b)^2/Q)\ \Delta H$ (we used $\Delta H = 0.01$, and the integration was carried out from $H = 0$ to $H = 10000$). We found the numerical values $\langle H\rangle = 1.29$, SD$H = 0.79$ for $b = 1.0$ and $\langle H\rangle = 2.06$, SD$H = 0.94$ for $b = 2$. In order to compute panels B and E, we fixed $\gamma/Q = 1.0$ and varied b in the range from 0 to 7. For panels C and F, we put $b = 1.0$ and $Q = 1.0$ and varied γ from 0.1 to 7.

REFERENCES

Bartlett, J.H. 1975. *Classical and modern mechanics*. Tuscaloosa: University of Alabama Press.

Beek, P.J., Rikkert, W.E.I., and P.C.W van Wieringen. 1996. Limit cycle properties of rhythmic forearm movements. *Journal of Experimental Psychology: Human Perception and Performance* 22: 1077–93.

Beek, P.J., R.C. Schmidt, A.W. Morris, M.-Y. Sim, and M.T. Turvey. 1995. Linear and nonlinear stiffness and friction in biological rhythmic movements. *Biological Cybernetics* 73: 499–507.

Beek, P.J., C.E. Peper, and D.F. Stegeman. 1995. Dynamic models of movement coordination. *Human Movement Science* 14: 573–608.

Bernstein, N.A. 1967. *The coordination and regulation of movements*. Oxford: Pergamon Press.

Beuter, A., Titcombe, M.S., F. Richer, C. Gross, and D. Guehl. 2001. Effect of deep brain stimulation on amplitude and frequency characteristics of rest tremor in Parkinson's disease. *Thalamus and Related Systems* 1: 203–11.

Daffertshofer, A., C. van den Berg, and P.J. Beek. 1999. A dynamical model for mirror movements. *Physica D* 132: 243–66.

Davids, K., C. Button, and S. Bennett. 2008. *Dynamics of skill acquisition: A constraints-led approach*. Champaign IL: Human Kinetics.

Delignieres, D., T. Nourrit, N.T. Deschamps, B. Lauriot, and N. Caillou. 1999. Effects of practice and task constraints on stiffness and friction functions in biological movements. *Human Movement Science* 18: 769–93.

Deuschl, G., J. Raethjen, R. Baron, M. Lindemann, H. Wilms, and P. Krack. 2000. *Journal of Neurology* 247(Suppl 5), V/33.

Dotov, D.G., D.G. Stephen, T.D. Frank, and M.T. Turvey. 2009. Dynamics of rhythms at resonance: Variability of unimanual pendulum oscillation at and away from resonance. Lecture given at New England Sequencing and Timing (NEST), Haskings Laboratories, New Haven, Connecticut.

Ebeling, W., and I.M. Sokolov. 2004. *Statistical thermodynamics and stochastic theory of nonequilibrium systems*. Singapore: World Scientific.

Eisenhammer, T., A. Hübler, N. Packard, J.A.S. Kelso. 1991. Modeling experimental time series with ordinary differential equations. *Biological Cybernetics* 65: 107–12.

Erdmann, U., W. Ebeling, L. Schimansky-Geier, and F. Schweitzer. 2000. Brownian particles far from equilibrium. *European Physical Journal B* 15: 105–13.

Erdmann, U., W. Ebeling, and A. Mikhailov. 2005. Noise-induced transition from translational to rotational motion of swarms. *Physical Review E* 71: 051904.

Feistel, R., and W. Ebeling. 1989. *Evolution of complex systems: Self-organization entropy and development*. Berlin: VEB Verlag.

Frank, T.D. 2003. Single particle dynamics of many-body systems described by Vlasov-Fokker-Planck equations. *Physics Letters A* 319: 173–80.

Frank, T.D. 2005a. Short-time correlations of many-body systems described by nonlinear Fokker-Planck equations and Vlasov-Fokker-Planck equations. *Physics Letters A* 337: 224–34.

Frank, T.D. 2005b. *Nonlinear Fokker-Planck equations: Fundamentals and applications*. Berlin: Springer.

Frank, T.D., and A. Daffertshofer. 2001. Multivariate nonlinear Fokker-Planck equations and generalized thermostatistics. *Physica A* 292: 392–410.

Frank, T.D., and S. Mongkolsakulvong. 2008. A nonextensive thermostatistical approach to the Haissinski theory of accelerator beams. *Physica A* 387: 4828–38.

Friedrich, R., S. Siegert, J. Peinke, S. Luck, M. Seifert, M. Lindemann, et al. 2000. Extracting model equations from experimental data. *Physics Letters A* 271: 217–222.

Glass, L., and M.C. Mackey. 1988. *From clocks to chaos*. Princeton NJ: Princeton University Press.

Goodman, L., M.A. Riley, S. Mitra, and M.T. Turvey. 2000. Advantages of rhythmic movements at resonance: Minimal active degrees of freedom, maximal noise, and maximal predictability. *Journal of Motor Behavior* 32: 3–8.

Graham, R. 1981. Onset of cooperative behavior in nonequilibrium steady-states. In *Order and fluctuations in equilibrium and nonequilibrium statistical mechanics*, eds., G. Nicolis, G. Dewel, and J.W. Turner, 235–88. New York: John Wiley.

Haken, H. 1973. Distribution functions for classical and quantum systems far from thermal equilibrium. *Zeitschrift für Physik* 263: 267–82.

Haken, H. 2004. *Synergetics: An introduction and advanced topics*. Berlin: Springer.

Kay, B.A., J.A.S. Kelso, E.L. Saltzman, and G. Schöner. 1987. Space-time behavior of single and bimanual rhythmic movements: Data and limit cycle model. *Journal of Experimental Psychology: Human Perception and Performance* 13: 178–92.

Kay, B.A., E.L. Saltzman, and J.A.S. Kelso. 1991. Steady-state and perturbed rhythmic movements: A dynamic analysis. *Journal of Experimental Psychology: Human Perception and Performance* 17: 183–97.

Kelso, J.A.S. 1995. *Dynamic patterns: The self-organization of brain and behavior*. Cambridge MA: MIT Press.

Lang, A.E., and A.M. Lozana. 1998a. Parkinson's disease – first of two parts. *New England Journal of Medicine* 339(15): 1044–53.

Lang, A.E., and A.M. Lozana. 1998b. Parkinson's disease – second of two parts. *New England Journal of Medicine* 339(16): 1130–43.

Lee, R.G., and R.B. Stein. 1981. Resetting of tremor by mechanical perturbations: A comparison of essential tremor and parkinsonian tremor. *Annals of Neurology* 10: 523–31.

Mackey, M.C., and L. Glass. 1977. Oscillation and chaos in physiological control systems. *Science* 197: 287–89.

Mottet, D., and R.J. Bootsma. 1999. The dynamics of goal-directed rhythmical aiming. *Biological Cybernetics* 80: 235–45.

Newell, K.M. 1986. Constraints on the development of coordination. In *Motor development in children. Aspects of coordination and control*, eds., MG Wade, HTA Whiting, 341–360. Dodrecht: Martinus Nijhoff.

Risken, H. 1989. *The Fokker-Planck equation: Methods of solutions and applications*. Berlin: Springer.

Schweitzer, F. 2003. *Brownian agents and active particles*. Berlin: Springer.

Schweitzer, F., W. Ebeling, and B. Tilch. 2001. Statistical mechanics of canonical-dissipative systems and applications to swarm dynamics. *Physical Review E* 64: 021110.

Silva, P., M. Moreno, M. Marisa, S. Fonseca, and M.T. Turvey. 2007. Steady-state stress at one hand magnifies the amplitude, stiffness, and nonlinearity of oscillatory behavior at the other. *Neuroscience Letters* 429: 64–68.

Strogatz, S.H. 1994. *Nonlinear dynamics and chaos*. Reading MA: Addison Wesley.

Tass, P., M.G. Rosenblum, J. Weule, J. Kurths, A. Pikovsky, J. Volkmann, et al. 1998. Detection of n:m phase locking from noisy data: Application to magnetoencephalography. *Physical Review Letters* 81: 3291–94.

Tass, P.A. 2002. Desynchronization of brain rhythms with soft phase-resetting techniques. *Biological Cybernetics* 87: 102–15.

Titcombe, M.S., L. Glass, D. Guehl, and A. Beuter. 2001. Dynamics of parkinsonian tremor during deep brain stimulation. *Chaos* 11: 766.

Van den Berg, C., P.J. Beek, R.C. Wagenaar, and P.C.W. van Wieringen. 2000. Coordination disorders in patients with Parkinson's disease: A study of paced rhythmic forearm movements. *Experimental Brain Research* 134: 174–86.

4

Observer-independent Dynamical Measures of Team Coordination and Performance

Silke M. Dodel, Ajay S. Pillai, Philip W. Fink, Eric R. Muth, Roy Stripling, Dylan D. Schmorrow, Joseph V. Cohn, and Viktor K. Jirsa

A common theme in research exploring the progression toward increasing levels of skill is that novices operate in a rule-based fashion (Benner 1984), with performance consisting of groups of individual actions based on a rigid and inflexible understanding of specific relationships, rather than on an integrated whole (McElroy et al. 1991; Glaser 1996), whereas experts operate in a more integrated and fluid manner (Benner 1984), with performance consisting of a single cohesive response (Dreyfus & Dreyfus 1980; Benner 1984; Benner 2004). Between these two extremes lies a transitional state, in which the novice gains knowledge to improve performance (Houldsworth et al. 1997) and learns to use this knowledge, coupled with past experience, to develop a more effective response (McElroy et al. 1991). Although it is commonly accepted that teams develop with time and experience (McIntyre & Salas 1995; Morgan et al. 1994), there is still much debate on how to quantify this evolution. Unlike individual performance, which focuses on acquiring task knowledge and applying it to problem-solving challenges, team performance emphasizes acquiring team coordination knowledge, which requires that individual team members learn each other's goal-related behaviors and, if necessary, adjust their own performance accordingly. We seek to explore the development of this team coordination by developing spatiotemporal measures that are based on team dynamics (i.e., team behavior over time), rather than on individual performance. We propose that team dynamics can be represented by a low-dimensional task-dependent manifold. Our approach is motivated in part by the uncontrolled manifold hypothesis (UCM) (Schöner 1995; Scholz & Schöner 1999; Salas & Fiore 2004; see also Latash, this volume) in movement sciences. There, the parameters of a perfect task performance span a task-dependent manifold in the *parameter space*, reflecting the fact that, for tasks with a high number of degrees of freedom, a multitude of different task executions are equally successful. For instance, in a dart game, a variety of possible arm movements all lead to hitting the bull's eye. In contrast, the manifolds spanned in *phase space* are the regions along which trajectories evolve in time. The phase space is defined by the set of variables that unambiguously define the state of a system (hence they are also called *state variables*, and the phase space is sometimes called *state space*). As parameters change, there may be a certain variation in the phase-space manifolds, which corresponds to the variation captured by the UCM. To gain insights into team coordination, we take the following approach: for a fixed set of parameters, a manifold in phase space exists that captures a "perfect" team dynamics. By assumption, variations of the trajectories within the manifold will not affect the performance of the team, since by definition this manifold is composed of trajectories that correspond to perfect task execution. Deviations from the manifold, however, are a sign of reduced team performance either via reduced skill or lack of coordination. With this approach, we are able to derive objective measures of team performance while taking into account the high number of degrees of freedom in the task.

Team dynamics may take any number of forms, ranging from the rule-based defense/offense pattern common to many sports, to the ruleless patterns observed in recurring combat operations in urban settings (e.g., Military Operations in Urbanized Terrain (MOUT; United States Marine Corps 1998). To better understand how team performance develops and how individual members contribute to underlying team dynamics, we developed a paradigm similar to *room clearing*, a basic urban combat scenario. Room clearing requires four individuals to enter a room after lining up outside the entryway in a single column (a "stack"), move in a predefined path into a room, and search and identify threats. A room is considered cleared when all four members have searched, accounted for, and removed any identified threats. For the current effort, a facility was constructed with multiple rooms of different sizes and shapes, and instrumented with cameras that collected information on the position and orientation of each team member (Fig. 4.1). Three teams with different skill levels (novices, intermediates, and experts) participated in the study. For the purpose of this study, the expert team was considered the gold standard for team performance. As a consequence, the set of expert team trajectories spans parts of the expert team manifold, which allows us to measure the extent of this particular manifold. The performance of the other teams was then quantified as the degree of deviation from the expert manifold. We performed the experiment in two different rooms (small and large L-shaped). The analysis of the data from both rooms provided qualitatively identical results, hence only the small-room data are discussed in detail and the results of the large-room data is provided in Appendix B. The data used in this study were the horizontal positions and velocities of each team member.

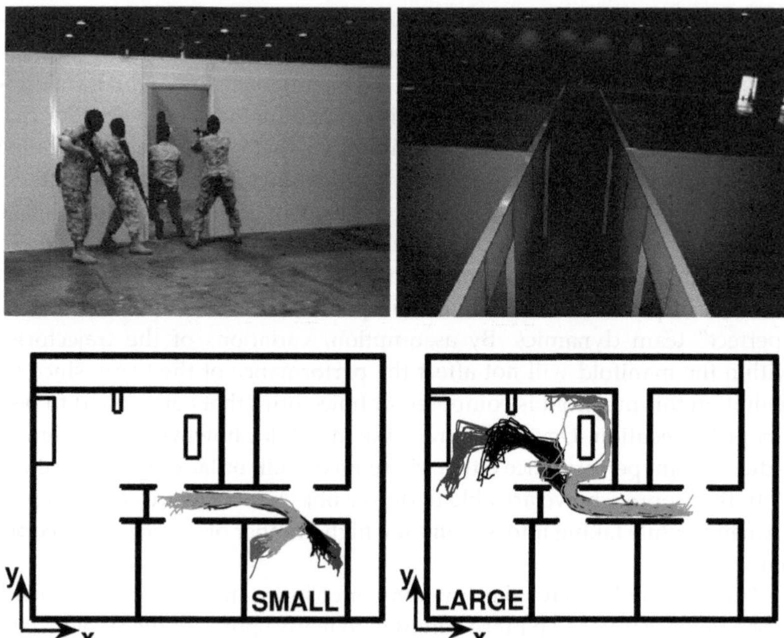

Figure 4.1 **Team dynamics experiment: Facility and team trajectories. Top left:** The four team members enter the room from an initial 'stack' formation, performing the room clearing task. **Top right:** MOUT facility at Clemson University. **Bottom left:** Map of the MOUT facility and the trajectories (in various gray shades) of the individual team members 1–4, respectively. **Bottom right:** The trajectories for the large room with the same conventions as in the small room.

EXPERIMENT: ROOM-CLEARING TASK IN A MOUT FACILITY

The room-clearing task was performed in the MOUT facility (Fig. 4.1) in the rooms marked "small" and "large." The small room was a 12-by-12 foot rectangular room, and the large room consisted of three 12-by-12 foot squares arranged in an L pattern. Position data for the team members was sampled at 30 Hz using a network of 36 cameras, calibrated to a common coordinate system, wired to a rack of seven computers to track positions in real time (Hoover & Olsen 1999). Raw video recordings were used to manually override errors in the automatic tracking. Data were collected on the room-clearing task from three teams of different skill levels (novice, intermediate, and expert), all males. The novice group was composed of four Clemson University undergraduate students with no prior room-clearing experience. The intermediate team was composed of four Clemson Army ROTC students with varying levels of room-clearing experience. The novice and intermediate teams had not completed room-clearing exercises together as a team prior to the experiment. The expert team was composed of four active-duty enlisted Marines (three lance corporals and one corporal) who had seen combat together as members of the same squad. Intermediate and Novice team members participated in a training exercise led by a former Marine team leader. Experts were provided with a basic familiarization of the facility but otherwise received no training during this experiment. To keep the initial condition of the team dynamics invariant, the team was asked to form a stack according to marked spots on the ground. After a "go" signal, the team entered the room. Team members were instructed to follow a single room entry pattern—the crossover entry pattern—but were otherwise not constrained (Fig. 4.1). The end of a trial was reached when each subject verbally signaled "all clear." No time constraints were imposed on the duration of the task. Each team performed the prescribed room-clearing task 48 times. To maintain alertness, eight of the trials contained one or two enemies in the room. These trials were excluded from further analysis to keep the task in all trials the same.

Team Behavior as a Flow on Task-dependent Manifolds in Phase Space

We propose to analyze team behavior based on the geometry of the dynamics of task variables (e.g., the positions of the team members over time). The ensemble of task variables that take on numerical values can be cast in a high-dimensional space, which is assumed to be the phase space in the ideal case, else a subspace thereof. More specifically, at each point in time, the task variables can be arranged to form a vector that gives the coordinates of a point in phase space. This vector, which we will refer to as *team vector*, contains the whole information about the behavior of the entire team at each point in time. Non-numerical task variables (e.g., oral communication between team members) are beyond the scope of the present chapter, but could, in principle, be mapped on numerical values and be included in the analysis. As the trial progresses, the team vector traces out a trajectory in phase space. Mathematically, the ensemble of the trajectories traced out by the team vector in phase space can be described as a manifold. The trajectories from different trials are distributed in a manner characteristic of the task, reflecting the degrees of freedom of the task, as well as the constraints imposed by the task. In other words, the manifold reflects the fact that the same task can be executed in multiple manners (e.g., a ball can be thrown from different positions to hit the goal) but at the same time is restricted by the nature of the task (e.g., a room can be entered only through the door, not through the wall). Due to the constraints imposed by the task, we expect the manifold to be low-dimensional, meaning that although the manifold "lives" in a high-dimensional phase space, it can be locally described by using only a few (appropriately chosen) coordinates. Figure 4.2 shows an illustration of a two-dimensional manifold spanned by trajectories in a three-dimensional phase space. The manifold

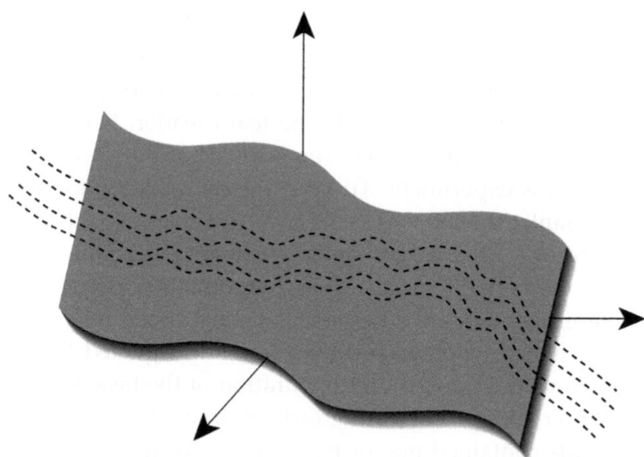

Figure 4.2 **Illustration of the manifold concept.** Team dynamics for a given task and skill level of a team is represented as a manifold in phase space (*gray surface*). Each dotted line represents one realization of the task over time by the team as a trajectory of the team vector in a 16-D phase space (here, 3-D space for illustration purposes) spanned by the horizontal positions and velocities of the four team members. Note that this figure is a cartoon and does not represent real data.

is two-dimensional because we could warp a two-dimensional coordinate system such that it fits on the manifold and hence could describe each point on the manifold by two coordinates.

The trajectories of the team vectors (from a set of trials) follow the flow on the manifold as they evolve in time and, as such, trace out the shape of the manifold. The flow prescribes the time evolution of the state vector. Noise omnipresent in biological signals introduces a stochastic component into the state vector's trajectory and gives the manifold a certain "thickness." Nonstationarities of the signal will generally influence the dynamics also, but can be considered to take part in the constitution of the manifold. This assumption appears to be reasonable, at least for the expert manifold, where the highly skilled experts perform their dynamics along the manifold following a brief transient after the start.

Measuring Task Performance from the Task-dependent Manifold

In the context of the UCM hypothesis in the movement sciences (Schöner 1995; Scholz & Schöner 1999; Salas & Fiore 2004), the hypothesized uncontrolled manifold consists of the configurations of the task variables (in case of movement, for instance, the configurations of the joints) that lead to the same set of values of the putative controlled variables (i.e., the same outcome). In other words, variations in task execution for which the corresponding variables stay within the manifold do not change the outcome and hence lead to the same level of performance. We adapt this concept to measure team performance, but expand it to the manifolds in the phase space, along which the team dynamics is assumed to evolve. Since the task in the MOUT experiment has no objective performance measure, we use the manifold generated from the data of the expert team as the gold standard and compare the manifolds of the other teams (novices and intermediates) against it (see also the contribution of Ting & Chvatal, this volume for other approaches toward the quantification of synergy among coordinated elements). Thus, here, we take the approach to define that the expert manifold is the task-dependent manifold for "perfect" task execution. In analogy to the UCM, we posit that variations *within* the manifold do not lead to a deterioration of task performance, but variations that result in a departure *from* the manifold do, and hence can be used to assess team performance (with respect to the expert team). We extend the concept of the UCM further in that we apply it not only to a single subject, but to a *team* of subjects. Furthermore, we assume that a manifold exists for each skill level. This allows us to go beyond the comparison of single trials (or their mean) and assess patterns by which task execution differs among teams of different skill levels.

Low-dimensional Representation of the Manifolds

Although team dynamics occurs in a high-dimensional phase space, task-related constraints usually confine the manifold to lower dimensions. The intrinsic dimension of the manifold (see Appendix C) over time informs about the degree of confinement of team behavior and was measured by performing a principal component analysis (PCA) across trials at each time point. In addition to giving the values of the variance in the various dimensions, PCA also informs about the directions of maximum variance across trials by means of the principal eigenvectors. They also serve as an approximation of the tangent spaces to the manifold. If the first principal eigenvectors (i.e., those that account for most of the total variance) are reasonably stationary over time, this indicates that there is a low-dimensional (equal to the intrinsic dimension of the manifold at these points in time) representation of the manifold in a *fixed subspace*. Note that the stationarity of the eigenvectors is a sufficient, but not a necessary condition for the existence of a fixed low-dimensional subspace, in which the manifold can be represented. The eigenvectors constitute a basis of this subspace, but even if the eigenvectors differ over time, they may span the same subspace. To determine whether the manifold or part of it lies in a stationary fixed subspace, we employed a procedure outlined in Appendix C.

In Appendix A, we give proof of concept for the measures presented in this section by analyzing synthetic data obtained from a flow on a planar manifold and on a spherical manifold, respectively. In both cases, the intrinsic dimension was correctly determined to be two and three dimensions, respectively (cf. Figs. 4.A2 and 4.A3 in Appendix A), and a reconstruction of the flow in a fixed two- and three-dimensional subspace, respectively, retrieved all essential features of the original flow (cf. Fig. 4.A4 in Appendix A).

Dynamical Measures of Team Coordination and Performance

From what has been presented so far, we can derive a dynamical measure for *team performance* by determining at each point in time the deviation of the nonexpert manifold (i.e., the manifold in which the nonexpert trajectories lie) to the expert manifold. Small deviations thereby correspond to almost perfect team performance and large deviations to poor team performance. However, team performance is dependent on both the skill of the individual team members, as well as on the coordination of the team. To derive a measure for team coordination we created *surrogate data*, in which the skill of each team member (i.e., his individual ability to execute the task as a team member) was maintained, but the coordination among the team members was removed (see Appendix C). By creating a number of trajectories of surrogate data, we created task-dependent manifolds in which team coordination is absent. These surrogate manifolds can be used to quantify *team coordination* of the team as a whole over time (see Appendix C). This was done by determining how much the original manifold is perturbed by removing team coordination at each point in time. In addition to the coordination of a team as a whole, we were also interested in *patterns of team coordination*. These are defined by the coordination between each pair of team members. We derived a measure for the coordination between each pair of team members by measuring how much of the original manifold is maintained if, in the surrogate manifold, the coordination between two team members is kept intact (see Appendix C).

To summarize, we have presented here a theoretical approach that allows deriving objective (i.e., observer-independent) dynamical measures of team performance and team coordination. In the next section, we will present the results of applying this approach to experimental data.

Team Performance and Team Coordination in the MOUT Experiment

Here, we present the results of applying the approaches outlined earlier and in Appendix C on the data of the room-clearing task in the MOUT experiment. The results presented in this section are from the data on the room-clearing task in the small room (see Fig. 4.1, *bottom left*); the results for the data on the room-clearing task in the large L-shaped room (see Fig. 4.1, *bottom right*) are qualitatively very similar and are presented in Appendix B.

Extraction of the Manifold

First, an abstract representation of team dynamics in terms of team manifolds was created as follows. For each trial, team dynamics was assessed in terms of the evolution of a team vector composed of positions and velocities of individual team members (i.e., x-position, x-velocity, y-position, y-velocity of team member 1, team member 2, etc.). As the trial progresses, this vector traces out a trajectory in a 16-dimensional phase space. Unlike the trajectories in the physical space shown in Figure 4.1 (*bottom*), each trajectory of the team vector represents the behavior of the entire team in a trial. The trajectories in phase space of the team vectors from the 40 trials are distributed in a manner characteristic of the task and the skill-level of the team and span a manifold (Fig. 4.2). For the given task, there are three manifolds, one for each team level. The manifold of the expert team serves as the gold standard (i.e., is taken as the manifold of perfect task execution against which the other two manifolds are compared).

Data Preprocessing and Characterization of the Manifolds

The data were arranged into an array by temporally aligning them to the entry point of the first stack member and truncating them to the same number of time points in all trials. After alignment and truncation, novice and expert data had a trial length of 3.7 s, and intermediates 4.3 s. The total variance of velocity was normalized to the total variance of position to account for the different nature of the two variables. Dimensionality and shape of the manifolds were analyzed by performing a PCA at each point in time. The eigenvectors serve as an approximation of the tangent spaces to the manifold and inform about directions of maximum variance across trials.

Properties of the Team Manifolds

Although team dynamics occur in a high-dimensional phase space, team coordination and other task- and team-related constraints usually confine the manifold to lower dimensions. To determine the degree of confinement of team behavior, we measured the intrinsic dimension of the manifold over time by performing a PCA across trials at each time point. The mean percent variance quantifies how much of the team dynamics is explained by the PCA for a given dimension. Figure 4.3 (*top*) shows that the mean percent variance saturates around four to five dimensions with no significant differences between team skill levels. Note that the confinement of the manifold to lower dimensionality is not a direct measure of team coordination, and the similarity of the dimensionality of the manifolds could indicate that here the confinement is mainly due to task constraints.

The principal eigenvectors yielded by PCA give information about the orientation of the manifolds in phase space and hence (for the expert manifold which serves as a gold standard) the directions of those variations in task execution that do not lead to decreased task performance. The first eigenvector over time of the expert manifold is shown in Figure 4.3 (*middle*). We see that the primary orientation of the expert manifold before the entry

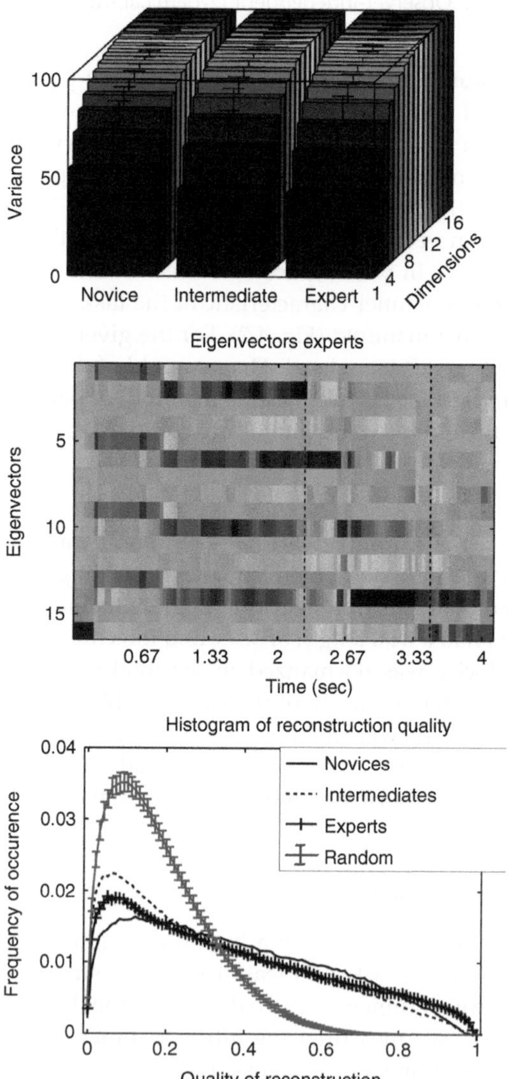

Figure 4.3 **Properties of the team manifolds. Top**: Mean percent variance (average over time) explained by the respective number of dimensions for the novice, intermediate and expert manifolds (*error bars*: 90% confidence interval). **Middle**: First principal component vector of the expert manifold over time. PCA was performed at each point in time over all trials. Ordering of the 16 elements: x-position, x-velocity, y-position, y-velocity for team member 1, team member 2, etc. (*vertical lines*: entry period). **Bottom:** Histogram of reconstruction quality of the team manifolds using subspaces from the expert manifold in contrast to randomly generated subspaces (n = 1,000). *Horizontal axis*: reconstruction quality values, vertical axis: relative frequency of occurrence (normalized). *Solid, marked, and dashed curves*: histograms of reconstruction quality of novice, intermediate, and expert manifolds, respectively, using subspaces of the expert manifold. *Gray curve with error bars* (1 SD): histogram of reconstruction quality using random subspaces (all team levels).

is dominated by variations of the x-position and x-velocity of the entire team, indicating that these variations that affect the whole team, but not the relative positions or velocities among the individual team members, do not negatively affect team performance. In addition, the first eigenvector is stationary during considerably long time intervals, indicating that during these time intervals the manifold is evolving essentially in a fixed subspace of the phase space. We used this finding to create a low-dimensional representation of the three team manifolds by projecting them onto a fixed three-dimensional subspace spanned by the first three principal eigenvectors of the expert manifold at $t = 1.13$ s, where the subspace in which the manifold evolves is reasonably stationary (see Appendix C). When using random subspaces for the representation, they captured on average only 10% of the team dynamics, whereas the fixed subspace yielded considerably higher reconstruction qualities (see Appendix C) of the team manifolds for all teams, regardless of team level (Fig. 4.3, *bottom*). This validates our choice of a three-dimensional representation of the manifolds in a fixed subspace of the expert manifold.

Team Coordination and Team Performance

We evaluated the degree of team coordination for each team by comparing the original team manifolds to team manifolds created from surrogate data sets in which team coordination was removed while retaining the individual performance level of each team member (see Appendix C). This allows assessing the evolution of team coordination over time. Below, we evaluate team coordination both for the team as a whole, as well as for individual pairs of team members, the latter allowing an analysis of the coordination patterns within a team (see Appendix C). Team performance is then assessed by comparing the respective measures of the nonexpert teams to those of the expert team.

We visualized the original team manifolds for each skill level by plotting the team trajectories in the fixed subspace defined earlier (Fig. 4.4, *first column*). Figure 4.4, second column, shows the corresponding manifolds of the surrogate data using the same subspace. No statistically significant difference was found between manifolds of the original and surrogate team data using Euclidean distances between the manifolds (see Appendix C), thus indicating that team coordination does not change the overall shape of the projected manifolds. However, removing team coordination significantly reduced the reconstruction quality of the manifolds with respect to the fixed subspace. A poor reconstruction quality with respect to this subspace signifies a deviation from the expert manifold and a deterioration of task performance. Team coordination is thus important for the successful execution of the task. To understand at which point in time coordination matters the most, we plotted the reconstruction quality in the fixed subspace as a function of time for the original manifolds and a set of surrogate

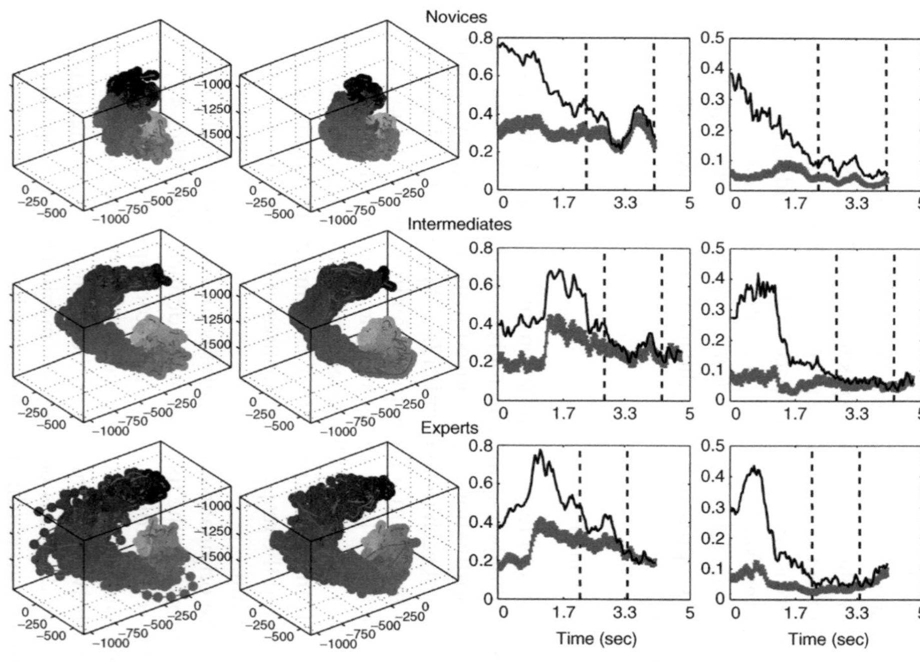

Figure 4.4 **Visualization of the manifolds and effect of removal of team coordination. First column:** Manifolds projected onto the 3-D fixed subspace of the expert manifold. *Top to bottom*: Novice, intermediate, and expert team manifold, respectively. Gray scale codes time (from black to light gray). **Second column:** Manifolds of surrogate data without team coordination, same order and gray scale code. **Third column:** Time evolution of reconstruction quality using the fixed subspace for original data (*black*) and surrogate data (*gray*, $n = 1{,}000$, *error bars*: 1 SD). *Vertical dashed lines*: entry of first and last stack member, respectively. **Fourth Column:** Team coordination over time using a measure that is independent of a fixed subspace. Original data (*black*) and surrogate data (*gray*, $n = 100$, *error bars*: 1 SD), the latter serving as baseline for team coordination.

manifolds (Fig. 4.4, *third column*). The difference between the reconstruction qualities of the original and the surrogate manifolds provides a measure of importance of team coordination for correct task execution at each point in time. During the initial phase of the trials, much variance in the surrogate data is not captured by the fixed subspace. The entry and the later phases of the trials are affected to a much smaller degree by the loss of team coordination. This result is largely independent of the choice of the fixed subspace, as is shown in Figure 4.B5 in Appendix B. A more direct measure of team coordination, which does not involve the choice of a fixed subspace, is defined by comparing each original team manifold with its surrogate manifold and assessing how much the original team manifold is perturbed by removing team coordination (see Appendix C). Since this measure does not refer to the expert manifold (for the nonexpert teams), it allows the analysis of team coordination independently of team performance. When applying this measure to the data, our results confirmed that team coordination is generally high during the initial phase of the trials, but lower during the later phases of the trial (Fig. 4.4, *last column*). In particular, expert and intermediate teams build up and maintain a high coordination during the initial phase of the trials, which abruptly falls off toward the entry. The novice team starts off with a similarly high coordination as the more advanced teams, which however immediately decays essentially monotonously toward the entry. Thus, while the importance of team coordination in the preparatory and initial phase of the team task is found in all teams regardless of skill level, time evolution of team coordination differs across skill levels.

Comparing teams across skill levels is a prerequisite to gain insight into team development and assess team performance. Assessing similarity between expert and non-expert manifolds by their Euclidean distance in the fixed subspace (see Appendix C) showed that the intermediate manifold is similar to the expert manifold, whereas the novice manifold is considerably different (Fig. 4.5, *top*). Again, this result is largely independent of the choice of the fixed subspace (see Fig. 4.B5 in Appendix B).

We also evaluated the degree of coordination between every pair of individual team members (see Appendix C). In particular, we compared coordination between nearest neighbors and non-nearest neighbors across skill levels. Nearest neighbors are team members who stand and move right next to each other in the stack. Because the immediate neighborhood relations change as the task evolves, this classification is valid only for certain time windows; here, before and at entry. We found that, for all skill levels, coordination is higher among nearest neighbors than among non-nearest neighbors (Fig. 4.5, *bottom two panels*). However, although this effect is relatively weak in the intermediate and expert teams, it is considerably stronger in the novice team. This indicates that the novice team relies in a disproportionate way on nearest-neighbor coordination. Together with the earlier finding of quickly decaying coordination of the novice team as a

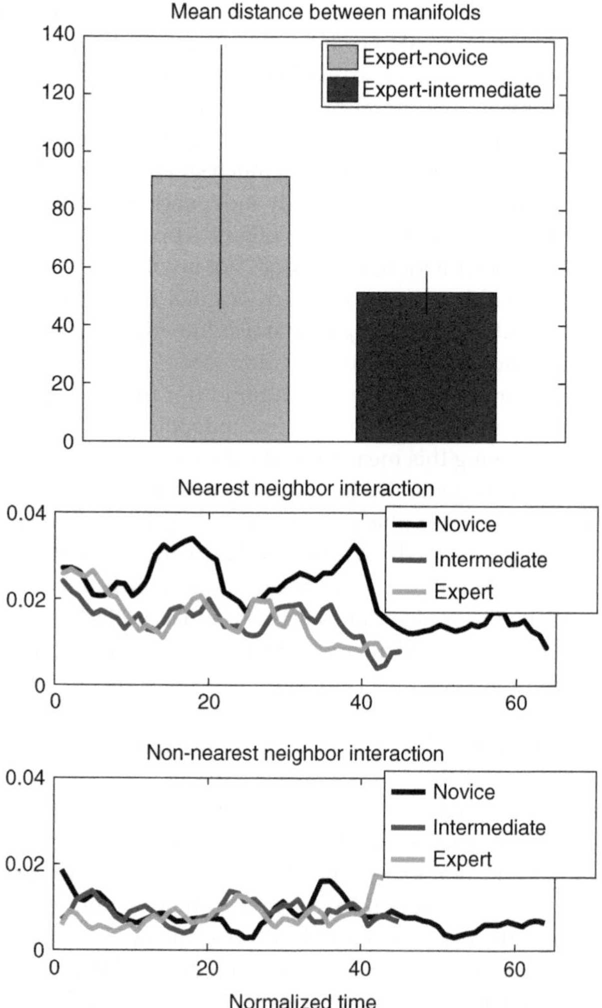

Figure 4.5 **Distance between manifolds and team coordination patterns. Top:** Euclidean distance between novice/intermediate and expert manifolds in the fixed subspace projection (mean over all fixed subspaces, *error bars*: 1 SD). **Bottom two panels:** Average team coordination between all nearest neighbors in a team (*upper panel*) and between all non-nearest neighbors in a team (*lower panel*) during the entry phase as a function of time (*black*: novices; *gray*: intermediates; *light gray*: experts). The normalized time corresponds to the entry phase in units of points in time from the beginning of the entry phase. One time point corresponds to 30.3 ms.

whole, this suggests that relying too much on nearest-neighbor coordination may disrupt coordination of the team as a whole and hence deteriorate task performance, as compared with the expert team.

CONCLUSION

We have analyzed team dynamics during a room-clearing task that involved teams of three skill levels. We provide a new approach for dynamically measuring team processes independently of a human observer by representing the dynamics of each team as a manifold in phase space. Our approach allows quantifying and tracking important features of team dynamics, such as team coordination and team performance over time. This revealed that, in all skill levels, team coordination is most prominent during the initial phases of the task and contributes to optimal team performance, as represented by the expert manifold. In the novice team, however, this coordination is quickly decaying, whereas in the intermediate and expert teams, coordination is maintained at the beginning of the task. Also, the dynamics of novice teams (as captured by their manifolds) differed significantly from the dynamics of the expert team in the same task, whereas the difference was much reduced for the intermediate team. Analyzing the coordination patterns within each team further showed that the novice team relies much more on nearest-neighbor coordination in the beginning of the trials than do intermediate and expert teams. This finding indicates that more advanced teams distinguish themselves by more homogeneous team coordination that extends across multiple team members and points toward heightened team awareness. Our results reveal significant differences between novice teams and more advanced teams in terms of team coordination and performance. Although coordination may be necessary for successful team performance, it cannot make up for poor individual team member performance; individual skill levels impact team skill levels (McIntyre & Salas 1995). In our setting, the effect of skill on team performance is more difficult to assess than the effect of team coordination since, as a team evolves, it improves both skill and team coordination. A possible assessment of the effects of skill of the individual team members could be done by additional experiments in which teams that have already acquired some team coordination are confronted with an unfamiliar task. In this case, the previously acquired team coordination may still be present, while the individual team members have to develop the skills to execute the new task. In our present study, the main differences were found between the novice team and more advanced teams, whereas within the advanced skill levels, the intermediate and expert teams showed similar features. Since our current data comprised only positions and velocities of the team members, it is possible that to reliably differentiate between intermediate and expert teams additional information may be required about the teams, such as head or body orientation or even oral communication between the team members. Once such information is available, it is easily included in our approach. Although in our study we used the expert team as a gold standard for team performance, user-defined performance measures and/or coordination patterns of interest could be automatically and reliably detected by our methods as well. For instance, if there were two expert teams, our method could detect differences in their coordination patterns; however, in the absence of additional performance criteria, it could not rank the expert teams with respect to each other. Whereas at this stage our methods certainly do not replace a human observer in a training situation, they could be of valuable assistance in the training process, for instance by dynamically detecting deviations from an optimal performance, as well as in the a posteriori analysis of the trials.

ACKNOWLEDGMENTS

This work was supported by DARPA grant NBCH1020010. VKJ acknowledges support by ATIP (CNRS) and the JS McDonnell Foundation. Per 5 C.F.R. 3601.108 and DoD JER 5500.7-R, 2-207 "The views, opinions, and/or findings contained in this article/presentation are those of the author/presenter and should not be interpreted as representing the official views or policies, either expressed or implied, of the Defense Advanced Research Projects Agency or the Department of Defense."

APPENDIX A: PROOF OF CONCEPT—ANALYSIS OF SYNTHETIC DATA

In this section, we provide proof of concept for determining the intrinsic dimensionality as well as the low-dimensional representation of a manifold (determined by the trajectories on the manifold) in a fixed subspace. To this end, we use two synthetic data sets in which the underlying structure and dynamics is known beforehand. The data sets are that of a planar manifold and a spherical manifold with limit cycle dynamics on it. Each of these systems is 16 dimensional. In the first data set, the dynamics will collapse onto a planar manifold and perform limit-cycle oscillations; the second data set is a spherical manifold with limit-cycle dynamics. Figure 4.A1 shows the three-dimensional phase space and the corresponding time series for both. Each data set is made up of 40 trajectories simulated with additive noise in which the initial conditions were slightly jittered.

Here, we briefly discuss how to create a low-dimensional representation of the manifold and show proof of concept of the approach. As mentioned earlier, to estimate the intrinsic dimensionality of the manifold we performed a PCA of the data at each point in time. Figure 4.A2 shows the evolution of the first principal eigenvector over time for both data sets. After the initial transient, the first two components of the eigenvector for the planar manifold and the first three components of the eigenvector for the spherical manifold are mostly invariant over time.

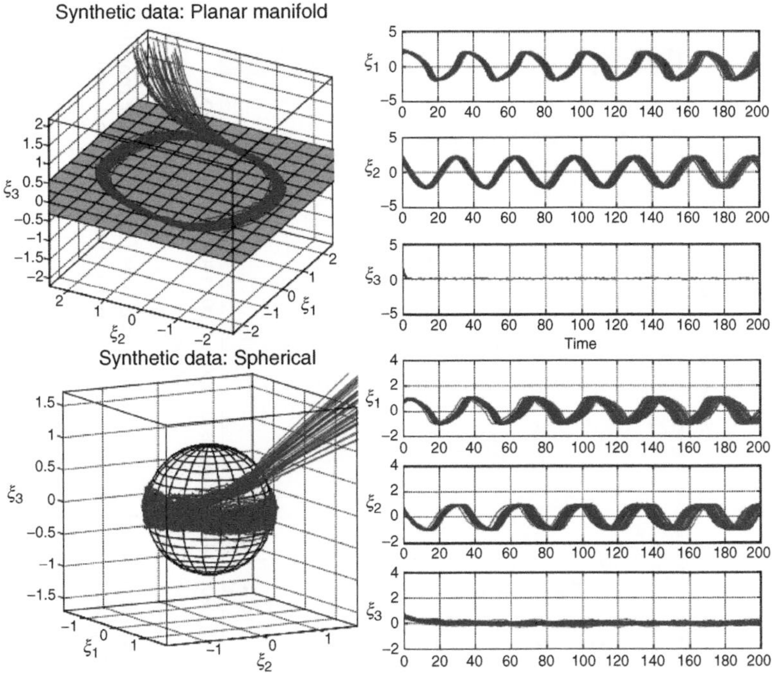

Figure 4A.1 Two synthetic data sets and the corresponding time series for the first three dimensions. The first data set is 40 trials of a 16-dimensional system in which the dynamics collapses onto a planar manifold and performs limit cycle oscillations. The second data set is a 16-dimensional system in which the manifold is spherical and the flow is in the limit cycle regime. The initial conditions are slightly jittered and the system is simulated with additive noise.

To create a low-dimensional representation of the manifold from the data, we project the 16-dimension data set onto a three-dimensional space. Here, the choice of subspace used to project the data was made by visual inspection of the invariance of the eigenvectors over time ($t = 500$), but for the real data we used a systematic approach for choosing the fixed subspace (see Appendix C). The left panel of Figure 4.A3 shows the intrinsic dimensionality of the data sets collapsed over time. It can be seen from that figure that, by using two dimensions for the planar and three dimensions for the spherical manifold, well over 90% of the variance in data is accounted for. To ascertain the validity of the reconstruction, we compared the reconstruction quality (see Appendix C) using the chosen fixed subspaces with the reconstruction quality using 1,000 randomly generated subspaces. Figure 4.A3 shows the histogram of the results of these reconstructions. It can be seen that the reconstruction quality using the invariant subspace is significantly different and higher compared to the reconstruction using the random subspaces.

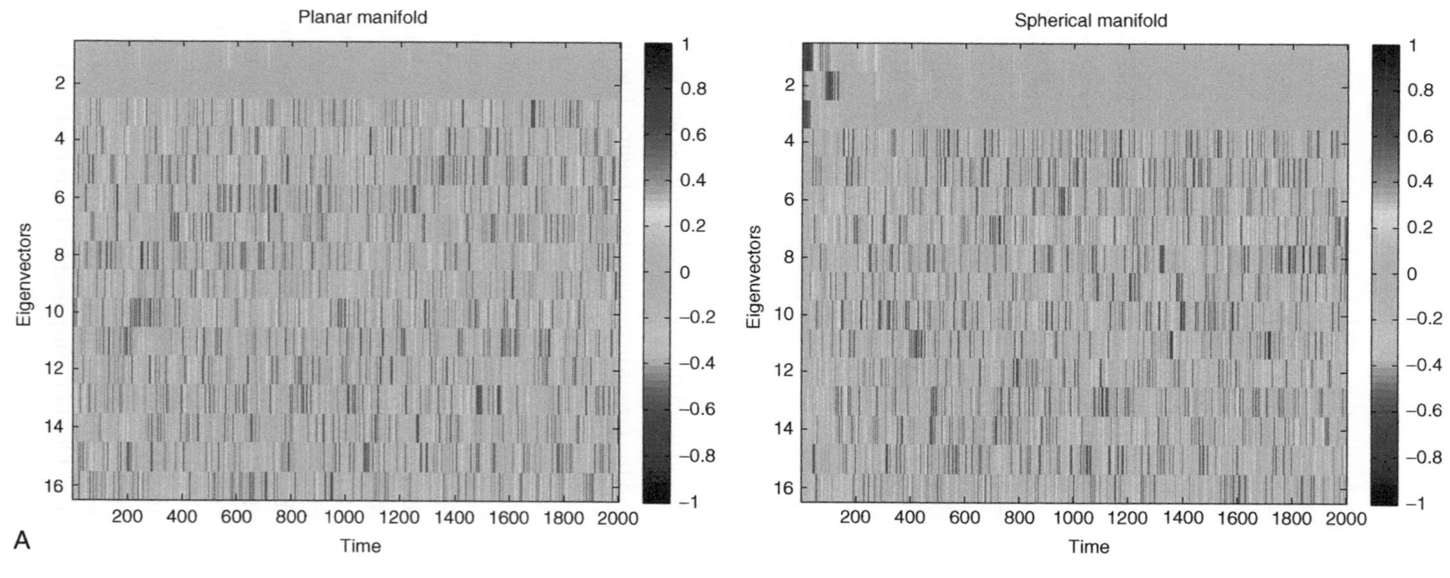

Figure 4A.2 **Top row**: Eigenvectors over time of the synthetic data sets. Top left panel shows the eigenvectors for the planar manifold and right panel the eigenvectors for the spherical manifold. After the initial phase, the first two eigenvectors for the planar and first three for the spherical manifolds are quite invariant over time.

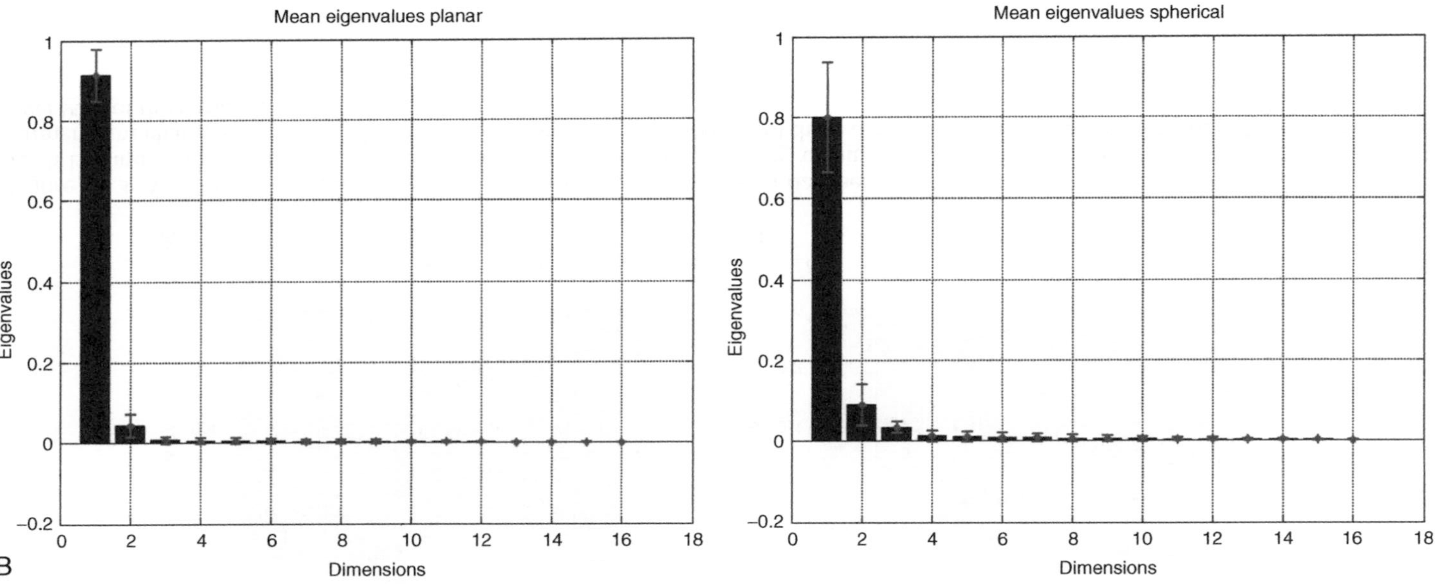

Figure 4A.2 (*Continued*)**Bottom row**: The mean eigenvalues over time for the synthetic data sets. Bottom left panel shows the mean eigenvalues over time for the planar manifold and the bottom right panel shows the mean eigenvalues for the spherical manifold. Corresponding to the eigenvectors, for the planar manifold, the first two eigenvalues capture most (over 90%) of the variance. For the spherical manifold, the first three eigenvalues capture most (over 90%) of the variance.

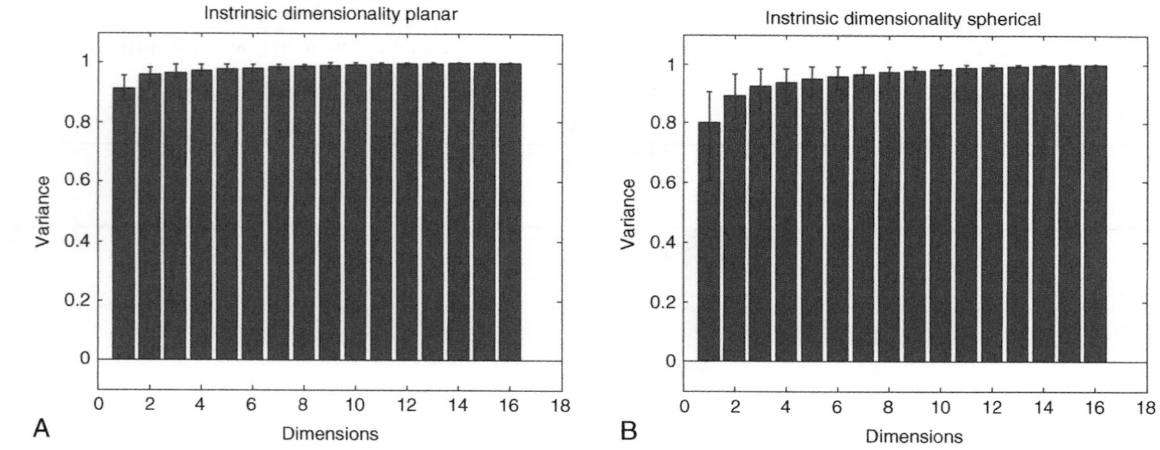

Figure 4A.3 **A** and **B**: Intrinsic dimensionality of the spherical and planar data set. The vertical axis shows the fraction of total variance. Each bar indicates the fraction of total variance that is accounted for by using the number of dimensions corresponding to the bar (dimensions changes from 1–16). With two dimensions for the planar and three dimensions for the spherical manifolds, we can capture over 90% of the variance.

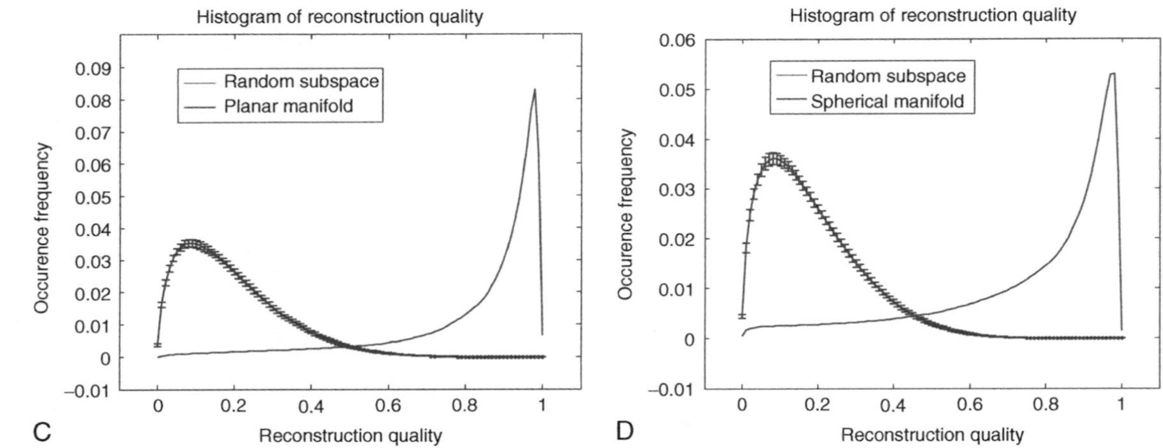

Figure 4A.3 (*Continued*) **C** and **D**: Histogram of the reconstruction quality of the synthetic data. Using subspaces from the actual data and randomly generated subspaces the synthetic data was reconstructed. This was done to ascertain the validity of the subspace used to reconstruct the data (see Figure A4). The gray solid curves show the histograms of reconstruction quality using the subspaces from the data. The curves with error bars show the reconstruction quality of the data using random subspaces. The vertical axis gives the relative frequency of occurrence of a particular value of reconstruction quality which is given along the horizontal axis. The reconstruction using random subspaces was performed 1,000 times each. The mean is plotted in gray with error bars. It can be seen that the subspaces chosen from the synthetic data explain the data much better than the random subspaces. The gray solid curve (using subspaces from data) has a higher frequency of occurrence of larger reconstruction quality values.

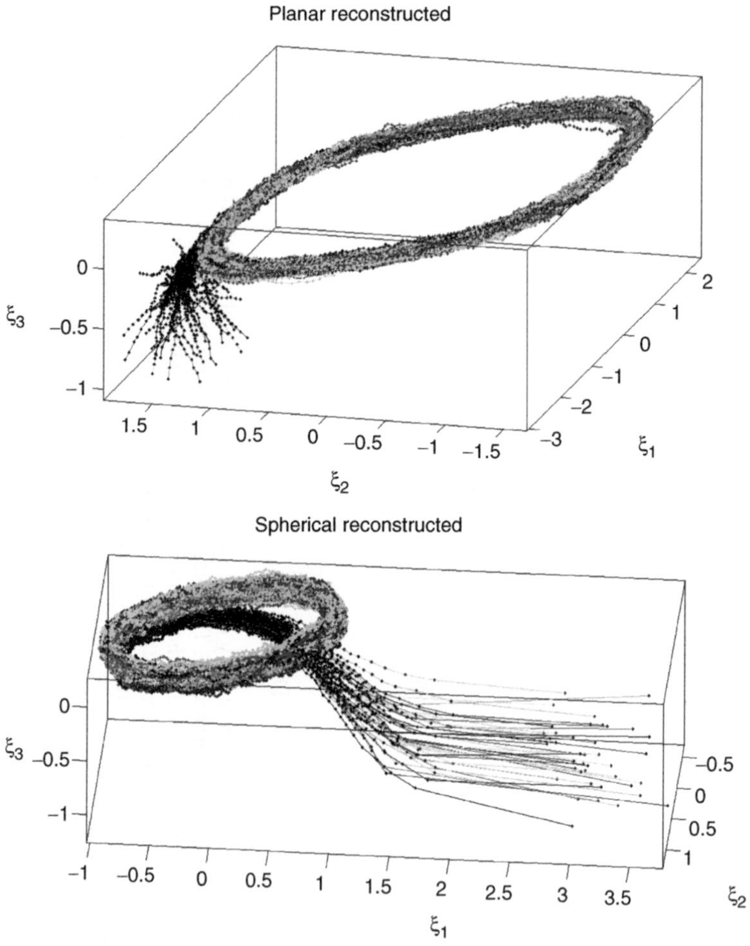

Figure 4A.4 **Top**: The top panel shows the reconstructed planar manifold in 3-D space using a subspace at time point t = 500. **Bottom**: The bottom panel shows the reconstructed spherical manifold in 3D space. The reconstructions have captured the shape of the manifold rather well. The gray scale coding indicates the change of time with black at the start and light gray at the end of the simulation.

Figure 4.A4 shows the low-dimensional representation of the manifolds in the three-dimensional fixed subspace at t = 500. We can see that the manifold shapes are clearly identifiable and correspond to the original simulations. The grayscale coding indicates the evolution of time, with black close to the initial condition and light gray close to the final time point of the simulation.

We conclude from our simulations using synthetic data that the intrinsic dimensionality of the manifold can be measured by PCA at each point in time, and a faithful low-dimensional reconstruction of the manifold can be achieved in a fixed subspace of the phase space.

APPENDIX B: RESULTS OF THE MOUT EXPERIMENT IN THE LARGE ROOM

Here, we show results from the large L-shaped room. Although the results for the small room and the L-shaped room are qualitatively identical, some minor differences reflect the higher complexity of the room-clearing task in the L-shaped room. These differences are indicated in the figure captions (Figs. 4.B1–5).

APPENDIX C: METHODS AND MEASURES

Intrinsic Dimensionality of the Manifolds

We determined the intrinsic dimensionality of the manifolds by performing a PCA across trials at each time point. PCA determines the variance that is accounted for by each dimension. The total variance is the sum of the variances in each dimension. The intrinsic dimension of the manifold at each point in time can be found by setting a threshold, for instance 90% of the total variance, and determining the number of dimensions needed to account for this level of total variance. Note that, to avoid thresholding effects (such as, e.g., determining the intrinsic dimension to four when three dimensions account for 89% of the total variance), we chose to depict the percent of the total variance that the various dimensions account for (cf. Fig. 4.3).

Reconstruction Quality

The *reconstruction quality* R of a vector v with respect to a given subspace is defined as $R = \| \mathbf{Pv} \|^2 / \| v \|^2$, where P is a projection matrix to the subspace. R has values between 0 and 1, the latter indicating perfect reconstruction.

Fixed Subspace

To determine whether the manifold or part of it lies in a stationary fixed subspace, we computed a matrix of reconstruction qualities. Each row of this matrix represents the temporal evolution of reconstruction quality (averaged over trials) of the data using a given fixed subspace of the expert manifold. The maximum value of the mean column serves as a measure of the subspace that best represents the data in a given dimension over time and was used to determine the fixed subspace.

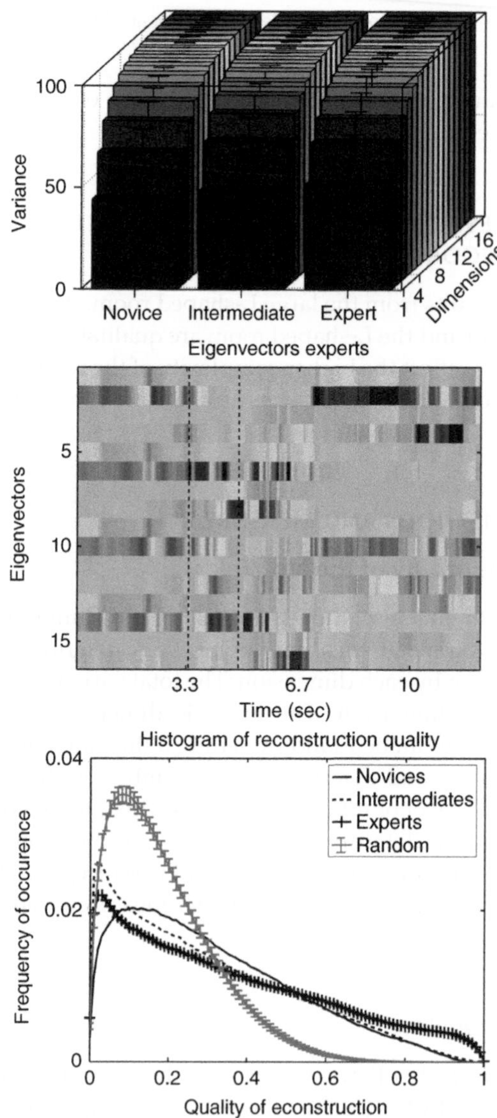

Figure 4B.1 Large room results corresponding to Figure 4.3. **Top:** Mean percent variance that is explained by the respective number of dimensions obtained from the principal component analysis for the expert, intermediate, and novice data sets. The mean is taken over time. Four to five components capture almost 90% of the entire team signal. The error bars indicate a 90% confidence interval. **Middle:** First principal component vector of the expert manifold over time. Ordering of the 16 elements: x-position, x-velocity, y-position, y-velocity for team member 1; then the same for team member 2, etc. As for the expert data of the small room, the vector is stationary over wide ranges of time. In contrast to the small room, the main variability of the expert team in the large room occurs in the x-velocity of the whole team essentially during the entire time interval before the entry. **Bottom:** Histogram of the reconstruction quality of the real data. Using subspaces from the expert manifold and randomly generated subspaces, the team dynamics data was reconstructed to ascertain the validity of the subspace used to reconstruct the data. See main text and Figure 4.3 for more details.

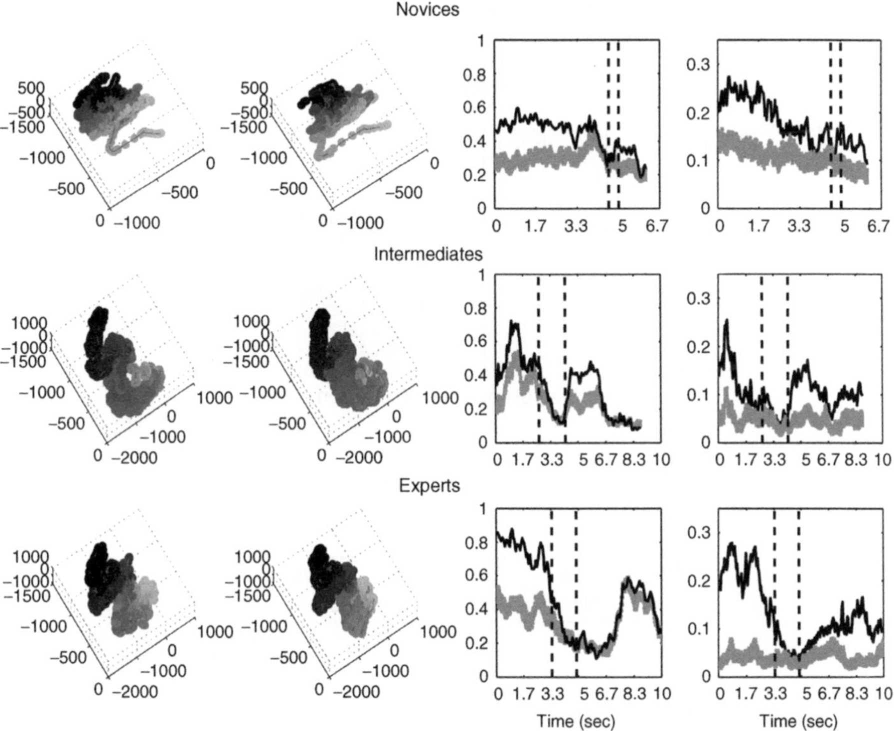

Figure 4B.2 Large room results corresponding to Figure 4. **First column:** Manifolds projected onto the 3-D fixed expert subspace at t = 1s. From top to bottom: novices, intermediates, experts. The gray scale codes evolution of time (from black through light gray). **Second column:** Manifolds for surrogate data, ordered and gray scale coded same as the original data. **Third column:** Reconstruction quality obtained from using the fixed subspace is plotted over time for original data (*black*) and surrogate data (*gray*), n = 1,000 with error bars of one standard deviation. The greater the difference between the two, the greater the importance of team coordination at the respective time point. Vertical bars indicate the entry of the first and last stack member, respectively. As in the small room data, team coordination in the large room plays the highest role before the entry, but does occur after the entry as well, although to a lesser extent. **Fourth column:** Team coordination over time using a measure that is independent of a fixed subspace. Original data (*black*) and surrogate data (*gray*), n = 100 with error bars of one standard deviation. The values for the surrogate data are given as a baseline. In contrast to the small room data, the team coordination measure of the large room data shows significant team coordination also after the entry (albeit lower than before the entry).

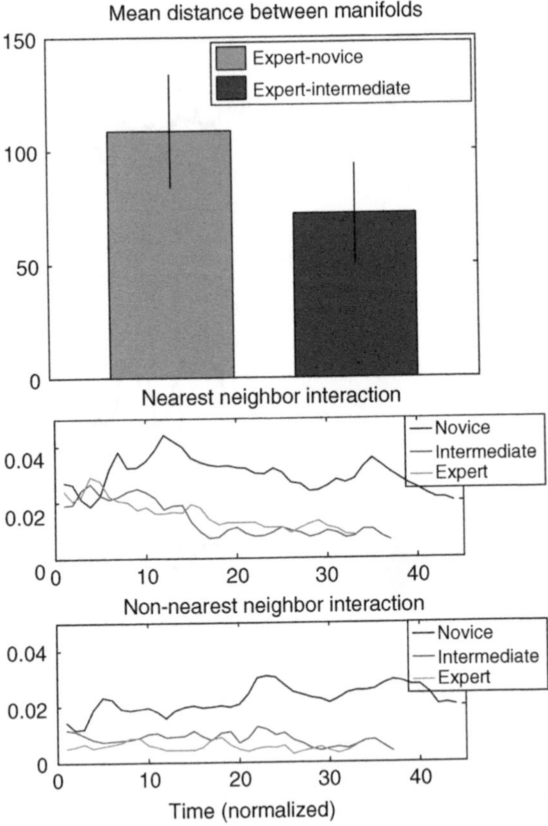

Figure 4B.3 Large room results corresponding to Figure 4.5. **Top:** Euclidean distance between novice/intermediate and expert manifolds in the fixed subspace projection (mean over all fixed subspaces, *error bars*: 1 SD). The Euclidean distance is significantly higher for the novice–expert distance than for the intermediate–expert distance $t(362)=58.7138$, $p < .0001$. **Bottom:** Degree of coordination between team members within a team. Here, only the entry phase of the room clearing task is shown along the horizontal axes. The vertical axes show the measure of team coordination patterns given in the methods section. The upper row shows the average coordination between nearest neighbors (i.e., team members 1 – 2, 2 – 3, and 3 – 4) during entry. These team members constitute the nearest neighbors during the entry phase. The lower row shows the average interaction between team members 1 – 3, 1 – 4, and 2 – 4 during entry. They are the non-nearest neighbors during the entry phase. Each team level is plotted in a different gray scale with black for novices, medium gray for intermediates, and light gray for experts.

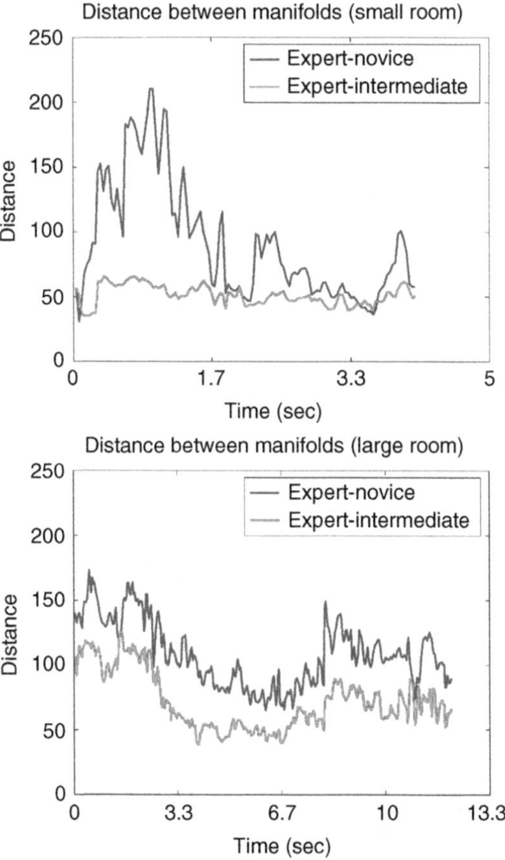

Figure 4B.4 Euclidean distance between expert and non-expert manifolds (projected onto a 3-D fixed subspace composed of the first three eigenvectors from the expert manifold at a given time point) as a function of the fixed subspace. For both small room (*top*) and large room (*bottom*), the distance between expert and novice manifold tends to be larger than the distance between expert and intermediate manifold. This effect is to a large extent independent of the subspaces. In the small room, the effect is strongest for fixed subspaces at the beginning of the trial, whereas in the large room the size of the effect is about the same for all fixed subspaces.

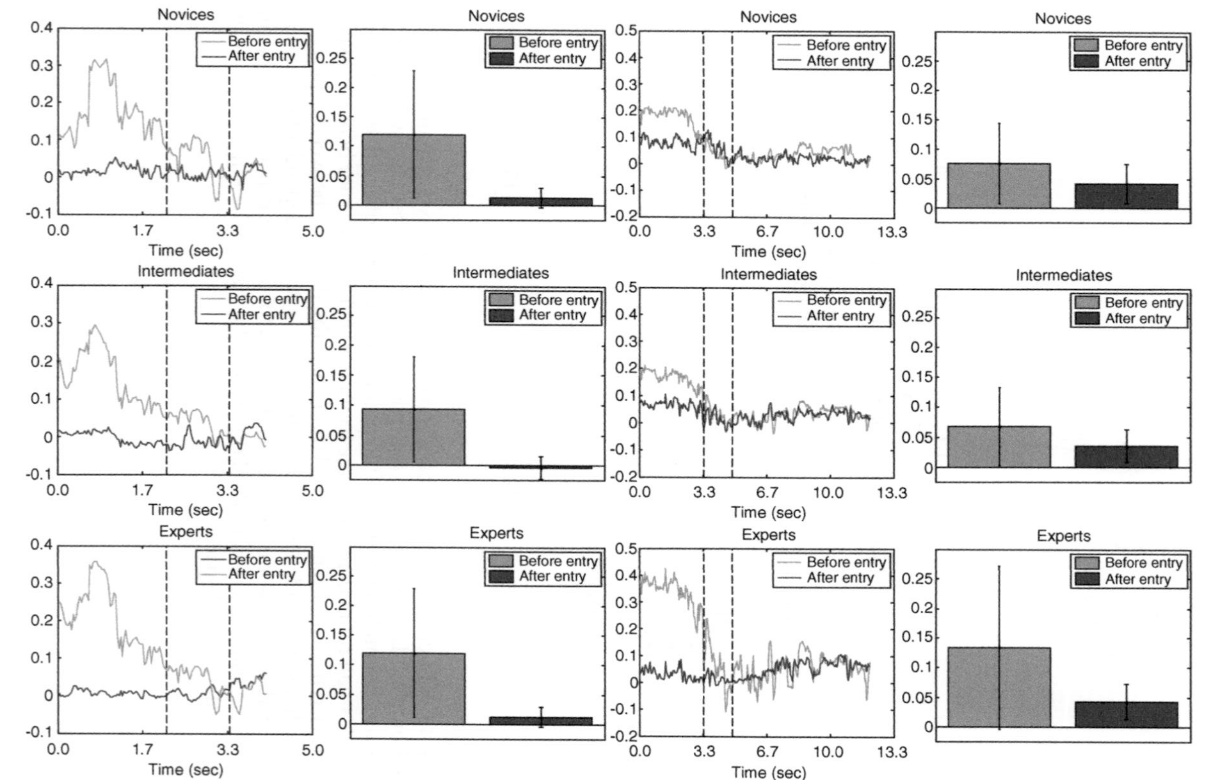

Figure 4B.5 Importance of team coordination at the beginning of the trial is largely independent of the choice of the fixed subspace.

Surrogate Data Without Team Coordination

We created a set of surrogate team manifolds (n = 1,000) in which we removed team coordination between the team members (see Müller & Sternad 2003 for other surrogate methods). Each surrogate team manifold was created by assembling 40 trajectories in phase space, in which the data from each team member was taken from a different trial. Through this operation, we remove the effect of coordination among the team members, but maintain the correct positions of the members within the team, as well as the correct individual motor execution of the task for each team member.

Team Coordination of a Team as a Whole

To quantify team coordination *C(t)* of the team as a whole over time, we determined how much the team manifold is perturbed by removing team coordination at each point in time. This was determined by computing the quantity $C(t) = 1/N\sum_{k=1}^{N}(M^{(k)}(t) - S^{(k)}(t))/M^{(k)}(t)$, where N = 16 is the dimension of the phase space, and $M^{(k)}(t)$ and $S^{(k)}(t)$ are the mean reconstruction qualities (averaged over trials) of the original and surrogate data, respectively, with respect to the first k dimensions of the original subspace at time t. The order of the dimensions is determined by the order of the principal eigenvectors.

Team Coordination Patterns Within a Team

Patterns of team coordination are defined by the coordination between each pair of team members. Coordination between a pair of team members *(i,j)*

Figure 4B.5 (*Continued*) The result is reproduced consistently for fixed subspaces before the entry, while for fixed subspaces after the entry no effect of team coordination is found. **First column:** Mean difference in reconstruction quality between original and surrogate data as a function of the fixed subspace (small room). *Dark gray curves*: mean difference in reconstruction quality when using fixed subspaces before the entry. *Light gray curves*: mean difference in reconstruction quality when using fixed subspaces after the entry. *From top to bottom*: novices, intermediates, experts. **Second column:** The mean differences in reconstruction quality (taken over all fixed subspaces) are significantly greater before than after the entry, indicating a higher importance of team coordination at the beginning of the trials. **Third column:** Corresponds to first column, but for the data from the large room. **Fourth column:** Corresponds to second column, but for the data from the large room.

is quantified by $G_{ij}(t) = 1/N\sum_{k=1}^{N}(Q_{ij}^{(k)}(t) - S^{(k)}(t))/M^{(k)}(t)$, where N = 16 is the dimension of the phase space, and $S^{(k)}(t)$ and $M^{(k)}(t)$ are as in the previous paragraph, and $Q_{ij}^{(k)}(t)$ is the reconstruction quality of particular surrogate data, in which the coordination between team members *i* and *j* has been left intact (i.e., the data for these two team members are taken from the same trial), whereas the data of the other team members are taken from different trials, respectively. $G_{ij}(t)$ is a measure of how much of the original team dynamics manifold is maintained by keeping the coordination between team members *i* and *j* intact, in comparison to keeping no coordination at all.

Team Performance Measure: Similarity of Two Team Manifolds

Similarity of the nonexpert manifolds to the expert manifold (projected to the fixed subspace) was assessed as follows. For each point on the expert manifold, the Euclidean distances to all points on the nonexpert manifold was computed and the fifth smallest distance (to reduce the effect of outliers) to each given point was retained. The distance between the two manifolds was then defined as the average over all fifth smallest distances.

REFERENCES

Benner, P. 1984. *From novice to expert: Excellence and power in clinical nursing practice.* Menlo Park, CA: Addison-Wesley.

Benner, P. 2004. Using the Dreyfus model of skill acquisition to describe and interpret skill acquisition and clinical judgment in nursing practice and education. *Bulletin of Science Technology & Society* 24, 3, 189–99.

Brannick, M.T., R.M. Roach, and E. Salas. 1993. Understanding team performance: A multimethod study. *Human Performance* 6, 287–308.

Buller, P.F. 1986. The team building-task performance relation: Some conceptual and methodological refinements. *Group & Organizational Studies* 11, 147–68.

Dreyfus, H.C., and S.E. Dreyfus. 1980. A five-stage model of the mental activities involved in directed skill acquisition Air Force Office of Scientific Research: United States Air Force, ORC 80-2 F49620-79-C-0063. Bolling, AFB, Washington, DC: United States Air Force.

Dyer, J.C. 1984. Team research and team training: A state of the art review. In *Human factors review,* ed., F.A. Muckler, 285–323. Santa Monica, CA: Human Factors Society.

Ericsson, K.A., R.T. Krampe, and C. Tesch-Romer. 1993. The role of deliberate practice in the acquisition of expert performance. *Psychological Reviews,* 700, 379–84.

Fitts, P.M. 1964. Perceptual motor skills learning. In *Categories of human learning,* ed., A.W. Melton, 243–85. New York: Academic Press.

Fowlkes, J.E., N.E. Lane, E. Salas, T. Franz, and R. Oser. 1994. Improving the measurement of team performance: The TARGETs methodology. *Military Psychology* 6, 47–61.

Glaser, R. 1996. Changing the agency for learning: Acquiring expert performance. In *The road to excellence*, ed., K.A. Ericsson, 303–11. Mahwah, NJ: Lawrence Erlbaum.

Hoover, A., and B.D. Olsen. 1999. A real-time occupancy map from multiple video streams. *Proceedings of the IEEE International Conference on Robotics and Automation* 3, 2261–66.

Houldsworth, B., J. O'Brien, J. Butler, and J. Edwards. 1997. Learning in the restructured workplace: A case study. *Education and Training* 39, 6, 211–18.

McElroy, E., D. Greiner, and M. de Chesnay. 1991. Application of the skill acquisition model to the teaching of psychotherapy. *Archives of Psychiatric Nursing* 5, 2, 113–17.

McIntyre, R.M., and E. Salas. 1995. Measuring and managing for team performance: Emerging principles from complex environments. In *Team effectiveness and decision making in organizations*, eds., R. Guzzo and E. Salas, 149–203. San Francisco: Jossey-Bass.

Modrick, J.A. 1986. Team performance and training. In *Human productivity enhancement: Training and human factors in systems design* Vol. 1, ed. J. Zeidner. New York: Praeger.

Morgan, B.B., E. Salas, and A.S. Glickman. 1994. An analysis of team evolution and maturation. *The Journal of General Psychology* 120, 277–91.

Müller, H., and D. Sternad. 2003. A randomization method for the calculation of covariation in multiple nonlinear relations: Illustrated with the example of goal-directed movements. *Biology and Cybernetics* 89, 1, 22–33.

Offermann, L.R., and R.K. Spiros. 2001. The science and practice of team development: Improving the link. *The Academy of Management Journal* 44, 2, 376–92.

Salas, E., and S. Fiore, eds. 2004. *Team cognition: Understanding the factors that drive process and performance*. Washington DC: American Psychological Association.

Schöner, G. 1995. Recent developments and problems in human movement science and their conceptual implications. *Ecology and Psycholgy* 8, 291–314.

Scholz, J.P., and G. Schöner. 1999. The uncontrolled manifold concept: identifying control variables for a functional task. *Experimental Brain Research* 126, 289–306.

United States Marine Corps. 1998. *Military operations in urbanized terrain*. Marine Corps Logistics Base, Albany, GA.

5

Decomposing Muscle Activity in Motor Tasks

Methods and Interpretation

Lena H. Ting and Stacie A. Chvatal

How do humans and animals move so elegantly through unpredictable and dynamic environments? Why does this question continue to pose such a challenge? During any motor task, many physiological elements throughout the body must be coordinated, such as limbs, muscles, neurons, etc. A major question in motor control is: How do the overall functions and characteristics of movements arise from the functional arrangement and coordination of both neuromuscular elements and environmental interactions? Although modern technology allows us to collect an unprecedented amount of data on the activity of neurons, muscles, and limbs during a wide variety of behaviors, we still lack an understanding of how individual elements of the body interact to produce the many movements we perform, let alone characteristics such as grace or clumsiness.

Interpreting both structure and variability in the motor system and relating it to the resulting biomechanical and behavioral outputs remains a grand challenge in understanding how we move. Nikolai Bernstein noted the fact that motor behaviors never repeat themselves exactly, even when the same task is performed in succession (Bernstein 1967). On the other hand, he also noted that characteristic output patterns occur even when a motor task is performed by different sets of muscles, such as when drawing shapes or letters on a piece of paper versus on a blackboard, or with a different appendage. Similarly, more recent studies also demonstrate that the performance of a motor task, such as reaching to a target, can occur quite consistently even when there is a great deal of variability in the underlying joint motions or torques contributing to that task (Newell and Carlton 1988; Latash et al. 2002; Ko et al. 2003; Reisman and Scholz 2006). These findings highlight the fact that our bodies have a large number of degrees of freedom in the joints, muscles, and neurons that allow them to be flexible and functionally reconfigured to perform the same task, as well as different tasks (see Kelso, Sternad, this volume). During any so-called coordinated movement, synchrony and similarity are observed across many different kinematic, kinetic, electromyographic, and neural signals (Bernstein 1967; Macpherson 1991). But, when looking across a wide behavioral repertoire, the synchrony and coordination observed in one movement may be abolished in another, such that fluctuations in the spatiotemporal dynamics of the multiple measures may appear coordinated in one instance and independent in another (Bernstein 1967; Macpherson 1991). Such differences are potentially due to both changes in the neural control of muscles, as well as to changing interactions of the body with the environment under various conditions.

Controlling movements requires not only organizing physiological processes for movement, but also requires consideration of the complex interactions of forces acting between the organism and the environment. Bernstein defined the coordination of movement as: "the process of mastering redundant degrees of freedom of the moving organ, in other words, its conversion to a controllable system" (Bernstein 1967). By "controllable" Bernstein meant that coordinated motor activity causes predictable biomechanical events, such as force generation and motion, that allow us to reliably perform a motor task. Thus, understanding movement requires characterizing the degrees of freedom of the physiological system that are used in the performance of any particular movement, the reconfiguration of such degrees of freedom in the performance of divergent movements (see Latash, this volume), and the relationships of these degrees of freedom to the biomechanical interactions that ultimately generate the movement (see Prilutsky, this volume). Gathering large sets of data during natural movements is becoming increasingly easier, thus allowing us to characterize coordination across many variables at different levels of the motor system; however, interpreting such large data sets and analyzing them to test motor control hypotheses remains a challenge.

Computational methods for analyzing large sets of data are now easily accessible and available; however, the utility of such methods for providing insight into motor control is debated. Can such techniques help us to understand increasingly large data sets? Can quantitative analysis provide further insight than that which scientists have gathered from observation? Are automated pattern-recognition techniques able to reveal that which an experienced scientist can see when examining raw data? What are the potential benefits and pitfalls of using such techniques? These questions will be addressed in this chapter.

Here, our goal is to provide instructive tutorials to provide an intuitive guide to the similarities and differences between two primary techniques used for the analysis and decomposition of multiple signals in motor control and neuroscience, as well as in engineering fields: principal components analysis (PCA) and non-negative matrix factorization (NMF) (Lee and Seung 1999). Although comprehensive texts on the quantitative aspects of these techniques are readily available (Ramsay and Silverman 2005), we present methods for understanding how the properties of each technique affect the decomposition and physiological interpretation of muscle activation patterns in a simple example and in actual data from postural control and walking. We have chosen two commonly used linear decomposition techniques that render the most divergent results; however, similar principles could be used as a basis for comparing other decomposition techniques, such as independent components analysis (ICA) or k-means analysis (Tresch et al. 2006). We will discuss the interpretations and implications of the results and how such techniques might be used to understand principles of motor coordination, as well as give insight into the function of the nervous system in translating goal-level intentions into specific muscle activation patterns for movement.

BASIC PROPERTIES AND DIFFERENCES BETWEEN PCA AND NMF: A SIMPLE EXAMPLE

Although PCA and NMF are similar in their underlying concept and mathematical representations, there are key differences in their implementation and in the resulting components. Both PCA and NMF are linear decomposition techniques that assume that the set of measured data is composed of linear combinations of a smaller number of underlying elements (Fig. 5.1A). That is, given a number of simultaneous observations of multiple data channels, any particular observation could be represented as:

$$M_j = c_{1j}W_1 + c_{2j}W_2 + \ldots + c_{nj}W_n + \text{error} \qquad \text{(Eq. 1)}$$

Here, M_j is a vector that represents measurements of multiple channels of data (Fig. 5.1B); for example, the activity of *m* muscles at a given time point, arranged in a column. On the right side of the equation, the components or basis functions W_i are vectors, also of length *m*, that represent invariant patterns of activity across those different channels. The pattern of muscle activity can be described by *n* scalar values c_{ij}, each of which specifies the contributions of each component to the measured muscle activation pattern M_j. If there are *m* muscles and $n<m$ components, then the representation of M_j in terms of the components W_i and the weight or scaling factors c_{ij} is lower-dimensional than simply stating the value of each element of M_j. Such linear decomposition techniques therefore test the hypothesis that, over a large number of observations of M_j, the components W_i remain fixed, but the scaling factors c_{ij} are allowed to change and are sufficient to account for all of the variations of the data measured across different conditions. When analyzing muscle activation patterns, the modules W_i are often referred to as muscle synergies (Tresch et al. 1999; Cheung et al. 2005; Ting and Macpherson 2005; Torres-Oviedo and Ting 2007) or M-modes (Danion et al. 2003; Krishnamoorthy et al. 2004; Latash et al. 2007). In this context, the hypothesis

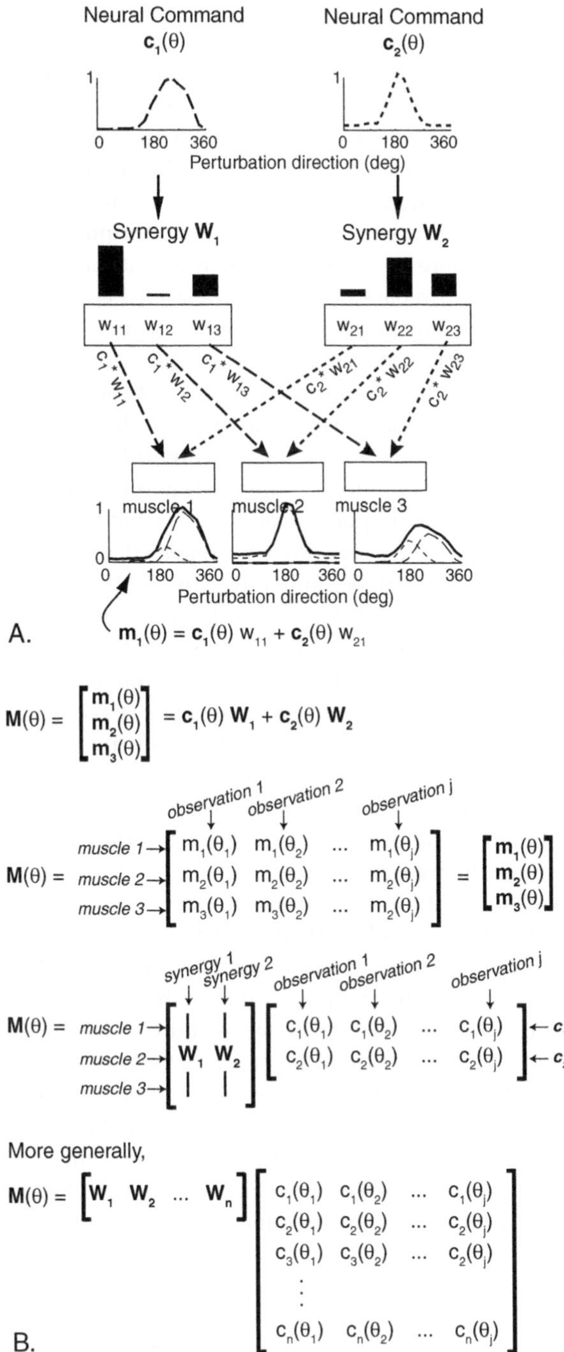

Figure 5.1 Electromyography (EMG) data decomposition schematic and muscle synergy concept. **A**: Any pattern of multiple muscle activation can be represented as a linear combination of the activations of that muscle by each

(Continued)

is that muscle synergies remain fixed, but activation of these synergies can vary, resulting in observed variations in individual muscle activity.

Although similar in concept, in practice, PCA and NMF are quite different; each method decomposes the variability within a given data set in very different ways. PCA is an analytical technique, meaning that the components are found through a straightforward set of computations. Therefore, it is easy to use and there are readily available algorithms included in most data processing software packages. This is possible because PCA requires that the components be orthogonal (e.g., perpendicular) to each other, creating a unique solution to any decomposition. Furthermore, it is relatively straightforward to select the appropriate number of components needed to explain a given data set based on a cutoff value for the variance accounted for. In contrast, NMF is found using a search algorithm, which means that it has to start with a set of random components and iteratively improve on them until an adequate proportion of the variability in the dataset is accounted for. Components generated by repeated searches will not be numerically identical but will be similar. Because NMF constrains both the weights c_i, as well as all of the elements of the components W_i to be non-negative, the problem is what is called *convex*. That is, there are no local minima for the search to be "stuck" in, therefore components from multiple searches are numerically similar. In a non-negative space, it is not possible for the components to be orthogonal; however, they must be independent, meaning that no component can be defined as a linear combination of the other components. The iterative technique also requires that the number of components be specified in advance, so that multiple searches must be done to determine the right number.

In the following set of tutorials, we use a simple two-dimensional example of a simulated dataset to illustrate the differences in how PCA and NMF decompose variability in the dataset. For all three examples, simulated muscle activity data are fabricated by assuming that there are two underlying components, which can be interpreted as muscle synergies, W_1 and W_2 that each define a different ratio between the activity of two muscles (Fig. 5.2A, *gray bars*). These components can also be drawn as vectors on a two-dimensional plot (Fig. 5.2A, *gray arrows*). A set of data, M, is created by randomly assigning the activation level of each component (c_1 and c_2) from a uniform distribution between 0 and 1. Each data point, or observation M_j, can be represented as a vector $[m_{1j}m_{2j}]$, and plotted as a single point on a set

Figure 5.1 (*Continued*) muscle synergy component. In this example, there are $n = 2$ components and $m = 3$ muscles, thus $M(\theta)$ can be represented in terms of the lower-dimensional combination of muscle synergies (components, W_i) and activation commands ($c_i(\theta)$). B) Organization of the data matrix and the structure of the W and c matrices.

of axes representing the level of activation of muscle 1 versus muscle 2 (Fig. 5.2A). The tutorials are available for download as part of the supplementary materials, at http://neuro.gatech.edu/groups/ting/PMCtutorial.html.

Orthogonality Versus Independence

The constraints of orthogonality and independence in PCA, and independence without orthogonality in NMF, account for the large differences between the components extracted by each technique. In this example, the activity of each component was equally weighted, so that the data is scattered evenly between the two vectors, W_1 and W_2, used to create the data (Fig. 5.2A). When PCA is applied to the data, two components are extracted (Fig. 5.2B). The first aligns with the center of the long axis of the data and accounts for 87% of the variability. Because the scaling factors can be positive or negative, the direction that W_1 points does not matter, only the line it defines. The second component must be at a right angle to the first component to satisfy orthogonality. It accounts for a much smaller portion of the variability, only 13%. Neither PCA component looks like the original components used to generate the data. Using NMF, the extracted components are similar to the original components, W_1 and W_2, used to generate the data, appearing at the edges of the data points (Fig. 5.2C). The variability accounted for by each component is similar, 49% and 51%, respectively. Although the components are not orthogonal, the addition of a second component nonetheless increases the set of possible patterns of muscle activation between muscles 1 and 2.

PCA Is Descriptive; NMF Is Prescriptive

PCA, much like a multiple regression, describes the mean and residual variance from the mean in successive principal components. Before identifying the components, the original dataset is typically demeaned; if this is not done, then the first principal component represents the mean value of each variable across the dataset. Otherwise, as in this example, the first principal component in PCA describes the largest deviation from that mean in each muscle across a given dataset. Each additional component describes the orthogonal direction containing the next largest deviations from that mean. In our two-dimensional example, it means that if the first component changes, then the second component must also change. The percentage of variability accounted for by each component decreases monotonically, describing the degree to which the dataset varies in the corresponding direction. Because PCA allows for both negative and positive values for the scaling factors, it is possible to describe any point on the plane with two independent components derived from data in that plane, regardless of the direction that they point (Fig. 5.2B). Data with multiple dimensions can be restricted to a plane by choosing only the first two principal components.

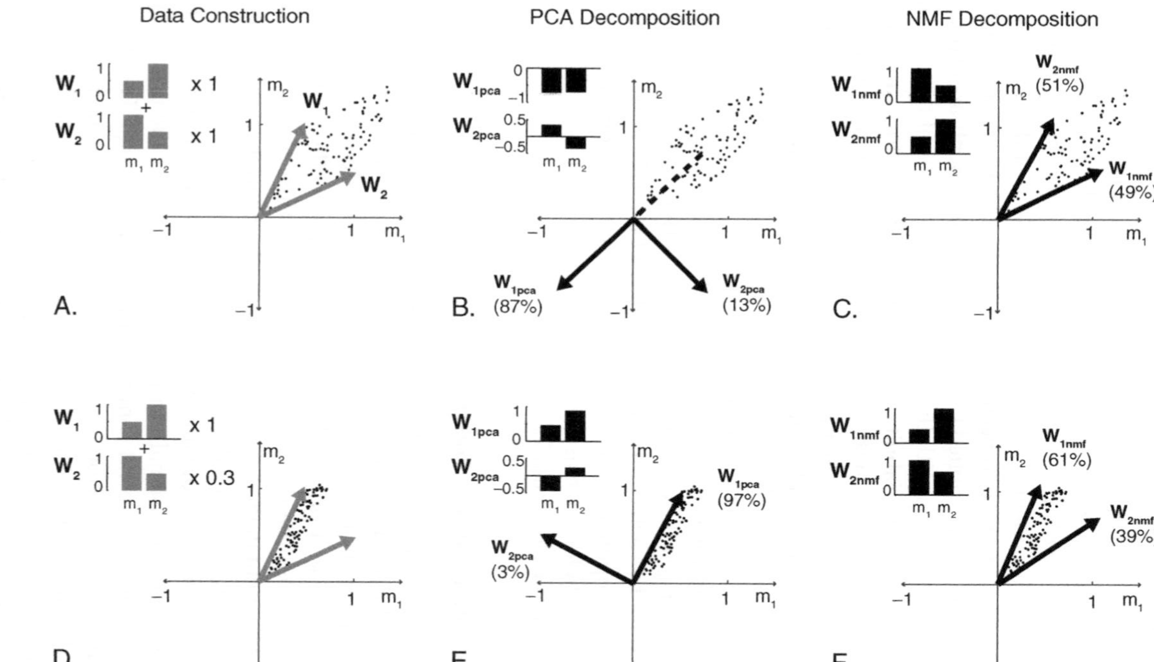

Figure 5.2 A 2-D example illustrating differences between components identified using principal components analysis (PCA) and non-negative matrix factorization (NMF). **A**: Data is constructed using two components specifying fixed ratios of muscle activation

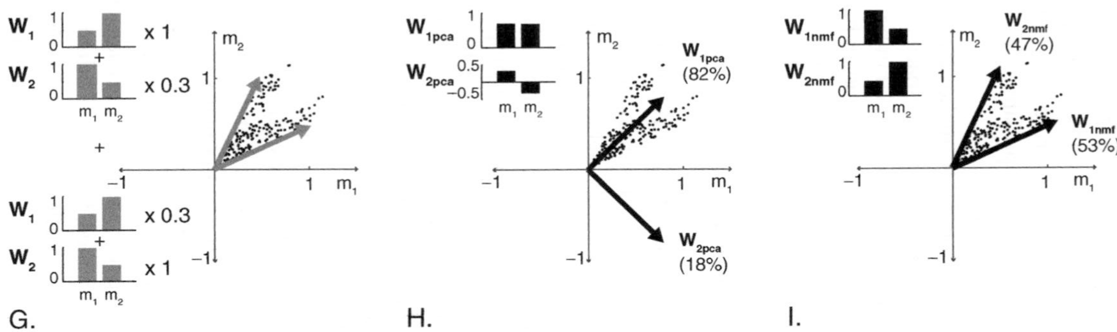

Figure 5.2 (*Continued*) between two muscles, W_1 (m_1=0.5*m_2) and W_2 (m_1=2*m_2). The contribution of each component for a given observation, or data point, is found by multiplying each component by a scaling factor (c_1 and c_2) selected from a uniform distribution ranging from 0–1. **B**: Components identified using PCA to decompose the data from A. The percentage of total data variability that each component accounts for is shown beside each vector. The first component is directed along the long axis of the data cloud, and the second is constrained to be in the orthogonal direction. C: Components identified using NMF to decompose the data from A. Components are found near the edges of the data cloud. Note the similarity to the original components (W_1 and W_2) used to generate the data. **D**: Data is constructed using the same two components as in A, except now it is weighted towards using W_1. In order to generate this data, c_1 was taken from a uniform distribution between 0 and 1, whereas c_2 was taken from a uniform distribution between 0 and 0.3. **E**: Components identified using PCA to decompose the data from D. W_{1pca} looks similar to W_1, reflecting the bias towards W_1 in the generation of the data set, but W_{2pca} is different from W_2. **F**: Components identified using NMF to decompose the data from D. Despite the bias in the generation of the data set, these components are similar to those used to generate the data, as well as the components identified in C. **G**: Data is constructed using the same two components as in A and D, except now part of the data is weighted towards using W_1 and part is weighted towards using W_2. To generate this data, c_1 was taken from a uniform distribution between 0 and 0.3, whereas c_2 was taken from a uniform distribution between 0 and 1, and this was included along with the data from D. **H**: Components identified using PCA to decompose the data from G. W_{1pca} passes between the two "clouds" of data where the mean values of m_1 and m_2 lie, and the components look similar to those identified in B. **I**: Components identified using NMF to decompose the data from G. Again the components are similar to those used to generate the data.

In NMF, the components prescribe a subspace within which all data points must lie. Because of the non-negativity constraints, only the points lying between the two components can be described (e.g., Fig. 5.2A). Thus, components from NMF tend to identify the edges of the dataset and define a convex hull, or polygon, within which all of the feasible data points lie (e.g., Fig. 5.2C). The condition of independence requires that each additional component increase the allowable subspace, as no two components can be represented as a linear combination of other components. Because there is no constraint on orthogonality, it is also possible for one component to change and the others to remain the same.

Therefore, the non-negativity constraints within NMF make it more restrictive than PCA, delimiting regions of the low-dimensional space that cannot be reached. Although dimension reduction can be achieved in both techniques by examining only the first few components, NMF imposes further restrictions. Components derived from PCA tend to *describe* the major direction of the data without imposing restrictions within the space defined by those components. In contrast, NMF *prescribes* a subspace in which possible combinations of muscle activity lie, restricting the expressible data points using those components.

Consider an example using the same components, W_1 and W_2, as in the previous tutorial, except this time the data are preferentially weighted toward using W_1 (Fig. 5.2D, data construction). This dataset was created from sampling the same muscle activation components as in the prior example, but with a higher activation of W_1 over W_2. Using PCA, both components changed direction compared to the previous tutorial (compare Fig. 5.2E and 2B). The first PCA component (W_{1pca}) rotated closer to the mean of the observed pattern of muscle activity and now looks qualitatively similar to the original W_1 used to construct the data (Fig. 5.2A), accounting for 97% of the variance. The second component must rotate a similar amount to maintain orthogonality (compare Fig. 5.2B and 2E). Both components identified in this case look different from those identified using PCA in the previous example. Thus, PCA describes the data in a similar sense to a mean and standard deviation. In contrast, both components found using NMF (Fig. 5.2F) were similar to the components W_1 and W_2 used to generate the data (Fig. 5.2D) and to those identified in the previous tutorial (Fig. 5.2C). There was a slight shift in the second component simply because there is less variance in that direction, and therefore a larger confidence interval. Thus, the components obtained from NMF identify vectors that prescribe the same space of possible solutions using those two components as in the prior tutorial, even when one component is more heavily weighted than the other.

Physiological Interpretability of PCA Versus NMF Components

In PCA, a component, W_i, can contain positive and negative numbers representing relative muscle activation levels, as well as positive and negative weightings, c_i. This means that positive and negative relationships can be inverted easily by negative weighting values. In the context of muscle activation patterns, this equal relationship between positive and negative activation is inconsistent with the transformation between motorneuron action potentials and muscle activity. Although motoneurons no doubt receive inhibitory as well as excitatory neural activity, the inhibitory effect can only be seen on motor output if there is also a high background level of muscle activity. That is, if inhibition occurs when muscles are quiescent, they have no effect on muscle activity due to the rectifying properties of neural transmission. Moreover, excitatory pathways and effects cannot be made inhibitory, and vice versa, so that there is no reason to think that an excitatory pattern would be identical to an inhibitory one. In contrast, in NMF, the components are constrained to be non-negative, which is physiological for neural and muscle output, since neurons are either firing action potentials (positive signal) or else in a resting state (zero signal).

One interesting result of the non-negativity constraint in NMF is that the underlying components resemble a "parts-based" decomposition, in which a series of parts are summed to create a whole. Since each component, or part, that is added cannot be subtracted out through the contributions of another component, the parts must resemble identifiable features of the output. In contrast, allowing negative numbers in PCA means that a given data point is created by addition and subtraction of contributions from different components to a given muscle's activity. The first component describes the mean, and the next components can add or subtract activity from that mean. Therefore, the resulting data point may bear no resemblance to the identified principal components.

Here, we demonstrate the different ways in which PCA and NMF deal with data that are not evenly distributed. Consider an example using data constructed from the same components, W_1 and W_2, from the first two tutorials, except now part of the data is skewed toward using W_1 and part skewed toward using W_2 (Fig. 5.2G). The components identified using PCA are similar to those found in the first tutorial: The first component passes between the two main "clouds" of data, and the second is orthogonal to the first (compare Fig. 5.2H to 2B). In contrast, components extracted using NMF look very similar to the original $W_1$and W_2 used to generate the data, as well as to those identified in the first two tutorials (compare Fig. 5.2I to 2F and 2C). The components lie along the edges of the data "clouds," and therefore can be used to describe any data points between them.

In this example, the components from PCA are directed in similar directions as in first example, with the first component aligned along the mean values of m_1 and m_2 across the dataset (Fig. 5.2H). Most of the data points are reached by scaling the contribution of the first component and adding or subtracting a contribution of the second component. However, these components do not resemble the two-armed "parts" of the dataset. In contrast, the components from NMF are again similar to those used to generate the data, and similar to the components found from the two other data sets (Fig. 5.2I). Here, the two components from NMF clearly identify two of the underlying "parts" that are obvious in the dataset (similar results can also be achieved through independent components analysis [ICA] in combination with PCA [Hyvärinen 2001; Tresch et al. 2006]).

Similarly, in the original paper describing differences between PCA and NMF, the components underlying decomposition of an image of a face were compared (Lee and Seung 1999). All of the PCA components look like entire faces, which are then added and subtracted together to generate a given face. To generate a face with a medium nose, large eyes, and small mouth, one might imagine starting with the mean face expressed by the first principal component and adding a component with a large nose, large eyes, and medium mouth, then subtracting another component with a small nose, medium eyes, and small mouth. The NMF components, however, are characterized by face parts such as the nose, eyes, and mouth. A face would be generated by selecting a component nose, scaling it by a medium number, selecting a component eyes and scaling it by a larger number, and selecting a component mouth and scaling it by a smaller number. Interestingly, this kind of parts-based decomposition is similar to the type of neural representations observed in the visual and other sensory encoding systems (Olshausen and Field 2004). Accordingly, there has been a shift from the use of PCA to NMF in visual system research (Simoncelli and Olshausen 2001).

IDENTIFYING COMPONENTS USING PCA AND NMF: A POSTURAL CONTROL EXAMPLE

Taken together, these three tutorials illustrate key differences in how PCA and NMF describe and partition the variability in a given data set, which are relevant to how they can be used to test motor control hypotheses. Although all of the data were generated from the same set of underlying components, the components identified by PCA changed when the mean levels of muscle activation changed, and all of the components changed simultaneously. NMF has the ability to identify components that are stable across different conditions, but combined differently. This demonstrates how different conclusions regarding the robustness and generality of components might be drawn depending on which decomposition algorithm is used.

In the literature, both PCA and NMF have been used to examine whether stable motor modules are used for generating movements. Several studies have addressed muscle coordination in standing balance control, because muscles in various regions of the body tend to act synchronously, and patterns of muscle activation can be easily related to a direction of body motion. During postural body sway, PCA has been used to identify components, called *M-modes*, that correspond to the direction of center of pressure changes used to stabilize the body (Aruin et al. 1998; Krishnamoorthy et al. 2003a). Similarly, in responses to different directions of perturbation during standing balance control, components from NMF, referred to as *muscle synergies*, have been identified that correspond to the direction of force applied at the ground to stabilize the body (Ting and Macpherson 2005; Torres-Oviedo et al.2006). However, as the number of postural conditions is increased, the underlying M-modes from PCA are found to change (Krishnamoorthy et al. 2004), whereas the muscle synergies from NMF remain consistent (Torres-Oviedo et al. 2006; Torres-Oviedo and Ting 2010).

Rarely are both techniques used in the same study, so that it is difficult to know whether the differences in the literature reflect the techniques used, the experimental design, or the particular motor tasks tested. Moreover, since NMF requires several decisions on the part of the investigator, choosing the right number of muscle synergies is not necessarily straightforward, which may also lead to different conclusions being drawn. Here, we provide examples where both PCA and NMF are performed on actual data from one subject during postural responses to multidirectional perturbations.

Introduction to Postural Responses

In order to maintain balance in light of an unexpected perturbation of the support surface, humans and animals must keep the projection of their center of mass (CoM) within the limits of their base of support. Various strategies may be used when balance is disrupted, requiring the activation of different muscles, such as taking a step, grabbing a handrail, or maintaining the feet in place to restore balance. When standing balance is disturbed with a discrete perturbation, first the direction of falling is sensed, and then the appropriate muscles are activated to restore balance. The initial change in muscle activity in the lower limbs does not occur until approximately 100 ms following the onset of a perturbation, and this initial muscle activity is called the *automatic postural response* (APR). Variations are observed even in responses to the same perturbation direction due to attention, expectation, and the like (Woollacott and Shumway-Cook 2002). When many trials and many perturbation directions are examined, the differences observed in individual muscle activations are difficult to interpret (Horak and Macpherson 1996; Henry et al. 1998). One hypothesis is that the nervous system activates these muscles in groups, and decomposition techniques such as PCA and NMF can be used to identify such groups and the relationships between the muscle activations (Krishnamoorthy et al. 2003a; Krishnamoorthy et al. 2003b; Torres-Oviedo and Ting 2007).

To generate the postural data examined here, subjects stood on a platform, which was suddenly moved in one of 12 different directions in the horizontal plane. Electromyographic (EMG) signals were collected from 16 lower trunk and leg muscles from the right side. For each trial, mean muscle activity during three time windows during the APR was calculated: 100–175 ms following perturbation onset (PR1), 175–250 ms (PR2), and

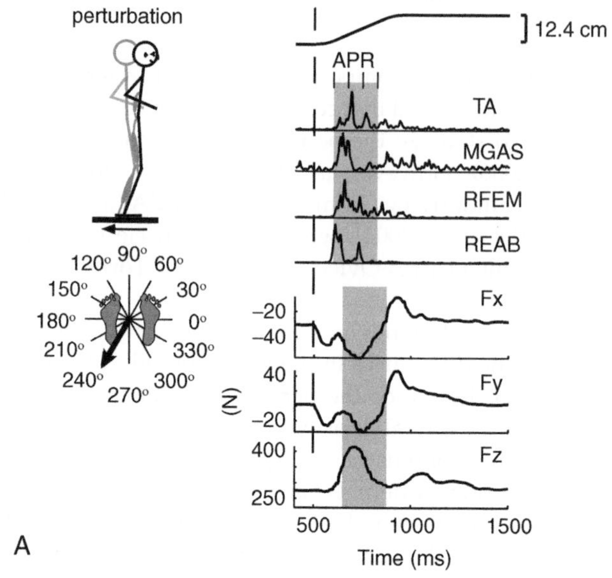

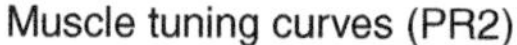

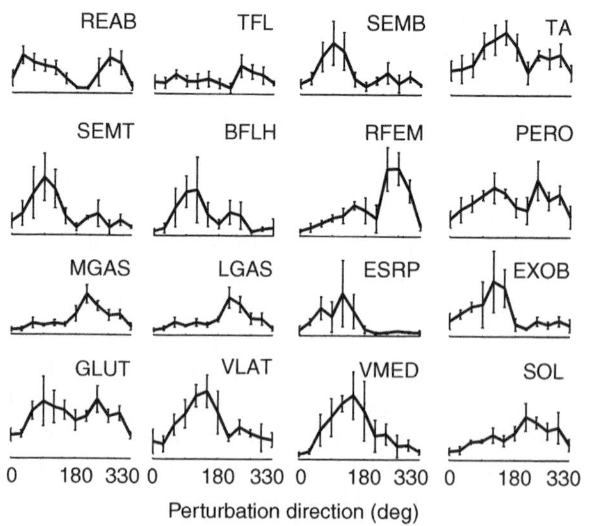

Figure 5.3 Example of postural responses to a backward and leftward perturbation of the support surface. **A**: Platform displacement during the ramp-and-hold perturbation. Electromyograph (EMG) responses occur 100 ms after the onset of platform motion (*vertical dashed line*). Shown here are tibialis anterior (TA), medial gastrocnemius (MGAS), rectus femoris (RFEM), and rectus abdominus (REAB) EMG responses. Mean EMG activity was calculated for three time bins during the APR (*shaded region*), beginning 100 ms (PR1), 175 ms (PR2), and 250 ms (PR3) following perturbation, as well as one background time period. Ground reaction forces under the right foot are also shown. **B**: Muscle tuning curves generated from 12 evenly spaced perturbation directions,

250–325 ms (PR3), as well as one background time window before the perturbation began (Fig. 5.3A). Therefore, this data set consisted of 16 muscles and 240 conditions (4 time windows × 12 perturbation directions × 5 trials in each direction). All of the data were arranged in a matrix in which each of the 16 rows contains the 240 observed values for a single muscle. The values in each row were normalized to the maximum value in that row, corresponding to the maximum level of muscle activity observed for that muscle across all conditions. Therefore, for each muscle all values ranged from 0 to 1. Before components are extracted using NMF, each muscle was also normalized to have unit variance, meaning that the sum of the squared values in the row equals 1. This allows the variations in each muscle to be considered with equal importance by the algorithm. One practical consideration is that, for NMF, the data should always be presented in the format N muscles × M conditions. However, PCA requires the data be transposed, in the format N conditions × M muscles.

In response to horizontal plane disturbances, each muscle was preferentially activated for particular perturbation directions (Fig. 5.3B). The muscle "tuning curves" demonstrate the directional sensitivity of the muscles. Each muscle is active maximally in a given direction, and less so for other directions. Some muscles have a single preferred direction (e.g., vastusmedialis, VMED), whereas others have multiple tuning directions (e.g., rectus abdominus, REAB). The muscle tuning curves demonstrate that each direction of perturbation evokes a different combination of muscle activity. The error bars on the muscle tuning curves also illustrate trial-to-trial variations observed in postural responses. Therefore, across perturbation directions, and even within a perturbation direction, different patterns of muscle activity are evoked. Does this mean that each muscle must have an independent neural command specifying its level of activation (Macpherson 1991)? Using NMF and PCA, we can test the hypothesis that the observed variations can be explained by the activation of a few muscle synergies (Fig. 5.1). In the following section, we will compare how NMF and PCA describe postural response data, address practical issues of selecting the appropriate number of components, and examine the robustness of the components across different postural tasks, specifically, two-legged versus one-legged perturbation responses.

Figure 5.3 (*Continued*) taken from time window PR2. Muscle tuning curves vary in magnitude over all perturbation directions, and their shapes vary from muscle to muscle. In addition to the four muscles shown in A, tensor fasciae latae (TFL), semimembranosus (SEMB), semitendinosus (SEMT), biceps femoris long head (BFLH), peroneus (PERO), lateral gastrocnemius (LGAS), erector spinae (ERSP), abdominal external oblique (EXOB), gluteus medius (GLUT), vastuslateralis (VLAT), vastusmedialis (VMED), and soleus (SOL) were also collected. Shown are the mean tuning curves ± standard deviations for five trials in each perturbation direction, presented randomly.

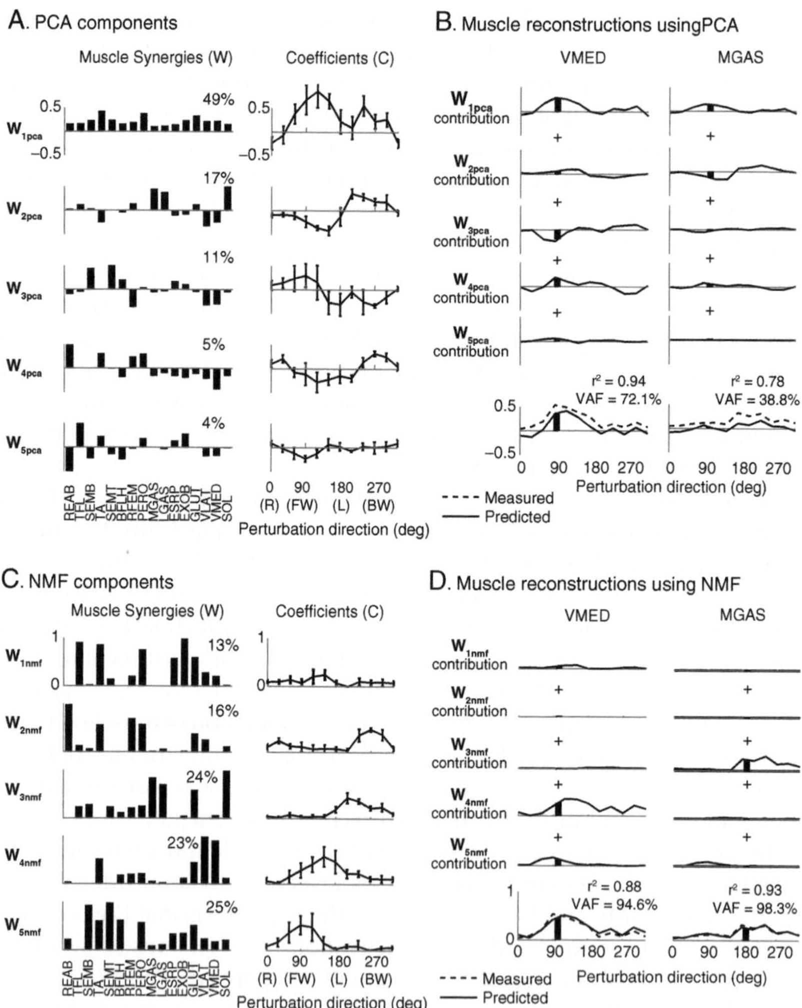

Figure 5.4 Components and activation coefficients identified from postural response data using principal components analysis (PCA) and non-negative matrix factorization (NMF). **A**: Components identified using PCA may have positive and/or negative muscle contributions and activation coefficients. Each bar represents the contribution of that muscle to that component. Percentages indicate the amount of total data variability accounted for by each component. Activation coefficient tuning curves from PR2 are shown as mean ± standard deviation of five trials. **B**: Tuning curves created from a single trial in each direction for two muscles reconstructed using the components identified in A. The contribution from each component is added or subtracted to form the reconstructed muscle tuning curve. The original data are shown with a dashed black line and the reconstructed data are shown with a solid black line. The variability accounted for (VAF) by the reconstruction as well as r^2 values are shown for each muscle tuning curve. **C**: Components identified using NMF have only positive muscle contributions and activation coefficients.

Components of Postural Responses Identified by PCA and NMF

Here, we compare five components selected by NMF and PCA to describe the postural response data for normal, two-legged stance (the procedure for selecting the number of components will be described in a later section).

The components identified by PCA are composed of muscle contributions that are both positive and negative, and are activated by weighting coefficients (or scaling factors) that may also be positive or negative (Fig. 5.4A). This example illustrates again that the components are identified in order of the percentage of variance that each explains. The first component describes the mean level of activity of the muscles across all conditions, and therefore has positive contributions from all of the measured muscles, with strong contributions from TA and PERO (Fig. 5.4A, W_{1pca}). The first component is also strongly activated for forward (90-degree) and backward (270-degree) perturbation directions, which evoke much more muscle activity than lateral perturbation (Henry et al. 1998). The subsequent components have contributions from fewer muscles, and these contributions are both positive and negative. Additionally, the activation coefficients may be positive or negative for different perturbation directions, and the magnitude of activation decreases with each subsequent component.

The way in which PCA decomposes data can best be illustrated by examining how the components contribute to an individual muscle tuning curve. Due to the positive and negative values taken both by the components and the activation coefficients in PCA, contributions from different components can be added and subtracted to obtain the total predicted muscle activity. An example of this can be seen in the reconstruction of the VMED tuning curve from the individual contributions from each component (Fig. 5.4B), which are found by multiplying the height of the VMED bar in each component with the activation coefficient for a given direction. Thus, each of the contributions resembles a scaled and possibly inverted version of the activation coefficient tuning curves of each component (Fig. 5.4A). The resulting tuning curve for VMED is generated by adding all five curves together (Fig. 5.4B, *bottom*). Although the peaks of the various contributions can vary, the resulting VMED tuning curve peaks near 90 degrees, and is roughly zero between 180 and 360 degrees. The response

---

Figure 5.4 (*Continued*) Percentages indicate the amount of total data variability accounted for by each component. Activation coefficient tuning curves from PR2 are shown here as mean ± standard deviation of 5 trials. **D**: Two muscle tuning curves reconstructed using the components identified in C. The contribution from each component is added to form the reconstructed muscle tuning curve. The original data are shown with a dashed black line and the reconstructed data are shown with a solid black line. The variability accounted for (VAF) by the reconstruction as well as r^2 values are shown for each muscle tuning curve.

of the VMED to the 90-degree perturbation is high, and is due to positive contributions from W_{1pca}, W_{2pca}, W_{4pca}, and W_{5pca} and a negative contribution from W_{3pca} (Fig. 5.4B, *bars*). Similarly, in the region between 180 and 360 degrees, negative and positive contributions from all the components cancel each other out, so that the resulting tuning curve is near zero. To reconstruct the tuning curve of MGAS, the same curves are scaled differently and added together. The near-zero activity of MGAS in the 90-degree perturbation direction results from the cancellation of positive and negative contributions, primarily from W_{1pca} and W_{2pca}. In general, when using components identified by PCA, the reconstructions tend to underpredict the recorded muscle activity.

In contrast to PCA, the components and activation coefficients identified by NMF contain only positive values, as constrained by the algorithm. They are identified in no particular order, as evidenced by the percentage of total variance accounted for by each component (Fig. 5.4C). Each component has large contributions from a few muscles, and smaller contributions from several other muscles, illustrating the multijoint coordination required for postural control. Each component has a corresponding activation coefficient that is tuned for a particular range of perturbation directions. These activations are also positive, and the magnitude of activation is similar across all five of the components.

The reconstruction of the individual muscle tuning curves illustrates the differences between PCA and NMF in the way the components are combined to predict the recorded data. As with PCA, the height of the VMED bar in each NMF component is used to scale the contribution of each component's tuning curve. In this case, since VMED is virtually zero in W_{2nmf} and W_{3nmf}, these components make essentially no contribution to the VMED tuning curve. In contrast to the case with PCA decomposition, the activity of VMED at 90 degrees is due to the additive contributions of three components W_{1nmf}, W_{4nmf}, and W_{5nmf} (Fig. 5.4D).

Using NMF, there is no cancellation of features (Fig. 5.4D). Each muscle's activity is reconstructed by adding the contributions from each muscle synergy, all of which are positive. Once a feature of the tuning curves is expressed in the contribution of a given component, it cannot be subtracted out. For MGAS, the tuning curve consists primarily of contributions from W_{3nmf}, which causes high activity of MGAS between 180 and 360 degrees, and W_{5nmf}, which is responsible for a low level of activity of MGAS between 0 and 180 degrees.

The separation of the contributions from each component makes it possible to use the patterns of muscle activity within each component to make predictions about the activity of other muscles. In this case, the activity of MGAS between 180 and 360 degrees can be attributed to W_{3nmf}, which coactivates high MGAS activity with high extensor activity in the LGAS, GLUT, and SOL. When MGAS is active between 0 and 90 degrees, its activity is due to W_{5nmf}, which coactivates small MGAS activity with high flexor and hamstring activity in SEMB, TA, and SEMT. This demonstrates that MGAS activity in different perturbation directions results from fundamentally different muscle coordination patterns. It may be a prime mover in 180- to 360-degree perturbations, and a stabilizer in 0- to 90-degree perturbations. The analysis demonstrated that MGAS is strictly covaried with SOL from 180 to 360 degrees, and strictly covaried with TA from 0 to 90 degrees. A traditional correlation analysis would reveal MGAS to be strongly correlated to SOL, and weakly correlated to TA, but it would not be able to decompose the different portions of MGAS activity to one or the other.

Here, the coefficient of determination (r^2) and variability accounted for (VAF), which are measures of goodness-of-fit between the predicted and recorded EMG signals, demonstrate that NMF components can explain the recorded muscle responses more closely than PCA components (NMF average r^2 for all muscles: 0.84, average VAF: 95.5%; PCA average r^2 for all muscles: 0.81, average VAF: 58.9%). Both r^2 and VAF are defined as the coefficient of determination, or percent variability accounted for in the dataset (1 – sum of squares error/total sum of squares). The Pearson correlation coefficient, r, is based on a linear regression with an offset and thus compares only shapes of two curves, allowing for their actual values to differ. VAF is based on a linear regression that must pass through the origin, and therefore requires that the actual values of the measurements be equal to have a high percent of variability accounted for. In the standard Pearson correlation coefficient (r^2), the sum of squares is taken with respect to the mean, whereas in the uncentered case (VAF), it is taken with respect to zero. In this postural example, PCA reconstructs the shape of the tuning curve well, but not the offset; as expressed by the reasonably high r^2 values, but much lower VAF. In contrast, NMF reconstructs the level of activity well, and allows for more differences in the shape of the curve, which is evidenced in the high VAF values.

Selecting the Appropriate Number of Components Using NMF

In both NMF and PCA, the investigator must determine the number of components required to sufficiently explain the data. With PCA, a cutoff of the total percent variability explained is typically chosen, and the components with the largest contributions are chosen to meet that criterion. A similar criterion can be used in NMF, in which the analysis is run multiple times, each with a different number of components, and VAF can be plotted as a function of component number (Fig. 5.5A). In this postural data example, a cutoff of 90% VAF selects four components. Note, however, that the VAF due to one component is very high, so that high VAF values can be misleading in the overall variability because generally they represent a small portion of the data having a large amplitude that contributes the most to the overall data variability.

Whether using PCA or NMF, using the overall variability accounted for to select the number of components may not generate adequate reconstructions of data, particularly when there are certain conditions in which

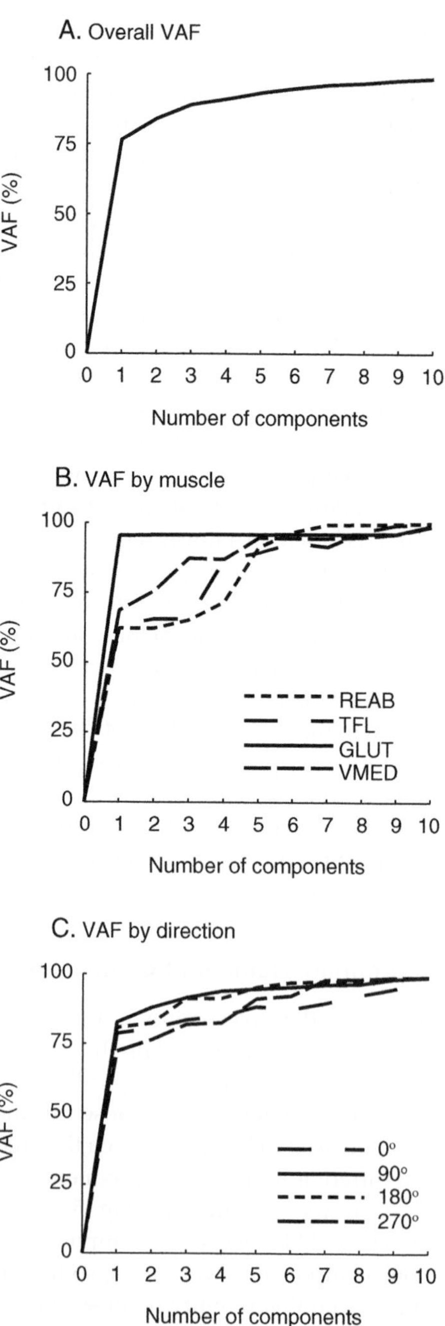

Figure 5.5 Scree plots showing variability accounted for (VAF) between the original data and the reconstruction using non-negative matrix factorization (NMF) components for the data shown in Figure 3. **A**: VAF for increasing

generally less activity occurs, but which nonetheless are an important feature of the dataset. In the postural control example, the overall level of muscle activity is higher in forward and backward directions. When choosing a smaller number of components, the muscle activity in forward and backward directions tends to be well-explained, whereas activity in lateral directions may not be well-reconstructed. Because muscle activity in lateral directions represents a small fraction of the total variability, it is difficult to discern from the overall VAF scree plot when such variations are accounted for. In both analyses, large differences in the magnitude of the variability across conditions always poses a problem when selecting components.

A number of additional criteria can be imposed to ensure that desired features of the dataset are reconstructed. For our postural control example, we further examined the variability accounted for within subsets of the data. We examined the VAF of each muscle, which ensures that each muscle's tuning curve is well-reconstructed. In certain cases, when a muscle's contribution to the overall variability is low, the features of its tuning curve may not be well reconstructed by the selected number of components, requiring additional components to be added. We then examined the data by perturbation direction, ensuring that the differences in the relative levels of activity by direction do not cause muscle activity in certain directions to be ignored. In these cases, rather than having a smooth increase in VAF as components are added, there tend to be jumps when the salient features are accounted for. Therefore, we specify a minimum %VAF that should be accounted for in all muscles and all perturbation directions, as well as require that the addition of the next component should not drastically improve the VAFs. Ultimately, however, only an experienced researcher examining the reconstructions of the original raw data traces can determine whether the features accounted for are physiological or are artifacts.

The scree plots from the postural response example demonstrate how five components were selected in this case (Fig. 5.5). Examining the overall VAF (Fig. 5.5A) reveals that one component seems sufficient to explain the variability in the data, using a 75% VAF criterion. However, examining the scree plots for individual muscles reveals that five components are

Figure 5.5 (*Continued*) number of components over the entire data set. **B**: VAF for increasing number of components for four individual muscles: REAB, TFL, GLUT, VMED. One component accounts for variability in GLUT relatively well, three components can explain VMED variability, but five is better at explaining variability in TFL and REAB. **C**: VAF for increasing number of components across individual perturbation directions. Shown here are the four cardinal directions, but the number of components needed was selected by looking at these types of plots for all muscles and all perturbation directions.

necessary in order for each of the muscles to achieve >75% VAF (Fig. 5.5B). These curves demonstrate that the activity of GLUT is well accounted for by the first component, but that activity of the other muscles is not. Three components are necessary for VMED to pass the 75% threshold. However, the addition of the second and third components does not change the VAF of TFL and REAB, as illustrated by the flat part of the lines. The fourth and fifth synergies account for the variability in TLF and REAB, respectively. Note that the addition of a sixth component does not drastically improve the VAF in any muscle. Therefore, five muscle synergies were chosen. Examining the variability accounted for across the various perturbation directions leads to a similar conclusion (Fig. 5.5C). Most directions have >75% VAF using only one or two components, but there is a sizeable improvement from four to five components for backward perturbations (270 degrees).

Finally, the composition of the components should be examined as additional components are added. The sharp jumps in the scree plots of VAF by muscle and by perturbation direction suggest that including an additional component may cause a previous component to split (Fig. 5.5B, sharp jump in REAB VAF from four to five components). The number of components selected as sufficient to explain the data should be high enough such that the components have stabilized, and the addition of new components does not significantly change the previous components. In this example, the composition of the components when six components (not shown) were used was compared with the five components identified here and shown not to alter the composition of the five components. Additionally, the reconstructions of the data and the activation coefficients of the sixth component can be used to deduce its contribution to features in the data. If the additional component accounts for a feature, such as a particular burst of muscle activity or tuning direction, that is unaccounted for by the other components, then it may be important; the investigator must decide whether this is a critical and/or physiological feature. If the activation coefficients appear to be evenly distributed across all perturbation directions, it is unlikely to account for a feature associated with muscle activation in a given direction, but is more likely noise.

USING NMF VERSUS PCA TO TEST MOTOR CONTROL HYPOTHESES: STANDING AND WALKING

Although it is possible to apply either PCA or NMF to any data matrix, the results may not necessarily provide insight into the underlying physiological mechanisms. It is important to ensure that the results are not artifacts of data collection or experimental design. Both techniques allow the dimension of the dataset to be identified. However, the maximum dimension is limited by the number of muscle signals analyzed, as well as by the number of disparate conditions examined. Therefore, it is critical that the data matrix itself be of high enough dimension such that a reduction in dimension is meaningful. The extraction of components relies on muscles being coordinated in different patterns. Therefore, the number of muscles recorded must be adequately high to capture different patterns of covariation, and the number of experimental conditions or possible variations observed must be of high enough dimension to capture different coordination patterns among the muscles. If muscle activation patterns are truly independent, this will also be reflected in the component analysis.

For example, the early studies of postural responses examined only two directions of perturbation (forward and backward). It was suggested that there were only two muscles synergies necessary, one active for forward perturbations, and another for backward perturbations (Nashner 1977; Horak and Macpherson 1996). However, these findings revealed experimental rather than physiological constraints. If NMF or PCA were applied only to forward and backward perturbations, they would arrive at a similar conclusion because the data only represent two conditions. By examining multiple perturbation directions, it becomes clear that more than two muscle synergies are needed to describe the full repertoire of postural responses (Macpherson 1988; Macpherson 1991; Henry et al. 1998), but a new muscle synergy is not necessary for each perturbation direction (Torres-Oviedo et al. 2006; Torres-Oviedo and Ting 2007). Similarly, the total number of components that can be extracted is limited by the number of muscles that are recorded. It also depends upon muscles being coactivated during certain conditions and not others. Therefore, if only a few muscles are recorded, it is possible that they would each comprise a single synergy if they are independently activated. Conversely, if they are always coactivated, then they will comprise only a single muscle synergy. Again, sufficient experimental conditions must be tested to demonstrate that the muscles could be coactive or independent, depending upon the condition. Such manipulations in pedaling revealed that certain muscles that are always coactive during forward pedaling may have different patterns of activation in backward pedaling (Ting et al. 1999).

Once it is established that the number of muscles and conditions is appropriate and can provide enough variability to extract a smaller number of components, the robustness of such components can then be tested across tasks (Krishnamoorthy et al. 2004; Cheung et al. 2005; d'Avella and Bizzi 2005; Torres-Oviedo et al. 2006). The generality of muscle synergies has been shown in a few studies in which synergies were shared between multiple tasks, such as frog kicking, jumping, and swimming, and in human walking/running, and pedaling forward and backward (Raasch and Zajac 1999; Ting et al. 1999; Cheung et al. 2005; d'Avella and Bizzi 2005; Cappellini et al. 2006; Torres-Oviedo et al. 2006). Although some synergies are used in multiple tasks, sometimes new synergies emerge when a new motor task is presented (Ivanenko et al. 2005) or the activation of the synergies may be adjusted (Cappellini et al. 2006).

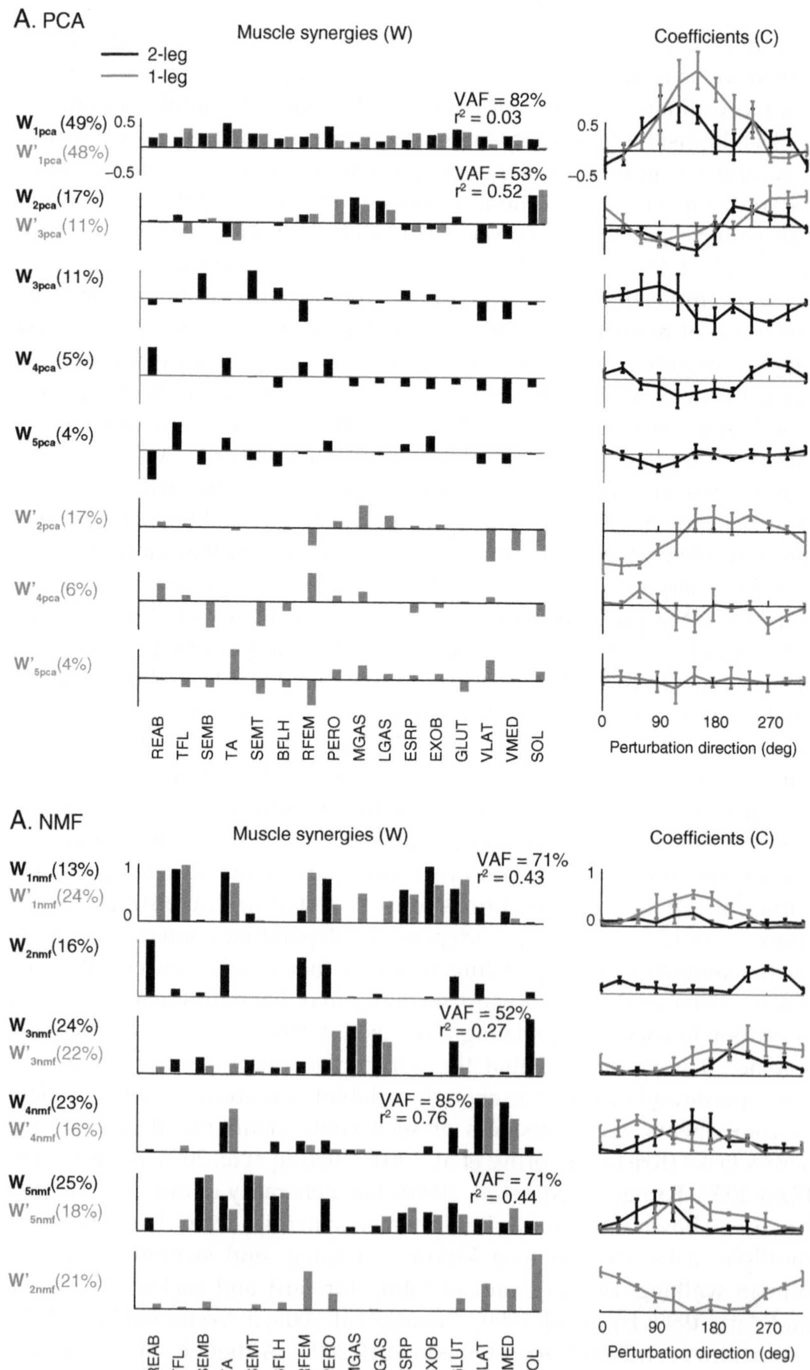

Figure 5.6 Comparison between components identified from one-leg postural responses compared to those identified from two-leg postural responses.

Here, we provide two examples of the differences between NMF and PCA when applied to test the robustness of muscle synergies (a) across postural tasks, and (b) during walking.

Are Muscle Synergies Stable or Artifact? Shared Versus Specific Components

Here, we used PCA and NMF to test whether muscle synergies are stable across postural tasks by comparing the components extracted from perturbations in two-legged stance extracted above (Fig. 5.4) to those from perturbations during one-legged stance. Subjects stood on their right leg and were subject to 12 directions of perturbations of smaller velocity and amplitude than in two-legged stance. One- and two-leg data were recorded in the same session, so that the activity of the 16 lower trunk and leg muscles from the stance side could be directly compared.

When PCA was applied to the one-leg data set to identify muscle synergies, two of the components extracted were similar to those identified from the two-leg postural responses (Fig. 5.6A). The first component (W'_{1pca}) is comprised of small contributions from all of the muscles, representing the average responses, so these would be expected to remain the same. Because the similarity between components from one- and two-legged stance are mainly based on the mean level of muscle activity, the VAF provides a better representation of the similarity than r^2 (r^2=0.0291, VAF = 82%). The third component from one-leg responses, W'_{3pca} (Fig. 5.6A, *gray bars*),

Figure 5.6 (*Continued*) **A**: Comparison of components and activation components identified using principal components analysis (PCA). Black bars and lines are two-leg responses (same as in Figure 5.4), and gray bars and lines are one-leg responses. Percentages on the left-hand side of each component represent the percent total variability that each component accounts for. Numbers to the right of each component are indicators of how closely the component from one-leg responses matches the one from two-leg responses. Both r^2 and uncentered r^2 (variability accounted for; VAF) are shown. The first component from one-leg (W'_{1pca}) and two-leg responses (W_{1pca}) matches fairly well, and the third component from one-leg responses (W'_{3pca}) matches the second component from two-leg responses (W_{2pca}). Subsequent components do not match; due to the orthogonality constraint of PCA, when one component changed, subsequent components changed also. **B**: Comparison of components and activation coefficients identified using non-negative matrix factorization (NMF). The same components are used in one-leg and two-leg responses, with the exception of one component that is specific to either condition. The additional component used in one-leg responses is tuned for 0-degree perturbations, which presumably are accounted for by the left leg in two-leg responses. The same components, or muscle synergies, can explain the different individual muscle activations observed between these two tasks, by only changing the activation of the muscle synergies.

looks similar to the second one identified from two-leg responses, W_{2pca} (Fig. 5.6A, *black bars*), suggesting it is more highly activated in two-leg responses. The other components, most of which account for a smaller percentage of variance, are quite different in the one-leg task compared to the two-leg task (max r^2 = 0.176, max VAF=17.5%). Therefore, if PCA were used to identify muscle synergies, the conclusion would be that different muscle synergies are used for one- and two-leg postural responses.

When NMF was applied to the one-leg data set to identify muscle synergies, however, four of the five components were very similar to those used during the two-leg balance responses (r^2=0.27 – 0.76, VAF=51%–85%, Fig. 5.6B). The muscle contributions to each of these four components was similar, and the activation coefficient tunings shifted slightly to account for differences in individual muscle tuning curves. The fifth component from two-leg stance (W_{2nmf}) had a large contribution from REAB, a hip flexor, whereas the fifth component in one-leg stance (W'_{5nmf}) has primarily SOL activity, an ankle extensor. This is likely because subjects were more likely to use a hip strategy in two-leg stance compared to one-leg stance. Further, the component used in one-leg stance (W'_{5nmf}) was strongly activated for rightward (0 degree) perturbations. Note that, in the two-leg stance, none of the five components were tuned for rightward perturbation directions (Fig. 5.6B). This suggests that when both legs can be used to respond to a rightward perturbation, subjects use muscles in the left leg to restore their balance, but when the left leg is not available, an additional component in the right leg must be activated to compensate for the loss of stability provided by the left leg. These results show that there are similar components that are used across postural tasks, suggesting that the muscle synergies derived from NMF are physiological constraints that the nervous system uses for muscle coordination, and not simply artifacts of the experiment or analysis.

Although the example demonstrates the possibility of stable components across tasks, thorough cross-validation tests should be performed to ensure that the components are indeed stable across tasks. Therefore, to draw stronger conclusions about the physiological basis of the components, the results of analyses across different subsets and combinations of the data should be compared (e.g., Torres-Oveido and Ting 2010). Apart from extracting components independently from control (e.g., two-leg) and test (e.g., one-leg) tasks, the components from the control condition can be used to reconstruct the test data. If they do not explain a sufficient percentage of the variability, then condition-specific components may be extracted from the remaining variability of the data (Cheung et al. 2005). Additionally, components extracted from the control and test data pooled into one large data set should render similar results. If the same components are identified in all of these cases, it is more likely that the technique has identified underlying physiological features of the data. In our example using NMF, the same components are identified in one-leg and two-leg stance using all

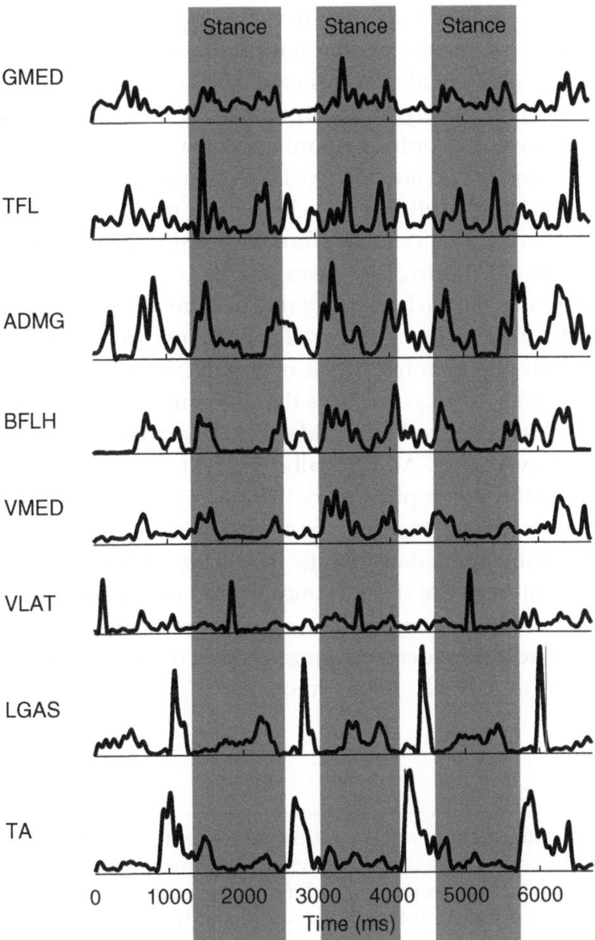

Figure 5.7 Example of muscle activity during a forward walking trial. Shown are eight muscles of the 16 recorded. The subject was walking at a speed of approximately 0.7 m/s. The shaded gray boxes indicate stance phase.

these different combinations (not shown). In contrast, PCA generates different components depending on which data combination is used.

Using Time As a Condition: Muscle Synergies During Walking

When applying PCA and NMF to a continuous motor task, such as locomotion, time can be considered to be a condition. Similar to the different directions of postural perturbations, different coordination patterns across muscles are observed at different timepoints in the locomotor cycle.

However, if muscles are activated in a similar pattern across time, such as in an isometric task, the use of time as a condition may not provide enough variability in the data to allow for meaningful interpretation. In this example, subjects walked freely at a slow (0.7 m/s) pace for at least ten steps each trial. Data were recorded beginning at heel strike of the third to fourth step, so that subjects had already reached a steady-state gait, and each trial includes at least three full stride cycles. Seven trials were included in the data matrix. Sixteen EMG signals were recorded in one leg (Fig. 5.7).

To create the data matrix, the mean activity was computed in 10 ms bins over the three steps in each trial. *Binning* has the advantages of smoothing the data, reducing the total number of conditions, thus reducing computation time, while maintaining much of the detail in the variations of the EMG within and across cycles. Note that the muscle activation patterns do not resemble the idealized sinusoidal EMG patterns often found due to smoothing or averaging. Additionally, the pattern of muscle activity and the duration of the stance phase vary from step to step, as does the number of bins. There is no need to stretch or shorten the data across time to obtain a consistent number of data points per stride. When creating the data matrix, different trials are simply concatenated end to end.

It is important to distinguish between two mutually exclusive hypotheses that can be tested by decomposing walking data into muscle synergies. For both PCA and NMF, the components W_i are assumed to be fixed,

Figure 5.8 Components and activation coefficients identified from walking data using principal components analysis (PCA) and non-negative matrix factorization (NMF). **A**: Components identified using PCA may have positive and/or negative muscle contributions and activation coefficients. Percentages indicate the amount of total data variability accounted for by each component. The shaded gray boxes indicate stance phase. Activation coefficients from one trial of walking (the same trial as in Figure 5.7) are shown. Components from PCA have contributions from many muscles. The first few components have activation patterns that are aligned with particular phases of the gait cycle, whereas the last few have less identifiable patterns. **B**: TA muscle activity from a single trial reconstructed using the PCA components identified in A. The original data are shown with a dashed black line and the reconstructed data are shown with a solid black line. Variability accounted for (VAF) and r^2 indicate goodness-of-fit. **C**: Components identified using NMF have only positive muscle contributions and activation coefficients. Components from NMF tend to have strong contributions from only a few muscles. Activations coefficients for some components (W_{1nmf}, W_{2nmf}, W_{3nmf}, and W_{6nmf}) are aligned with particular phases of the gait cycle, whereas others may be stabilizing components since they are active throughout the entire trial (W_{4nmf} and W_{5nmf}). **D**: TA muscle activity from a single trial reconstructed using the NMF components identified in C. The original data are shown with a dashed black line and the reconstructed data are shown with a solid black line. VAF and r^2 indicate goodness-of-fit.

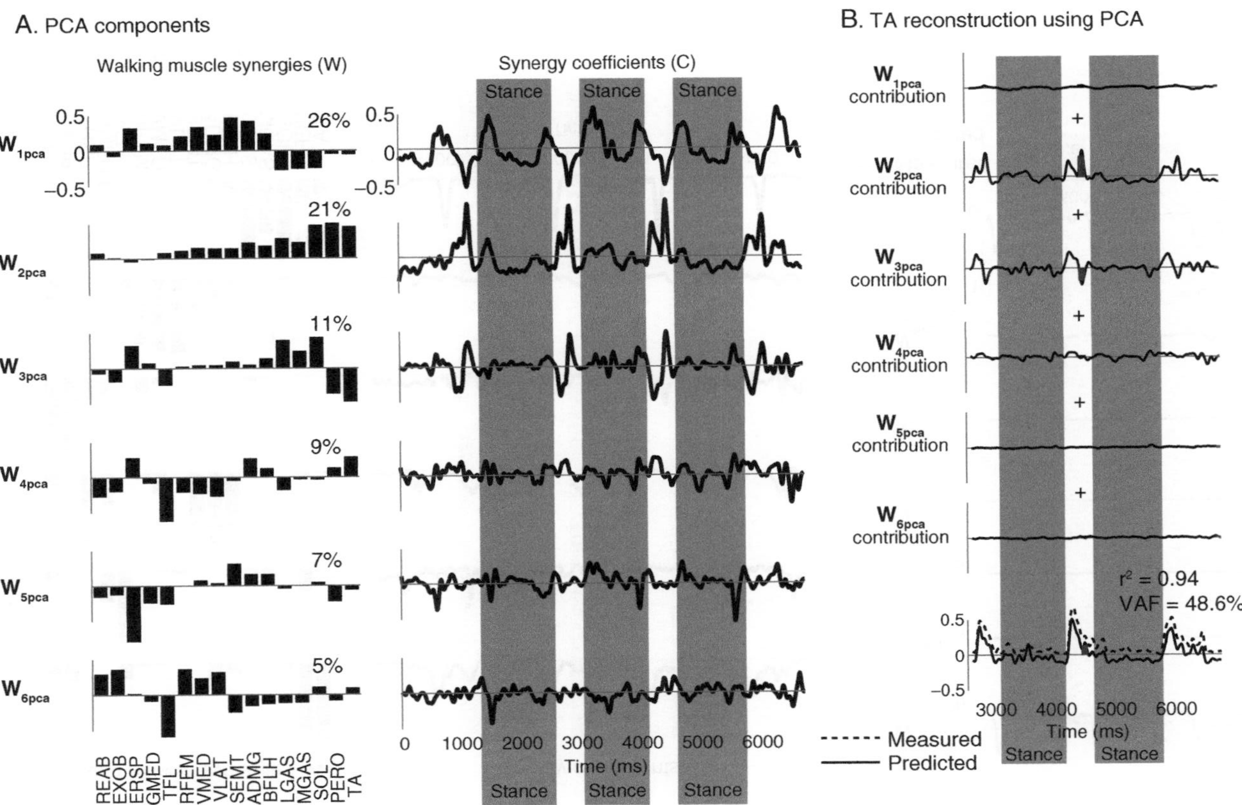

Figure 5.8 See figure caption on p. 128

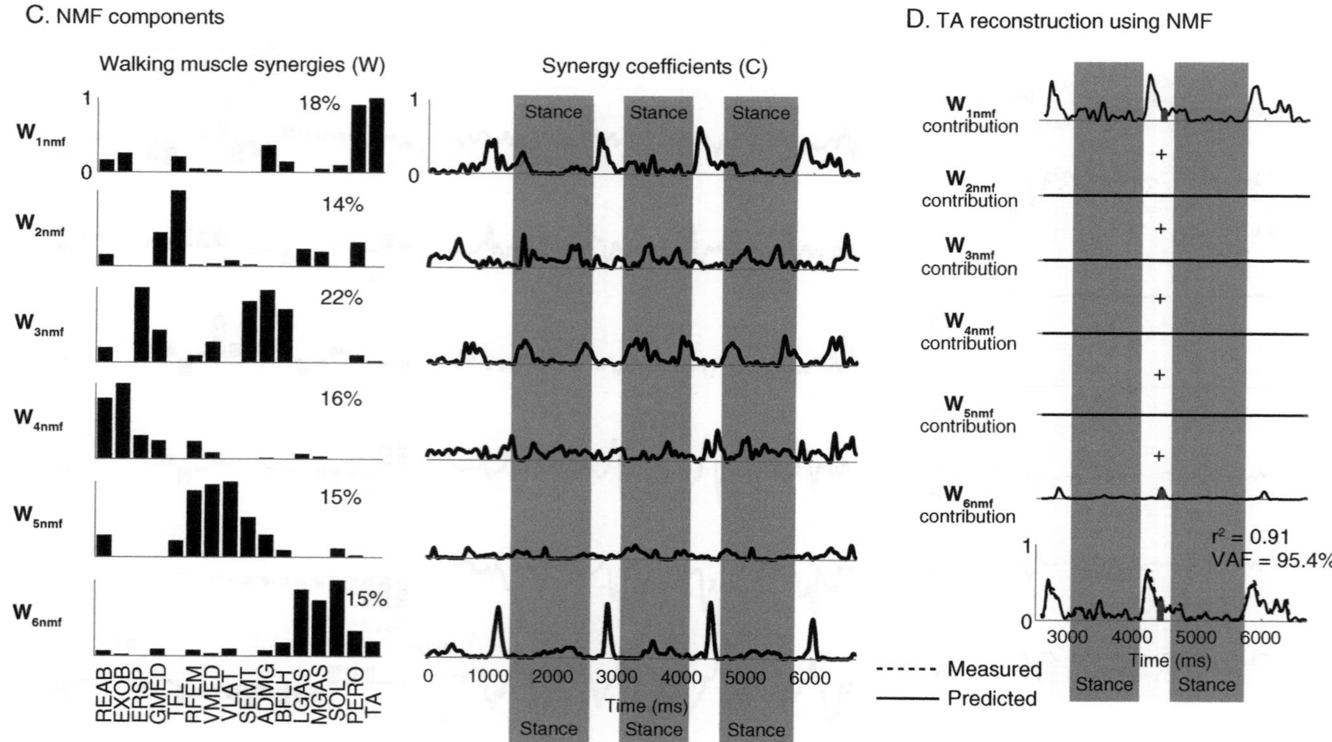

Figure 5.8 See figure caption on p. 128

whereas the activation coefficients or scaling factors c_i are allowed to vary (Clark et al. 2010). Here we choose W's to refer to fixed muscle activation patterns, whereas we allow c's to vary across time. The data must be structured such that the muscles are the observations (rows for NMF, columns for PCA) and the time windows are the conditions (columns for NMF, rows for PCA). Conversely, it is possible to hypothesize that the timing patterns are stereotypical across cycles, and that the muscle coordination patterns vary (Ivanenko et al. 2004; Cappellini et al. 2006). Fixed timing patterns might be generated by a central pattern-generating neural circuit, with their muscle targets changing with phase. In this case, it is necessary to stretch the cycles in time so that they all have the same number of points. In this case, the data should be transposed, such that the time points are the observations, and the muscles are the conditions, with repeated trials or cycles concatenated. However, in neither analysis can both the components and the timing patterns vary. Either muscular coactivation patterns or timing patterns must be assumed to be the same across all conditions.

Here, we compare six components extracted from one subject's walking data using PCA and NMF (Fig. 5.8).

Similar to the postural response example, the first component identified using PCA primarily describes the mean level of muscle activity, and the later ones described deviations from that mean. The first two components contained primarily positive contributions from nearly all of the muscles. The first component was activated positively at the beginning and end of stance and activated negatively in swing, whereas the second component was positively activated in swing but negatively activated in stance. The subsequent components all had both negative and positive contributions from different muscles, and their activation coefficients over time decreased in amplitude, but increased in frequency. Although the first three components had peaks that corresponded to identifiable events in the gait cycle and various EMG activity (Fig. 5.7), the last three had high-frequency oscillations that were not localized to a particular phase in the locomotor cycle. Reconstructing the TA EMG signal reveals that the activity during swing phase is composed of contributions from two components primarily, although there are small contributions from all components (Fig. 5.8B). Both components contribute to the large peak in TA activity. However, the smaller, secondary burst is due to a positive contribution from W_{2pca}that is largely cancelled by a negative contribution from W_{3pca}. (Fig. 5.8B). Note that the r^2 value is quite high, indicating a good match of shape, whereas the VAF level is low, indicating that the predicted EMG amplitudes do not match measured values.

The six components extracted using NMF were quite different from those found using PCA. Each component consists of large contributions from a small number of muscles, and the muscles tend to be grouped according to joint or function. Some of the components were activated at specific points during the gait cycle, such as W_{3nmf} being activated at early stance and again at late stance, W_{1nmf} activated during early swing, and W_{6nmf} during late swing. Other muscle synergies were activated throughout both stance and swing, suggesting that they may be used for stabilization (W_{4nmf} and W_{5nmf}). As in the postural example, the bursts of activity appearing in the activation coefficients resemble the bursts observed in the original EMG data (Fig. 5.7). Only two NMF components contribute to TA EMG activity (Fig. 5.8D). W_{1nmf} contributes most of the TA activity, including the large burst in early swing phase. The contribution from W_{6nmf} adds a small secondary burst.

Again, the components extracted during walking must also be cross-validated over a number of different test extractions to be sure that they are stable and not artifacts of the way the data are represented. In our NMF analyses, we find components to be stable across time bins sizes of 10 to 100 ms during walking. Components are also stable if fewer trials are analyzed, or if faster walking speeds are analyzed. Moreover, the components extracted from one speed can account for variations in EMG occurring with changes in walking speed (Clark et al. 2010). However, the components change if EMGs are averaged across strides, and less of the variability from stride to stride is accounted for by components extracted from averaged data.

CONCLUSION

Are linear decomposition techniques useful for understanding motor control (Macpherson 1991; Tresch and Jarc 2009)? Ultimately, no decomposition technique is perfect, and much discretion and interpretation must be exercised on the part of the investigator when drawing conclusions from any such analysis. Computational analyses cannot replace the judgment and intuition of the researcher, and ultimately the results must make sense in a physiological context. Therefore, it is critical that the implicit hypotheses, assumptions, and constraints inherent in any technique be understood in order to use it usefully in motor control or other scientific research. In the best-case scenario, a linear decomposition can be a tool that can formally test a hypothesis that the researcher formulates by looking at the raw data and observing the synchrony and variability across multiple EMG signals. It allows different periods of activity within a muscle to be attributed to different underlying components. In the end, the relationship between the derived components and the original data may potentially allow a researcher to draw conclusions about the underlying neural mechanisms if the components do not represent limitations of the recordings, experimental conditions, or other data artifact. Ultimately, to make any sort of physiological conclusion, the extracted components must be interpreted in terms of the known underlying physiological mechanisms and biomechanical outputs. The examples presented here demonstrate intuitively the workings of NMF and PCA, with the aim of informing and aiding in the interpretation of data. Such exercises can be performed to better understand any kind of decomposition technique, each with its own advantages and disadvantages (Tresch et al. 2006).

Is the added computation useful for understanding motor tasks? In some cases, the answer may be "no," particularly for any kind of initial analysis of a motor task or experimental condition. The technique must appropriately match the hypothesis. Component decompositions can be useful when examining the detailed workings of complex multimuscle coordination. It is useful for comparing complex muscle coordination across different tasks or trials in which muscle activity changes, but the underlying coordination principles may be the same, as we have shown in fast and slow walking (Clark et al. 2010), or one- and two-legged postural control (Torres-Oviedo and Ting 2010). In cases in which repeated measures are not possible, such as in patient populations, highly variable motor patterns are difficult to analyze from traditional techniques that rely on averaging. In this case, a component decomposition can identify whether common underlying elements are being activated across different trials or tasks (Clark et al. 2010). Similarly, the underlying components may provide a better measure of similarity or differences across individuals than the comparison of individual EMG traces (Ting 2007; Ting and McKay 2007). It is possible to identify whether individuals with different EMG patterns have similar underlying components but activate them differently, or if instead they have different numbers or composition of underlying components (Torres-Oviedo and Ting 2007; Clark et al. 2010).

Decomposition can also be useful for understanding the function of the underlying components. These analyses are difficult and do not always work. They require many practical considerations to accommodate limitations of the analysis techniques, and require the investigator to guess at the correct variables that are being controlled. But if a relationship is not found, it does not mean that there is no functional role for that component. Previous work in postural control has shown in cats that muscle synergies are recruited to control forces at the ground (Ting and Macpherson 2005; Torres-Oviedo et al. 2006). Such an analysis includes biomechanical variables as additional observations (rows) in the data matrix and extracts functional muscle synergies, which are composed of both muscles and functional variables (Torres-Oviedo et al. 2006). However, the application of NMF to biomechanical variables poses a challenge because negative and positive changes in forces necessarily result from different muscle groups requiring them to be partitioned physiologically (Ting and Macpherson 2005; Torres-Oviedo et al. 2006; Valero-Cuevas 2009). Because changes in velocity and position require the integration of forces, the relationship between muscle activity and kinematics is highly redundant, and also difficult to predict without explicit models (Gottlieb et al. 1995; Lockhart and Ting 2007). This redundancy is evident in studies relating the activation of components found using PCA to center-of-pressure shifts in human balance control using the uncontrolled manifold hypothesis (Latash et al. 2002; Krishnamoorthy et al. 2003a; Ting and Macpherson 2005). These studies demonstrate that, although functional roles of individual components may be identified, the variability in their activation may not be reflected in the variability of the output because they are precisely coordinated by higher mechanisms in the nervous system to reduce variations in the desired motor task. Alternately, biomechanical simulation and analysis techniques allow the functional role of the muscle coordination patterns identified by the extracted components to be explicitly tested (Raasch et al. 1997; Berniker et al. 2009; Neptune et al. 2009). Additionally, the feasibility of robustly using such components to coordinate a repertoire of movement can also be explored (Raasch and Zajac 1999; Valero-Cuevas 2000; Valero-Cuevas et al. 2003; Kargo and Giszter 2008; McKay and Ting 2008). However, it is difficult to build appropriate dynamics models and to record from all of the muscles involved in a movement to use such techniques. Moreover, models of the neural control mechanisms that shape and use the components effectively need to be explored (Berniker et al. 2009). Again, in order for any of these techniques to be useful in relating muscle activity to functional variables, the investigator must have a good understanding of their raw data and the underlying physiological and biomechanical mechanisms in order to interpret the results of the component analysis appropriately.

Do the identified components extracted using computational techniques reflect the organization of neural circuits for movement? One of the attractive features of components from NMF is that they generate a parts-based type of representation that appears similar to both neurophysiological observations, as well as to predictions from "sparse-coding" algorithms in sensory systems (Olshausen and Field 2004). The idea is that in a retinotopic, somatotopic, or other sort of spatial sensory map in the nervous system, only a small region is activated for any given stimulus, such as a location in space, or a part of the body. This "sparse" coding means that a minimum of neurons is used to encode a particular feature from among all of the information contained in that map. But, as in PCA, it is also possible to imagine a system in which neurons in the entire map are activated given a particular stimulus, and their net output results in the identification of a particular stimulus. The sparseness property has also been proposed for motor system, and is proposed to improve energetic expenditure by reducing the number of neurons involved in any given behavior, as well as improving computational efficiency, thus reducing the total number of elements that need to be modified during motor adaptation (Olshausen and Field 2004; Fiete et al. 2007; Ting and McKay 2007). Accordingly, localized regions of motor cortex are activated to perform a given movement, and muscle synergies for reaching have been proposed to result from cortico-motoneuronal cells that project to multiple muscles (Scott and Kalaska 1997; Graziano and Aflalo 2007). Similarly, reticulospinal neurons active during postural control (Schepens and Drew 2004; Schepens and Drew 2006; Schepens et al. 2008; Stapley and Drew 2009) also project to multiple muscles in the limbs and trunk, and interneurons in the spinal cord may facilitate coordination of muscles within and between the limbs during locomotion (Quevedo et al. 2000; McCrea 2001; Drew et al. 2008).

Although, NMF components may provide one computational tool among the many needed to understand the sensorimotor transformations involved in determining how we move, much research is warranted before any of the questions about the utility and interpretability of the resulting components can be resolved. Component decompositions allow large datasets of EMG data and other variables to be decomposed into components that must be interpreted and compared to the organization of neural control systems upstream, and their functional biomechanical outputs downstream. NMF is especially useful for examining neural and muscle activity signals that are inherently non-negative. PCA may prove more useful for analyzing biomechanical variables that take on both positive and negative values without consideration for muscle activity. The continued development of physiologically relevant decomposition techniques combined with experimental and computational studies may eventually allow us to better understand how learning, adaptation, and rehabilitation occurs in the motor system.

ACKNOWLEDGMENTS

Supported by NIH NS 053822 and HD 46922.

REFERENCES

Aruin, A.S., W.R. Forrest, and M.L. Latash. 1998. Anticipatory postural adjustments in conditions of postural instability. *Electroencephalography and Clinical Neurophysiology* 109:350–59.

Berniker, M., A. Jarc, E. Bizzi, and M.C. Tresch. 2009. Simplified and effective motor control based on muscle synergies to exploit musculoskeletal dynamics. *Proceedings of the National Academy of Sciences of the USA* 106:7601–06.

Bernstein, N. 1967. *The coordination and regulation of movements*. New York: Pergamon Press.

Cappellini, G., Y.P. Ivanenko, R.E. Poppele, and F. Lacquaniti. 2006. Motor patterns in human walking and running. *Journal of Neurophysiology* 95:3426–37.

Cheung, V.C., A. d'Avella, M.C. Tresch, and E. Bizzi. 2005. Central and sensory contributions to the activation and organization of muscle synergies during natural motor behaviors. *Journal Neuroscience* 25:6419–34.

Clark, D.J., L.H. Ting, F.E. Zajac, R.R. Neptune, and S.A. Kautz. 2010. Merging of healthy motor modules predicts reduced locomotor performance and muscle coordination complexity post-stroke. *Journal of Neurophysiology* 103(2): 844–57.

d'Avella, A., and E. Bizzi. 2005. Shared and specific muscle synergies in natural motor behaviors. *Proceedings of the National Academy of Sciences of the USA* 102:3076–81.

Danion, F., G. Schoner, M.L. Latash, S. Li, J.P. Scholz, and V.M. Zatsiorsky. 2003. A mode hypothesis for finger interaction during multi-finger force-production tasks. *Biological Cybernetics* 88:91–98.

Drew, T., J. Kalaska, and N. Krouchev. 2008. Muscle synergies during locomotion in the cat: A model for motor cortex control. *Journal of Physiology* 586:1239–45.

Fiete, I.R., M.S. Fee, and H.S. Seung. 2007. Model of birdsong learning based on gradient estimation by dynamic perturbation of neural conductances. *Journal of Neurophysiology* 98:2038–57.

Gottlieb, G.L., C.H. Chen, and D.M. Corcos. 1995. Relations between joint torque, motion, and electromyographic patterns at the human elbow. *Experimental Brain Research* 103:164–67.

Graziano, M.S., and T.N. Aflalo. 2007. Rethinking cortical organization: Moving away from discrete areas arranged in hierarchies. *Neuroscientist* 13:138–47.

Henry, S.M., J. Fung, and F.B. Horak. 1998. EMG responses to maintain stance during multidirectional surface translations. *Journal of Neurophysiology* 80:1939–50.

Horak, F.B., J.M. Macpherson. 1996. Postural orientation and equilibrium. In *Handbook of physiology*, Section 12, 255–92. New York: American Physiological Society.

Hyvärinen, A., J. Karhunen, and E. Oja. 2001. *Independent component analysis*. New York: John Wiley & Sons.

Ivanenko, Y.P., G. Cappellini, N. Dominici, R.E. Poppele, and F. Lacquaniti. 2005. Coordination of locomotion with voluntary movements in humans. *Journal of Neuroscience* 25:7238–53.

Ivanenko, Y.P., R.E. Poppele, and E. Lacquaniti. 2004. Five basic muscle activation patterns account for muscle activity during human locomotion. *Journal of Physiology* 556:267–82.

Kargo, W.J., and S.F. Giszter. 2008. Individual premotor drive pulses, not time-varying synergies, are the units of adjustment for limb trajectories constructed in spinal cord. *Journal of Neuroscience* 28:2409–25.

Ko, Y., J. Challis, J. Stitt, and K. Newell. 2003. Organization of compensatory postural coordination patterns. *Journal of Motor Behavior* 35:325–42.

Krishnamoorthy, V., S. Goodman, V. Zatsiorsky, and M.L. Latash. 2003a. Muscle synergies during shifts of the center of pressure by standing persons: Identification of muscle modes. *Biological Cybernetics* 89:152–61.

Krishnamoorthy, V., M.L. Latash, J.P. Scholz, and V.M. Zatsiorsky. 2003b. Muscle synergies during shifts of the center of pressure by standing persons. *Experimental Brain Research* 152:281–92.

Krishnamoorthy, V., M.L. Latash, J.P. Scholz, and V.M. Zatsiorsky. 2004. Muscle modes during shifts of the center of pressure by standing persons: Effect of instability and additional support. *Experimental Brain Research* 157:18–31.

Latash, M.L., J.P. Scholz, and G. Schoner. 2002. Motor control strategies revealed in the structure of motor variability. *Exercise and Sport Sciences Reviews* 30:26–31.

Latash, M.L., J.P. Scholz, and G. Schoner. 2007. Toward a new theory of motor synergies. *Motor Control* 11:276–308.

Lee, D.D., and H.S. Seung. 1999. Learning the parts of objects by non-negative matrix factorization. *Nature* 401:788–91.

Lockhart, D.B., and L.H. Ting. 2007. Optimal sensorimotor transformations for balance. *Nature Neuroscience* 10:1329–36.

Macpherson, J.M. 1988. Strategies that simplify the control of quadrupedal stance. II. Electromyographic activity. *Journal of Neurophysiology* 60:218–31.

Macpherson, J.M. 1991. How flexible are muscle synergies? In *Motor control: Concepts and issues*, eds., D.R. Humphrey and H.-J. Freund, 33–47. New York: Wiley Press.

McCrea, D.A. 2001. Spinal circuitry of sensorimotor control of locomotion. *Journal of Physiology* 533:41–50.

McKay, J.L., and L.H. Ting. 2008. Functional muscle synergies constrain force production during postural tasks. *Journal of Biomechanics* 41:299–306.

Nashner, L.M. 1977. Fixed patterns of rapid postural responses among leg muscles during stance. *Experimental Brain Research* 30:13–24.

Neptune, R.R., D.J. Clark, and S.A. Kautz. 2009. Modular control of human walking: A simulation study. *Journal of Biomechanics* 42:1282–87.

Newell, K.M., and L.G. Carlton. 1988. Force variability in isometric responses. *Journal of Experimental Psychology. Human Perception and Performance* 14: 37–44.

Olshausen, B.A., and D.J. Field. 2004. Sparse coding of sensory inputs. *Current Opinion in Neurobiology* 14:481–87.

Quevedo, J., B. Fedirchuk, S. Gosgnach, and D.A. McCrea. 2000. Group I disynaptic excitation of cat hindlimb flexor and bifunctional motoneurones during fictive locomotion. *Journal of Physiology* 525:549–64.

Raasch, C.C., and F.E. Zajac. 1999. Locomotor strategy for pedaling: Muscle groups and biomechanical functions. *Journal of Neurophysiology* 82:515–25.

Raasch, C.C., F.E. Zajac, B. Ma, and W.S. Levine. 1997. Muscle coordination of maximum-speed pedaling. *Journal of Biomechanics* 30:595–602.

Ramsay, J.O., B.W. Silverman. 2005. *Functional data analysis*. Berlin: Springer.

Reisman, D.S., and J.P. Scholz. 2006. Workspace location influences joint coordination during reaching in post-stroke hemiparesis. *Experimental Brain Research* 170:265–76.

Schepens, B., and T. Drew. 2004. Independent and convergent signals from the pontomedullary reticular formation contribute to the control of posture and movement during reaching in the cat. *Journal of Neurophysiology* 92: 2217–38.

Schepens, B., and T. Drew. 2006. Descending signals from the pontomedullary reticular formation are bilateral, asymmetric, and gated during reaching movements in the cat. *Journal of Neurophysiology* 96:2229–52.

Schepens, B., P. Stapley, and T. Drew. 2008. Neurons in the pontomedullary reticular formation signal posture and movement both as an integrated behavior and independently. *Journal of Neurophysiology* 100:2235–53.

Scott, S.H., and J.F. Kalaska. 1997. Reaching movements with similar hand paths but different arm orientations. I. Activity of individual cells in motor cortex. *Journal of Neurophysiology* 77:826–52.

Simoncelli, E.P., and B.A. Olshausen. 2001. Natural image statistics and neural representation. *Annual Review of Neuroscience* 24:1193–1216.

Stapley, P.J., and T. Drew. 2009. The pontomedullary reticular formation contributes to the compensatory postural responses observed following removal of the support surface in the standing cat. *Journal of Neurophysiology* 101: 1334–50.

Ting, L.H. 2007. Dimensional reduction in sensorimotor systems: A framework for understanding muscle coordination of posture. *Progress in Brain Research* 165: 299–321.

Ting, L.H., S.A. Kautz, D.A. Brown, and F.E. Zajac. 1999. Phase reversal of biomechanical functions and muscle activity in backward pedaling. *Journal of Neurophysiology* 81:544–51.

Ting, L.H., and J.M. Macpherson. 2005. A limited set of muscle synergies for force control during a postural task. *Journal of Neurophysiology* 93:609–13.

Ting, L.H., and J.L. McKay. 2007. Neuromechanics of muscle synergies for posture and movement. *Current Opinion in Neurobiology* 17:622–28.

Torres-Oviedo, G., and L.H. Ting. 2010. Subject-specific muscle synergies in human balance control are consistent across different biomechanical contexts. *Journal of Neurophysiology*.

Torres-Oviedo, G., J.M. Macpherson, and L.H. Ting. 2006. Muscle synergy organization is robust across a variety of postural perturbations. *Journal of Neurophysiology* 96:1530–46.

Torres-Oviedo, G., and L.H. Ting. 2007. Muscle synergies characterizing human postural responses. *Journal of Neurophysiology* 98:2144–56.

Tresch, M.C., V.C. Cheung, and A. d'Avella. 2006. Matrix factorization algorithms for the identification of muscle synergies: Evaluation on simulated and experimental data sets. *Journal of Neurophysiology* 95:2199–212.

Tresch, M.C., A. Jarc. 2009. The case for and against muscle synergies. *Current Opinion in Neurobiology* 19(6):601–7.

Tresch, M.C., P. Saltiel, and E. Bizzi. 1999. The construction of movement by the spinal cord. *Nature Neuroscience* 2:162–67.

Valero-Cuevas, F.J. 2000. Predictive modulation of muscle coordination pattern magnitude scales fingertip force magnitude over the voluntary range. *Journal of Neurophysiology* 83:1469–79.

Valero-Cuevas, F.J. 2009. A mathematical approach to the mechanical capabilities of limbs and fingers. *Advances in Experimental Medicine and Biology* 629:619–33.

Valero-Cuevas, F.J., M.E. Johanson, and J.D. Towles. 2003. Towards a realistic biomechanical model of the thumb: The choice of kinematic description may be more critical than the solution method or the variability/uncertainty of musculoskeletal parameters. *Journal of Biomechanics* 36:1019–30.

Woollacott, M., and A. Shumway-Cook. 2002. Attention and the control of posture and gait: A review of an emerging area of research. *Gait &Posture* 16:1–14.

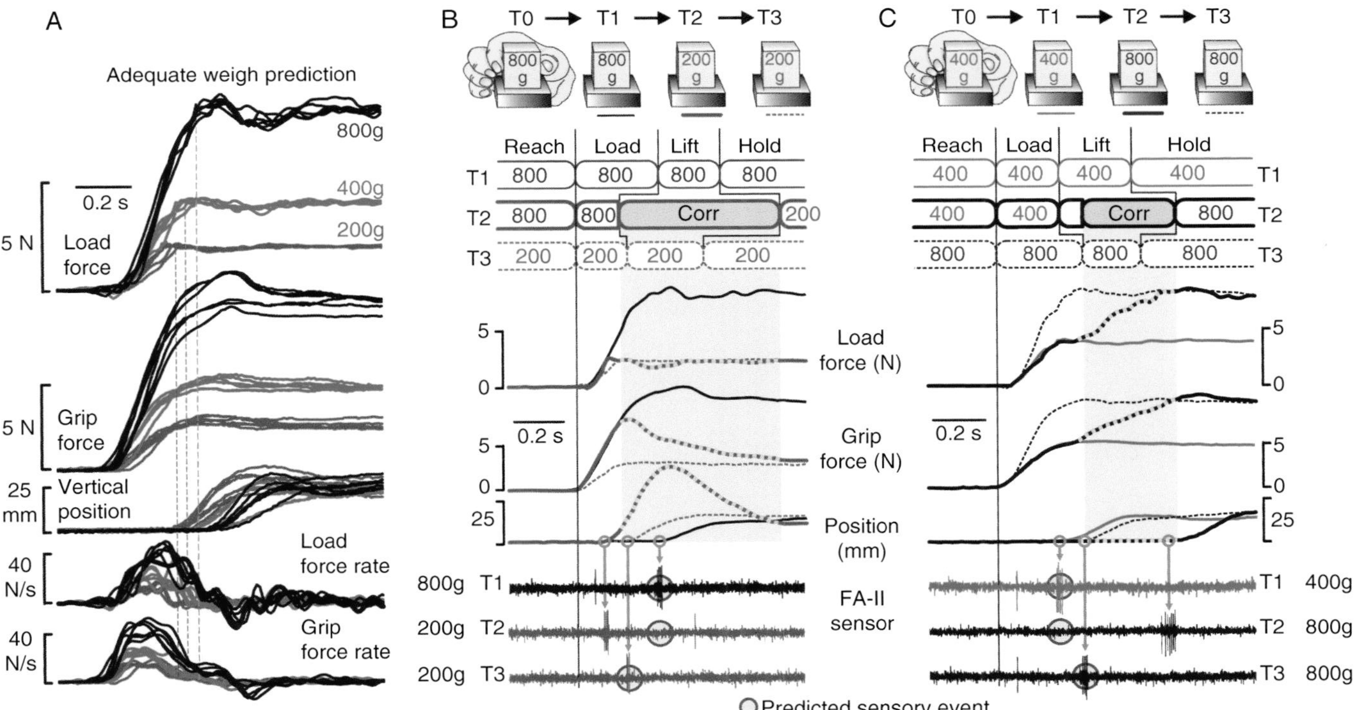

Figure 2.1 Adaptation of motor output to object weight. **A**: Fingertip forces and object position during the initial part of adequately programmed lifts with three objects of different weights (data from 24 single trials from a single participant superimposed). **B** and **C**: Force adjustments and single unit tactile afferent responses to unexpected changes in object weight. Gray circles and vertical lines (*Continued*)

Figure 2.1 (*Continued*) indicate the instance of lift-off for each trial and the arrowheads point at the signals generated by the lift-off in a FA-II (Pacinian) afferent. The circles behind the nerve traces indicate the corresponding predicted sensory events. **B**: Three successive trials (T1–3) in which the subject lifted an 800 (*blue curves*), a 200 (*red solid curves*), and then the 200 g object again (*red dashed curves*). The forces in T1 were adequately programmed for the prevailing weight because the participant had previously lifted the 800 g object (T0). The forces in T2 were erroneously programmed for the previously lifted 800 g object. In T2, sensory information indicating lift-off occurred earlier than expected, which triggered a corrective action (*yellow-dashed red curves*) terminating the strong force drive and bringing the object back to the intended position. **C**: Three successive trials (T1–3) in which the subject lifted a 400 (*green curves*), an 800 (*blue solid curves*), and then an 800 g object again (*blue dashed curves*). The forces in T2 were erroneously programmed for a 400 g object and the absence of sensory information at the expected lift-off time elicited a corrective action (*yellow-dashed blue curves*) that involved additional force increases until terminated by sensory input signaling lift-off. **B** and **C**: The top diagrams represent sequential action-phase controllers parameterized for different weights. Corrective actions ("Corr") were triggered about 100 ms after a mismatch between predicted and actual sensory information related to lift-off and were linked to an updating of weight parameterization in the remainder of the trial and the next trial. Modified from Johansson, R.S., and J.R. Flanagan. 2009. Coding and use of tactile signals from the fingertips in object manipulation tasks. *Nature Reviews Neuroscience* 10: 345–59, with permission of the publisher.

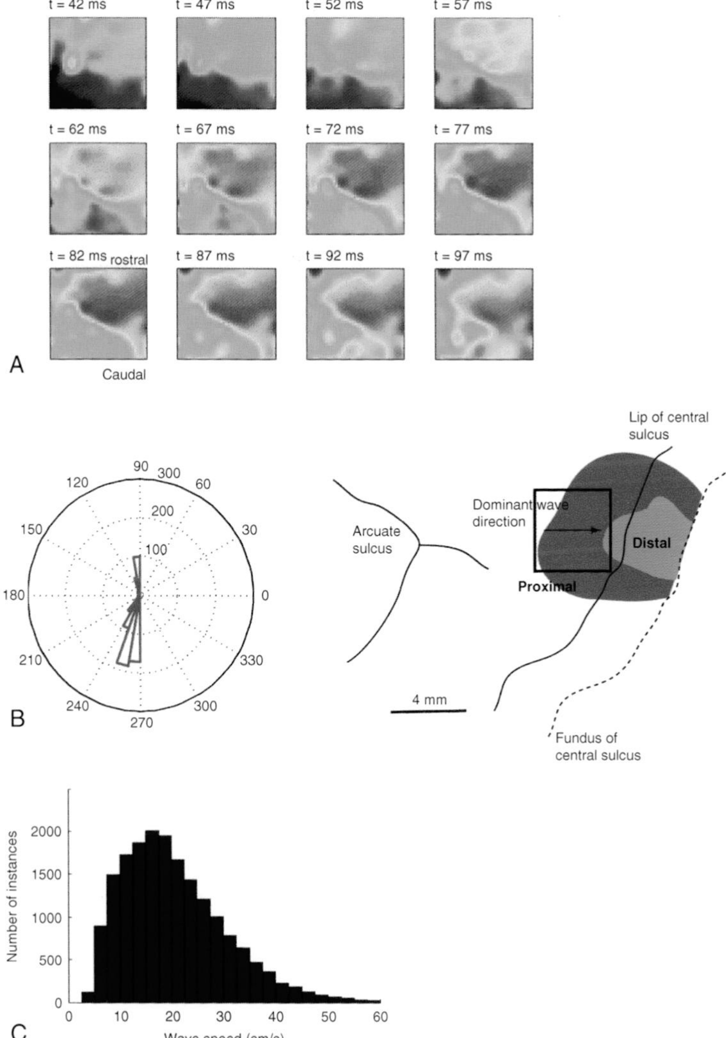

Figure 7.5 Wave propagation in the beta frequency range of the local field potential (LFP) across MI during the reach-to-grasp task. **A**: An example of one instance of an LFP wave propagating across the primary MI in the rostral to caudal direction (i.e., downward). To visualize this wave, the voltage signal on each channel was band pass-filtered between 10–45 Hz, normalized such that the maximum and minimum voltage values were set to 1 and –1, respectively, and then color coded, where red is a positive value and blue is a negative value. Time is measured with respect to the visual onset of the object (i.e., removal of the opaque screen). **B:** Left, the distribution of wave directions across many instances of linear wave propagation using a threshold PGD value of 0.5 (see Methods). Right, the direction of the dominant wave direction plotted on a schematic of the flattened motor cortex showing the proximal and distal topography. The square box represents the 4 × 4 mm multielectrode array. **C**: The distribution of wave speeds across many samples of linear wave propagation using the same PGD threshold.

Part 2

Cortical Mechanisms of Motor Control

6

Dynamics of Motor Cortical Networks

The Complementarity of Spike Synchrony and Firing Rate

Alexa Riehle, Sébastien Roux,
Bjørg Elisabeth Kilavik, and Sonja Grün

One of the most fascinating processes involved in motor behavior is movement preparation. It is based on central processes responsible for the maximally efficient organization of motor performance (for a review, see Requin et al. 1991; Riehle 2005). Both contextual and sensory information have to be assembled and integrated to shape the motor output. A strong argument in favor of the efficiency hypothesis of preparatory processes is the fact that providing prior information about movement parameters and/or removing time uncertainty about when to move significantly shortens reaction time. The notion of uncertainty, which is related to the manipulation of contextual information, is at the core of preparatory processes. The best-suited paradigm for studying such processes is the so-called *preparation paradigm*. In this paradigm, two signals are presented successively to the subject in each trial: the first, the preparatory signal (PS), provides prior information about what to do after occurrence of the second, the GO signal, and/or about when the GO signal will occur. By means of such prior information, the context in which the subject is placed can be experimentally manipulated. The subject knows with more or less precision both *what* to do and *when* to initiate the requested movement, and has to adjust movement preparation accordingly.

Recently, the topic of motor cortical activity involved in movement preparation was reviewed in great detail (Riehle 2005). Here, we restrict our efforts to a description of the dynamical interaction of cortical spiking activity involved in movement preparation by investigating the complementarity of precise spike synchrony and firing rate in the same cortical networks. We will first summarize the principles of the dynamics of synchronous precise spiking activity by describing in more detail that synchronous spiking activity is short-lasting, no longer than a few hundreds of milliseconds (Fig. 6.1–4, and Fig. 6.6). It modulates in time (Fig. 6.1) and can by no means be predicted from firing rate modulation (Figs. 6.1, 6.4, 6.6). Neurons may participate in different cell assemblies at different moments in time by changing partners (Fig. 6.3). We then will describe the direct relationship between synchronous spiking activity and firing rate modulation of the same neurons and their relation to behavior. In particular, synchrony occurs in relation to signal expectancy (Figs. 6.1, 6.5, 6.7). There is a clear structure in population synchrony (i.e., neurons in an entire population tend to be synchronized at behaviorally relevant moments in time; Figs. 6.5, 6.7). Synchrony becomes more structured with learning and practice along with an improvement of behavioral performance, whereas firing rate mainly decreases (Fig. 6.5). Synchrony may provide an internally triggered switch signal to modify directional movement preparation (Figs. 6.5, 6.7), and movement direction may be represented by one coding scheme, but not the other (Figs. 6.6, 6.7).

In order to detect and evaluate the occurrence of coincident spikes we used the *unitary events* analysis[1] (Grün et al. 1999, 2002a,b, 2003a; for a review see Grün 2009). Basically, this technique detects time epochs that contain a significant amount of excess spike synchrony (i.e., synchrony

---

[1] Dynamic changes in the temporal relations between the occurrences of spikes in simultaneously recorded pairs of neurons were analyzed offline by an extended version of the *unitary event* method (Grün et al. 2002a). It enables researchers to capture the temporal precision of spike synchronization and does not require cross-trial stationarity (see Grün 2009 and Maldonado et al. 2008 for a detailed description). The unitary event method allows us to detect spike synchronization that occurs in excess, compared to a chance synchronization given by the firing rates. The basic operation is to compare the detected coincidence counts (*empirical coincidences*, Fig. 6.1B, *squares*, and average across trials; see Fig. 6.1C, *black curve*) to the expected number given by the product of the firing probabilities of the involved neurons (*predicted coincidences*, Fig. 6.1C, *gray curve*). Significance of the empirical coincidence counts is evaluated by calculating the probability of getting such an amount or an even larger one (*p*-value, P), assuming a Poisson distribution, with the mean being the predicted number. The larger the number of excess coincidences, the closer P is to zero, and conversely, the larger the number of lacking coincidences, the closer its complement, 1–P, is to zero, while P approaches 1. Coincidences that compose an empirical number that surpasses the significance level (p <0.05 or 0.01) are called unitary events (see Fig. 6.1E, *squares*). For a better visualization, we use a logarithmic function $\log_{10}[(1-P)/P]$ (*joint-surprise measure*, Grün et al. 2002a, cf. Fig. 6.1D), expressing the surprise value of the outcome.

To account for nonstationarity of the firing rates in time, the evaluation of unitary events is performed in a sliding window of 100 ms duration that is shifted along the data (Grün et al. 2002b), here in steps of 5 ms. Within each window, the expected number of coincidences is calculated as the sum of the trial-by-trial expectancies, each calculated as the product of the marginal firing probabilities (Grün et al. 2003a). This procedure considers differences in the trial-by-trial firing rates and therefore accounts for nonstationarities across trials. A window identified to contain significantly more coincidences than expected by chance contains a combination of chance coincidences and the excess coincidences.

occurring more often than expected by the firing rates of the involved neurons). Their occurrence violates the assumption of independence and is interpreted as a signature of an activation of a functional cell assembly (Aertsen et al. 1991). The null hypothesis is formulated in terms of statistical independence on the basis of the individual firing probabilities of the neurons. By means of this null hypothesis, it is possible to calculate the number of predicted coincidences. As a result of calculating the statistical significance of the difference between predicted and empirical coincidences, one obtains both the strength and the occurrence time of significant excess coincident spiking activities (unitary events). This technique allows one to describe a detailed relationship between spike synchronization, rate modulation, and behaviorally relevant events (Riehle et al. 1997, 2000; Grammont and Riehle 1999, 2003; Kilavik et al. 2009).

DYNAMICS OF SYNCHRONOUS SPIKING ACTIVITY

It is well accepted that sensorimotor functions, including preparatory processes, are based on cooperative processing in neuronal networks, which are widely distributed over various brain structures. However, it is much less clear how these networks organize their spiking activity dynamically in space and time to cope with momentary computational demands. Based on theoretical considerations, the concept emerged that computational processes in the brain could also rely on the relative timing of spike discharges among neurons within such functional groups (von der Malsburg 1981; Abeles 1982, 1991; Gerstein et al. 1989; Palm 1990; Singer 1999), commonly called *cell assemblies* (Hebb 1949). To critically test if such a temporal scheme is actually implemented in the central nervous system, it is necessary to simultaneously observe the spiking activities of many neurons, and to analyze them for signs of temporal coordination. One type of temporal coordination consists of coincident spiking activities. Indeed, it has been argued that the synaptic influence of multiple neurons converging onto others is much stronger if they fire in coincidence (Abeles 1982; Rudolph and Destexhe 2003), making synchrony of firing ideally suited to raise the saliency of responses and to express relations among neurons with high temporal precision.

If cell assemblies are involved in cortical information processing, they should be activated in a systematic relation to the behavioral task. We simultaneously recorded the activity of small samples of individual neurons in motor cortex of monkeys performing delayed multidirectional pointing tasks. The question we then addressed was whether or not the level of synchrony (i.e., the interaction among neurons) remains constant over time. In other words, does the synchronization strength, expressed by the number of coincident spikes per second, depend only on the firing rate of the participating neurons, or is the level of synchrony context-dependent? In Figure 6.1, an example of a pair of neurons is shown.

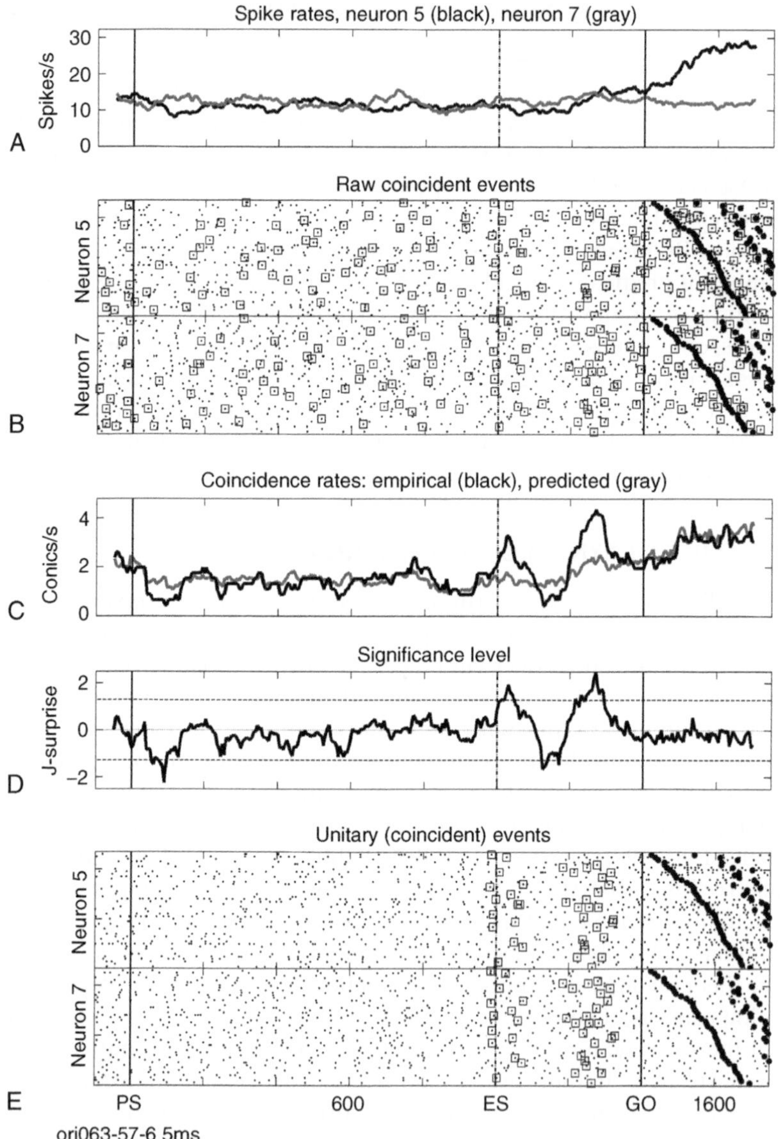

Figure 6.1 Dynamics of synchronous spiking activity 1. **A**: Firing rate profiles, averaged across trials, of two simultaneously recorded neurons. **B**: Synchronous spikes were detected with a precision of up to 5ms and visualized by squares in the raster displays of the two neurons. Each small dot corresponds to a spike and each line to a trial. Trials were arranged according to increasing reaction times from top to bottom. First range of large dots following GO indicate movement onset (reaction time), and the second range the end of movement. **C**: Empirical (*black*) and predicted (*gray*) coincidence rates. **D**: Time resolved statistical significance expressed by the joint-surprise measure. The horizontal dashed lines correspond to a statistical significance level of $p = 0.05$. **E**: Unitary Events (*squares*) indicate coincident spikes detected within a significant window. PS, preparatory signal; ES, expected GO signal; GO, GO signal. Time in milliseconds, starting at PS. Data are from task 1.

During movement preparation, that is, during the delay between preparatory (PS) and GO signal, both neurons do virtually not change their activity, except at the end of the delay, when neuron 5 progressively increases its activity in anticipation of the GO signal and continues to increase after GO during movement performance (Fig. 6.1A). Since the number of predicted coincidences is calculated trial by trial in sliding windows (for the analysis technique, see Footnote 1) on the basis of the instantaneous firing rate of the participating neurons estimated within each window, the rate of the predicted coincidences (*gray curve* in Fig. 6.1C) necessarily reflects the combined discharge rates of the two neurons. Surprisingly, when comparing the average rate of the predicted coincidences (*gray curve* in Fig. 6.1C) with the average rate of the empirical coincidences (*black curve*), it can clearly be seen that the actual coincidence rate modulates strongly, thereby at some instances largely exceeding and at others largely undershooting the chance level. The modulation of synchrony, independent of the firing rate, is expressed by the joint-surprise measure shown in Fig. 6.1D. If its value is equal to zero, the spiking activities of the two neurons are not correlated; that is, neurons fire independently from each other such that the synchrony is at a level as one would expect by taking into account their instantaneous firing rates. If its value becomes positive, more synchrony occurs than expected, and vice versa, if it becomes negative, there is less synchrony than expected. The modulation of precise synchrony (Fig. 6.1D) is thus by no means predictable simply by inspecting the modulation of the firing rates of the neurons over time (Fig. 6.1A). It is interesting to note that the modulation of synchrony starts at the moment when the animal expected the occurrence of a GO signal[2] (expected signal, ES), which may occur at that moment in 50% of the trials, but did not occur during the long delay trials as selected here. Furthermore, epochs containing unitary events

---

[2] Task 1: We trained three Rhesus monkeys in a task that was explained in detail in Roux et al. (2003, 2006). The monkeys were trained to execute movements in two opposite directions from a common center position (see sketch in Fig. 6.5A). On a vertical panel, three touch-sensitive targets with light-emitting diodes (diameter: 3 cm) were mounted in a horizontal line, 10 cm apart. The animal self-initiated each trial by touching the center target with the active hand. After a fixed delay of 500 ms, a preparatory signal (PS) was presented. Both peripheral targets were presented simultaneously as PS, one in red and the other in green. The animal learned to attribute to each color one of two possible delay durations. If the (directionally noninformative) auditory GO signal occurred after a short delay, the monkey had to select the red target, whereas after a long delay he had to select the green one. Both the laterality of the colored targets and the presentation of the two durations were varied at random with equal probability. Thus, the probability for the GO signal to occur after the short delay was 0.5. Once this moment passed and GO did not occur (in long delay trials), the probability for the occurrence of GO after the long delay became 1. The animals learned to discriminate between two delay durations. Durations were either 600 and 1,200 ms, or 1,000 and 1,400 ms, respectively.

never last longer than a few hundreds of milliseconds, and usually last a much shorter time.

Another important observation of synchronous spiking activity is that its temporal precision may change over time. If such changes occur, temporal precision typically increases during the preparatory period and is highest toward its end (cf. Riehle et al. 2000; Grün et al. 2003b). Figure 6.2 shows the epochs during which the spiking activity of the same two neurons as presented in Figure 6.1 were significantly synchronized for various coincidence widths (y-axis) (i.e., precision of synchrony). We analyzed temporal precision of spike synchrony between 1 and 10 ms, corresponding to the temporal window in which synchronous excitatory inputs have been shown to be most efficient (Abeles 1982; Destexhe and Paré 1999; Azouz and Gray 2000; Azouz 2005). One possible interpretation of our results is that the increase of temporal precision of synchronous activity facilitates the efficiency of the motor output.

CELL ASSEMBLIES

An essential ingredient of the notion of coordinated ensemble activity within a cell assembly is its flexibility and dynamic nature. This logically implies that neurons may participate in different cell assemblies at different times, depending on stimulus context and behavioral demands.

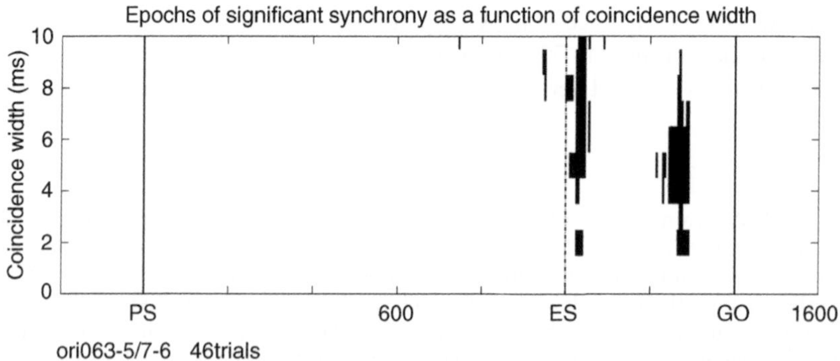

Figure 6.2 Dynamics of synchronous spiking activity 2. The epochs of significant synchrony (p <0.05) are indicated for coincidence widths between 1 and 10 ms (y-axis) (same data as presented in Figure 6.1). Data were analyzed using a sliding window of 100 ms that was shifted in steps of 5 ms along the data during the behavioral trial. If the result of the analysis in a window was statistically significant, the center of the window was marked in black. The two neurons synchronized significantly their activity right after a GO was expected (ES) with a temporal precision of about 4–10 ms, whereas about 150 ms before GO another epoch of significant synchrony occurred, but with increased temporal precision (about 3–6 ms).

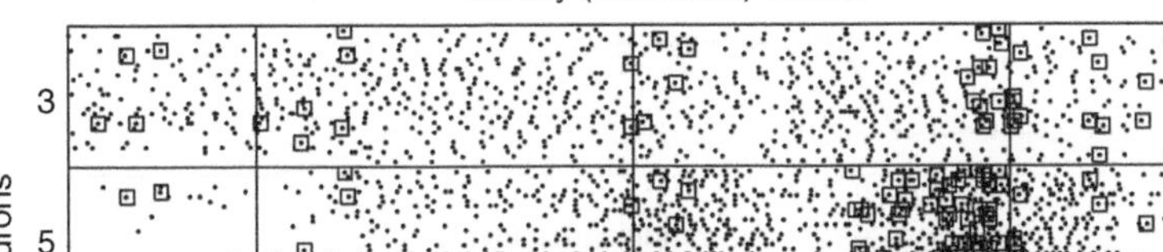

Figure 6.3 Cell assemblies. Spiking activity of three simultaneously recorded neurons in task 1 is shown. Each dot corresponds to a single spike time, and each line to a behavioral trial. Coincident spikes with a temporal precision of up to 5 ms occurring in statistically significant (p <0.05) windows are marked by squares (*Unitary Events*). For details see Figure 6.1. Data are from task 1.

Figure 6.3 shows an example of three simultaneously recorded neurons. Each of the three panels shows a raster display of the spiking activity of a single neuron. The squares indicate those coincident spikes that were detected within statistically significant analysis windows with a temporal precision of up to 5 ms (as in Fig. 6.1E). Concretely, around PS, neurons 3 and 5 significantly synchronized their activity, then around ES all three neurons were significantly synchronized; before GO, neurons 5 and 7 were synchronized, and right after GO, neurons 3 and 5 were synchronized. In other words, Figure 6.3 suggests a successive activation of different cell assemblies during the behavioral trial, determined by the coincident partner neurons, and neuron 5 may belong to all assemblies by changing partners. The main message that we have to retain from this figure is that the lifetime of assemblies is rather short, and that assemblies are mainly formed at particular behaviorally relevant moments in time.

BINDING BY SYNCHRONY

Neurons in motor cortex change their activity in relation not only to movement execution, but also to movement preparation (for review, see Riehle 2005). The next question we addressed was if any relationship existed between neurons (or populations of neurons) that were involved in one of these aspects. Do (groups of) preparation-related neurons interact with (groups of) execution-related neurons? A surprising result revealed that, indeed, many neurons—which were classified on the basis of their firing rate to be functionally involved in different processes, for instance the one related to movement preparation (neuron 1 in Fig. 6.4A) and the other to movement execution (neuron 3)—significantly synchronized their spiking

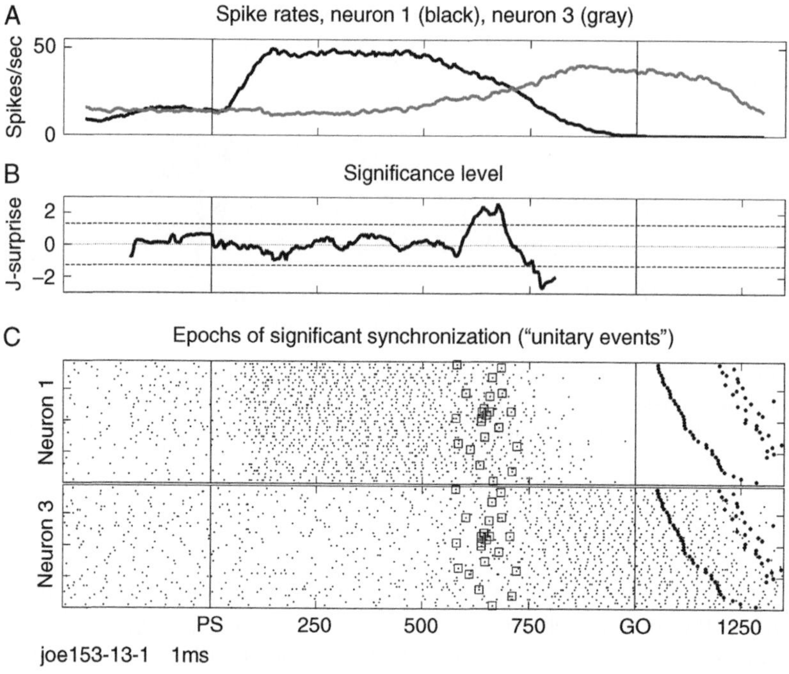

Figure 6.4 Binding by synchrony. The significant synchrony between the spiking activities of two neurons recorded in task 2 is shown for a coincidence precision of 1ms. For details see Figure 6.1, especially A, D, and E. The two neurons synchronize significantly their activity only during a short epoch in time. Data from Grammont, F., and A. Riehle. 1999. Precise spike synchronization in monkey motor cortex involved in preparation for movement. *Experimental Brain Research* 128: 118–22.

activity at a specific instant in time (Grammont and Riehle 1999; task 2[3]). Interestingly, they did not continuously synchronize their activity during the whole task, but they were transiently "connected" by synchrony during the transition from preparation to execution. The classification of the two neurons forming the pair, based on their firing rate, would by no means

---

[3] Task 2: Two Rhesus monkeys were trained to perform pointing movements in six directions (for details, see Grammont and Riehle 1999; Bastian et al. 2003). The animal sat in a primate chair in front of a vertical panel on which seven touch-sensitive, light-emitting diodes (LEDs) were mounted, one in the center and six equidistantly in a circle around it. The center target was lit, and the animal had to touch it to initiate the trial. Then, after a fixed delay of 500 ms, during which the animal had to continue to press the target, a preparatory signal (PS) was presented consisting of the illumination of one of the peripheral targets in green. After a fixed delay of 1 s, the green target turned red, serving as GO signal. It instructed the animal to release the center target and to point at the specified target as quickly as possible. During a session of about 150 trials, all six movement directions were presented at random with equal probability.

allow one to describe the functional link between them, which can only be detected by means of the synchronization pattern.

Transient synchronization of spiking activity in ensembles of coactive neurons may help to strengthen the effectiveness within such groups and thereby help, for instance, to increase performance speed, in conjunction with the increase in firing rate during movement preparation, which is partly correlated, on a trial-by-trial basis, with behavioral reaction time (cf. Riehle and Requin 1993; review: Riehle 2005). Indeed, it has been demonstrated that both the strength of synchronous activity (Riehle et al. 1997) and the temporal precision of statistically significant synchrony (Fig. 6.2; Riehle et al. 2000) increased toward the end of the preparatory period. Moreover, time-resolved cross-correlation studies have shown that neurons strongly synchronized their activity at the end of the preparatory period in trials with short reaction times, but synchronized less precisely or not at all in trials with long reaction times (Riehle 2005; Roux S, Riehle A, unpublished observations).

SYNCHRONY AND BEHAVIORAL PRACTICE

The timing of the modulation of synchrony and firing rate at the population level in motor cortex suggests that synchrony may be preferentially involved in early preparatory and cognitive processes, whereas rate modulation may rather control movement initiation and execution (Riehle et al. 2000; Grammont and Riehle 2003). This finding raised the question of whether the structure of spike synchrony and firing rate is formed by learning or intensive practice. Therefore, we examined the temporal structure of the activity of motor cortical neurons as a function of daily practice. We found in three monkeys that the timing of the behavioral task is clearly represented in the temporal structure of significant spike synchrony (Kilavik et al. 2009; task 1, see Footnote 2), and this temporal structure is shaped by practice. We were able to show this effect by evaluating the strength of synchrony of the entire neuronal population by summing the empirical coincidence counts across all pairs of neurons and comparing this number to the sum of the predicted pair-by-pair and trial-by-trial numbers in sliding windows. The result showed that population synchrony emerged by practice at a time instance relevant for the behavior in late experimental sessions. Synchrony increased in strength, along with an improvement of the behavior as measured by decreasing reaction time. In contrast, the firing rate of the same neurons mainly decreased at this behaviorally relevant moment in time.

Figure 6.5 shows the results from recording sessions in one of the three analyzed monkeys during 6 weeks of daily performance. In Figure 6.5B, the performance in terms of behavioral reaction times is shown to significantly decrease with time ($p < 0.01$). For the neuronal activity, data were split into two populations corresponding to the first (in gray, 42 pairs of neurons) and the second half (in black, 45 pairs of neurons) of the

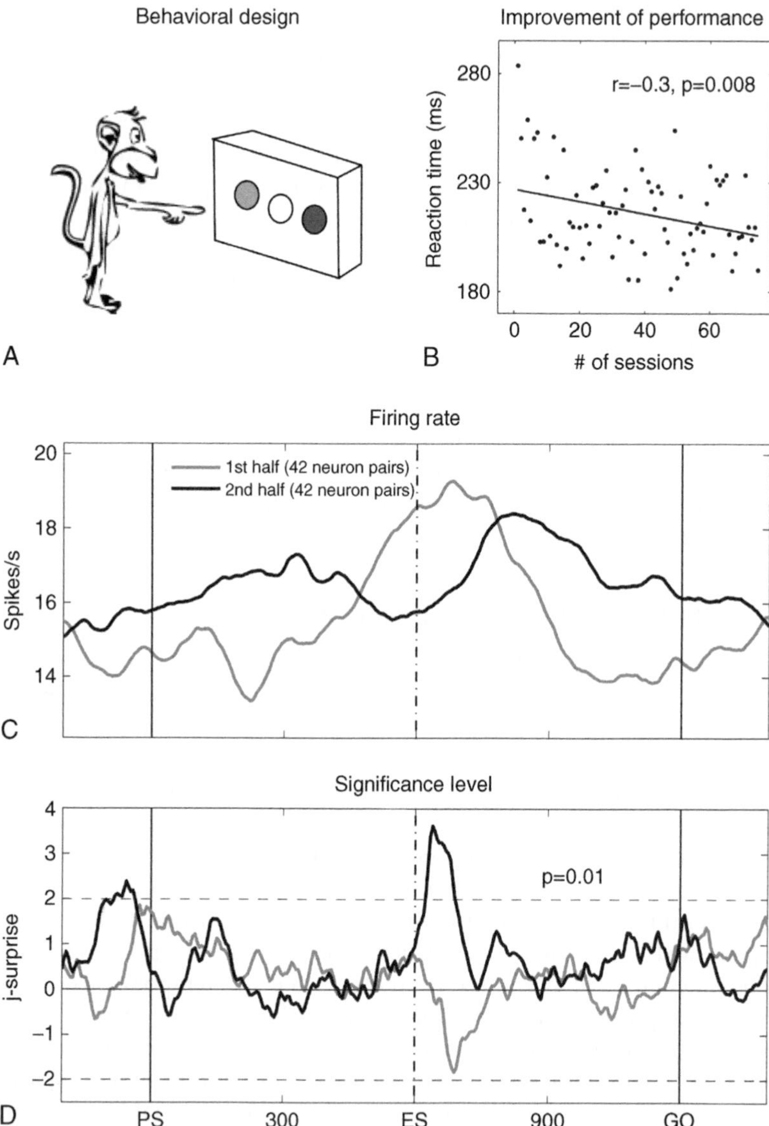

Figure 6.5 Synchrony and behavioral practice. **A**: Sketch of the design of task 1 (for details, see footnote 2). **B**: Mean behavioral reaction times during successive recording sessions. The solid line shows the regression line and indicates improvement of performance as statistically significant ($p = 0.008$). **C** and **D**: Quantification of population activity. **C**: Average firing rate profiles obtained during the first half (42 neuron pairs; *gray line*) and second half (45 neuron pairs; *black line*) of the recording sessions. **D**: Joint-surprise function calculated from the difference between the empirical and predicted numbers of coincidences in each sliding window for each of the populations of neuron pairs of the first and the second half of the sessions (*gray and black line*, respectively). The horizontal dashed lines correspond to a significance level of $p = 0.01$ for excess (*top line*) and lacking (*bottom line*) coincidences.

recording sessions. In Figure 6.5C, the averaged firing rates of the neurons are shown. Then, the number of coincident spikes per analysis window (100 ms, shifted in steps of 5 ms) is summed across all trials of all pairs of neurons and for coincidence widths of 2 and 3 ms (for more details of the analysis technique, see Kilavik et al. 2009). The difference between empirical and predicted coincidences is then tested by calculating the joint surprise (Fig. 6.5D). This value indicates the modulation of the strength of synchrony during the trial. The striking result is that synchrony increased and became more structured with practice (Fig. 6.5D), whereas the collective firing rate mainly decreased at the moment when synchrony increased (Fig. 6.5C). In particular, synchrony increased strongly in relation to signal expectancy. Indeed, in the first half of the sessions (*gray curve*), synchrony never reached the significance level of $p = 0.01$ (*dashed lines* in Fig. 6.5D), whereas during the second half of sessions (*black curve*), it largely exceeded this level. In addition, we find a total inversion of the resulting synchrony around ES—in the first half of the sessions there was less synchrony than expected by chance, albeit not significant, whereas in the second half, a high amount of excess synchrony is found at this particular moment in time. During the remaining time in the delay period, the joint-surprise is close to zero in both populations, reflecting that coincidences are occurring at chance level. Thus, our results clearly demonstrate an increase of spike synchrony with task practice at behaviorally relevant moments in time. Indeed, we obtained similar results in two other animals showing an increase of synchrony with practice accompanied by an overall decrease in firing rate and an improvement of behavioral performance (Kilavik et al. 2009).

This systematic increase in synchrony is not related to an external signal, but must be internally driven by the estimation of the elapsed time during the trial (for the task, see Footnote 2). As the behavioral output in this task was strictly tied to the task timing, the improved performance with practice suggests an improved estimation of the moment in time of a possible GO signal occurrence (Riehle et al. 1997, 2000; Grammont and Riehle 2003). It is thus tempting to speculate that the increase in synchrony related to this specific moment reflects a cognitive state, an internal representation of (the nonappearance of) an expected event. Alternatively, it could be related to a shift in the cognitive state necessary for movement reprogramming, as in this specific task the time of GO also indicates movement direction (see also Sakamoto et al. 2008).

SYNCHRONY AND MOVEMENT DIRECTION

This led us to analyze the same neuronal data in relation to movement direction. We found that the spiking activity of more than 65% of the neurons recorded in task 1 (see Footnote 2) was selectively modulated during the second part of long trials by movement direction (Roux et al. 2003).

This is in agreement with the fact that movement direction is one of the (spatial) movement parameters that is most represented in motor cortical activity during movement preparation (Riehle 2005; cf. Georgopoulos 1995). This is best described in studies in which the execution of movements was required in more than two movement directions. For instance, 76% of motor cortical neurons that were recorded in a delayed center-out reaching task including six directions from a common home position were significantly directionally selective (Grammont and Riehle 2003). Furthermore, preferred directions of directionally selective neurons were homogeneously distributed across all movement directions (Grammont and Riehle 2003; see also Georgopoulos et al. 1982). On the other hand, we found in many pairs of neurons recorded in task 1 that spike synchrony was also directionally selective. During this task, pointing movements had to be performed in two opposite directions, which had to be selected as a function of the correct estimation of the delay duration (Roux et al. 2003, 2006, see Footnote 2). In long trials, the moment when a GO signal was expected at the end of a short trial (ES) was of crucial importance for this task. During the first half of the delay, corresponding to the short delay, the monkey may prepare a movement to the red target, albeit weakly, because the probability of its execution was only 0.5. Once this moment passed and no signal was presented, the probability to execute a movement to the opposite (green) target became 1. In other words, after the ES in long trials, preparation may switch from one movement direction to the opposite. Note that the GO signal did not contain any directional information; it only indicated when to move. The selection of the target, and thus movement direction, was a function of both the color of the targets presented by PS and the duration between PS and GO.

Figure 6.6 shows an example of synchronous spiking activity in relation to movement direction. In Figure 6.6A, the PS indicated a movement to the right ("red" target, corresponding to the gray circle in the inset), if a GO signal would have occurred after a short delay. However, in this behavioral condition, the GO signal only occurred after a long delay and, thus, a movement to the left ("green" = black circle) target had to be executed. Toward the end of the short delay, when the monkey did not yet know whether or not to execute the movement, the neurons significantly synchronized their activity. But the significance level of synchrony was rather low, reaching barely the threshold for $p = 0.05$ (*dashed line*). In Figure 6.6B, a right movement had to be executed after a long delay (*black circle*, see inset). The conditional probability to do so was 1 at the end of the delay, reflected in the strong synchrony that occurred just before GO, whose joint-surprise measure exceeds the value 2 ($p < 0.01$). Furthermore, it can clearly be seen that the directionally selective synchrony pattern can by no means be predicted by the firing rate of the two neurons. In this example, only neuron 5 exhibits directionally selective changes in firing rate during movement preparation. It increased its activity at the end of the delay for a

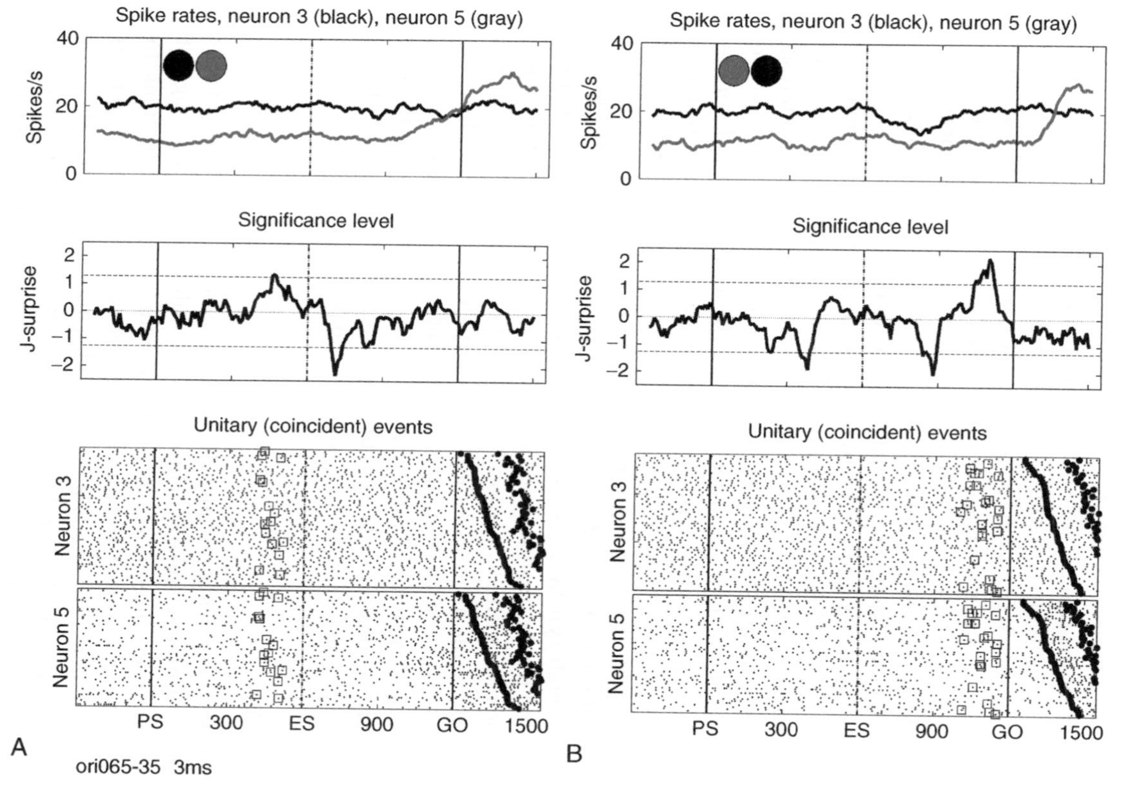

Figure 6.6 Synchrony related to movement direction. Synchronous spiking activity of one pair of neurons recorded in task 1 in relation to the two opposite movement directions (coincidence precision of up to 3 ms). For more details see Figure 6.1. **A**: Movement to the left. **B**: Movement to the right. The insets in A and B show the constellations of PS, see text.

leftward movement (Fig. 6.6A), and only during movement execution for a rightward movement (B), whereas neuron 3 did not change its activity in relation to either movement direction.

In order to study directionally selective synchronous activity and to compare it with the firing rate, we analyzed population data. In many pairs of neurons, we found a pattern of synchrony around ES that turned out to be reciprocal for the two possible behavioral conditions in long trials. This is shown for an individual example in Figure 6.7C with an increase of synchrony for the switch from the left to the right movement (in black, "preferred direction"), and a decrease in synchrony for the other condition (in gray, "anti-preferred direction"). Remember, this specific moment in time (ES) depends exclusively on correct time estimation, corresponding to an internally triggered switching signal (see, for details, Roux et al. 2003; Footnote 2). The firing rates of the two neurons in the two conditions are presented in Figure 6.7A (preferred direction, as determined by synchrony) and 6.7B (anti-preferred direction). We then performed the same analysis as already presented in Figure 6.5 for an entire population of neurons. We selected 36 out of 56 (64%) recorded pairs of neurons that showed, for the two possible long delay trial types, a synchrony pattern like that presented in Figure 6.7C. For each pair of neurons, data were split in trials of the preferred movement direction (significant increase in synchrony around ES) and trials in the anti-preferred direction (decrease in synchrony). We found that even though synchrony was reciprocal around ES (as requested for being selected for the analysis, see Figure 7.7E), the mean firing rate of the same neurons was virtually identical in the two populations (Fig. 6.7D). We performed the same analysis for a second monkey and obtained the same results (34/59 pairs, 58%). Note that the data sets were selected according the synchronous activity of individual pairs of neurons, and individual neurons may be directionally selective (see earlier discussion), but this selectivity might be lost by averaging across the population.

CONCLUSION

The modulation of firing rate and the modulation of neuronal cooperativity in terms of precise spike synchrony (in the millisecond range) suggest that the brain uses different strategies in different contextual situations. In order to deal with internal and purely cognitive processes, such as expecting an event, increasing motivation, or modifying an internal state, neurons may preferentially synchronize their spike occurrences without necessarily changing their firing rates. In contrast, when processing external, behaviorally relevant events, such as the occurrence of a signal providing prior information and/or cueing the execution of the requested movement, neurons may preferentially modulate their firing rates (Riehle et al. 1997; Grammont and Riehle 2003). Thus, both a temporal code (e.g., the precise spike synchrony) and a rate code (firing rate modulation) may

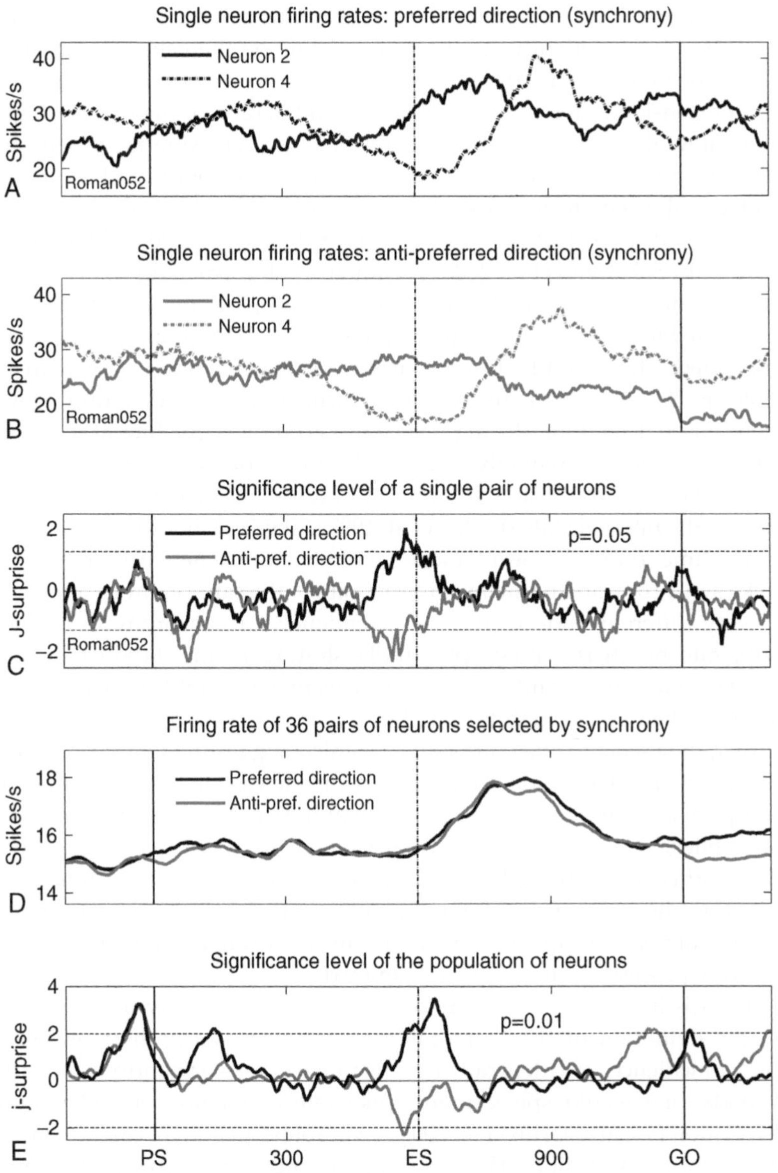

Figure 6.7 Synchrony related to movement direction. **A–B**: Mean firing rate of two neurons during the two long delay trial types in opposite movement directions (task 1). **C**: Strength of synchrony. For one movement direction, synchrony increased significantly above the expected level around ES (*black line*, "preferred" direction), whereas for the other movement direction, the same neurons exhibited at the same behavioral event (ES) significantly less spike synchrony than expected (*gray line*, "anti-preferred" direction). **D–E**: Quantification of firing rate (D) and synchrony (E) of 36 pairs of neurons, exhibiting the same characteristics as those shown in A–C. For more details see Figure 6.5 and text.

serve different and complementary functions, acting in concert at some times and independently at others, depending on the behavioral context. Thus, one may consider the temporal code not as an alternative, but rather as an extension to the rate code. Such a combination of the two strategies may allow the extraction of more information from patterns of neuronal activity and thereby increase the dynamics, the flexibility, and the representational strength of a distributed system such as the cerebral cortex (Riehle et al. 1997; Hatsopoulos et al. 1998; Baker et al. 2001, Maldonado et al. 2008; Sakamoto et al. 2008, Tsujimoto et al. 2008). During movement preparation, in motor cortex particularly, abrupt changes in firing rate (transient bursts) are probably deliberately kept to a minimum, if not totally prevented. This could be to prevent accidental activation of downstream motor nuclei. Most often, the changes in firing rate are gradual until movement onset. Therefore, during preparation, phasic signalling at a precise time would be preferentially mediated by a temporal code, such as transitory spike synchronization, in order to indicate internal events and/or to modify the internal state (Riehle et al. 1997; Kilavik et al. 2009).

The time courses of the interaction within neuronal networks in terms of spike synchrony and of the mean firing rate of the same neurons appear to be very different. Indeed, there is a tendency for synchrony to precede firing rate, but there is no simple parallel shifting in time of these two measures (cf. Grammont and Riehle 2003). This makes it unlikely that the two coding schemes are tightly coupled by a stereotyped transformation. Rather, they seem to obey different dynamics, suggesting that the coherent activation of cell assemblies may trigger the increase in firing rate in large groups of neurons. For instance, the preparatory coherent activation of cell assemblies, by way of synchrony, may generate the increase in firing rate in large cortical networks, which in turn communicate with the periphery for initiating the movement (cf. Grammont and Riehle 2003). However, the functional relationship between synchrony and firing rate involved in preparatory processes remains to be examined.

The distinction between rate and synchronous activity also depends on the definition of the temporal precision of a synchronous event. If the "coincidence" width is rather in the range of tens or hundreds of milliseconds, one would speak about spike rate correlation or spike count correlation (see also Grün et al. 2003b). We found that there can be considerable rate covariation. However, interestingly, rate covariation may occur simultaneously but independently from spike synchronization (Grün et al. 2003a). Both time scales seem to be relevant for cortical processing; measures derived from the different temporal scales seem to indicate context-specific and complementary processes (Riehle et al. 1997). In this study, we have shown that, in motor cortex, internal processes seem to be reflected by synchronous activity on a fine temporal scale, whereas stimulus-related synchrony is accompanied by rate changes. Whether this principle can be generalized to other cortical areas remains to be explored.

ACKNOWLEDGMENTS

We thank Marc Martin for animal welfare. This work was supported by the French government (ANR-05-NEUR-045-01), UE grant 15879 (FACETS), BMBF Grant 01GQ0420 to the BCCN, and the Initiative and Networking Fund of the Helmholtz Association within the Helmholtz Alliance on Systems Biology.

REFERENCES

Abeles, M. 1982. Role of cortical neuron: integrator or coincidence detector? *Israeli Journal of Medical Science* 18: 83–92.

Abeles, M. 1991. *Corticonics: Neural circuits of the cerebral cortex*. Cambridge: Cambridge University Press.

Aertsen, A., Vaadia, E., M. Abeles, E. Ahissar, H. Bergman, B. Karmon, et al. 1991. Neural interactions in the frontal cortex of a behaving monkey: Signs of dependence on stimulus context and behavioral state. *Journal für Hirnforschung* 32: 735–43.

Azouz, R. 2005. Dynamic spatiotemporal synaptic integration in cortical neurons: Neuronal gain, revisited. *Journal of Neurophysiology* 94: 2785–96.

Azouz, R., and C.M. Gray. 2000. Dynamic spike threshold reveals a mechanism for synaptic coincidence detection in cortical neurons in vivo. *Proceedings of the National Academy of Science USA* 97: 8110–15.

Baker, S.N., R. Spinks, A. Jackson, and R.N. Lemon. 2001. Synchronization in monkey motor cortex during a precision grip task. I. Task-dependent modulation in single-unit synchrony. *Journal of Neurophysiology* 85: 869–85.

Bastian, A., G. Schöner, and A. Riehle. 2003. Preshaping and continuous evolution of motor cortical representations during movement preparation. *European Journal of Neuroscience* 18: 2047–58.

Destexhe, A., and D. Paré. 1999. Impact of network activity on the integrative properties of neocortical pyramidal neurons in vivo. *Journal of Neurophysiology* 81: 1531–47.

Georgopoulos, A.P. 1995. Current issues in directional motor control. *Trends in NeuroScience* 18: 506–10.

Georgopoulos, A.P., J.F. Kalaska, R. Caminiti, and J.T. Massey. 1982. On the relations between the direction of two-dimensional arm movements and cell discharge in primate motor cortex. *Journal of Neuroscience* 2: 1527–37.

Gerstein, G.L., P. Bedenbaugh, and A.M.H.J. Aertsen. 1989. Neural assemblies. *IEEE Transactions on Bio-medical Engineering* 36: 4–14.

Grammont, F., and A. Riehle. 1999. Precise spike synchronization in monkey motor cortex involved in preparation for movement. *Experimental Brain Research* 128: 118–22.

Grammont, F., and A. Riehle. 2003. Spike synchronization and firing rate in a population of motor cortical neurons in relation to movement direction and reaction time. *Biological Cybernetics* 88: 360–73.

Grün, S. 2009. Data-driven significance estimation for precise spike correlation. *Journal of Neurophysiology* 101: 1126–40.

Grün, S., M. Diesmann, and A. Aertsen. 2002a. 'Unitary Events' in multiple single-neuron activity. I. Detection and significance. *Neural Computation* 14: 43–80.

Grün, S., M. Diesmann, and A. Aertsen. 2002b. 'Unitary Events' in multiple single-neuron activity. II. Non-stationary data. *Neural Computation* 14: 81–119.

Grün, S., M. Diesmann, F. Grammont, A. Riehle, and A. Aertsen. 1999. Detecting Unitary Events without discretization of time. *Journal of Neuroscience Methods* 94: 67–79.

Grün, S., A. Riehle, A. Aertsen, and M. Diesmann. 2003b. Temporal scales of cortical interactions. *Nova Acta Leopoldina* NF 88, Nr. 332: 189–206.

Grün, S., A. Riehle, and M. Diesmann. 2003a. Effect of cross-trial nonstationarity on joint-spike events. *Biological Cybernetics* 88: 335–51.

Hatsopoulos, N.G., C.L. Ojakangas, L. Paninski, and J.P. Donoghue. 1998. Information about movement direction obtained from synchronous activity of motor cortical neurons. *Proceedings of the National Academy of Science USA* 95: 15706–11.

Hebb, D.O. 1949. *The organization of behavior*. New York: Wiley and Sons.

Kilavik, B.E., S. Roux, A. Ponce-Alvarez, J. Confais, S. Grün, and A. Riehle. 2009. Long-term modifications in motor cortical dynamics induced by intensive practice. *Journal of Neuroscience* 29: 12653–63.

Maldonado, P., C. Babul, W. Singer, E. Rodriguez, D. Berger, and S. Grün. 2008. Synchronization of neuronal responses in primary visual cortex of monkeys viewing natural images. *Journal of Neurophysiology* 100: 1523–32.

Palm, G. 1990. Cell assemblies as a guideline for brain research. *Concepts in Neuro-Science* 1: 133–48.

Requin, J., J. Brener and C. Ring. 1991. Preparation for action. In *Handbook of Cognitive Psychophysiology: Central and autonomous nervous system approaches*. eds., R.R. Jennings and M.G.H Coles, 357–448. New York: Wiley & Sons.

Riehle, A. 2005. Preparation for action: one of the key functions of the motor cortex. In *Motor cortex in voluntary movements: A distributed system for distributed functions*, eds., A. Riehle and E. Vaadia, 213–240. Boca Raton FL: CRC-Press.

Riehle, A., F. Grammont, M. Diesmann, and S. Grün. 2000. Dynamical changes and temporal precision of synchronized spiking activity in monkey motor cortex during movement preparation. *Journal of Physiology Paris* 94: 569–82.

Riehle, A., S. Grün, M. Diesmann, and A. Aertsen. 1997. Spike synchronization and rate modulation differentially involved in motor cortical function. *Science* 278: 1950–53.

Riehle, A., and J. Requin. 1993. The predictive value for performance speed of preparatory changes in activity of the monkey motor and premotor cortex. *Behavioural Brain Research* 53: 35–49.

Rudolph, M., and A. Destexhe. 2003. Tuning neocortical pyramidal neurons between integrators and coincidence detectors. *Journal of Computational Neuroscience* 14: 239–51.

Roux, S., M. Coulmance, and A. Riehle. 2003. Context-related representation of timing processes in monkey motor cortex. *European Journal of Neuroscience* 18: 1011–16.

Roux, S., W.A. MacKay, and A. Riehle. 2006. The pre-movement component of motor cortical local field potentials reflects the level of expectancy. *Behavioural Brain Research* 169: 335–51.

Sakamoto, K., H. Mushiake, N. Saito, K. Aihara, M. Yano, and J. Tanji. 2008. Discharge synchrony during the transition of behavioral goal representations encoded by discharge rates of prefrontal neurons. *Cerebral Cortex* 18: 2036–45.

Singer, W. 1999. Neural synchrony: A versatile code for the definition of relations. *Neuron* 24: 49–65.

Tsujimoto, S., A. Genovesio, and S.P. Wise. 2008. Transient neuronal correlations underlying goal selection and maintenance in prefrontal cortex. *Cerebral Cortex* 18: 2748–61.

von der Malsburg, C. 1981. *The correlation theory of brain function*. Göttingen: Internal Report 81-2: Abteilung Neurobiologie, MPI für Biophysikalische Chemie.

7

Proximal-to-Distal Sequencing Behavior and Motor Cortex

Nicholas G. Hatsopoulos, Leonel Olmedo, and Kazutaka Takahashi

Since the advent of single-unit cortical recordings in awake, behaving primates in the 1960s (Evarts 1964; Evarts 1966), extensive research has investigated the physiological properties in single cortical neurons as they relate to sensory stimuli, motor behavior, and cognition. In the context of motor control, the encoding properties of neurons in several frontal and parietal cortical areas, including the primary motor cortex, have been examined. The activity of single motor cortical neurons has been shown to correlate with a variety of movement-related features including force, direction, speed, and position (Evarts 1968; Smith et al. 1975; Cheney and Fetz 1980; Georgopoulos et al. 1982; Georgopoulos et al. 1984; Taira et al. 1996; Moran and Schwartz 1999; Paninski et al. 2004). However, very little is known about spatiotemporal activity patterns that emerge across large neuronal ensembles that may encode and mediate complex, coordinated behavior. This is largely due to the fact that, until recently, few studies have employed multielectrode electrophysiological methods to simultaneously record from large neuronal ensembles.

Psychophysically, it is known that a variety of motor behaviors such as throwing, jumping, and hitting share a particular coordination pattern referred to as proximal-to-distal (P-D) sequencing, in which the more proximal muscles activate prior to the distal muscles and the associated proximal joints begin moving before the distal joints. This sequential coordination pattern may also subserve more fundamental behaviors, including reach-to-grasp and climbing, that trace their evolutionary roots to primate foraging for food in arboreal environments. In this chapter, we describe a recently discovered spatiotemporal pattern of neural activity in the primary motor cortex that may mediate this proximal-distal sequencing pattern of coordination. Specifically, we hypothesize that traveling waves of activity propagate along a rostral-to-caudal axis in the motor cortex in order to facilitate sequential activation of proximal and distal segment representations. At the end of the chapter, we discuss recent experiments looking at the kinematics of reach-to-grasp behaviors and the potential role of propagating activity waves in coordinating shoulder, elbow, and wrist joint motions.

PROXIMAL-TO-DISTAL SEQUENCING

Proximal-to-distal sequencing is a ubiquitous coordination pattern that has been observed in both upper and lower limb segments. The sequencing pattern has been extensively documented in terms of joint motion (i.e., timing of peak velocity), as well as in terms of muscle activation measured using electromyographic (EMG) electrodes (Table 7.1). With respect to

Table 7.1 List of motor behaviors that exhibit proximal to distal sequencing along with the time delay between proximal and distal limb segmental motion or muscle activity

Behavior	Measurement	Time Delay (ms) between Proximal & Distal Component	Author
Throwing			
baseball	EMG onset	94 (AD vs. FCU)	(Hirashima et al. 2002)
handball	Peak ang. velocity	41 (elbow vs. wrist)	(Joris et al. 1985)
Striking			
Golf swing	Peak ang. velocity	~100 (shoulder vs. wrist)	(Milburn 1982)
Kicking	Peak ang. velocity	~72 (hip vs. knee)	(Putnam 1993)
Expert Pianists	Peak ang. velocity	~150 (shoulder vs. wrist)	(Furuya and Kinoshita 2007)
Jumping	EMG peak	~160 (GM vs. soleus)	(Bobbert and van Ingen Schenau 1988)
Dancing	Kinematic onset	~120 (hip vs. ankle)	(Bronner and Ojofeitimi 2006)
Reach to touch	EMG onset	~60 (deltoids vs. EDC)	(Murphy et al. 1985)

AD, anterior deltoid; FCU, flexor carpi ulnaris; GM, gluteus maximus; EDC, extensor digitorum communis; Deltoids correspond to both anterior and posterior deltoid muscles.

upper limb motor behavior, P-D sequencing of the shoulder, elbow, and wrist has perhaps been most thoroughly studied in the context of throwing behavior (Atwater 1979) in baseball (Pappas et al. 1985; Hirashima et al. 2002), handball (Joris et al. 1985), water polo (Elliott and Armour 1988), and track and field sports such as javelin (Bartlett et al. 1996) and shot put (Zatsiorsky et al. 1981). Motor behaviors whose goal it is to strike or hit an object often exhibit P-D sequencing as well. These behaviors include the tennis serve (Elliott et al. 1995), the tennis and squash forehand strokes (Elliott and Marsh 1989; Elliott et al. 1996), the golf swing (Milburn 1982), and even piano playing (Furuya and Kinoshita 2007). As for the lower-limb, ball kicking (Putnam 1993) and jumping (Bobbert and van Ingen Schenau 1988) have been shown to generate sequencing of the hip, knee, and ankle joints and muscles.

One of the important goals of many if not all of the behaviors just described is to impart maximal kinetic energy on a distal object or body part. To accomplish this, the summation of speed principle in biomechanics states the speed at the end of a distal segment (and, therefore, the kinetic energy of an object being thrown or struck) can be maximized by summing the velocity contributions of more proximal segments to which it is attached (Putnam 1993). This principle is often used to explain the sequential onset times of proximal-to-distal limb segments. However, by itself, it does not uniquely specify such a sequential pattern. For example, to maximize the Cartesian speed of the fingertips, the joint velocities of the shoulder, elbow, wrist, and fingers should reach a peak speed at the same time at a fully extended orientation. However, what is actually observed in P-D sequencing behaviors is that peak joint velocity of a distal joint occurs when the neighboring, proximal joint is decelerating. A kinetic account of P-D sequencing of throwing and striking suggests that interaction torques acting on a joint based on the velocity and acceleration of neighboring joints can largely explain this sequencing pattern (Putnam 1993). Finally, a third account of this pattern comes from the idea that sequencing naturally follows from the transfer of momentum from the proximal-to-distal limb segments just as the cracking of a whip results from a traveling wave of momentum and energy from the handle to the tip (Alexander 1991). Regardless of whether or not there is a clear mechanical explanation for this pattern, what is crucial for our argument is that muscle activation also follows this sequential pattern, as has been shown in throwing, kicking, and jumping (Bobbert and van Ingen Schenau 1988; Putnam 1993; Hirashima et al. 2002). Interestingly, computer modeling studies of overarm throwing have demonstrated that maximal throwing speed occurs at a specific delay between proximal and distal muscle activation: approximately 100 ms between shoulder flexor and rotator muscles (Alexander 1991), and approximately 50 ms between elbow extensors and wrist flexors (Chowdhary and Challis 1999).

TOPOGRAPHY OF PRIMARY MOTOR CORTEX

The topographic organization of the primary motor cortex has been extensively debated for decades and is still not completely resolved. Although a gross somatotopy segregates leg, arm, and face representations in the medial to lateral direction, it is still controversial whether a more refined somatotopy exists within the arm area that defines distinct representations of the shoulder, elbow, wrist, and fingers. Some studies in humans as well as nonhuman primates have suggested highly distributed, overlapping representations of different parts of the forelimb (Donoghue et al. 1992; Schieber and Hibbard 1993; Sanes et al. 1995). On the other hand, several intracortical microstimulation studies have indicated a horseshoe-like representation such that distal representations of the fingers and wrist are represented within a central core region surrounded by proximal representations of the shoulder and elbow joints. An early study that supported this organization monitored overt movement of the joints due to electrical stimulation (Kwan et al. 1978). More recently, another group performed a more quantitative and detailed analysis using stimulation-evoked EMG activity from 24 muscles of the arm and hand and found a similar organization of proximal and distal muscles within the motor cortex (Park et al. 2001; Park et al. 2004). For the purposes of this chapter, what is particularly interesting about this somatotopic organization lies mid-laterally along the rostral to caudal axis, such that proximal limbs are represented more rostrally on the precentral gyrus and extending into area 6 (i.e., the premotor cortex), whereas distal limb representations occur more caudally into the rostral bank of the central sulcus. For the broad class of motor behaviors that involve P-D sequencing as described earlier, this fine-scale somatotopic organization implies that more rostral portion of the motor cortex will be recruited before the more caudal portion buried within the central sulcus.

β LOCAL FIELD POTENTIAL OSCILLATIONS AND PROPAGATING WAVES

Oscillatory activity in the β frequency range (i.e., approximately between 13 and 35 Hz) is a prominent feature of motor cortical physiology that was observed by Berger in his early electroencephalograph (EEG) recordings but then well documented by Jasper (Jasper and Andrews 1936, 1938). More recently, local field potential (LFP) recordings from penetrating microelectrodes have recorded β oscillations in the primary and premotor cortices of nonhuman primates (Murthy and Fetz 1992; Sanes and Donoghue 1993). In contrast to single-neuron action potentials, LFPs represent the aggregate synaptic potentials from a spherical volume of neural tissue surrounding the electrode tip. Recent evidence suggests that the radius of this recording volume is relatively local (i.e., approximately 250 microns; Katzner et al. 2009). Oscillatory LFP activity arises when synaptic potentials in that volume synchronize with respect to each other on a fine time scale and oscillate on a broader time scale. Despite the extensive study of this phenomenon, the functional role, if any, of β oscillations remains elusive.

Two prevailing viewpoints exist, which ironically have very little to do with movement control per se. One hypothesis states that β oscillations signal a heightened level of attention or task engagement (Murthy and Fetz 1992; Donoghue et al. 1998; Saleh et al. 2010). Early evidence for this hypothesis came from the work of Murthy and Fetz, who observed short bouts (lasting between 100 and 200 ms each) of β LFP oscillations while monkeys either explored for raisins placed in recessed wells of a so-called Kluver board or were over-trained to perform a wrist flexion-extension task (Murthy and Fetz 1992, 1996). Although neither the amplitude nor the frequency of the β oscillations within each bout varied with task conditions, the frequency of occurrence of these bouts increased during the exploratory task as compared to the over-trained task, thus suggesting that β oscillations indicate a heighten level of attention, vigilance, or task engagement. A second hypothesis argues that β oscillations play a role in maintaining a fixed postural state and preventing movement based on experiments with normal monkeys and humans, as well as patients with Parkinson disease (Baker et al. 1999, 2001; Gilbertson et al. 2005; Kuhn et al. 2008; Williams and Baker 2009).

We propose an alternate hypothesis that β oscillations serve to facilitate the sequential recruitment of proximal and distal limb representations in motor cortex. Our hypothesis stems from our recent discovery that LFP oscillations in the β frequency range exhibit systematic phase shifts across different primary motor cortical (MI) sites horizontally, such that propagating waves of activity travel across the motor cortex. We employed microelectrode arrays that were implanted on the precentral gyri of nonhuman primates. Among a variety of complex wave patterns observed, we documented a common, linearly traveling wave pattern that propagates across the motor cortex along a rostral-to-caudal axis (Rubino et al. 2006). By sampling the wave directions at multiple time points in a data set, we often observed a bimodal distribution of wave directions, with a dominant peak corresponding to a rostral-to-caudal direction and a weaker, secondary peak corresponding to the caudal-to-rostral direction. Occasionally, a unimodal distribution was observed whose peak corresponded to the rostral-to-caudal direction. The distribution of propagation speeds was always unimodal, with a mean speed ranging from 10 to 50 cm/s depending on the animal and task.

Although we have not documented whether these waves travel across the entire primary motor cortex, we can speculate what implications a rostral-to-caudal wave would have for P-D sequencing. Assuming an average wave speed of approximately 20 cm/s and a motor cortical spatial extent of approximately 1 cm, each wave would travel from the rostral extent of MI near the border of area 6 to the caudal extent near the fundus of the central sulcus in approximately 50 ms. Because the LFP represents the aggregate synaptic potentials of neuropil surrounding the electrode tip, such a wave would facilitate the sequential recruitment of MI neurons representing shoulder and elbow movements on the precentral gyrus, followed by distal representations of the wrist and fingers buried in the central sulcus (see the section "Topography of Primary Motor Cortex") in 50 ms, which is, interestingly, the period of the β oscillation.

This time delay of approximately 50 ms is consistent with a study that examined sequential activation of distinct motor cortical populations in a monkey performing a button press task (Murphy et al. 1985). Using intracortical microstimulation, the authors first identified each electrode site as one that evoked proximal (i.e., shoulder or elbow) movements or distal (wrist and fingers) movements. They then recorded single units from these electrodes while the monkey reached out and pressed a button. They found that the mean modulation latency of units recorded from proximal electrode sites occurred approximately 60 ms earlier than that of units recorded on distal electrode sites. More importantly, in a few cases, the authors were able to simultaneously record from two units using paired electrodes, one of which evoked proximal movements while the other evoked distal movements via electrical stimulation. They found that the trial-by-trial modulation onset times of the two units were usually positively correlated, such that when one unit initiated its modulation later, the other would also and vice versa.

REACH-TO-GRASP

We have recently conducted a number of experiments involving unconstrained three-dimensional reaching and grasping to investigate whether P-D sequencing is also present in a more natural behavior such as reach-to-grasp and whether propagating waves of activity may play a role in facilitating this recruitment pattern. It should be noted that the propagating waves described earlier were observed in constrained behaviors in two dimensions that involved only the shoulder and elbow joints.

Method

Task

A female monkey (*Macaca mulatta*) was trained to reach out and grasp one of four possible objects: a sphere requiring a whole-hand grasp; a small, thin plate requiring a key grip; a small D-ring requiring a precision grip; and a large D-ring in two different orientations that involved a power grip. Each object was presented in one of seven different locations and distances from the monkey via a robot. On each trial, the monkey's hand pressed a button next to its body while an opaque screen blocked its vision as the robot moved the object to a specified location. As soon as the screen was removed, the monkey reached out to grasp the object and pull it, at which point the monkey was rewarded with juice.

Recordings

A six-camera Vicon 460 motion capture system recorded the kinematics (sampled at 250 Hz) of reflective markers placed on the upper torso, arm, and wrist in order to determine the joint angular position trajectories during the reach to grasp. We developed a right arm skeletal model using OpenSim (software developed by the National Institutes of Health [NIH] Center for Biomedical Computing and located at www.Simtk.org) to estimate the following seven different joint angle trajectories based on the marker trajectories: shoulder adduction/abduction, shoulder flexion/extension, shoulder rotation, elbow flexion/extension, forearm pronation/supination, wrist flexion/extension, and wrist adduction/abduction. The origin of the seven angle trajectories corresponds to a posture of the arm down by the body, such that the upper arm is adducted; the forearm is fully extended and semipronated, such that the palm is facing into the body; and the thumb is oriented toward the front. Increasing shoulder rotation and forearm pronation angles are in the counter-clockwise direction looking down from the shoulder. A third-order Butterworth low-pass filter with 30 Hz cutoff frequency was applied bidirectionally to each of the joint angle trajectories, which were then differentiated to compute the corresponding joint velocities. Local field potentials were recorded continuously at 2 KHz from a 100-electrode Utah microelectrode array (Blackrock Microsystems, Salt Lake City, UT) implanted in the primary motor cortex contralateral to the right arm. Each electrode was coated with iridium oxide at its tip and was 1.5 mm in length. The inter-electrode spacing of the array was 400 μm. Signals from up to 96 electrodes from each array were amplified (gain of 5,000), digitized, band-pass filtered between 0.3 and 500 Hz, and stored on disk using a Cerebus acquisition system (Blackrock Microsystems, Inc., UT).

Frequency Domain Analysis

Local field potential data were preprocessed first by removing all channels with errant means or clear movement artifacts and were then down sampled to 1 kHz. For each reach and grasp trial, unless otherwise noted, the LFP signal from each channel from 200 ms prior to the removal of the screen and 200 ms after the monkey grasped an object was analyzed. A sixth-order Butterworth low-pass filter with cutoff frequency of 100 Hz was applied bidirectionally for all valid channels. The mean power spectrum and spectrogram across all trials over all valid channels were computed using the multitaper method (Mitra and Pesaran 1999) with the time-bandwidth product of 2 and 3 tapers. To compute the mean spectrogram, LFP signals from 500 ms prior and 1,000 ms after a removal of the screen were used, and a 500 ms moving window with a 2 ms window step size were used.

Phase Calculations

We applied the Hilbert transform to extract the instantaneous phase of the LFP (Le Van Quyen et al. 2001). The Hilbert transform (*Hb*) of a real signal can be computed by convolving the signal with $1/\pi t$ in the time domain or by performing the equivalent operations in the frequency domain. $s(t)+iHb[s(t)]=a(t)e^{i\varphi(t)}$ is called the analytic signal of a real signal $s(t)$. The instantaneous phase of $s(t)$ is $\varphi(t)$, the instantaneous amplitude is $a(t)$, and the instantaneous frequency is $d\varphi/dt$.

For each trial, we band-pass filtered each channel of the LFP to obtain $V(x,y,t)$, the local β field potential at point (x, y) on the array at time t. We applied the Hilbert transform to the signal on each (x, y) channel to obtain the instantaneous amplitude, $a(x,y,t)$, and the instantaneous phase, $\varphi(x, y, t)$:

$$V(x,y,t)+i\,Hb[V(x,y,t)]=a(x,y,t)e^{i\varphi(x,y,t)} \quad \text{(Eq. 1)}$$

Velocity

We defined the velocity of coherent activity to be the velocity of the contours of constant phase (Fleet and Jepson 1990). Let $\varphi(x,y,t)$ be the phase of β activity at time t and coordinates x and y of the multielectrode array. The velocity, $v = (dx/dt, dy/dt)$ was computed by taking the total derivative of $\varphi(x,y,t)$ with respect to time:

$$d\varphi/dt=\nabla\varphi\cdot\mathrm{v}+\partial\varphi/\partial t=0 \quad \text{(Eq. 2)}$$

The velocity direction, which is perpendicular to the phase contours, is $-\nabla\varphi$. The velocity magnitude or speed is $\frac{\partial\varphi}{\partial t}/\|\nabla\varphi\|$. Velocity is only well-defined when the phase gradient is not zero and when the signal exhibits a "coherent" propagation direction. We define the phase gradient directionality, *PGD*(*t*), to measure how well phase gradients align across the array at each time point:

$$PGD(t)=\|\overline{\nabla\varphi}\|/\overline{\|\nabla\varphi\|} \quad \text{(Eq. 3)}$$

The bar denotes the spatial average at a fixed time. If the phase gradients at all spatial points on the array align at time *t*, *PGD*(*t*) will be 1. On the other hand, if the phase gradients are randomly distributed, *PGD* will be close to zero. Estimates of wave direction and speed were based on times for which

$PGD(t) > 0.5$ for at least 10 ms continuously. When the phase gradients are well-aligned across the array, the direction of the velocity is well-estimated by $-\overline{\nabla\varphi}$ and the speed by:

$$speed(t) = \left|\overline{(\partial\varphi / \partial t)}\right| / \left\|\overline{\nabla\varphi}\right\| \quad \text{(Eq. 4)}$$

Results

We focused our analysis on data from one recording session involving a total of 52 reach-to-grasp trials to four of the seven possible locations, involving between two and four objects per location. We observed stereotyped temporal patterns in the joint angle trajectories of seven degrees of freedom of the arm and wrist during the reach-to-grasp task (Fig. 7.1). The mean (standard deviation) reaction time (i.e., the time from the removal of the opaque screen and movement onset defined as button release) was 226 (109) ms and the mean (standard deviation) movement time (i.e., time from movement onset to object contact) was 404 (74) ms. We focused our analysis on shoulder, elbow, and wrist flexion/extension joint velocities for reach-to-grasp movements. By examining the relative timing in peak velocity across these three joint angles, a proximal-to-distal sequence is evident for reach-to-grasp to one object in one location (Fig. 7.2A). Shoulder flexion velocity reaches a peak value at approximately 100 ms after the onset of movement, followed by peak elbow extension velocity at 150–200 ms after movement onset, and finally peak wrist flexion velocity at between 200 and 250 ms after movement onset. This pattern remained relatively invariant despite variations in object type and location (Fig. 7.2B). The median time delay between shoulder and elbow flexion/extension peak velocities was 48 ms, and between elbow and wrist flexion peak velocities was 60 ms. The total median time delay between shoulder and wrist peak velocities was 112 ms (Fig. 7.3A). More importantly, trial-by-trial comparisons in timing between peak joint velocities indicated a significant positive correlations between all pairs of joints ($p < 0.05$, t-test on Fisher z-transformed correlation) (Fig. 7.3B). That is, if the shoulder peak velocity occurred later with respect to its mean on a given trial, the elbow and wrist peak velocities likewise occurred later than their respective means. The mean time differences, together with the significant correlations, constitute a sequential coordination pattern that we speculate may have a cortical origin.

To begin to test the hypothesis that cortical wave propagation plays a role in this coordination pattern, we examined LFP oscillations that occurred during the reach-to-grasp task. The power spectrum of the LFP recorded during the task on all electrodes reveals a local peak in power at 20 Hz residing in the β frequency range (Fig. 7.4A). A spectrogram aligned on removal of the opaque screen reveals that β power begins before movement onset and continues throughout the movement, with an attenuation at object grasp (Fig. 7.4B).

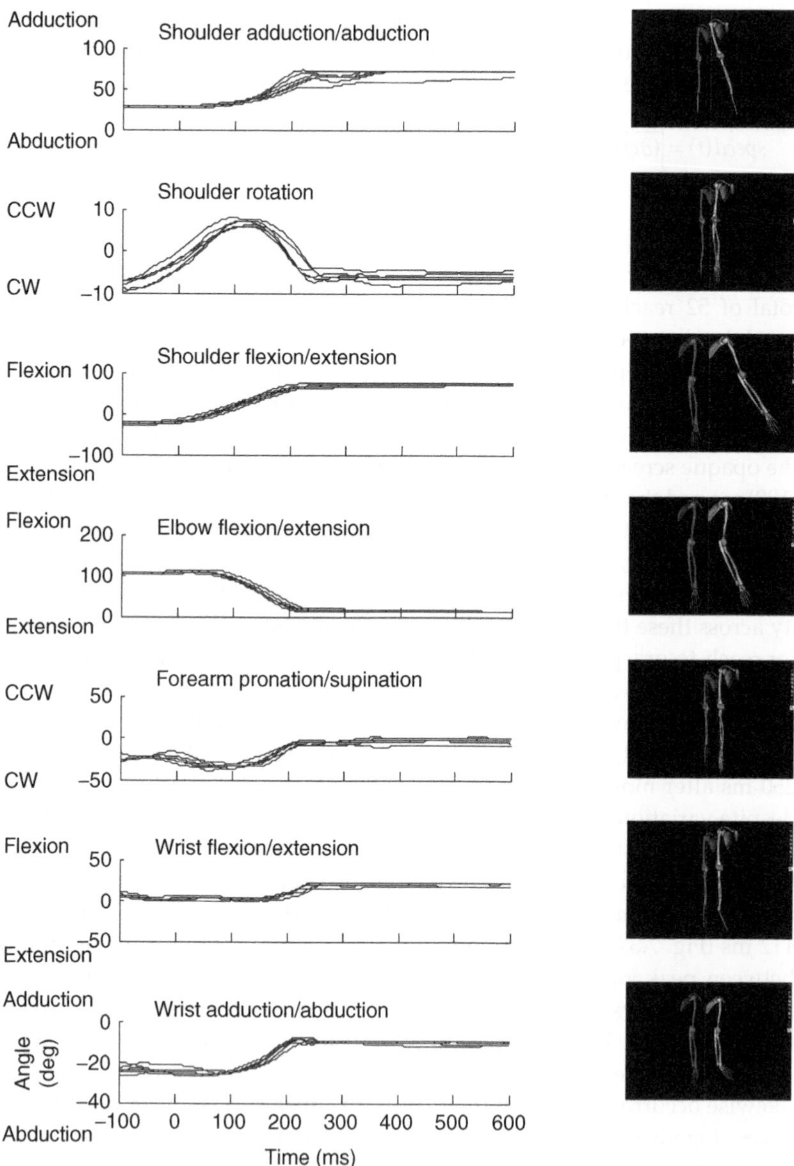

Figure 7.1 **Left panels**: Seven trials of joint angle trajectories for seven degrees of freedom during the reach and grasping of one object placed in one location. **Right panels**: For each joint angle, the arm posture at the origin of the joint angle coordinate system is shown as well as a posture corresponding to a positive value for that joint angle.

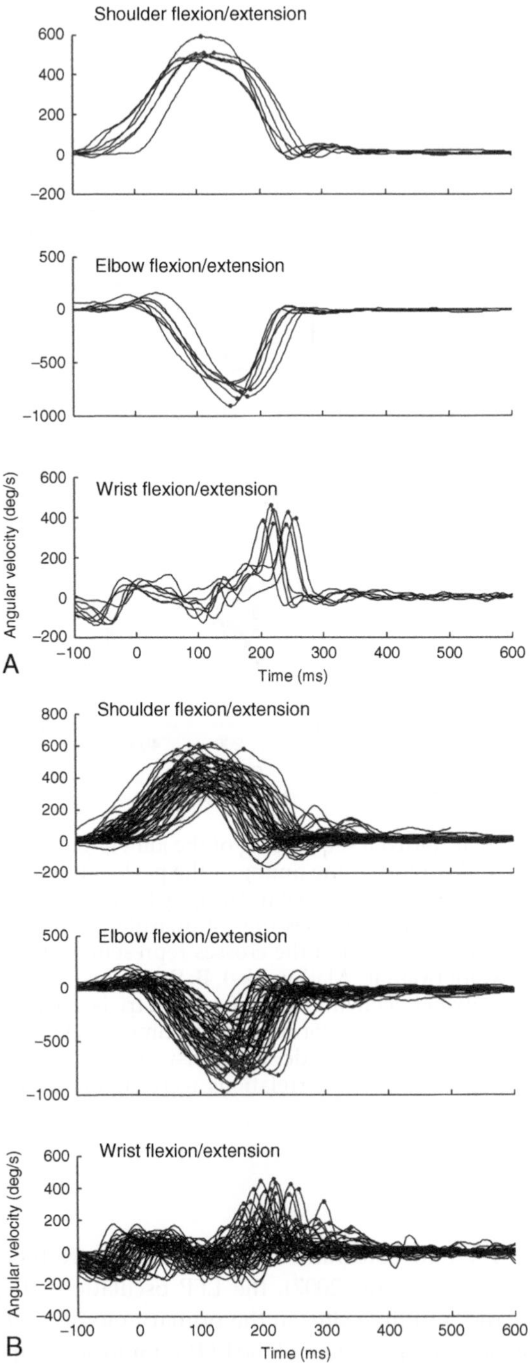

Figure 7.2 Shoulder, elbow, and wrist flexion/extension velocity trajectories to **A**, one object in one location and **B**, to many objects (up to five objects) in four locations. The black dots indicate the peak velocities on each trial. Positive angular velocities correspond to the flexion direction.

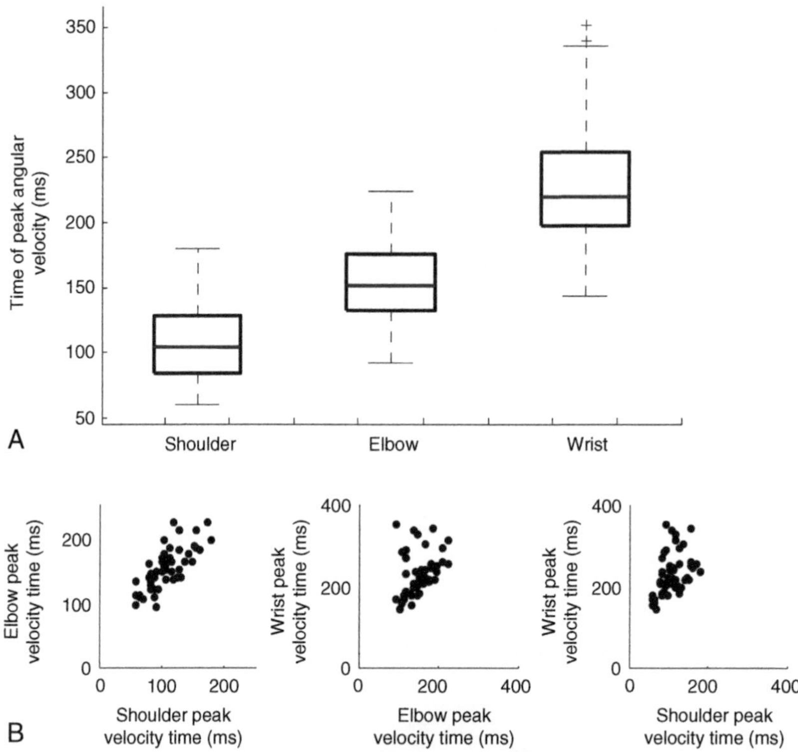

Figure 7.3 Proximal-to-distal sequencing of the joint angular velocities during reach-to-grasp. **A**: Box plots of the timing of the peak joint velocities for shoulder, elbow, and wrist flexion/extension. The gray horizontal line represents the median, the black box encompasses the 1st quartile around the median, the whiskers plot the data range, and the crosses represent outliers as defined by the function, Boxplot (Matlab, Mathworks). **B**: Scatter plots relating the timing in peak joint velocity between limb joints for all 52 trials. Each point represents a single trial. The trial-by-trial correlations in timing between shoulder and elbow, elbow and wrist, and shoulder and wrist joint peak velocities was 0.75, 0.34, and 0.42, respectively. All correlations were significantly different from zero ($p < 0.05$, t-test).

As we observed in constrained reaching tasks (Rubino et al. 2006; Takahashi and Hatsopoulos 2007), the LFP oscillations displayed wave propagation across multiple sites in the primary motor cortex (Fig. 7.5A). By computing the spatial gradient of the LFP at multiple sample time points and using a measure of linear wave propagation (PGD or phase gradient directionality; see "Methods"), we found that most samples of linear wave propagation travelled along one dominant direction (i.e., 270 degrees on the array) corresponding to a rostral-to-caudal direction along the

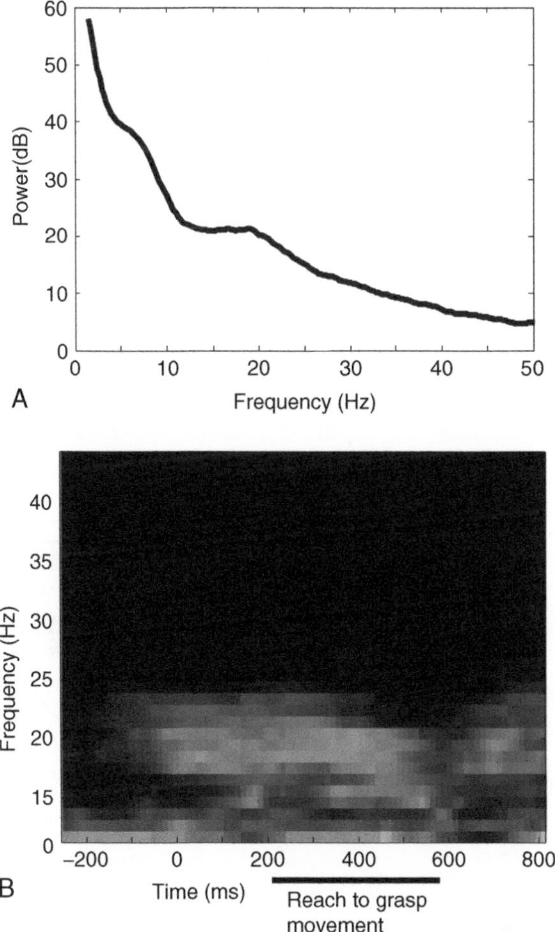

Figure 7.4 Spectral analysis of the local field potential (LFP) recorded in MI. **A**: The LFP power spectrum computed by averaging the spectra over multiple trials of the reach-to-grasp task and then averaging over 61 electrode sites. Data were taken from movement onset to object grasp. **B**: A gray-scale spectrogram averaged over trials and channels showing the temporal dynamics of power of the reach-to-grasp behavior. White indicates higher power than black. Time zero represent the time at which the opaque screen is removed. The horizontal line denotes the approximate duration of the reach-to-grasp movement from movement onset to object grasp.

precentral gyrus (Fig. 7.5B). These linear waves traveled over a narrow range of speeds from less than 10 cm/s up to 60 cm/s, with a median speed of 19 cm/s (Fig. 7.5C). Assuming that these waves propagate at that median speed across the entire motor cortex, a given wave would traverse the entire arm area of MI in approximately 50 ms.

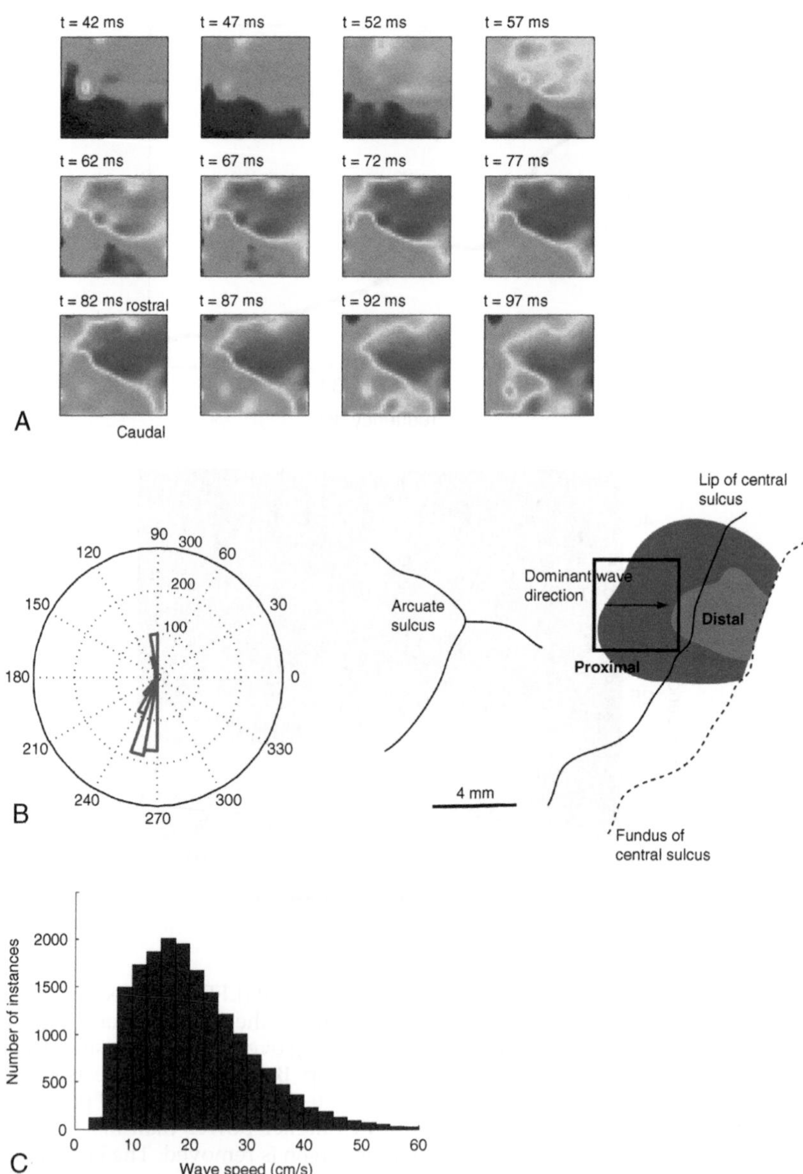

Figure 7.5 Wave propagation in the beta frequency range of the local field potential (LFP) across MI during the reach-to-grasp task. **A**: An example of one instance of an LFP wave propagating across the primary MI in the rostral to caudal direction (i.e., downward). To visualize this wave, the voltage signal on each channel was band pass-filtered between 10–45 Hz, normalized such that the maximum and minimum voltage values were set to 1 and –1, respectively, and then color coded, where red is a positive value and blue is a negative value. Time is measured with respect to the visual onset of the object (i.e., removal of the opaque screen). **B:** Left, the distribution of wave directions across many

CONCLUSION

We have put forth a hypothesis that propagating wave activity in the MI may play a role in sequentially recruiting proximal and distal representations at the cortical level, resulting in the pervasive P-D sequencing pattern in motor behavior. We have documented that such a sequencing pattern occurs in reach-to-grasp behavior and that concurrently propagating LFP waves in MI travel predominantly in the rostral-to-caudal direction. Given the proximal/distal topography in the MI described earlier, this provides indirect evidence that these waves may recruit proximal representations before distal ones. Moreover, the speed of wave propagation results in a time delay of approximately 50 ms between the rostral and caudal portions of the MI, which is consistent with the delay in onset times of proximal versus distal cortical sites (Murphy et al. 1985).

We are still missing, however, more direct evidence that these propagating waves participate in P-D sequencing. First, if there exists a direct relationship between cortical wave propagation and this coordination pattern, it will be more clearly seen by measuring muscle activity via EMG electrodes as opposed to joint kinematics. The motor cortex ultimately affects muscle activation and does not uniquely specify the motions of the joints because of a variety of biomechanical complexities at the periphery, including interaction torques, external torques and forces, and the length- and velocity-tension characteristics of muscles. Our analysis of the timing in peak joint velocities emphasizes this point by indicating that the time delay between the shoulder and wrist motions is over 80% slower than the time it takes the propagating wave to traverse the entire motor cortex.

Secondly, a moment-by-moment correspondence between the LFP wavefront and muscle activities of the shoulder, elbow, and wrist would provide more direct evidence for our hypothesis. For example, does the cortical wave speed vary with the recruitment delay between shoulder and wrist muscles on a trial-by-trial basis? Can the wave direction be altered by setting up different coordination patterns, such as the distal-to-proximal sequencing that is observed during postural reactions to perturbations (Latash et al. 1995)?

Last, the LFP is an aggregate measure of subthreshold, synaptic potentials near the electrode tip and, therefore, is not a direct measure of output spiking from individual MI neurons that would ultimately be responsible for exciting those motor units in the spinal cord that activate proximal and

Figure 7.5 (*Continued*) instances of linear wave propagation using a threshold PGD value of 0.5 (see Methods). Right, the direction of the dominant wave direction plotted on a schematic of the flattened motor cortex showing the proximal and distal topography. The square box represents the 4 × 4 mm multielectrode array. **C**: The distribution of wave speeds across many samples of linear wave propagation using the same PGD threshold. (See color plate.)

distal musculature. Therefore, it will be important to demonstrate that motor cortical neurons fire in a sequential order matching the temporal dynamics of the LFP wave.

Understanding the neural basis of motor coordination, in general, remains a fundamental challenge in motor control. Of particular interest is the cortical contribution to planning and execution of voluntary coordination patterns. In this chapter, we have focused on a relatively simple sequencing pattern of the arm and restricted our attention to cortical waves with linear wave fronts. However, in the future, it will be important to explore other more complex arm coordination patterns, as well as coordination of the fingers, of both arms, and other body segments. Characterizing more complex spatiotemporal patterns of cortical activity will be made possible with more sophisticated mathematical and statistical methods, as well as with advances in recording technologies that include higher-density multielectrode arrays and optical recording.

REFERENCES

Alexander, R.M. 1991. Optimum timing of muscle activation for simple models of throwing. *Journal of Theoretical Biology* 150: 349–72.

Atwater, A.E. 1979. Biomechanics of overarm throwing movements and of throwing injuries. *Exercise and Sport Science Review* 7: 43–85.

Baker, S.N., J.M. Kilner, E.M. Pinches, and R. Lemon. 1999. The role of synchrony and oscillations in the motor output. *Experimental Brain Research* 128: 109–17.

Baker, S.N., R. Spinks, A. Jackson, and R.N. Lemon. 2001. Synchronization in monkey motor cortex during a precision grip task. I. Task-dependent modulation in single-unit synchrony. *Journal of Neurophysiology* 85: 869–85.

Bartlett, R.M., E. Muller, S. Lindinger, F. Brunner, and C. Morriss. 1996. Three-dimensional evaluation of the kinematic release parameters for javelin throwers of different skill levels. *Journal of Applied Biomechanics* 12: 58–71.

Bobbert, M.F., and G.J. van Ingen Schenau. 1988. Coordination in vertical jumping. *Journal of Biomechanics* 21: 249–62.

Bronner, S., and S. Ojofeitimi. 2006. Gender and limb differences in healthy elite dancers: passe kinematics. *Journal of Motion and Behavior* 38: 71–79.

Cheney, P.D., and E.E. Fetz. 1980. Functional classes of primate corticomotoneuronal cells and their relation to active force. *Journal of Neurophysiology* 44: 773–91.

Chowdhary, A.G., and J.H. Challis. 1999. Timing accuracy in human throwing. *Journal of Theoretical Biology* 201: 219–29.

Donoghue, J.P., S. Leibovic, and J.N. Sanes. 1992. Organization of the forelimb area in squirrel monkey motor cortex: Representation of digit, wrist, and elbow muscles. *Experimental Brain Research* 89: 1–19.

Donoghue, J.P., J.N. Sanes, N.G. Hatsopoulos, and G. Gaal. 1998. Neural discharge and local field potential oscillations in primate motor cortex during voluntary movements. *Journal of Neurophysiology* 77: 159–73.

Elliott, B., and T. Marsh. 1989. A biomechanical comparison of the topspin and backspin forehand approach shots in tennis. *Journal of Sports Science* 7: 215–27.

Elliott, B., R. Marshall, and G. Noffal. 1995. Contributions of upper limb segment rotations during the power serve in tennis. *Journal of Applied Biomechanics* 11: 433–42.

Elliott, B., R. Marshall, and G. Noffal. 1996. The role of upper limb segment rotations in the development of racket-head speed in the squash forehand. *Journal of Sports Science* 14: 159–65.

Elliott, B.C., and J. Armour. 1988. The penalty throw in water polo: a cinematographic analysis. *Journal of Sports Science* 6: 103–14.

Evarts, E.V. 1964. Temporal patterns of discharge of pyramidal tract neurons during sleep and waking in the monkey. *Journal of Neurophysiology* 27: 152–71.

Evarts, E.V. 1966. Pyramidal tract activity associated with a conditioned hand movement in the monkey. *Journal of Neurophysiology* 29: 1011–27.

Evarts, E.V. 1968. Relation of pyramidal tract activity to force exerted during voluntary movement. *Journal of Neurophysiology* 31: 14–27.

Fleet, D.J., and A.D. Jepson. 1990. Computation of component image velocity from local phase information. *International Journal of Computer Vision* 5: 77–104.

Furuya, S, and H. Kinoshita. 2007. Roles of proximal-to-distal sequential organization of the upper limb segments in striking the keys by expert pianists. *Neuroscience Letters* 421: 264–69.

Georgopoulos, A.P., R. Caminiti, and J.F. Kalaska. 1984. Static spatial effects in motor cortex and area 5: Quantitative relations in a two-dimensional space. *Experimental Brain Research* 54: 446–54.

Georgopoulos, A.P., J.F. Kalaska, R. Caminiti, and J.T. Massey. 1982. On the relations between the direction of two-dimensional arm movements and cell discharge in primate motor cortex. *Journal of Neuroscience* 2: 1527–37.

Gilbertson, T., E. Lalo, L. Doyle, V. Di Lazzaro, B. Cioni, and P. Brown. 2005. Existing motor state is favored at the expense of new movement during 13–35 Hz oscillatory synchrony in the human corticospinal system. *Journal of Neuroscience* 25: 7771–79.

Hirashima, M., H. Kadota, S. Sakurai, K. Kudo, and T. Ohtsuki. 2002. Sequential muscle activity and its functional role in the upper extremity and trunk during overarm throwing. *Journal of Sports Science* 20: 301–10.

Jasper, H., and H. Andrews. 1936. Human brain rhythms. I. Recording techniques and preliminary results. *Journal of General Psychology* 14: 98–126.

Jasper, H., and H. Andrews. 1938. Electroencephalography. III. Normal differentiation of occipital and precentral regions in man. *Archives of Neurology and Psychiatry* 39: 96–115.

Joris, H.J., A.J. van Muyen, G.J. van Ingen Schenau, and H.C. Kemper. 1985. Force, velocity and energy flow during the overarm throw in female handball players. *Journal of Biomechanics* 18: 409–14.

Katzner, S., I. Nauhaus, A. Benucci, V. Bonin, D.L. Ringach, and M. Carandini. 2009. Local origin of field potentials in visual cortex. *Neuron* 61: 35–41.

Kuhn, A.A., F. Kempf, C. Brucke, L. Gaynor Doyle, I. Martinez-Torres, A. Pogosyan, et al. 2008. High-frequency stimulation of the subthalamic nucleus suppresses oscillatory beta activity in patients with Parkinson's disease in parallel with improvement in motor performance. *Journal of Neuroscience* 28: 6165–73.

Kwan, H.C., W.A. MacKay, J.T. Murphy, and Y.C. Wong. 1978. Spatial organization of precentral cortex in awake primates. II. Motor outputs. *Journal of Neurophysiology* 41: 1120–31.

Latash, M.L., A.S. Aruin, I. Neyman, and J.J. Nicholas. 1995. Anticipatory postural adjustments during self inflicted and predictable perturbations in Parkinson's disease. *Journal of Neurology, Neurosurgery, and Psychiatry* 58: 326–34.

Le Van Quyen, M., J. Foucher, J. Lachaux, E. Rodriguez, A. Lutz, J. Martinerie, and F.J. Varela. 2001. Comparison of Hilbert transform and wavelet methods for the analysis of neuronal synchrony. *Journal of Neuroscience Methods* 111: 83–98.

Milburn, P.D. 1982. Summation of segmental velocities in the golf swing. *Medicine and Science in Sports and Exercise* 14: 60–64.

Mitra, P.P., and B. Pesaran. 1999. Analysis of dynamic brain imaging data. *Biophysical Journal* 76: 691–708.

Moran, D.W., and A.B. Schwartz. 1999. Motor cortical representation of speed and direction during reaching. *Journal of Neurophysiology* 82: 2676–92.

Murphy, J.T., Y.C. Wong, and H.C. Kwan. 1985. Sequential activation of neurons in primate motor cortex during unrestrained forelimb movement. *Journal of Neurophysiology* 53(2): 435–45.

Murthy, V.N., and E.E. Fetz. 1992. Coherent 25- to 35-Hz oscillations in the sensorimotor cortex of awake behaving monkeys. *Proceedings of the National Academy of Science U S A* 89: 5670–74.

Murthy, V.N., and E.E. Fetz. 1996. Oscillatory activity in sensorimotor cortex of awake monkeys: synchronization of local field potentials and relation to behavior. *Journal of Neurophysiology* 76: 3949–67.

Paninski, L., M.R. Fellows, N.G. Hatsopoulos, and J.P. Donoghue. 2004. Spatiotemporal tuning of motor cortical neurons for hand position and velocity. *Journal of Neurophysiology* 91: 515–32.

Pappas, A.M., R.M. Zawacki, and T.J. Sullivan. 1985. Biomechanics of baseball pitching. A preliminary report. *American Journal of Sports Medicine* 13: 216–22.

Park, M.C., A. Belhaj-Saif, and P.D. Cheney. 2004. Properties of primary motor cortex output to forelimb muscles in rhesus macaques. *Journal of Neurophysiology* 92: 2968–84.

Park, M.C., A. Belhaj-Saif, M. Gordon, and P.D. Cheney. 2001. Consistent features in the forelimb representation of primary motor cortex in rhesus macaques. *Journal of Neuroscience* 21: 2784–92.

Putnam, C.A. 1993. Sequential motions of body segments in striking and throwing skills: descriptions and explanations. *Journal of Biomechanics* 26 Suppl 1: 125–35.

Rubino, D., K.A. Robbins, and N.G. Hatsopoulos. 2006. Propagating waves mediate information transfer in the motor cortex. *Nature Neuroscience* 9: 1549–57.

Saleh, M., Reimer, J., Penn, R.D., Ojakangas, C.L., Hatsopoulos, N.G. 2010. Fast and slow oscillations in human primary motor cortex predict oncoming behaviorally relevant cues. *Neuron*, 65: 461–471.

Sanes, J.N., and J.P. Donoghue. 1993. Oscillations in local field potentials of the primate motor cortex during voluntary movement. *Proceedings of the National Academy of Science U S A* 90: 4470–74.

Sanes, J.N., J.P. Donoghue, V. Thangaraj, R.R. Edelman, and S. Warach. 1995. Shared neural substrates controlling hand movements in human motor cortex. *Science* 268: 1775–77.

Schieber, M.H., and L.S. Hibbard. 1993. How somatotopic is the motor cortex hand area? *Science* 261: 489–92.

Smith, A.M., M.C. Hepp-Reymond, and U.R. Wyss. 1975. Relation of activity in precentral cortical neurons to force and rate of force change during isometric contractions of finger muscles. *Experimental Brain Research* 23: 315–32.

Taira, M., J. Boline, N. Smyrnis, A.P. Georgopoulos, and J. Ashe. 1996. On the relations between single cell activity in the motor cortex and the direction and magnitude of three-dimensional static isometric force. *Experimental Brain Research* 109: 367–76.

Takahashi, K., and N.G. Hatsopoulos. 2007. Copropagating waves of local field potentials and single-unit spiking in motor cortex. 37th Annual Meeting of the Society for Neuroscience, San Diego, CA.

Williams, E.R., and S.N. Baker. 2009. Circuits generating corticomuscular coherence investigated using a biophysically based computational model. I. Descending systems. *Journal of Neurophysiology* 101: 31–41.

Zatsiorsky, V.M., G.E. Lanka, and A.A. Shalmanov. 1981. Biomechanical analysis of shot putting technique. *Exercise and Sport Sciences Review* 9: 353–89.

Part 3

Lessons from Biomechanics

8

The Biomechanics of Movement Control

Walter Herzog

One of the most basic problems in biomechanics is the *distribution problem* (Crowninshield and Brand 1981a). The distribution problem deals with the determination of the individual muscle forces that contribute to movements. For example, what are the lower limb muscle forces that produce human locomotion? On the surface, such a question seems straightforward and an answer easy to obtain, but that is not the case, because human and animal musculoskeletal systems tend to be redundant. That is, they contain many more muscles than are strictly necessary to accomplish a task.

Misiaszek and Pearson (2002) nicely demonstrated *redundancies* of the cat hindlimb musculature. They found that cat locomotion was not altered by elimination of the soleus muscle through botulinum toxin injections, and also showed that eliminating the soleus, plantaris, and lateral gastrocnemius simultaneously, although producing an observable gait alteration initially, could be compensated for by increased medial gastrocnemius activity and full gait recovery within days. This is just one of many examples demonstrating that elimination of selected muscles might not produce visible alterations in a movement, or, in other words, movements can be produced with a variety of different muscle activation strategies. One of the key questions then becomes: What is the true muscle activation strategy chosen by the neuromusculoskeletal system for a given movement under normal circumstances, and what is the underlying reason for that choice?

For human locomotion, it has been argued for more than a century that minimizing the *metabolic cost* of transport is likely the basic principle that governs muscle coordination patterns (Weber and Weber 1836). From an evolutionary point of view, this is an appealing proposal, and it is supported to a certain degree by the observation that constraints imposed on free human gait, such as artificially changing the preferred stride length or stride frequency for a given speed of walking or running, is typically associated with an increase in metabolic cost (Bertram and Ruina 2001). Further evidence for this notion comes from animal and human studies in which gait transitions (for example, from walking to running), appear to occur at speeds at which one gait pattern (walking) becomes metabolically more costly than another pattern (running) when speed is increased (Hoyt and Taylor 1981; Alexander 1989).

However, when analyzing how movements are executed and, perhaps more importantly in the context of this chapter, how they are controlled, we must never forget the *mechanics* of the target system. After all, when we move, we interact with the outside world either by moving objects or by exerting forces on our static environment. When walking, humans and animals produce characteristic patterns of ground reaction forces. These forces vary in magnitude and direction during the stance phase of locomotion, and they represent the combined action of the muscular forces of the whole system. For a given leg geometry at a distinct phase of stance during gait, activation of a single muscle produces a ground reaction force in a precisely defined direction (Kaya et al. 2006). However, that direction will typically not coincide with that of the total ground reaction force required for smooth gait, thus other muscles must be activated to not only control the magnitude but also the direction of the ground reaction force. Thus, locomotion is not only accomplished by producing a set of net joint moments, but also by controlling the forces we impose on the ground. A given ankle moment can be achieved with a variety of different combinations of muscle forces, but these combinations do not necessarily produce the same ground reaction force. Similarly, when we analyze arm movements, as is often done in motor control studies, and the direction of arm movement is described along the plane of a table, the muscles that can contribute to that motion (rather than hindering it) are not arbitrary, and some muscles, when activated, will produce a force vector more aligned with the intended movement direction than other muscles. It seems intuitive that muscles that have a "mechanical" advantage would be recruited more readily than those whose movement direction is far from that of the desired movement.

Finally, muscles have different functional and mechanical *properties*. For example, the force-length (Gordon et al. 1966) and force-velocity properties (Hill 1938) determine a muscle's instantaneous force capabilities, and must be considered when analyzing movement control. Imagine a muscle that is perfectly suited to perform a certain movement based on its anatomical location, but it is shortening so fast during a given movement task, or might be so short, that it cannot produce any force. Therefore, its contribution to that movement is zero even if it was activated maximally, and the metabolic cost of activating a muscle that cannot produce force or work is wasted.

So, how can we analyze movements and learn about movement control strategies? In biomechanics, there have been two basic approaches to this problem: the first is by direct *measurement of the muscle forces* during movements, and inferring underlying control strategies from those measurements; and the second is by theoretical modeling and *predictions of individual muscle forces* during movement. In this chapter, I briefly discuss both of these approaches and attempt to summarize some of the lessons learned. In the discussion of muscle force measurements, I will primarily focus on those involving the hindlimb musculature of the cat, as this is the most extensively studied experimental system. For the discussion of theoretical approaches used to predict individual muscle forces, I will concentrate on mathematical optimization, as this is the most often used and most heavily discussed theoretical approach in the biomechanics field dealing with movement control. The lessons learned from both these approaches are that the mechanics of muscle action and the mechanical properties of muscles are strong determinants on how force-sharing occurs among synergistic muscles.

DIRECT MUSCLE FORCE MEASUREMENTS

Probably the first systematic measurements of muscle forces in a freely moving system were the recordings of soleus and medial gastrocnemius (MG) forces in the freely moving cat by Walmsley et al. (1978). They used buckle-type tendon force transducers on the separated tendons of soleus and MG and indwelling, fine wire electromyographic (EMG) electrodes to measure the forces and activation patterns for standing still, walking, trotting, galloping, and jumping. They demonstrated that peak soleus forces remained nearly constant across speeds of locomotion ranging from 0.6 to 3.0 m/s, and were slightly decreased from the locomotion values for standing still and jumping (Fig. 8.1). In contrast, MG forces increased steadily with increasing speeds of locomotion, as expected, and quadrupled during jumping from the values observed at the highest running speeds (Fig. 8.1). They interpreted this force-sharing behavior in view of the fiber type distribution of these two muscles: the soleus being composed virtually 100% of slow (Ariano et al. 1973; Burke et al. 1974) and the MG being primarily composed of fast twitch motor units (Burke and Tsairis 1973; Ariano et al. 1973). They argued that the slow soleus muscle was primarily responsible for static and slow movement tasks, and was recruited near its maximum even for slow locomotion, whereas the MG was primarily recruited for fast and powerful bursts of activity and was only recruited to a small degree during walking and slow running. Hodgson (Hodgson 1983) repeated the study by Walmsley et al. (1978) and interpreted the finding that soleus forces become smaller with increasing movement speed or power production (Fig. 8.2), with the idea that the slow motor units of the soleus muscle might be selectively deactivated at fast speeds of movements, and he implicated rubrospinal and cutaneous pathways for producing this selective inhibition.

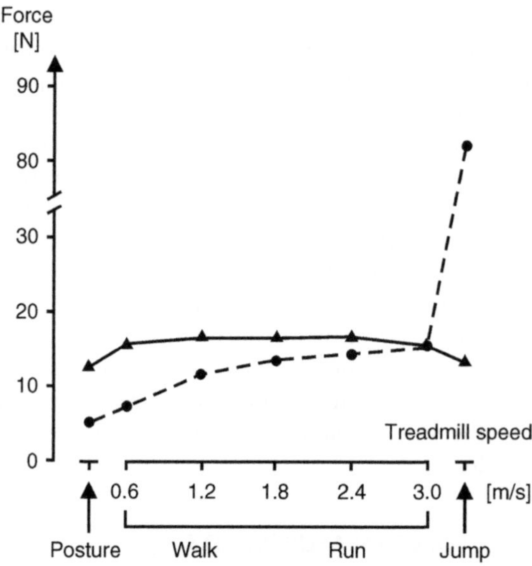

Figure 8.1 Forces in the cat soleus (▲ solid line) and medial gastrocnemius (• dashed line) for postural, locomotor and jumping activities). The soleus forces remain relatively constant across all locomotor tasks, while the medial gastrocnemius forces increase continuously with increasing speeds of locomotion and quadruple from running to jumping. Note how the force contribution is greater for soleus for "slow, static" movement conditions, while force contributions are dominated by the medial gastrocnemius for the "powerful" jumping activities. Adapted from Walmsley, B., J.A. Hodgson, and R.E. Burke. 1978. Forces produced by medial gastrocnemius and soleus muscles during locomotion in freely moving cats. *Journal of Neurophysiology* 41: 1203–15, with permission of the publisher.

While analyzing the force-sharing behavior of the soleus, MG, plantaris, and tibialis anterior in the cat hindlimb (Herzog et al. 1993), we found that force sharing in the ankle extensor group could vary from one extreme to the other. For standing still, it was possible to observe soleus forces and EMG activity in the absence of MG forces and activation, whereas for paw-shaking, a response elicited in cats by either attaching a piece of sticky tape to the toes of the hindlimb or immersing the foot into water, soleus activation was typically small, sometimes completely absent, whereas MG (Herzog 1998) or lateral gastrocnemius forces/EMG were high (Smith et al. 1980) (Fig. 8.3).

Another example of a counter-intuitive behavior of synergistic musculature can be observed during cat jumping, and measuring the contributions of soleus and MG to this motion. As the cat prepares for jumping, soleus forces are relatively high, whereas MG forces are intermediate (Fig. 8.4). At the onset of the propulsive phase of jumping, soleus activation is dramatically decreased, and soleus force becomes zero approximately 40 ms prior

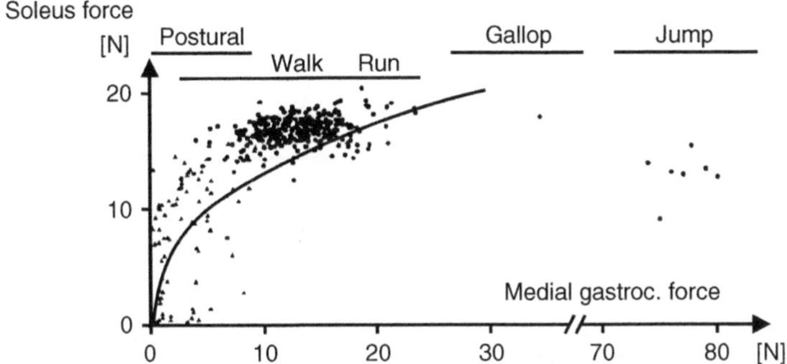

Figure 8.2 Peak soleus versus medial gastrocnemius forces for a variety of locomotor activities of the cat. Note the dominant soleus forces for postural tasks and slow walking and the decrease in soleus forces for jumping. Furthermore, note the dramatic increase in medial gastrocnemius forces with increasing speeds of locomotion and jumping. The solid line approximating the experimental data points is an attempt to predict the force sharing between cat soleus and gastrocnemius using a "minimization" of fatigue cost function that accounts for the fiber type distribution of these two muscles in the cost function as proposed by Dul et al. (1984). Adapted from Walmsley, B., J.A. Hodgson, and R.E. Burke. 1978. Forces produced by medial gastrocnemius and soleus muscles during locomotion in freely moving cats. Journal of Neurophysiology 41: 1203–15.

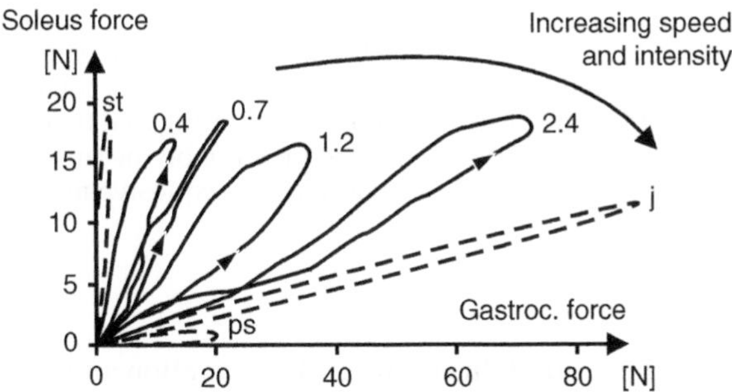

Figure 8.3 Force sharing curves for the cat soleus and medial gastrocnemius. The solid lines represent different locomotor speeds: 0.4, 0.7, and 1.2 m/s walking and 2.4 m/s trotting, whereas the dashed lines represent postural tasks (st = standing still), jumping (j), and paw shake response (ps). Note how for postural tasks, medial gastrocnemius forces are virtually silent and soleus forces are high, whereas for paw shaking, soleus forces are silent (there is no electromyographic activity and the small forces observed are passive) and medial gastrocnemius forces are substantial.

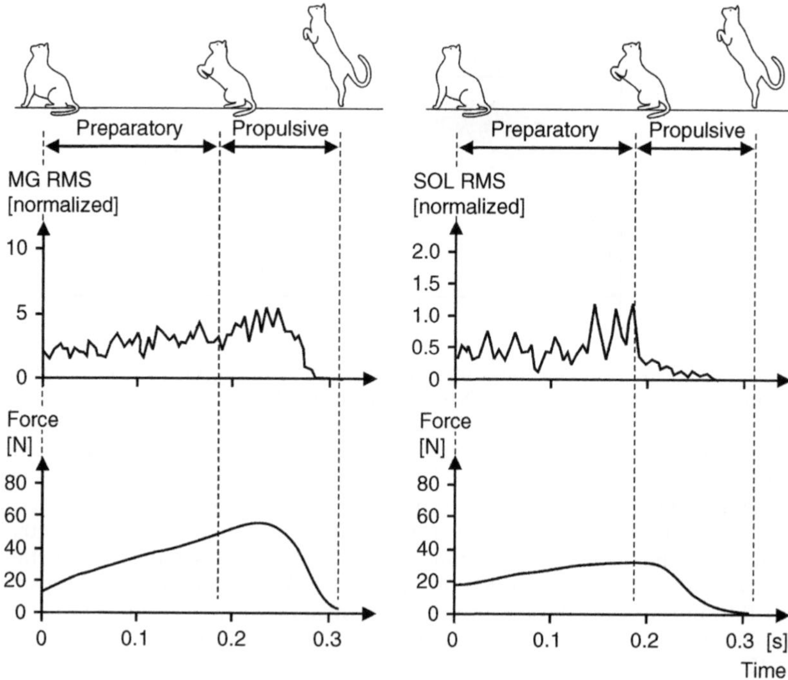

Figure 8.4 Root mean square (RMS) values of the electromyographic activity and force-time histories for cat medial gastrocnemius (MG, *left panel*) and soleus (Sol, *right panel*) during the preparation and propulsive phase of cat jumping. Note that MG activity is increased initially and then maintained for most of the propulsive phase whereas soleus activity is abolished at the beginning of the propulsive phase. Similarly, MG force becomes zero at the end of the propulsive phase, as one would expect, whereas soleus force becomes nearly zero much before the end of the propulsive phase, indicating that there is a deactivation of soleus during the propulsive phase presumably because soleus would not be able to contribute to ankle extension in this explosive movement.

to take-off from the ground. In contrast, MG activation and forces increase for a good part of the propulsive phase, and deactivation occurs in such a way that MG forces become zero at the instant of take-off. Therefore, the soleus exhibits a highly nonintuitive behavior, in that it is deactivated and force becomes zero at a time when high ankle extensor moments are required. Kaya et al. (2008) proposed that deactivation of the soleus occurred because it was shortening so quickly during the propulsive phase of jumping that even maximal activation would not result in muscle force. Therefore, it appears that there are neural pathways that inhibit wasteful muscle activation in anticipation of contractile conditions that do not allow for force and work production in the muscle.

Aside from the mechanical and physiological properties of muscles, it has been argued that their multijoint nature might also be a determinant for how muscles contribute to movements. Van Ingen Schenau et al. (1992) argued that one-joint muscles are primarily activated when they are shortening during a movement task and therefore contribute positive work, whereas bi- and multiarticular muscles were primarily recruited to control the direction of the external forces exerted on the environment; for example, the ground reaction forces during locomotion. In order to address this issue quantitatively, Kaya et al. (2006) developed a musculoskeletal model of the cat hindlimb and determined the direction of ground reaction force for each muscle at any given instant in time during the stance phase of locomotion (Fig. 8.5). They then measured soleus, MG, plantaris, and vastus lateralis muscle forces and/or activations during cat locomotion, simultaneously with the corresponding ground reaction forces. They argued that, if a muscle was primarily activated to control the direction of the ground reaction force vector, its force would be high if the muscle produced a ground reaction force with a direction that was well aligned with the instantaneous direction of the resultant ground reaction force, and that the muscle force would be small or zero if this alignment was bad. In contrast, a muscle whose force was not associated with the control of the ground

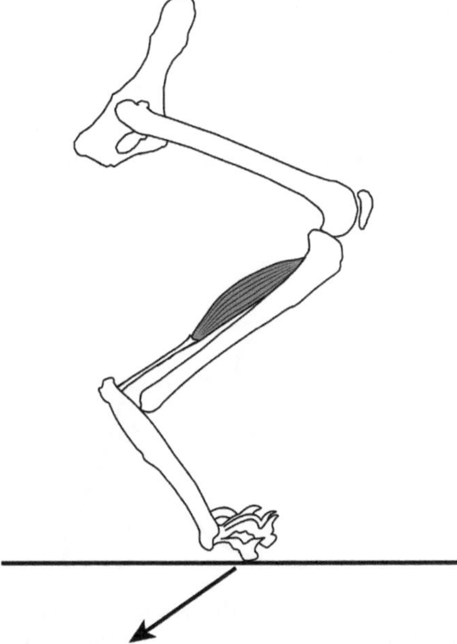

Figure 8.5 Schematic illustration of the point that a given muscle (such as the cat soleus shown here) provides a ground reaction force with a direction that is uniquely determined by the configuration of the hind limb.

reaction force direction would produce force magnitudes that were independent of the alignment of the muscle's and the system's ground reaction force vectors. Within this theoretical frame work, Kaya and colleagues (2006) identified that the MG and plantaris were primarily activated to control the direction of the ground reaction forces, whereas the soleus and vastus lateralis were not. Since the MG and plantaris are two-joint, and the soleus and vastus lateralis are one-joint muscles in the cat, the idea was supported that bi- or multiarticular muscles might preferably be recruited so as to finely control the direction of the external ground reaction forces during locomotion.

For locomotion, ground reaction force patterns are similar for different people. This has to be the case, as the ground reaction forces, together with the gravitational force, are the only external forces acting on a person, and therefore they determine the center of mass path during locomotion. Since all people walk similarly, the ground reaction forces have to be similar. However, for other movements, for example bicycling, the situation can (at least theoretically) be quite different. Bicyclists exert forces on the pedals to propel the bike forward. The pedal is constrained to follow a circular path around its axis of rotation, and as long as there is a component of the resultant force vector pointing along the circular path of the pedal, the pedal will follow that path because of its constrained movement (Fig. 8.6). Any forces perpendicular to the path are absorbed and do not contribute to propulsion. Thus, pedaling can be achieved with a variety of pedal force profiles, and although it appears optimal if muscles were recruited in such a way as to produce a pedal force direction that is always tangential (or nearly so) to the pedal's path, that is not what happens in real bicycling. The constraints of a bicycle's crank and pedal system produce a muscle activation pattern that maximizes cycling performance while producing

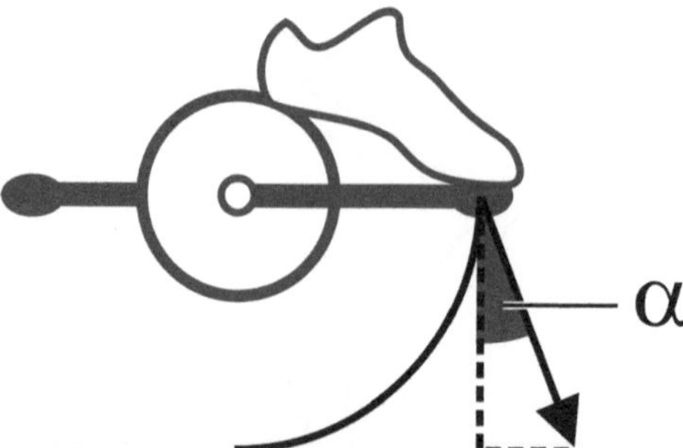

Figure 8.6 Schematic illustration of the resultant pedal force. Although it appears of advantage to exert a force on the pedal that is tangential to the circular path of the pedal, this typically does not happen. In the power phase of bicycling, the resultant pedal force typically has a tangential and radial component, as shown.

substantial nontangential forces that do not contribute to the work and power output of cycling. Imagine a bicycle in which the pedal can move in the direction of the resultant applied force (that is, the pedal is not constrained along a circular path but can move along the axis of the crank). For such a crank design, cycling performance would decrease compared to the constrained situation, emphasizing the somewhat counter-intuitive notion that a constrained system allows for better performance than an unconstrained system. The fact that, in cycling, we do not have to worry about maintaining a circular path of the pedal, as that is constrained to occur independently of the detailed forces we apply on the pedal, allows for greater variability in how cyclists apply forces to pedals and results in better performance.

Summarizing, research involving direct force measurements from multiple synergistic muscles has led to the following conclusions:

- Force sharing between synergistic muscles is highly task specific and can occupy the entire quadrant of a force sharing plot (Fig. 8.3)
- Force sharing directly depends on the mechanics of the movement and the anatomical, mechanical, and physiological properties of the muscles involved.
- Agonistic muscles (muscles whose joint moment is the same as the required resultant joint moment) may not contribute to a movement if the contractile conditions are such that force and work production would be small (or zero) even if fully activated.

MUSCLE FORCE PREDICTIONS

Although direct muscle force measurements allow for ultimate insight into how movements are organized, they are often impractical and have significant limitations. Human muscle forces have been measured for selected movement conditions (Komi et al. 1987; Dennerlein et al. 1998); however, calibration of the buckle-type tendon transducers used in these situations cannot be performed easily, as the tendon would need to be released from the bone and attached to a force transducer. Such a procedure has never been performed in research involving humans, thus the voltage signals from the human tendon transducers have been "calibrated" indirectly either using an artificial tendon or using a theoretical inverse dynamics approach (Andrews 1974). Both of these approaches are fraught with limitations and thus defy the invasive efforts necessary for direct muscle force measurements. Other limitations of direct muscle force measurements in human movement are the ethical considerations and the invasiveness of the procedure that would likely affect movement execution and control and thus the validity of the results.

For these reasons, much of the work aimed at determining individual muscle force-time histories during human movement has been performed using theoretical approaches. Theoretical approaches have the great advantage in that they are easy to implement, are noninvasive and can be used for large numbers of subjects and complex systems. However, as discussed at the beginning of the chapter, human (and animal) musculoskeletal systems tend to be redundant—that is, the number of muscles crossing a joint typically exceeds the degrees of freedom of the joint and thus the equations of motion that can be written for the system of interest. For example, consider the human knee (Fig. 8.7). Aside from the bony contact areas and ligamentous force transmission, at least ten muscle units can be identified as independent force producers across the joint. Typically, bony contact forces are assumed to act perpendicularly to the contact surfaces, and their

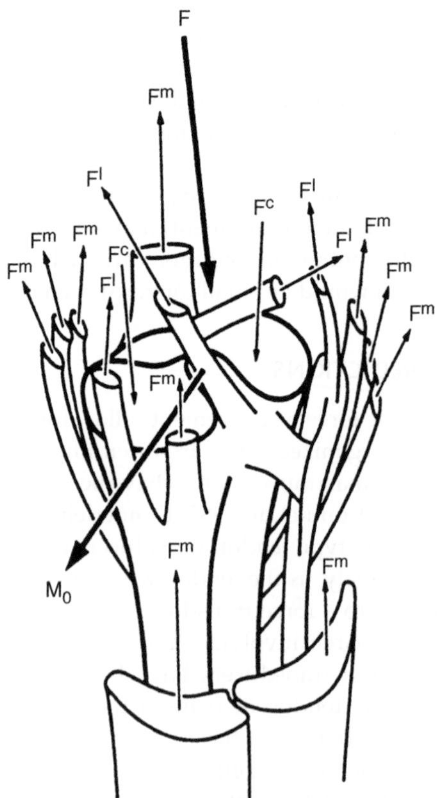

Figure 8.7 Schematic illustration of the structures crossing the human knee. Muscle forces are indicated as F^m, ligamentous forces as F^l, bony contact forces as F^c, whereas the bold arrows indicate the equivalent resultant joint force (F) and joint moment (M_0). Adapted from Crowninshield, R.D., and R.A. Brand. 1981a. The prediction of forces in joint structures: Distribution of intersegmental resultants. *Exercise and Sport Science Review* 159–181.

lines of action are assumed to run through the joint center of rotation (or close to it), so that any moments about the joint are zero (or small) and can be neglected (Andrews 1974). Similarly, ligamentous forces are thought to contribute little (if anything) to joint moments within the normal physiological range of motion, and thus are typically neglected, leaving the muscle forces as the only forces that contribute significantly to joint moments (Crowninshield and Brand 1981a and b). If we agree with these assumptions, the resultant joint moment, M_o, which can be readily obtained using standard inverse dynamics analysis (Andrews 1974), is equivalent to the sum of the moments produced by all muscle forces, or:

$$M_o = \sum_{i=0}^{n} (r_{i/o} \times F_i^m) \qquad \text{(Eq. 1)}$$

Where $r_{i/o}$ is the location vector for the ith muscle force and F_i^m is the ith muscle force vector.

It is feasible to assume that the location vector described in Equation 1 can be determined through anatomical investigation, and so can the lines of action of the various muscle forces. Therefore, Equation 1, expressed for the knee (Fig. 8.7), becomes a vector equation with ten unknown muscle force magnitudes; or equivalently, Equation 1 can be expressed as three independent scalar equations with ten unknowns. This represents a mathematically indeterminate system with an infinite number of possible solutions. The trick now is to find the solution that is actually chosen by the neuromusculoskeletal system and to verify that this solution is not only mathematically but also experimentally unique.

When asking the question, "Are 'identical' movements executed with 'identical' force-sharing patterns among muscles?," the answer is clearly "No." Overwhelming evidence in the literature suggests that EMG patterns or ground reaction forces during locomotion vary slightly from step cycle to step cycle, thus it would be prudent to expect that variations also occur in how muscles contribute to a given "prescribed" movement. In one of few studies aimed at addressing this question directly, forces in the cat soleus, gastrocnemius, and plantaris were measured for repeat step cycles at given nominal speeds of treadmill locomotion (Herzog et al. 1994). As expected, it was found that, indeed, a given locomotor task (walking at 1.2 m/s on a motor-driven treadmill) was associated with a fair amount of variability in the muscles' force-time histories (Fig. 8.8) and the associated force-sharing patterns (Fig. 8.9). Therefore, when attempting to determine how animal or human neuromusculoskeletal systems solve a given movement problem, it must be kept in mind that movement execution and the associated muscle force-sharing patterns are variable. Nevertheless, Figures 8.8 and 8.9 illustrate that this variability is confined and that the general muscle coordination patterns for a movement seem preserved. It appears that, when executing a movement, a general force-sharing pattern is associated with the task, but that this pattern has some

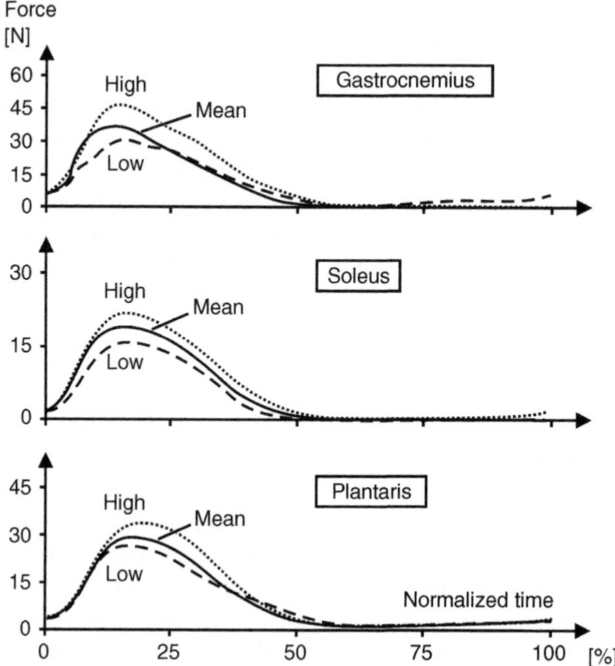

Figure 8.8 Force–time histories of gastrocnemius, soleus and plantaris for cat walking at 1.2 m/s. The mean curves (*solid lines*) represent the mean force–time history for 43 consecutive steps from a single animal. The high curves (*dotted lines*) represent the average of the three-step cycles giving the highest peak forces, and the low curves (*dashed lines*) represent the average of the three-step cycles giving the lowest peak forces. Note the variability in force-time traces for a well-controlled walking speed with essentially identical movement patterns.

distinct slack. My interpretation of this observation is that it would be very hard to control a system that has a rigid movement execution pattern and that the variability that is seen in the performance of a given movement allows for flexibility in execution and adaptability upon sudden perturbations.

Keeping this in mind, it is still very much accepted, and probably rightly so, that movements are executed in a fairly standard, although not a perfectly stereotypical, way. Theoretical approaches aimed at studying the control of muscle force-sharing patterns are aimed at identifying the underlying mechanisms that determine movement control. Probably the most common approach in biomechanics has been to search for optimal movement control parameters that satisfy all the constraints of movement execution. Mathematical optimization theory allows for the testing of such approaches and has been widely used for approximately the past four decades to gain insight into human and animal movement control

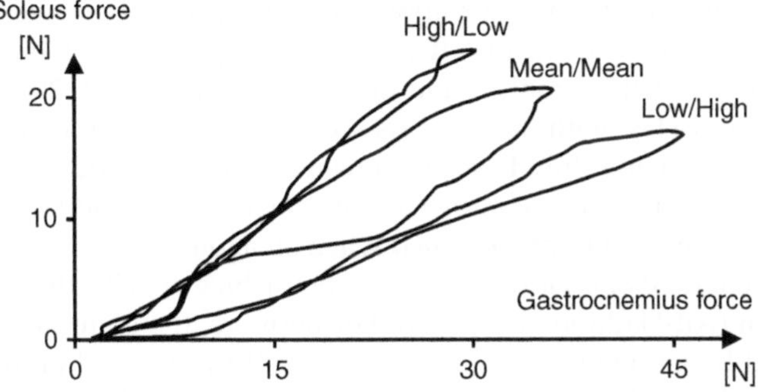

Figure 8.9 Force-sharing between cat soleus and gastrocnemius. The high/low curve shows the mean force-sharing loop of three (out of 43) step cycles with the highest soleus forces, the low/high curve is the corresponding mean force-sharing loop for the three step cycles with the highest gastrocnemius forces, and the mean/mean curve represents the mean force-sharing loop for all 43 consecutive step cycles of this one cat walking at a nominal speed of 1.2 m/s on a motor-driven treadmill.

(Crowninshield and Brand 1981a; Herzog 1996; Tsirakos et al. 1997; Erdemir et al. 2007). For technical and computational reasons, such optimization approaches were restricted to linear optimization theory prior to 1978, but these will not be discussed here as there is common consensus that these approaches are much too limited to capture any realistic force-sharing patterns during voluntary movements.

The first nonlinear optimization approach aimed at predicting individual muscle forces was proposed by Pedotti et al. in 1978. These scientists proposed a quadratic optimization scheme aimed at minimizing forces in the lower limb musculature during locomotion. Constraints included that the resultant joint moments needed to be satisfied by the sum of the moments produced by the muscle forces and that all muscle forces needed to be tensile. Crowninshield and Brand (1981b) extended the nonlinear optimization approach proposed by Pedotti and colleagues beyond quadratic programming, and more importantly, associated a physiological criterion for the force-sharing patterns during movement. Specifically, they proposed that muscle forces during human locomotion are selected in such a manner as to maximize endurance time: that is, the time the task (walking, for example) could be maintained. In order to achieve this objective they proposed that the cubed sum of the muscle stresses needed to be minimized, as this was argued to be equivalent to maximizing endurance.

$$\min \theta \text{ and } \theta = \sum_{i=1}^{N} (F_i^m / \text{pcsa}_i)^3 \qquad \text{(Eq. 2)}$$

Where F_i^m is the ith muscle force, and pcsa_i is the ith muscular physiological cross-sectional area.

This nonlinear optimization approach had several advantages over earlier linear approaches in that it tended to keep muscle stresses low by involving all of the agonistic muscles (Ait-Haddou et al. 2004), and by favoring muscles with large cross-sectional areas and moment arms (Crowninshield and Brand 1981b). However, it is straightforward to show that, in a model as proposed by Crowninshield and Brand (1981b), maximum endurance times are obtained when all agonistic muscle stresses are equal (Denoth 1987). However, this is not achieved with their proposed algorithm (Ait-Haddou et al. 2004). Furthermore, the endurance criterion proposed by Crowninshield and Brand (1981b) was based on the known inverse relationship between muscle stress and endurance time, and although muscles have very different endurance times depending on the distribution of fibre types, such considerations were not part of their proposed force-sharing predictions.

To improve on the force-sharing predictions obtained earlier, Dul et al. (1984) proposed that muscles contribute to movements such that fatigue is minimized. To represent a fatigue criterion properly, and account for differences in endurance between different muscles, fibre type content of the muscles was a required input into the optimization model. They compared their theoretical predictions of force-sharing to experimental results obtained for the cat soleus and medial gastrocnemius discussed earlier (Walmsley et al. 1978). Their predictions agreed well with experimental findings (Fig. 8.2), however the following caveats apply. First, force-sharing among synergistic muscles is always considered for a given instant in time, but the comparison of soleus and MG forces in the cat were made for the peak forces obtained during locomotion (Fig. 8.2), which do not occur at the same time (Walmsley et al. 1978; Hodgson 1983; Abraham and Loeb 1985; Herzog and Leonard 1991; Gregor et al. 2001). Second, although the predictions by Dul et al. (1984) approximate the force-sharing patterns of cat soleus and MG fairly well for static tasks and slow speeds of locomotion, they inherently cannot predict the decrease in soleus force with simultaneously increasing MG forces as speed of locomotion is increased (Fig. 8.2).

The first direct comparisons of force-sharing patterns predicted using nonlinear optimal control strategies with directly measured muscle forces was performed for the soleus, gastrocnemius, and plantaris muscles in the freely walking cat (Herzog and Leonard 1991). For a one-degree-of-freedom system (ankle flexion/extension), the predicted force-sharing patterns lacked many of the experimentally observed behaviors, including the "loop-type" force-sharing behavior and the ability to predict increasing forces in one agonist while simultaneously predicting decreasing forces in another agonist muscle. Therefore, it was concluded that the most frequently used optimal control strategies proposed in the biomechanics literature (Crowninshield and Brand 1981a; Herzog 1996; Erdemir et al. 2007) were not particularly useful in predicting movement control strategies and the recruitment patterns of synergistic muscles.

One of the limitations of all previous optimization approaches was that either the solutions to the force-sharing problem were obtained using numerical modeling of large-scale and complex systems that did not allow for generalization of the findings, or the solutions were based on analytical approaches that inherently would allow for generalizations of the findings, but they were obtained for simplistic models with limited degrees of freedom and a small number of muscles (Herzog and Binding 1992, 1993).

However, in 2004, a general, graphical solution of the Crowninshield and Brand-type optimization algorithms was published and allowed for conceptual analysis of the mathematical behavior of the theoretical approaches used in the past and comparison with available experimental data (Ait-Haddou et al. 2004). These investigations led to the conclusion that, aside from fibre type distribution and structural parameters, the instantaneous contractile properties of the target muscles, as well as their force-, length-, velocity-, and history-dependent mechanical properties, were of utmost importance in the prediction of individual muscle forces. This led to the creation of cost functions in optimal control strategies that accounted for contractile conditions and mechanical properties. One such approach, in which force-velocity and contractile conditions were included, allowed for conceptual force-sharing predictions that had been observed experimentally but could not be predicted theoretically: for example, the "loop-type" force-sharing behavior of agonistic muscles in a one-degree-of-freedom model, or the deactivation of an agonistic muscle (Schappacher-Tilp et al. 2009). We believe that, with these newly developed optimal control strategies, it might be possible, after 40 years of investigation, to predict accurate force-sharing patterns and real control strategies for voluntary human and animal movements.

CONCLUSION

The control of joint moments and movements through muscles typically represents a mathematically redundant problem; that is, there are more muscles than are strictly required to perform a given movement. Animal research has clearly demonstrated that this is not only a theoretical phenomenon but one that also holds true for actual movements (Misiaszek and Pearson 2002). However, despite the apparent redundancy, voluntary movements are performed with stereotypical muscle activation patterns accompanied by characteristic variations (Herzog et al. 1994). When measuring these force-sharing patterns in free animal movements, it becomes apparent that the mechanical properties of the muscles, and their mechanics of action, are strong determinants of the recruitment order and magnitude of muscle contraction (Walmsley et al. 1978; Hodgson 1983; Herzog and Leonard 1991; Abraham and Loeb 1985; Fowler et al. 1993). Mathematical optimization, in conjunction with biomechanical modeling of the target systems, has been employed frequently to determine the force-sharing patterns of muscles with little success initially. However, the recent publication of the general solution of the optimization problem associated with the classic distribution problem in biomechanics (Ait-Haddou et al. 2004) has allowed for validation of synergistic force-sharing without the need for direct muscle force measurements and musculoskeletal modeling (Jinha et al. 2009). Furthermore, incorporation of the contractile properties and instantaneous contractile conditions into optimal design problems allows for realistic predictions of force-sharing patterns observed during voluntary movement (Schappacher-Tilp et al. 2009).

REFERENCES

Abraham, L.D., and G.E. Loeb. 1985. The distal hindlimb musculature of the cat. *Experimental Brain Research* 58: 580–93.

Ait-Haddou, R., A. Jinha, W. Herzog, and P. Binding. 2004. Analysis of the force-sharing problem using an optimization model. *Mathematical Biosciences* 191: 111–22.

Alexander, R.M. 1989. Optimization and gaits in the locomotion of vertebrates. *Physiology Review* 69: 1199–1227.

Andrews, J.G. 1974. Biomechanical analysis of human motion. *Kinesiology* 4: 32–42.

Ariano, M.A., R.B. Armstrong, and V.R. Edgerton. 1973. Hindlimb muscle fiber populations of five mammals. *Journal of Histochemistry and Cytochemistry* 21(1): 51–55.

Bertram J.E., and A. Ruina. 2001. Multiple walking speed-frequency relations are predicted by constrained optimization. *Journal of Theoretical Biology* 209: 445–53.

Burke, R.E., D.N. Levine, M. Saleman, and P. Tsairis. 1974. Motor units in cat soleus muscle: physiological, histochemical and morphological characteristics. *Journal of Physiology (London)* 238: 503–14.

Burke, R.E., and P. Tsairis. 1973. Anatomy and innervation ratios in motor units of cat gastrocnemius. *Journal of Physiology (London)* 234: 749–65.

Crowninshield, R.D., and R.A. Brand. 1981a. The prediction of forces in joint structures: Distribution of intersegmental resultants. *Exercise and Sport Science Review* 159–181.

Crowninshield, R.D., and R.A. Brand. 1981b. A physiologically based criterion of muscle force prediction in locomotion. *Journal of Biomechanics* 14: 793–801.

Dennerlein, J.T., E. Diao, C.D. Mote, and D.M. Rempel. 1998. Tensions of the flexor digitorum superficialis are higher than a current model predicts. *Journal of Biomechanics* 31: 295–301.

Denoth, J. 1987. Methodological problems in prediction of muscle forces. In *Biomechanics 11A.* pp. 82–87. (Groot G., Hollander AP.,Huijing PA., van Ingen Schenau GJ., eds) Free University Press (Amsterdam)

Dul, J., G.E. Johnson, R. Shiavi, and M.A. Townsend. 1984. Muscular synergism–II. A minimum-fatigue criterion for load sharing between synergistic muscles. *Journal of Biomechanics* 17: 675–84.

Dul, J., M.A. Townsend, R. Shiavi, and G.E. Johnson. 1984. Muscular synergism – I. On criteria for load sharing between synergistic muscles. *Journal of Biomechanics* 17: 663–73.

Erdemir, A., S. McLean, W. Herzog, and A.J. van den Bogert. 2007. Model-based estimation of muscle forces exerted during movements. *Clinical Biomechanics (Bristol, Avon)* 22: 131–54.

Fowler, E.G., R.J. Gregor, J.A. Hodgson, and R.R. Roy. 1993. Relationship between ankle muscle and joint kinetics during the stance phase of locomotion in the cat. *Journal of Biomechanics* 26: 465–83.

Gordon, A.M., A.F. Huxley, and F.J. Julian. 1966. The variation in isometric tension with sarcomere length in vertebrate muscle fibres. *Journal of Physiology (London)* 184: 170–92.

Gregor, R.J., J.L. Smith, D.W. Smith, A. Oliver, and B.I. Prilutsky. 2001. Hindlimb kinetics and neural control during slope walking in the cat: Unexpected findings. *Journal of Applied Biomechanics* 17: 277–86.

Herzog, W. 1996. Force-sharing among synergistic muscles: theoretical considerations and experimental approaches. In *Exercise and sport sciences reviews*, ed. J.O. Holloszy, pp. 173–202. Baltimore: Williams & Wilkins.

Herzog, W. 1998. Force sharing among the primary cat ankle muscles. *European Journal of Morphology* 36: 280–87.

Herzog, W., and P. Binding. 1992. Predictions of antagonistic muscular activity using nonlinear optimization. *Mathematical Biosciences* 111: 217–29.

Herzog, W., and P. Binding. 1993. Cocontraction of pairs of antagonistic muscles: Analytical solution for planar static nonlinear optimization approaches. *Mathematical Biosciences* 118: 83–95.

Herzog, W., and T.R. Leonard. 1991. Validation of optimization models that estimate the forces exerted by synergistic muscles. *Journal of Biomechanics* 24S: 31–39.

Herzog, W., T.R. Leonard, and A.C.S. Guimaraes. 1993. Forces in gastrocnemius, soleus, and plantaris tendons of the freely moving cat. *Journal of Biomechanics* 26: 945–53.

Herzog, W., V. Zatsiorsky, B.I. Prilutsky, and T.R. Leonard. 1994. Variations in force-time histories of cat gastrocnemius, soleus, and plantaris muscles for consecutive walking steps. *Journal of Experimental Biology* 191: 19–36.

Hill, A.V. 1938. The heat of shortening and the dynamic constants of muscle. *Proceedings of the Royal Society of London* 126: 136–95.

Hodgson, J.A. 1983. The relationship between soleus and gastrocnemius muscle activity in conscious cats: A model for motor unit recruitment? *Journal of Physiology (London)* 337: 553–62.

Hoyt, D.F., and C.R. Taylor. 1981. Gait and the energetics of locomotion in horses. *Nature* 292: 239–40.

Jinha, A., R. Ait-Haddou, M. Kaya, and W. Herzog. 2009. A task-specific validation of homogeneous non-linear optimisation approaches. *Journal of Theoretical Biology* 259: 695–700.

Kaya, M., T.R. Leonard, and W. Herzog. 2006. Control of ground reaction forces by hindlimb muscles during cat locomotion. *Journal of Biomechanics* 39: 2752–66.

Kaya, M., T.R. Leonard, and W. Herzog. 2008. Premature deactivation of soleus during the propulsive phase of cat jumping. *Journal of the Royal Society, Interface* 5: 415–426.

Komi, P.V., M. Salonen, M. Järvinen, and O. Kokko. 1987. In vivo registration of Achilles tendon forces in man. I. Methodological development. *International Journal of Sports Medicine* (8 Supplement): 3–8.

Misiaszek, J.E., and K.G. Pearson. 2002. Adaptive changes in locomotor activity following botulinum toxin injection in ankle extensor muscles of cats. *Journal of Neurophysiology* 87: 229–39.

Pedotti, A., V.V. Krishnan, and L. Stark. 1978. Optimization of muscle-force sequencing in human locomotion. *Mathematical Biosciences* 38: 57–76.

Schappacher-Tilp, G., P. Binding, E. Braverman, and W. Herzog. 2009. Velocity-dependent cost function for the prediction of force sharing among synergistic muscles in a one degree of freedom model. *Journal of Biomechanics* 42: 657–60.

Smith, J.L., B. Betts, V.R. Edgerton, R.F. Zernicke. 1980. Rapid ankle extension during paw shakes: Selective recruitment of fast ankle extensors. *Journal of Neurophysiology* 43: 612–20.

Tsirakos, D., V. Baltzopoulos, and R. Bartlett. 1997. Inverse optimization: functional and physiological considerations related to the force-sharing problem. *Critical Reviews in Biomedical Engineering* 25: 371–407.

van Ingen Schenau, G.J., P.J.M. Boots, G. de Groot, R.J. Snackers, and W.W.L.M. van Woensel. 1992. The constrained control of force and position in multi-joint movements. *Neuroscience* 46: 197–207.

Walmsley, B., J.A. Hodgson, and R.E. Burke. 1978. Forces produced by medial gastrocnemius and soleus muscles during locomotion in freely moving cats. *Journal of Neurophysiology* 41: 1203–15.

Weber, W., and E. Weber. 1836. *Mechanik der menschlichen Gehwerkzeuge*. Göttingen: W. Fischer-Verlag.

9

Control of Locomotion

Lessons from Whole-body Biomechanical Analysis

Boris I. Prilutsky and Alexander N. Klishko

It has been recognized for a long time that limb motion-dependent dynamics (Bernstein 1935, 1947, 1967; Zajac and Gordon, 1989; Sainburg et al. 1999; Dounskaya 2005), joint geometry and kinematics (Flanders and Soechting 1990; Burkholder and Nichol 2004), and muscle–tendon mechanical properties (Feldman 1986; Mussa-Ivaldi et al. 1985; Brown et al. 1999; Sandercock and Heckman 1997; Lin and Rymer 2000; see also Herzog, this volume) must be accounted for by any motor control theory explaining how the nervous system plans, executes, and corrects movement. Even seemingly simple, fast one-joint movements to a specified joint angle demonstrate complex muscle activity patterns that grade with requirements for distance, speed, and accuracy, and include corrective reactions based on task performance (e.g., Gottlieb et al. 1992). The necessity to consider biomechanics of the motor system in any discussion of movement control is dictated by the fact that there is no one-to-one correspondence between a neural command and the resulting movement (Bernstein, 1935, 1947, 1967): Motor output depends on movement history, current state of the musculoskeletal system, intersegmental dynamics, current conditions of the changing external environment, neural noise (errors in neural commands), and more (for reviews, see Wetzel and Stuart 1976 and Latash, this volume).

So, the biomechanical properties of the musculoskeletal system during one-joint or one-limb movements considerably complicate motor control. Given that, how do quadrupedal animals operate their four extremities, casually switch between gaits (Hildebrand 1965); distribute loads between fore- and hindlimbs (Fung and Macpherson 1995; Hodson et al. 2000, 2001); divide labor among joints to generate the mechanical energy necessary for propulsion (Lee et al. 2008); select specific muscles around individual joints (Prilutsky et al. 1994; Gregor et al. 2006; Kaya et al. 2003; for reviews see Prilutsky 2000a; Prilutsky and Zatsiorsky 2002, and Herzog, this volume); and recruit selected compartments (English 1984) and groups of motor units within a muscle (Hodson-Tole et al., 2009) to meet various task demands? Note that this is all done in changing environmental conditions (such as slope of surface, changing accuracy demands, and perturbations). Available information on whole-body biomechanics of quadrupedal locomotion might help answer some of these questions.

In this chapter, we review some of our previous (Prilutsky et al. 2005; Gregor et al. 2006; Maas et al. 2007) and preliminary results (Prilutsky et al. 2001; Farrell et al. 2008) on whole-body movements during cat locomotion. Our experimental procedures have been described in the just-listed publications and are briefly outlined here. Prior to locomotion experiments, we train cats, using food awards (e.g., Prilutsky et al. 2005) 5 days a week for several months, to walk on a wooden walkway (2.5 m long and 0.5 m wide) with Plexiglas walls (0.6 m high) and with three small force plates (Bertec, OH; 0.16 m long and 0.11 cm wide) embedded in the walkway floor. This training also includes such locomotion tasks as walking on a sloped surface (50% or 27-degree upslope and downslope) or precise stepping on horizontal ladders with rungs of different width (Beloozerova and Sirota 1993a,b; 2010) or narrow and wide paths (Farrell et al. 2008). To describe whole-body locomotion, the cat body is typically represented as a planar system of 21 rigid segments (with known inertial properties, Hoy and Zernicke, 1985) interconnected by frictionless hinge joints (Fig. 9.1A). Joint positions indicated in Figure 9.1A by small black circles are recorded by means of 24 small (6 or 9 mm in diameter) reflective markers, which are attached to cat shaved skin by double-sided adhesive tape prior to motion capture experiments. Four additional markers are attached to the head, as indicated in Figure 9.1A. Marker positions during locomotion are recorded by a six-camera high-speed motion capture system Vicon (UK) with the sampling rate of 120 frames per second. Coordinates of the knee and elbow joints are recalculated based on recorded coordinates of adjacent joints and measured lengths of segments forming the knee and elbow, to minimize errors caused by skin movement. Recorded marker coordinates and ground reaction forces measured by three force plates allow for calculations of over 200 mechanical variables of locomotion as functions of step cycle time that include linear and angular displacements; velocities and accelerations of each body segment; angles, velocities, moments, and power at each joint; and displacement, velocity, and acceleration of the cat center of mass (Fig. 9.1B; for details, see Prilutsky et al. 2005; Gregor et al. 2006; Maas et al. 2007). In addition, negative, positive, and net mechanical work at each limb joint is calculated. Electromyographic (EMG) activity of up to nine major hindlimb muscles is recorded using implanted fine-wire electrodes (Teflon-insulated multistrand, 100 μm diameter, Cooner Wire, CA; for details of implantation and EMG analysis see Prilutsky et al. 2005; Gregor et al. 2006).

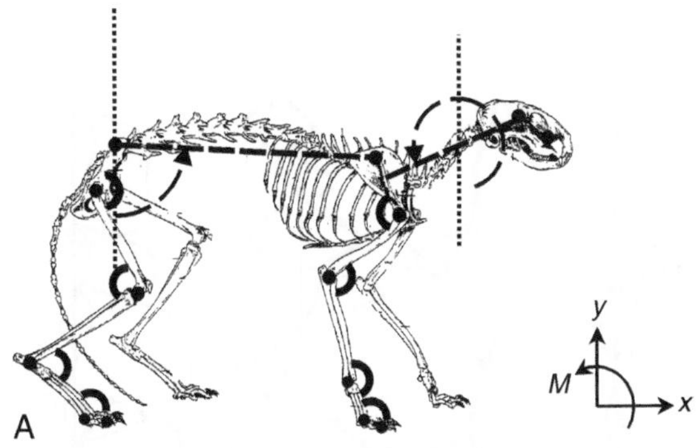

Figure 9.1 A cat body model (A) and selected mechanical variables of cat locomotion (B, C, D). **A**: Schematic representation of a cat model. The model consists of 21 rigid segments connected by frictionless hinge joints. Joint angles are defined as enclosed angles. Orientation of each segment is determined as the angle between the negative direction of the vertical axis and the longitudinal segment axis directed from the distal to the proximal end of the segment as indicated for the head/neck segment. **B**: Selected mechanical variables of the right forelimb (RF) obtained during whole-body walking in the cat. From top to bottom: (1) Cat stick figures (thicker solid lines show the right-side limbs, trunk and head; thinner solid lines show the left-side limbs; dashed thicker and thinner lines denote the ground reaction force vector applied to the right or left limb, respectively). (2) Angles at the metacarpophalangeal (*dashed line*), wrist (*thin line*), elbow (*dot-dashed line*), and shoulder (*thick line*) joints; see A for definition of angles. (3) Horizontal velocity and jerk of the toe of the RF. (4) Moments at the metacarpophalangeal, wrist, elbow, and shoulder joints (negative/positive values correspond to extension/flexion at the joints [plantar/dorsi flexion for the MCP and wrist]). (5) Power at the metacarpophalangeal, wrist, elbow, and shoulder joints (negative/positive power corresponds to absorption/generation of power). No joint moments and powers were calculated for the second step cycle because in this cycle, the cat RF did not touch the force plate. **Bottom**: Step diagrams, where stance is represented by black line and swing by no line; LF, left forelimb; LH, left hindlimb; RF, right forelimb; and RH, right hindlimb. Vertical solid lines indicate RF toe takeoff; interrupted lines indicate RF touchdown. **C**: Selected kinematic and kinetic variables of the right hindlimb (RH) during two consecutive cycles of walking. In all the panels, except where indicated, dashed lines represent MTP joints, thin lines represent ankle joints, dot-dashed lines represent knee joints, and thick lines represent hip joints. Other designations are as in B. **D**: Selected kinematic and kinetic variables of the left forelimb (LF), left hindlimb (LH), and the general center of mass during two consecutive cycles of walking. From top to bottom: (1) Cat stick figures. (2) Angular velocity of metacarpals, forearm, upper arm, and scapular of the LF (positive values correspond to counterclockwise segment rotation with respect to the proximal joint). (3) Horizontal acceleration of hind digits, metatarsals, shank, and thigh of the LH. (4) Horizontal (Vx) and vertical (Vy) velocity of the general center of mass. (5) Horizontal (subscript x) and vertical (subscript y) components of the ground reaction force vector applied to the right forelimb (RF), left forelimb (LF), right hindlimb (RH), and left hindlimb (LH). **Bottom**: Step diagrams for the LF, LH, RF, and RH limbs in which stance is represented by black line and swing by no line. Reproduced from Prilutsky, B.I., M.G. Sirota, R.J. Gregor, and I.N. Beloozerova. 2005. Quantification of motor cortex activity and full-body biomechanics during unconstrained locomotion. *Journal of Neurophysiology* 94:2959–69, with permission of the publisher.

(*Figure continues on next page*)

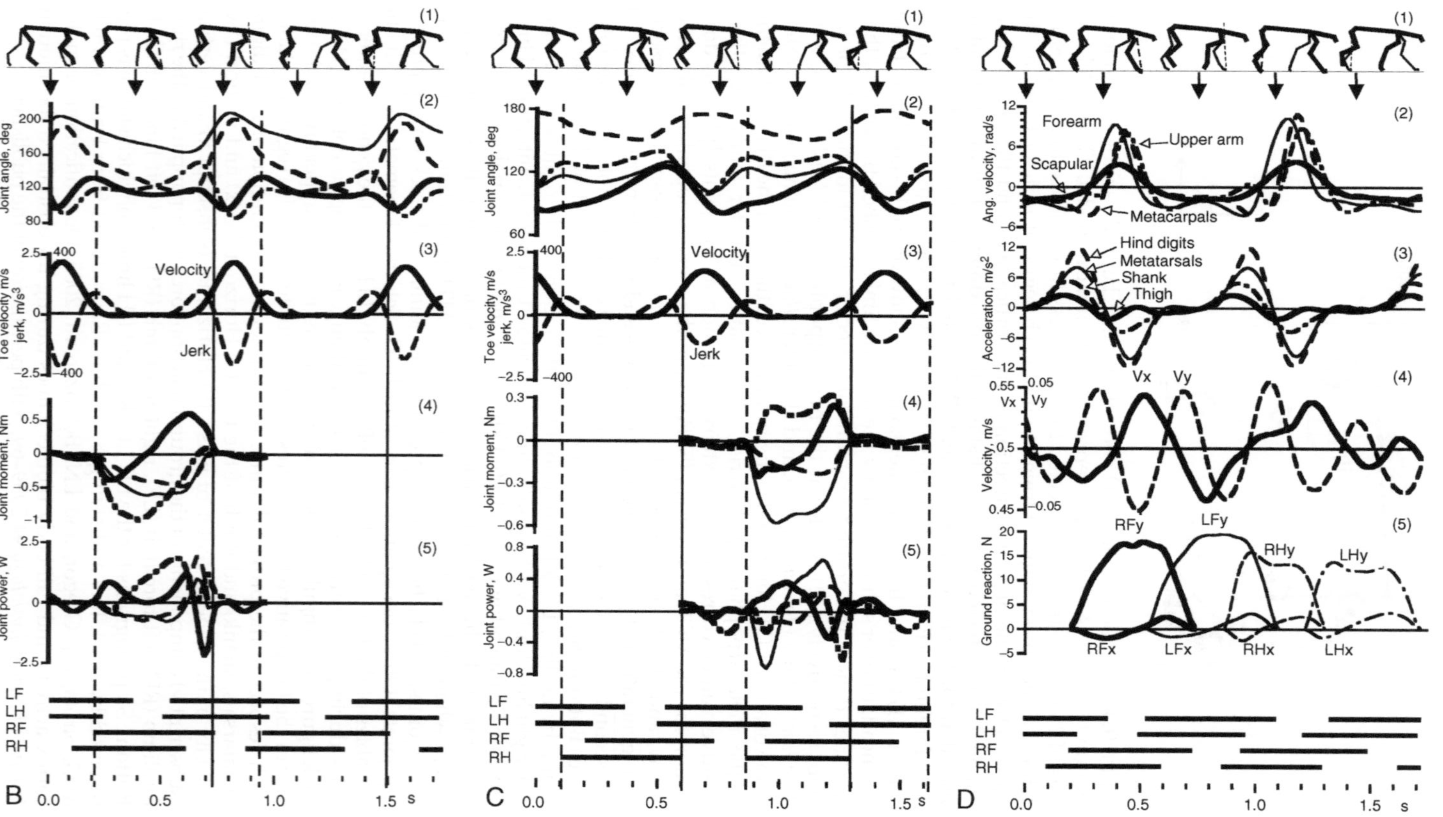
(1)
(2)
(3)
(4)
(5)
Joint angle, deg
Toe velocity m/s
jerk, m/s3
Velocity
Jerk
Joint moment, Nm
Joint power, W
LF
LH
RF
RH
B
C
D
s
Ang. velocity, rad/s
Forearm
Upper arm
Scapular
Metacarpals
Acceleration, m/s2
Hind digits
Metatarsals
Shank
Thigh
Velocity, m/s
Vx
Vy
Ground reaction, N
RFy
LFy
RHy
LHy
RFx
LFx
RHx
LHx

WHOLE-BODY LOCOMOTION AS A MODEL OF A MULTIELEMENT SYSTEM BEHAVIOR

If one considers the body of a quadrupedal animal as a multielement system (see a definition of such systems Latash, this volume), several levels of system mechanical organization can be identified that may or may not correspond to the levels of the corresponding neural control system. An analysis of the performance of elemental variables at identified levels of the musculoskeletal system can be considered the first step in understanding the control of whole-body locomotion.

Gait Redundancy and Gait Selection

We start with perhaps the highest organizational level of whole-body quadrupedal locomotion that gives rise to the different modes of locomotor behaviors typically referred to as gaits: for example, walk, trot, amble, pace, canter, gallop, and the like (Hildebrand 1965, 1989; Gambaryan 1974). Each gait is characterized by specific sequences of leg movements, duty factor (relative duration of stance phase to cycle time), and relative phase relationships between limbs, which can be expressed by a support diagram indicating duration of stance and swing phases of each leg (Fig. 9.2). According to Hildebrand (1989), there are over 400 theoretically possible quadrupedal gaits; however, only a relatively small number of them are used by individual species.

Cats, for example, choose walking gaits to move with speeds below approximately 1 m/s. During walking on level and sloped surfaces, and during highly trained precise stepping on narrow cross-bars of a horizontal ladder or along a narrow 5 cm wide path with self-selected speeds, cats typically use a support formula 2-3-2-3-2-3-2-3, which indicates the number of paws in contact with the ground in each of eight phases of the cycle (Figs. 9.1 and 9.2). When the animal is learning a novel complex locomotor task (stepping on a horizontal ladder, or walking along a narrow path) or walks very slowly, the support formula changes to 4-3-4-3-4-3-4-3 (Fig. 9.2). This change in gait is likely caused by the necessity to improve postural stability by placing the vertical projection of the general center of mass inside the area of support provided by four or three paws. Cats walking on a treadmill were reported to change their typical overground walking gait to a pace gait in which fore- and hindlimbs of the same side move in phase, with an increased stride length and a duty factor to cope with possible sudden stops of the treadmill (Blaszczyk and Loeb 1993). The authors associated these gait changes with the need to improve stability and the requirement to avoid collisions between ipsilateral hind- and forepaws during walking with increased stride length.

When the speed of locomotion increases beyond approximately 1 m/s, cats select running gaits; initially, a trot with diagonal step cycles in which

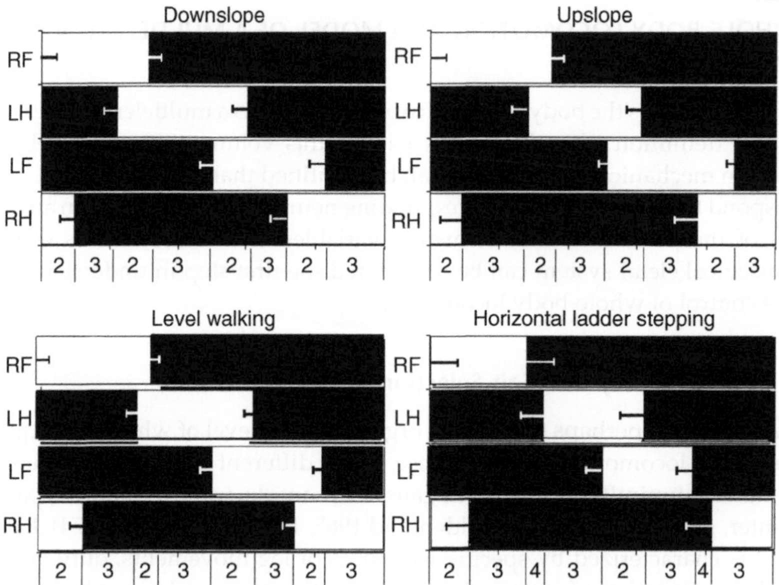

Figure 9.2 Support diagrams of level (five cats, speed 0.88 ± 0.07 m/s), –50% (–27°) downhill (two cats, speed 0.67 ± 0.08 m/s) and 50% (27°) uphill (two cats, speed 0.67 ± 0.11 m/s) walking and precise stepping on a horizontal ladder with 5 cm wide rungs (two cats, speed 0.58 ± 0.05 m/s). Black and white rectangles indicate the duration (mean ± SD) of stance swing phases.

support by diagonal pairs of legs—left hindlimb (LH)-right forelimb (RF) and left forelimb (LF)-right hindlimb (RH)—alternates with no support phases (Stuart et al. 1973). At speeds of locomotion higher than approximately 3 m/s, cats prefer the rotatory gallop, the transverse gallop, or the half bound (Stuart et al. 1973), which are characterized by asymmetrical patterns of leg movements. Several other transitional gaits used by cats for locomotion on flat surface have also been observed (English and Lennard 1982). Walking gaits do not change substantially when cats walk upslope or downslope (Fig. 9.2, see also Carlson-Kuhta et al. 1998 and Smith et al. 1998), except when they ascend very steep slopes (e.g., 100% [45 degrees]), in which case they sometimes switch to a half-bound gait (Carlson-Kuhta et al. 1998).

As can be seen from the presented data on gaits, cats prefer a limited number of gaits at slow, moderate, and fast speeds out of over 400 possible tetrapod gaits. What factors determine gait selection? Maintenance of balance and avoidance of collisions between fore- and hindlimbs are important factors, but they alone cannot explain why animal use different gaits that have similar support areas and no interference between limbs. Several other factors that likely determine the selection of preferred gaits include metabolic energy expenditure (Hoyt and Taylor 1981), loads exerted by limbs on the ground (Farley and Taylor 1991), certain constraints on joint kinematics (Hreljac 1995), excessive muscle activity (Prilutsky and Gregor 2001), and other factors (for review, see Alexander 1989).

Gaits are likely selected by the top levels of the motor control system. This assertion follows from experiments with decerebrate cats in which mild electrical stimulation of the mesencephalic locomotor region (MLR) in the midbrain resulted in walking gaits, and in trotting and galloping gaits at stronger stimulations (Shik et al. 1966; for review, see Orlovsky et al. 1999). Brain areas rostral to the MLR are capable of integrating sensory information about the external environment and the body physiological state, and of generating relatively simple commands to the MLR and other similar locomotor regions (Jordan 1991; Orlovsky et al. 1999) to initiate voluntary gait changes or start and stop locomotion. If voluntary selection of gaits is performed at the higher levels of the nervous system, the levels below the MLR, spinal pattern generators (CPGs), for example, must be capable of executing basic gait patterns autonomously, without detailed supervision of the higher centers. This has been shown to be the case as spinal cats after training are able to walk by engaging a CPG and motion-dependent feedback from muscles, skin, and joints (for review, see Frigon and Rossignol 2006). Central pattern generators in the spinal cord can also select gaits without supraspinal commands, based on afferent information from proprioceptive receptors in muscles, skin, and joints (for review, see Pearson 2008)—spinal cats and 7- to 12-month-old human babies select movement direction, walking speed, and the corresponding gait depending on speed and direction of moving treadmill belts (e.g., Yang et al. 2005; Frigon and Rossignol 2006). Motion-dependent information received by forelimbs as opposed by hindlimbs has a greater impact on phase relations between fore- and hindlimbs during locomotion (Akay et al. 2006) or corrective postural responses after perturbations (Deliagina et al. 2006).

Load Distribution Among Limbs in Tetrapods

A typical description of gaits using support formulas (Fig. 9.2) only considers time and positional information of moving limbs. However, within particular gaits with several limbs on the ground, the animal can choose from many possible combinations of forces exerted by limbs on the surface. During normal quiet standing, many quadrupedal mammals exert greater forces on the ground with the forelimbs than with the hindlimbs (Gray 1968; Macpherson 1988). This choice of posture could be explained by mass distribution along the animal body, with heavier segments (e.g., neck and head) located more rostrally. However, animals can still shift weight among the four limbs and maintain static equilibrium, as long as the projection of the general center of mass on the horizontal plane is within the paw support area (Fung and Macpherson 1995; Deliagina et al. 2006; for a review, see Duarte and Zatsiorsky, this volume, and Ting and Chvatal, this volume). Despite this redundancy, cats select a particular standing posture with the trunk oriented parallel to support surface, vertical forelimb orientation, and hindlimb configuration that creates a force component along the trunk (Fung and Macpherson 1995). In this typical posture, weight of the animal body is shifted toward the forelimbs. Such posture was shown to minimize the sum of squared three-dimensional joint moments in hindlimbs, reduce hindlimb muscle activity, and enhance stability (Fung and Macpherson 1995). After perturbations of standing posture, cat recovery responses are directed toward the unperturbed posture (Fung and Macpherson 1995; Ting and Macpherson 2004; Deliagina et al. 2006; Karayannidou et al. 2008). Thus, load distribution between fore- and hindlimbs during quiet standing in cats appears to be selected to enhance postural stability and minimize joint moments and muscle activity.

During locomotion on a flat surface, peaks of vertical forces exerted by the forelimbs of quadrupedal mammals on the ground also exceed those of the hindlimb. For example, during walking with a constant self-selected speed, peaks of cat forelimb vertical forces are about 20% greater than peaks of hindlimb vertical forces (Fig. 9.1D and Fig. 9.3, *top panel*). Similar results were reported for walking or running of other tetrapods: pigs (Thorup et al. 2008), dogs (Walter and Carrier 2007), goats (Pandy et al. 1988), and horses (Hodson et al. 2000, 2001; Dutto et al. 2004). This force distribution among fore- and hindlimbs is not a necessary condition for locomotion, because animals can be trained to locomote with weight shifted toward hindlimbs (e.g., Hildebrand 1989). Cats learning a difficult novel task of stepping between adhesive tape strips exert greater vertical forces with hindlimbs (Prilutsky et al. 2001).

During upslope and downslope walking, cats change the locomotor kinematics and kinetics of hindlimbs (Smith et al. 1998; Carlson-Kuhta et al. 1998; Gregor et al. 2006; Donelan et al. 2009; Kaya et al. 2003) and the distribution of loads between the fore- and hindlimbs (Fig. 9.3). During upslope walking, hindlimbs exert substantially greater normal and tangential forces on the ground compared to forelimbs (Fig. 9.3, *bottom panel*). During downslope walking, forelimb forces are almost two times higher than hindlimb forces (Fig. 9.3, *middle panel*). Again, this distribution of load between fore- and hindlimbs is not unique, and cats could apparently walk uphill using preferentially their forelimbs (climbing).

During walking or running on a flat surface with low to moderate constant speeds without slippage, the decelerating and accelerating force impulses exerted by limbs on the ground in each cycle should be about equal (e.g., Zatsiorsky 2002). As a consequence, during bipedal human running, the absolute values of the negative and positive impulses of anterior–posterior ground reaction forces are essentially equal (e.g., Cavagna et al. 1964). During quadrupedal level walking, constant speeds of locomotion can be maintained with a different distribution of decelerating and

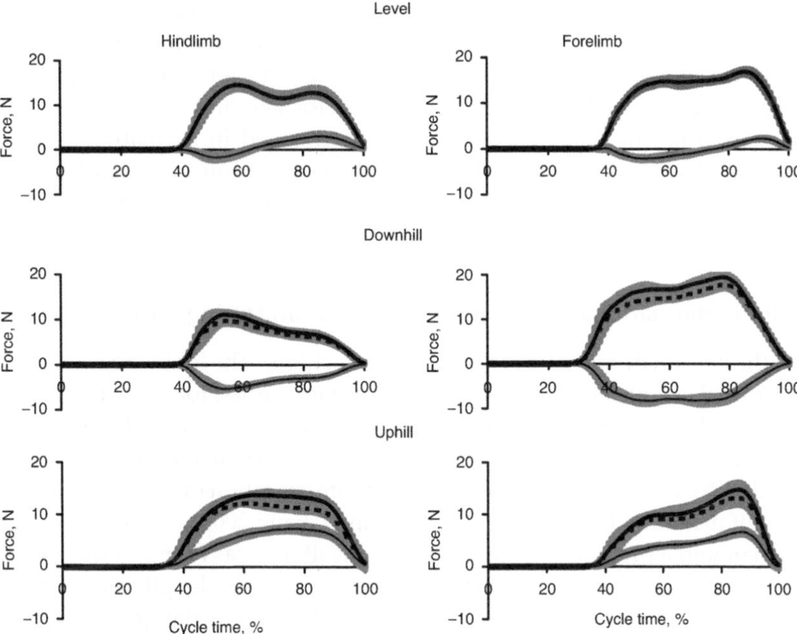

Figure 9.3 Ground reaction forces applied to hind- and forepaws during level, downhill (–50%) and uphill (50%) walking. Mean ± SD of multiple trials of one representative cat. Thick continuous line, the magnitude of ground reaction force vector; dashed line, the normal force component (perpendicular to walking surface); and thin continuous line, the tangential force component (positive values correspond to direction of progression).

accelerating actions between fore- and hindlimbs. Cats choose to accelerate themselves more (do more positive work) with hindlimbs and decelerate more (do negative work) with forelimbs during level walking (Fig. 9.1D and Fig. 9.3, *top panel*). This preference may be explained by relatively larger hindlimb muscles, since muscle force potential is proportional to muscle physiological cross-sectional area and maximal muscle work is proportional to muscle volume (e.g., Alexander and Ker 1990). Although forelimbs experience similar or greater forces (Fig. 9.3) and do a similar absolute amount of work during body deceleration (see below), the advantage of using relatively weaker forelimbs for body deceleration is that deceleration involves eccentric muscle action, which substantially enhances muscle force potential, reduces metabolic cost, and allows passive structures (ligaments, cartilage, bones) to absorb some of the body energy (for reviews, see Zatsiorsky and Prilutsky 1987; Prilutsky 2000b; Devita et al. 2008, and Herzog, this volume). Horses, which have a similar distribution of muscle mass across fore- and hindlimbs, also accelerate themselves more with hindlimbs and decelerate with forelimbs during trotting at constant speeds (Dutto et al. 2004).

Regulation of load distribution among legs of quadrupedal animals must involve afferent signals from load receptors in the feet and muscles. These receptors are essential for regulating stance-to-swing transitions (e.g., Ekeberg and Pearson 2005) and thus for gait and posture selection. Signals from the load receptors are also involved in regulation of CPG activity (Guertin et al. 1995; Rybak et al. 2006) and in the modulation of muscle activity in level and slope walking (Pearson 2008; Gregor et al. 2006; Donelan et al. 2009).

Joint Redundancy and Interjoint Coordination During Locomotion

At the next anatomical level of body organization—the limb—regulation of a particular limb length, its orientation, and its exerted force on the ground can be achieved with different joint angles and joint moments. For instance, during level walking, rats tend to maintain a particular length of the hindlimb over a cycle by using interjoint compensation even after denervation of major ankle extensors (Bauman and Chang 2009). Similar tendency to maintain a preinjury leg length during walking was found in cats (Maas et al. 2007; Chang et al. 2009). Stabilizing a typical leg length during locomotion allows the animal to keep its trunk parallel to the ground, a postural feature that was shown to decrease total hindlimb muscle activity and enhance stability (Fung and Macpherson 1995). Interjoint stabilization of leg length and orientation, and force exerted by the leg on the ground also occurs in human hopping (Auyang et al. 2009; Yen et al. 2009).

Interjoint coordination is provided by muscles crossing a joint. Net mechanical actions of muscles at joints can be quantified by determining the resultant joint moments (Manter 1938; Winter 1983; Zatsiorsky 2002) and their sum across joints of each leg, the so-called *support moment* (Winter 1983).

During the stance phase of cat level walking, hindlimb extensor moments dominate, with a greatest contribution of knee and ankle extensors to the total hindlimb support moment (Fig. 9.4, *top panel*). The forelimb support moment during the first half of stance is mostly provided by the elbow extensors, and during the second half of stance by shoulder flexors (Fig. 9.4, *top panel*).

Changing slope of locomotion from downslope to upslope modifies the contribution of joints to the total support moments of hind- and forelimbs. For example, the largest hindlimb muscle group, hip extensors (Sacks and Roy 1982), becomes dominant among hind- and forelimb joints in upslope walking (Fig. 9.4, *bottom panel*), whereas in downslope walking, the greatest contribution is provided by the large shoulder flexors (Fig. 9.4, *middle panel*).

This specific distribution of moments between hind- and forelimbs and between proximal and distal joints appears to be a common feature of quadrupedal (horses, Dutto et al. 2004; goats, Pandy et al. 1988; Lee et al. 2008;

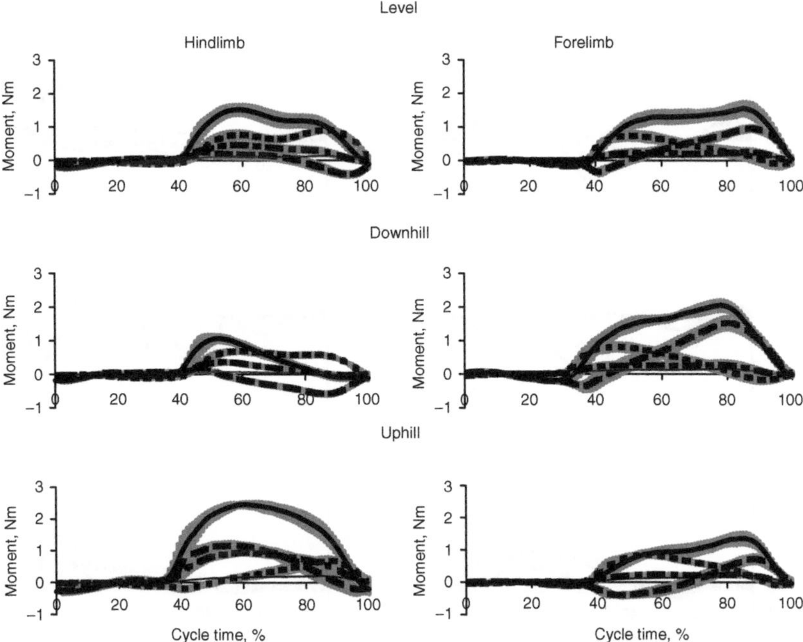

Figure 9.4 Resultant moments at hind- and forelimb joints during level, downhill (–50%) and uphill (50%) walking. Mean ± SD of multiple trials of one representative cat. Positive values correspond to extension moments (the shoulder anatomical flexors act as extensors during locomotion). **Left panels**: Thin continuous line, metatarsophalangeal (MTP) moment; dashed-dot line, ankle moment; dot line, knee moment; dashed line, hip moment; and thick continuous line, hindlimb support moment, i.e. the sum of moments across all hindlimb joints. **Right panels**: Thin continuous line, metacarpophalangeal (MCP) moment; dashed-dot line, wrist moment; dot line, elbow moment; dashed line, shoulder moment; thick continuous line, forelimb support moment.

dogs, Walter and Carrier 2007) and bipedal (birds, Roberts and Scales 2004; Rubenson and Marsh 2009 and humans, e.g. Winter 1983) locomotion and reflects a specific distribution of muscle mass across hind- and forelimbs and proximal and distal joints.

Greater muscle mass and volume of hindlimb joints may determine their preferential use by quadrupedal animals for generating mechanical energy during level and uphill locomotion. Cats, for example, generate most of the positive power and work during stance of level and upslope walking by ankle, knee, and hip joint moments that substantially exceed the power and work of forelimb joints, especially in upslope walking (Fig. 9.5, *top and bottom panels*). Although the maximum ability of a muscle to absorb mechanical energy and to do negative work also depends on muscle mass and volume, cats generate comparable values of negative

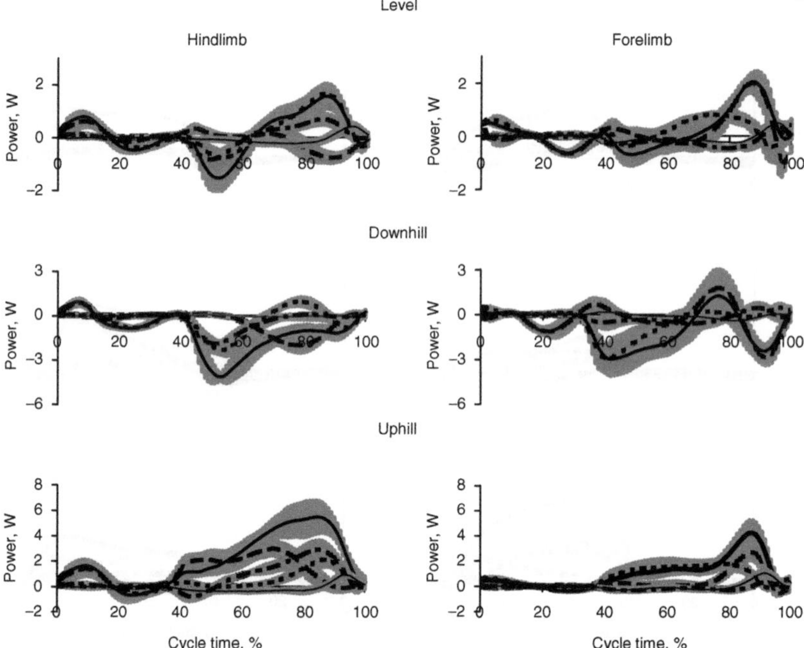

Figure 9.5 Mechanical power at hind- (*left panel*) and forelimb (*right panel*) joints during level, downhill (-50%) and uphill (50%) walking. Mean ± SD of multiple trials of one representative cat. Positive values correspond to energy generation, negative correspond to energy absorption. **Left panels**: Thin continuous line, MTP power; dashed-dot line, ankle power; dot line, knee power; dashed line, hip power; thick continuous line, total hindlimb power, i.e. the sum of powers across all hindlimb joints. **Right panels**: Thin continuous line, MCP power; dashed-dot line, wrist power; dot line, elbow power; dashed line, shoulder power; thick continuous line, total forelimb power.

power with fore- and hindlimbs during downslope walking, and substantial energy absorption occurs in the wrist and elbow joints (Fig. 9.5, *middle panel*), which are operated by muscles of relatively small size (e.g., Glenn and Whitney 1987). Energy absorption by distal forelimb joints during level and downslope locomotion can be aided by larger, more proximal muscles that could absorb additional energy transferred through multijoint muscles from distal to proximal joints (e.g., Bobbert and van Ingen Schenau 1988; Prilutsky and Zatsiorsky 1994; Prilutsky et al. 1996a; Gregersen et al. 1998). Passive body tissues also contribute to energy absorption during locomotion (e.g., Zatsiorsky and Prilutsky 1987; Devita et al. 2008).

The contributions of individual joints to total energy generation by hind- and forelimbs are consistent in general with muscle mass distribution along the limbs. Proximal joint moments (produced by proximal muscles) do generally more positive work during level and upslope locomotion in cats (Table 9.1), horses (Dutto et al. 2006), and goats (Lee et al. 2008).

Thus, the general features of interjoint coordination within and between hind- and forelimbs are (a) stabilization of leg length and orientation through interjoint coordination, (b) generally greater contribution of

Table 9.1 Positive, negative and total joint work done during level, downslope (–50%) and upslope (50%) walking in one representative cat (Mean ± SD, in J)

Downslope walking			
	Hindlimb		
Joint	Positive	Negative	Net
Mp	0.006 ± 0.003	-0.009 ± 0.005	0.003 ± 0.005
Ankle	0.007 ± 0.002	-0.21 ± 0.02	-0.20 ± 0.02
Knee	0.07 ± 0.03	-0.32 ± 0.02	-0.25 ± 0.03
Hip	0.06 ± 0.01	-0.26 ± 0.05	-0.21 ± 0.05
Sum 1	0.14 ± 0.03	-0.80 ± 0.05	-0.66 ± 0.03
Sum 2	0.06 ± 0.01	-0.71 ± 0.03	-0.66 ± 0.03
	Forelimb		
Joint	Positive	Negative	Net
Mc	0.014 ± 0.009	-0.05 ± 0.02	-0.04 ± 0.02
Wrist	0.03 ± 0.02	-0.13 ± 0.04	-0.11 ± 0.03
Elbow	0.06 ± 0.02	-0.32 ± 0.10	-0.26 ± 0.10
Shoulder	0.16 ± 0.09	-0.34 ± 0.07	-0.18 ± 0.14
Sum 1	0.26 ± 0.06	-0.85 ± 0.21	-0.58 ± 0.27
Sum 2	0.10 ± 0.11	-0.68 ± 0.16	-0.58 ± 0.27
Upslope walking			
	Hindlimb		
Joint	Positive	Negative	Net
Mp	0.04 ± 0.01	-0.09 ± 0.01	-0.05 ± 0.01
Ankle	0.44 ± 0.07	-0.06 ± 0.03	0.39 ± 0.05
Knee	0.24 ± 0.07	-0.04 ± 0.01	0.19 ± 0.07
Hip	0.69 ± 0.08	-0.02 ± 0.01	0.67 ± 0.08
Sum 1	1.41 ± 0.16	-0.21 ± 0.04	1.21 ± 0.12
Sum 2	1.25 ± 0.13	-0.05 ± 0.01	1.21 ± 0.12

(*Continued*)

Table 9.1 Positive, negative and total joint work done during level, downslope (–50%) and upslope (50%) walking in one representative cat (Mean ± SD, in J) (*Continued*)

Upslope walking			
	Forelimb		
Joint	Positive	Negative	Net
Mc	0.06 ± 0.01	-0.06 ± 0.01	0.000 ± 0.009
Wrist	0.012 ± 0.003	-0.08 ± 0.01	-0.06 ± 0.01
Elbow	0.49 ± 0.08	-0.003 ± 0.002	0.48 ± 0.08
Shoulder	0.23 ± 0.05	-0.05 ± 0.01	0.18 ± 0.05
Sum 1	0.78 ± 0.09	-0.18 ± 0.02	0.60 ± 0.07
Sum 2	0.62 ± 0.07	-0.03 ± 0.01	0.60 ± 0.07
Level walking			
	Hindlimb		
Joint	Positive	Negative	Net
Mp	0.03 ± 0.01	-0.04 ± 0.02	-0.02 ± 0.02
Ankle	0.10 ± 0.04	-0.06 ± 0.02	0.04 ± 0.02
Knee	0.21 ± 0.02	-0.10 ± 0.01	0.11 ± 0.01
Hip	0.08 ± 0.01	-0.10 ± 0.03	-0.01 ± 0.04
Sum 1	0.41 ± 0.06	-0.30 ± 0.02	0.12 ± 0.04
Sum 2	0.27 ± 0.07	-0.15 ± 0.03	0.12 ± 0.04
	Forelimb		
Joint	Positive	Negative	Net
Mc	0.019 ± 0.002	-0.04 ± 0.01	-0.03 ± 0.01
Wrist	0.013 ± 0.007	-0.07 ± 0.03	-0.05 ± 0.03
Elbow	0.13 ± 0.01	-0.03 ± 0.05	0.09 ± 0.05
Shoulder	0.13 ± 0.09	-0.09 ± 0.02	0.04 ± 0.11
Sum 1	0.29 ± 0.08	-0.23 ± 0.05	0.05 ± 0.05
Sum 2	0.16 ± 0.05	-0.11 ± 0.02	0.05 ± 0.05

Sum 1 is the sum of work values for individual joints within a particular leg. Sum 2 was calculated by first computing the total power of all joints within a leg and then computing work values from the leg power. Calculations of Sum 2 imply that simultaneous energy generation (positive power) and absorption (negative power) occurring at several joints at the same time are produced by the same multijoint muscles (Prilutsky et al. 1996b; Zatsiorsky 2002).

proximal moments to the total support moment of both hind- and forelimbs, and (c) greater contribution of proximal joints of hindlimbs to mechanical power and work production.

Muscle Redundancy and Muscle Coordination

In a simple one-degree-of-freedom joint actuated by two antagonistic muscles, there is an infinite number of ways to produce a given value of joint moment, or to change a joint trajectory by setting different levels of muscle coactivation. Typical multiaxial joints are operated by multiple muscles, which serve multiple degrees of freedom, thus resulting in much greater complexity and redundancy. This design feature of the musculoskeletal system provides the animal with a great variety of possible strategies for muscle actions. A large repertoire of available muscle functions is indispensable for the survival of animals in challenging surroundings and allows for flexible adaptations to novel environmental demands and injury. However, motor redundancy and muscle redundancy, in particular, complicate control of such a system, as was noticed many years ago (Bernstein 1935, 1947, 1967).

An intriguing characteristic of muscle coordination during locomotion is the relatively stereotypic patterns of muscle activity among individual subjects of the same species and across species (for reviews, see van Ingen Schenau and Bobbert 1993; Prilutsky 2000a; Prilutsky et al. 2009), despite muscle redundancy and the existence of many other possible muscle activation patterns that could accomplish the task. Several features of stereotypic muscle coordination during locomotion have been summarized (Prilutsky 2000a) and include (a) reciprocal activation of one-joint antagonistic muscles, (b) synergistic activation of agonists, (c) strong dependence of EMG magnitude of two-joint muscles on moments at the two joints the muscle crosses, (d) coactivation of one-joint muscles with their two-joint antagonists (e.g., one-joint knee extensor vastii and two-joint knee flexor and ankle extensor gastrocnemius are coactive in human [e.g., Prilutsky et al. 1996b], and cat [e.g., Smith et al. 1998; Krouchev et al. 2006] locomotion), and (e) inhibition of a one-joint muscle when its two-joint synergists are highly active (e.g., one-joint ankle extensor soleus and two-joint gastrocnemius during a cat paw shake, Smith et al. 1980).

There have been several explanations for why and how this muscle coordination takes place. The functional significance of the muscle activation strategy during locomotion and some other skilled behaviors has been proposed based on the fact that the just described features of muscle coordination are qualitatively predicted by the optimization of simple cost functions that minimize muscle fatigue, sense of effort, neural noise, and other similar functions (Crowninshield and Brand 1981; Prilutsky and Gregor 1997; Prilutsky and Zatsiorsky 2002; Pataky et al. 2004; Haruno and Wolpert 2005; however, see Herzog, this volume). Spinal pathways that could account for such muscle coordination include Ia inhibitory interneurons that mediate reciprocal inhibition of antagonists (Sherrington 1893; Eccles and Lundberg 1958a; Feldman and Orlovsky 1975) and length- and force-dependent heterogenic pathways that link together muscles across different joints (Eccles et al. 1957; Eccles and Lundberg 1958b; Nichols 1994, 1999).

The muscle coordination strategy observed in locomotion could be an emergent property of a motor control scheme in which parameters of the motor control system (e.g., thresholds of the tonic stretch reflexes) are regulated by the brain (e.g., Feldman 1986; Bullock and Grossberg 1988; see also Latash, this volume). The observed muscle coordination could also reflect a modular structure of the motor control system, as muscle activity patterns during locomotion and postural responses are represented by a small number of muscle synergies (Ting and Macpherson 2005; Cappellini et al. 2006; Berniker et al. 2009; see also Ting and Chvatal, this volume). Furthermore, the appropriate tuning of motion-dependent feedback has been proposed to contribute to the observed muscle coordination (Todorov and Jordan 2002; Pruszynski et al. 2009).

These and/or other neural mechanisms regulating muscle activity during various locomotor tasks must integrate motion-dependent information and adjust muscle activity to changes in the environment (slope of terrain, speed of locomotion, sudden perturbations, etc.). For example, during upslope walking in humans (Lay et al. 2007), cats (Smith et al. 1998; Carlson-Kuhta et al. 1998; Gregor et al. 2006; Donelan et al. 2009), and other animals (Roberts and Scales 2004; Rubenson and Marsh 2009), leg extensors increase their activity, whereas during downslope walking, the EMG activity is reduced. In both examples, muscle coordination generally retains the features outlined earlier. The modulation of muscle activity in slope walking has been partly attributed to force-dependent afferent signals from Golgi tendon organs, cutaneous afferents in the paws (Gregor et al. 2006; Donelan et al. 2008), and cat neck and head position and corresponding afferent signals from neck muscles and vestibular afferents (Gottschall and Nichols 2007).

CONCLUSION

Whole-body biomechanical analysis of locomotion is becoming more common and has recently provided new information on how animals coordinate individual elements of their musculoskeletal system. Quadrupedal animals of different sizes, from cats to horses, appear to employ similar motor strategies. They prefer walking gaits at slow locomotion speeds and switch to running at about the same relative speed (Froude number). During postural tasks and locomotion by healthy animals and after selected injuries, animals tend to stabilize specific orientations of the trunk and legs by distributing body weight between fore- and hindlimbs and by using interjoint compensation. Hindlimbs and proximal muscles are used preferentially for body acceleration in a gait cycle, whereas forelimbs contribute more to body deceleration. Individual joints and muscles tend to contribute to resultant support forces and moments in accordance with their ability to produce force and to generate and/or absorb mechanical energy. The neural control system appears to select appropriate motor strategies from a large number of possible variants, which might indicate optimization of some physiological goals and properties (e.g., stability, energy expenditure, mechanical stress, etc.). Any credible motor control theory should account for these whole-body behaviors and explain how they emerge. Attempts in this direction have been undertaken (see, for example, the reference configuration hypothesis, Feldman et al. 2007).

ACKNOWLEDGMENTS

We would like to thank Robert J. Gregor and Vladimir M. Zatsiorsky for fruitful discussions. Preparation of this chapter was partly supported by NIH grants HD-032571 and NS-048844 and by the Center for Human Movement Studies, Georgia Institute of Technology, Atlanta, GA, USA.

REFERENCES

Akay, T., D.A. McVea, A. Tachibana, and K.G. Pearson. 2006. Coordination of fore and hind leg stepping in cats on a transversely-split treadmill. *Experimental Brain Research* 175:211–22.

Alexander, R.M. 1989. Optimization and gaits in the locomotion of vertebrates. *Physiology Review* 69:1199–227.

Alexander, R.McN., and R.F. Ker . 1990. The architecture of the muscles. In *Multiple muscle systems, biomechanics and movement organization*, eds., J.M. Winters and S.L.Y. Woo, 568–77. New York: Springer.

Auyang, A.G., J.T. Yen, and Y.H. Chang. 2009. Neuromechanical stabilization of leg length and orientation through interjoint compensation during human hopping. *Experimental Brain Research* 192:253–64.

Bauman, J., and Y.H. Chang. 2009. Conservation of limb function after peripheral nerve injury in rat locomotion. [Abstract 118]. American Society of Biomechanics Annual Meeting. Penn State University. State College, PA.

Beloozerova, I.N., and M.G. Sirota. 1993a. The role of the motor cortex in the control of accuracy of locomotor movements in the cat. *Journal of Physiology* 461:1–25.

Beloozerova, I.N., and M.G. Sirota. 1993b. The role of the motor cortex in the control of vigour of locomotor movements in the cat. *Journal of Physiology* 461: 27–46.

Beloozerova, I.N., B.J. Farrell, M.G. Sirota, and B.I. Prilutsky. 2010. Differences in movement mechanics, electromyographic, and motor cortex activity between accurate and non-accurate stepping. *Journal of Neurophysiology* 103:2285–2300.

Berniker, M., A. Jarc, E. Bizzi, and M.C. Tresch. 2009. Simplified and effective motor control based on muscle synergies to exploit musculoskeletal dynamics. *Proceedings of the National Academy of Science U S A* 106:7601–06.

Bernstein, N.A. 1935. The problem of interrelation between coordination and localization. [In Russian.] *Archives of Biological Sciences* 38: 1–35.

Bernstein, N.A. 1947. *On the construction of movements.* [In Russian.] Moscow: Medgiz.

Bernstein, N.A. 1967. *The coordination and regulation of movements.* Oxford: Pergamon.

Blaszczyk, J., and G.E. Loeb. 1993. Why cats pace on the treadmill. *Physiology and Behavior* 53:501–07.

Bobbert, M.F., and G.J. van Ingen Schenau. 1988. Coordination in vertical jumping. *Journal of Biomechanics* 21:249–62.

Brown, I.E., E.J. Cheng, and G.E. Loeb. 1999. Measured and modeled properties of mammalian skeletal muscle. II. The effects of stimulus frequency on force-length and force-velocity relationships. *Journal of Muscle Research and Cell Motility* 20:627–43.

Bullock, D., and S. Grossberg. 1988. Neural dynamics of planned arm movements: emergent invariants and speed-accuracy properties during trajectory formation. *Psychology Review* 95:49–90.

Burkholder, T.J., and T. R. Nichols. 2004. Three-dimensional model of the feline hindlimb. *Journal of Morphology* 261: 118–29.

Cappellini, G., Y.P. Ivanenko, R.E. Poppele, and F. Lacquaniti. 2006. Motor patterns in human walking and running. *Journal of Neurophysiology* 95:3426–37.

Carlson-Kuhta, P., T.V. Trank, and J.L. Smith. 1998. Forms of forward quadrupedal locomotion. II. A comparison of posture, hindlimb kinematics, and motor patterns for upslope and level walking. *Journal of Neurophysiology* 79: 1687–1701.

Cavagna, G.A., F.P. Saibene, and R. Margaria. 1964. mechanical work in running. *Journal of Applied Physiology* 19:249–56.

Chang, Y.H., A.G. Auyang, J.P. Scholz, and T.R. Nichols. 2009. Whole limb kinematics are preferentially conserved over individual joint kinematics after peripheral nerve injury. *Journal of Experimental Biology* 212:3511–21.

Crowninshield, R.D., and R.A. Brand. 1981. A physiologically based criterion of muscle force prediction in locomotion. *Journal of Biomechanics* 14:793–801.

Deliagina, T.G., G.N. Orlovsky, P.V. Zelenin, and I.N. Beloozerova . 2006. Neural bases of postural control. *Physiology (Bethesda)* 21:216–25.

Devita, P., L. Janshen, P. Rider, S. Solnik, and T. Hortobágyi. 2008. Muscle work is biased toward energy generation over dissipation in non-level running. *Journal of Biomechanics* 41:3354–59.

Donelan, J.M., D.A. McVea, and K.G. Pearson. 2009. Force regulation of ankle extensor muscle activity in freely walking cats. *Journal of Neurophysiology* 101: 360–71.

Dounskaya, N. 2005. The internal model and the leading joint hypothesis: implications for control of multi-joint movements. *Experimental Brain Research* 166: 1–16.

Dutto, D.J., D.F. Hoyt, E.A. Cogger, and S.J. Wickler. 2004. Ground reaction forces in horses trotting up an incline and on the level over a range of speeds. *Journal of Experimental Biology* 207: 3507–14.

Dutto, D.J., D.F. Hoyt, H.M. Clayton, E.A. Cogger, and S.J. Wickler. 2006. Joint work and power for both the forelimb and hindlimb during trotting in the horse. *Journal of Experimental Biology* 209:3990–99.

Eccles, J.C., R.M. Eccles, and A. Lundberg. 1957. The convergence of monosynaptic excitatory afferents on to many different species of alpha motoneurons. *Journal of Physiology* 137: 22–50.

Eccles, R.M., and A. Lundberg. 1958a. The synaptic linkage of 'direct' inhibition. *Acta Physiol Scand* 43:204–15.

Eccles, R.M., and A. Lundberg. 1958b. Integrative patterns of 1a synaptic actions on motoneurons of hip and knee muscles. *Journal of Physiology* 144: 271–98.

Ekeberg, O., and K. Pearson. 2005. Computer simulation of stepping in the hind legs of the cat: an examination of mechanisms regulating the stance-to-swing transition. *Journal of Neurophysiology* 94:4256–68.

English, A.W. 1984. An electromyographic analysis of compartments in cat lateral gastrocnemius muscle during unrestrained locomotion. *Journal of Neurophysiology* 52:114–25.

English, A.W., and P.R. Lennard. 1982. Interlimb coordination during stepping in the cat: in-phase stepping and gait transitions. *Brain Research* 245:353–64.

Farrell, B.J., E.E. Stout, M.G. Sirota, I.N. Beloozerova, and B.I. Prilutsky. 2008. Accurate target stepping in the cat: the full-body mechanics and activity of limb muscles. [Abstract 658.11.] Society for Neuroscience Meeting, Washington, DC.

Farley, C.T., and C.R. Taylor. 1991. A mechanical trigger for the trot-gallop transition in horses. *Science* 253:306–08.

Feldman, A.G. 1986. Once more on the equilibrium-point hypothesis (λ-model) for motor control. *Journal of Motor Behavior* 18: 17–54.

Feldman, A.G., V. Goussev, A. Sangole, and M.F. Levin. 2007. Threshold position control and the principle of minimal interaction in motor actions. *Progress in Brain Research* 165:267–81.

Feldman, A.G., and G.N. Orlovsky. 1975. Activity of interneurons mediating reciprocal Ia inhibition during locomotion. *Brain Research* 84: 181–94.

Flanders, M., and J.F. Soechting. 1990. Arm muscle activation for static forces in three-dimensional space. *Journal of Neurophysiology* 64:1818–37.

Frigon, A., and S. Rossignol. 2006. Functional plasticity following spinal cord lesions. *Progress in Brain Research* 157: 231–60.

Fung, J., and J.M. Macpherson. 1995. Determinants of postural orientation in quadrupedal stance. *Journal of Neuroscience* 15:1121–31.

Gambaryan, P.P. 1974. *How mammals run: Anatomical adaptations*. New York: John Wiley & Sons/Israel Program for Scientific Translations.

Gregersen, C.S., N.A. Silverton, and D.R. Carrier. 1998. External work and potential for elastic storage at the limb joints of running dogs. *Journal of Experimental Biology* 201:3197–3210.

Glenn, L.L., and J.F. Whitney. 1987. Contraction properties and motor nucleus morphology of the two heads of the cat flexor carpi ulnaris muscle. *Journal of Morphology* 191:17–23.

Gottlieb, G.L., M.L. Latash, D.M. Corcos, T.J. Liubinskas, and G.C. Agarwal. 1992. Organizing principles for single joint movements: V. Agonist-antagonist interactions. *Journal of Neurophysiology* 67:1417–27.

Gottschall, J.S., and T.R. Nichols. 2007. Head pitch affects muscle activity in the decerebrate cat hindlimb during walking. *Experimental Brain Research* 182:131–35.

Gray, J. 1968. *Animal locomotion*. London: Weidenfield & Nicolson.

Gregor, R.J., D.W. Smith, and B.I. Prilutsky. 2006. Mechanics of slope walking in the cat: quantification of muscle load, length change, and ankle extensor EMG patterns. *Journal of Neurophysiology* 95:1397–409.

Guertin, P., M.J. Angel, M.C. Perreault, and D.A. McCrea. 1995. Ankle extensor group I afferents excite extensors throughout the hindlimb during fictive locomotion in the cat. *Journal of Physiology* 487: 197–209.

Haruno, M., and D.M. Wolpert. 2005. Optimal control of redundant muscles in step-tracking wrist movements. *Journal of Neurophysiology* 94:4244–55.

Hildebrand, M. 1965. Symmetrical gaits of horses. *Science* 150:701–08.

Hildebrand, M. 1989. The quadrupedal gaits of vertebrates. *BioScience* 39: 766–75.

Hodson, E., H.M. Clayton, and J.L. Lanovaz. 2000. The forelimb in walking horses: 1. Kinematics and ground reaction forces. *Equine Vet J* 32: 287–94.

Hodson, E., H.M. Clayton, and J.L. Lanovaz. 2001. The hindlimb in walking horses: 1. Kinematics and ground reaction forces. *Equine Vet J* 33: 38–43.

Hodson-Tole, E.F., H. Maas, B. Farrel, R.J. Gregor, and B.I. Prilutsky. 2009. Patterns of motor unit recruitment in feline ankle extensor muscles during different motor tasks. [Abstract A6.36.] Society of Experimental Biology Meeting, Glasgow, UK.

Hoy, M.G., and R.F. Zernicke. 1985. Modulation of limb dynamics in the swing phase of locomotion. *Journal of Biomechanics* 18:49–60.

Hoyt, D.F., and C.R. Taylor. 1981. Gait and the energetics of locomotion in horses. *Nature* 292: 230–40.

Hreljac, A. 1995. Determinants of the gait transition speed during human locomotion: Kinematic factors. *Journal of Biomechanics* 28:669–77.

Jordan, L.M. 1991. Brainstem and spinal cord mechanisms for the initiation of locomotion. In *Neurobiological basis of human locomotion*, eds., M. Shimamura, S. Grillner, and V.R. Edgerton, pp. 3–20. Tokyo: Japan Scientific Society Press.

Karayannidou, A., T.G. Deliagina, Z.A. Tamarova, M.G. Sirota, P.V. Zelenin, G.N. Orlovsky, and I.N. Beloozerova. 2008. Influences of sensory input from the limbs on feline corticospinal neurons during postural responses. *Journal of Physiology* 586:247–63.

Kaya, M., T. Leonard, and W. Herzog. 2003. Coordination of medial gastrocnemius and soleus forces during cat locomotion. *Journal of Experimental Biology* 206: 3645–55.

Krouchev, N., J.F. Kalaska, and T. Drew. 2006. Sequential activation of muscle synergies during locomotion in the intact cat as revealed by cluster analysis and direct decomposition. *Journal of Neurophysiology* 96:1991–2010.

Lay, A.N., C.J. Hass, T. Richard Nichols, and R.J. Gregor. 2007. The effects of sloped surfaces on locomotion: An electromyographic analysis. *Journal of Biomechanics* 40:1276–85.

Lee, D.V., M.P. McGuigan, E.H. Yoo, and A.A. Biewener. 2008. Compliance, actuation, and work characteristics of the goat foreleg and hindleg during level, uphill, and downhill running. *Journal of Applied Physiology* 104: 130–41.

Lin, D.C., and W.Z. Rymer. 2000. Damping actions of the neuromuscular system with inertial loads: soleus muscle of the decerebrate cat. *Journal of Neurophysiology* 83:652–58.

Maas, H., B.I. Prilutsky, T.R. Nichols, and R.J. Gregor. 2007. The effects of self-reinnervation of cat medial and lateral gastrocnemius muscles on hindlimb kinematics in slope walking. *Experimental Brain Research* 181:377–93.

Macpherson, J.M. 1988. Strategies that simplify the control of quadrupedal stance. I. Forces at the ground. *Journal of Neurophysiology* 60: 204–17.

Manter, J.T. 1938. The dynamics of quadrupedal walking. *Journal of Experimental Biology* 15: 522–40.

Mussa-Ivaldi, F.A., N. Hogan, and E. Bizzi. 1985. Neural, mechanical, and geometric factors subserving arm posture in humans. *Journal of Neuroscience* 5:2732–43.

Nichols, T.R. 1994. A biomechanical perspective on spinal mechanisms of coordinated muscular action: An architecture principle. *Acta Anatomie* 151: 1–13.

Nichols, T.R. 1999. Receptor mechanisms underlying heterogenic reflexes among the triceps surae muscles of the cat. *Journal of Neurophysiology* 81:467–78.

Orlovsky, G.N., T.G. Deliagina, and S. Grillner. 1999. *Neuronal control of locomotion: From mollusc to man*. New York: Oxford University Press.

Pandy, M.G., V. Kumar, N. Berme, and K.J. Waldron. 1988. The dynamics of quadrupedal locomotion. *Journal of Biomechanics Engineering* 110: 230–37.

Pataky, T.C., M.L. Latash, and V.M. Zatsiorsky. 2004. Prehension synergies during nonvertical grasping, II: Modeling and optimization. *Biological Cybernetics* 91: 231–42.

Pearson, K.G. 2008. Role of sensory feedback in the control of stance duration in walking cats. *Brain Research Review* 57:222–27.

Prilutsky, B.I. 2000a. Coordination of two- and one-joint muscles: Functional consequences and implications for motor control. *Motor Control* 4:1–44.

Prilutsky, B.I. 2000b. Eccentric muscle action in sport and exercise. In *Encyclopedia of sports medicine. Biomechanics in sport*, ed. V.M. Zatsiorsky, 56–86. Oxford, UK: Blackwell Science Ltd.

Prilutsky, B.I., I.N. Beloozerova, M.G. Sirota, and R.J. Gregor. 2001. Biomechanics of precise stepping in the cat. [Abstract 941.12.] Society for Neuroscience Annual Meeting. San Diego, CA.

Prilutsky, B.I., and R.J. Gregor. 1997. Strategy of coordination of two- and one-joint leg muscles in controlling an external force. *Motor Control* 1: 91–115.

Prilutsky, B.I., and R.J. Gregor. 2001. Swing- and support-related muscle actions differentially trigger human walk-run and run-walk transitions. *Journal of Experimental Biology* 204:2277–87.

Prilutsky, B.I., W. Herzog, and T.L. Allinger. 1994. Force-sharing between cat soleus and gastrocnemius muscles during walking: Explanations based on electrical activity, properties, and kinematics. *Journal of Biomechanics* 2: 1223–35.

Prilutsky, B.I., W. Herzog, and T. Leonard. 1996a. Transfer of mechanical energy between ankle and knee joints by gastrocnemius and plantaris muscles during cat locomotion. *Journal of Biomechanics* 29:391–403.

Prilutsky, B.I., A.N. Klishko, B. Farrell, L. Harley, G. Phillips, and C.L. Bottasso. 2009. Movement coordination in skilled tasks: Insights from optimization. In *Advances in neuromuscular physiology of motor skills and muscle fatigue*, ed. M. Shinohara, 139–71. Kerala, India: Research Signpost.

Prilutsky, B.I., L.N. Petrova, and L.M. Raitsin. 1996b. Comparison of mechanical energy expenditure of joint moments and muscle forces during human locomotion. *Journal of Biomechanics* 29:405–15.

Prilutsky, B.I., M.G. Sirota, R.J. Gregor, and I.N. Beloozerova. 2005. Quantification of motor cortex activity and full-body biomechanics during unconstrained locomotion. *Journal of Neurophysiology* 94:2959–69.

Prilutsky, B.I., and V.M. Zatsiorsky. 1994. Tendon action of two-joint muscles: Transfer of mechanical energy between joints during jumping, landing, and running. *Journal of Biomechanics* 27:25–34.

Prilutsky, B.I., and V.M. Zatsiorsky. 2002. Optimization-based models of muscle coordination. *Exercise and Sport Science Review* 30:32–38.

Pruszynski, J.A., I. Kurtzer, T.P. Lillicrap, and S.H. Scott. 2009. Temporal evolution of "automatic gain-scaling." *Journal of Neurophysiology* 102:992–1003.

Roberts, T.J., and J.A. Scales. 2004. Adjusting muscle function to demand: Joint work during acceleration in wild turkeys. *Journal of Experimental Biology* 207: 4165–74.

Rubenson, J., and R.L. Marsh. 2009. Mechanical efficiency of limb swing during walking and running in guinea fowl (*Numida meleagris*). *Journal of Applied Physiology* 106:1618–30.

Rybak, I.A., K. Stecina, N.A. Shevtsova, and D.A. McCrea. 2006. Modelling spinal circuitry involved in locomotor pattern generation: Insights from the effects of afferent stimulation. *Journal of Physiology* 577:641–58.

Sacks, R.D., and R.R. Roy. 1982. Architecture of the hind limb muscles of cats: functional significance. *Journal of Morphology* 173(2):185–95.

Sainburg, R.L., C. Ghez, and D. Kalakanis. 1999. Intersegmental dynamics are controlled by sequential anticipatory, error correction, and postural mechanisms. *Journal of Neurophysiology* 81:1045–56.

Sandercock, T.G., and C.J. Heckman. 1997. Force from cat soleus muscle during imposed locomotor-like movements: Experimental data versus Hill-type model predictions. *Journal of Neurophysiology* 77:1538–52.

Sherrington, C.S. 1893. Note on the knee-jerk and the correlation of action of antagonistic muscles. *Proceedings of the Royal Society B* 52:556–64.

Shik, M.L., F.V. Severin, and G.N. Orlovsky. 1966. Control of walking and running by means of electrical stimulation of the mid-brain. *Biophysics* 11: 756–65.

Smith, J.L., B. Betts, V.R. Edgerton, and R.F. Zernicke. 1980. Rapid ankle extension during paw shakes: selective recruitment of fast ankle extensors. *Journal of Neurophysiology* 43:612–20.

Smith, J.L., P. Carlson-Kuhta, and T.V. Trank. 1998. Forms of forward quadrupedal locomotion. III. A comparison of posture, hindlimb kinematics, and motor patterns for downslope and level walking. *Journal of Neurophysiology* 79: 1702–16.

Stuart, D.G., T.P. Withey, M.C. Witzel, G.E. Goslow Jr. 1973. Time constraints for inter-limb co-ordination in the cat during unrestrained locomotion. In *Control of posture and locomotion*, eds., R.B. Stein, K.G. Pearson, R.S. Smith, and J.B. Redford, 537–60. New York: Plenum.

Ting, L.H., and J.M. Macpherson. 2004. Ratio of shear to load ground-reaction force may underlie the directional tuning of the automatic postural response to rotation and translation. *Journal of Neurophysiology* 92:808–23.

Ting, L.H., and J.M. Macpherson. 2005. A limited set of muscle synergies for force control during a postural task. *Journal of Neurophysiology* 93:609–13.

Thorup, V.M., B. Laursen, and B.R. Jensen. 2008. Net joint kinetics in the limbs of pigs walking on concrete floor in dry and contaminated conditions. *Journal of Animal Science* 86:992–98.

Todorov, E., and M.I. Jordan. 2002. Optimal feedback control as a theory of motor coordination. *Nature Neuroscience* 5:1226–35.

van Ingen Schenau, G.J., and M.F. Bobbert. 1993. The global design of the hindlimb in quadrupeds. *Acta Anatomica (Basel)* 146:103–108.

Walter, R.M., and D.R. Carrier. 2007. Ground forces applied by galloping dogs. *Journal of Experimental Biology* 210:208–16.

Winter, D.A. 1983. Biomechanical motor patterns in normal walking. *Journal of Motor Behavior* 15:302–30.

Wetzel, M.C., and D.G. Stuart. 1976. Ensemble characteristics of cat locomotion and its neural control. *Progress in Neurobiology* 7:1–98.

Yang, J.F., E.V. Lamont, and M.Y. Pang. 2005. Split-belt treadmill stepping in infants suggests autonomous pattern generators for the left and right leg in humans. *Journal of Neuroscience* 25: 6869–76.

Yen, J.T., A.G. Auyang, and Y.H. Chang. 2009. Joint-level kinetic redundancy is exploited to control limb-level forces during human hopping. *Experimental Brain Research* 196:439–51.

Zajac, F.E., and M.E. Gordon. 1989. Determining muscle's force and action in multi-articular movement. *Exercise and Sports Science Review* 17:187–230.

Zatsiorsky, V.M. 2002. *Kinetics of human movement*. Champaign, IL: Human Kinetics.

Zatsiorsky, V.M., and B.I. Prilutsky. 1987. Soft and stiff landing. *International series on biomechanics Vol. 6B. Biomechanics X-B*, 739–43. Champaign, IL: Human Kinetics.

10

Control of Equilibrium in Humans

Sway over Sway

Marcos Duarte, Sandra M. S. F. Freitas, and Vladimir Zatsiorsky

In humans, the postural control of a segment or the whole body about a reference position is achieved by passive and active restoring forces applied to the system under control. Under this rationale, the control of whole-body posture during upright standing has been modeled as an inverted pendulum oscillating about a fixed position. This simple representation has been very useful for understanding many aspects of human postural control. However, some behaviors observed during upright standing are not well captured by this representation. For example, we conducted a series of studies on natural (unconstrained) prolonged (several minutes) upright standing and showed that individuals tend to oscillate about a moving reference position (Duarte and Zatsiorsky 1999; Duarte et al. 2000; Duarte and Zatsiorsky 2000; Duarte and Zatsiorsky 2001; Freitas et al. 2005b; Prado and Duarte 2009).

In fact, there are no mechanical or neural constraints requiring that humans regulate their upright posture around a reference position somewhat aligned with the vertical axis. An alternative idea is that humans simply adopt a strategy to maximize the safety margin for falling. For example, Slobounov and colleagues (1997) have proposed that we regulate our upright posture by maximizing the time the body center of pressure (COP) would take to contact the stability boundaries at any instant, given the instantaneous position, velocity, and acceleration of the COP at that instant (this time was termed the *virtual time to contact*). By maximizing the virtual time to contact, a standing person would avoid a fall. Although it remains to be shown to what extent virtual time to contact is incompatible with posture control around a reference point, this theory has not been disproved.

The concept of COP is very useful for understanding the regulation of postural control. The COP expresses the position of the resultant vertical component of the ground reaction force applied to the body at the ground surface. The COP is a two-dimensional position dependent on the acceleration of the body and its segments (because it is related to the forces applied to the body). A related concept to COP is the center of gravity (COG). The COG is defined as a specific point in a system of particles (or segments for the human body) that behaves as if the weight of all particles were concentrated at that point. From simple mechanics, if the vertical projection of the COG (COGv) steps out of the base of support (the area at the floor that circumscribes the region of contact of our body with the ground, e.g., for the bipedal posture, it is the area circumscribing the feet), the body will be unable to apply restoring forces to maintain the upright posture. In this sense, the contour of the base of support can be viewed as the stability boundaries for controlling posture.

In fact, the limits of stability that standing humans are able to use are smaller than the physical limits given by the contours of the feet. Figure 10.1 presents mean values for the limits of the base of support, limits of stability the adults can voluntarily reach during standing, COP area of sway during prolonged natural (unconstrained) standing for 30 minutes, and COP area of sway during standing still for 40 seconds. Figure 10.1 shows that, while standing still, humans occupy a very small area of the base of support and that during unconstrained standing this area is much larger. With regards to the amount of sway produced during standing, in general, it is assumed that more sway means more instability and is an indication of a deteriorated posture control system. This rationale is based on many experiments on aging and pathological conditions that showed increased sway in those conditions (see for example, the reviews of Horak et al. 1989; Bonnet et al. 2009). However, this is not always the case. Patients with Parkinson disease in some cases demonstrate reduced postural sway compared to elderly adults, despite the fact that patients with Parkinson disease do present severe problems of postural control (Romero and Stelmach 2003). Another proposition for postural control is that at least part of the sway during upright posture is, in fact, an intentional sway (Riccio et al. 1992; Riley et al. 1997; Riley and Turvey 2002; Stoffregen et al. 2005; Bonnet et al. 2009). In this view, more sway does not necessarily imply more instability; neither it is an indication of a deteriorated posture control system. In addition, although elderly persons, when asked to stand as still as possible for a short period of time, commonly show increased postural sway during standing compared to younger persons, elderly persons show the opposite behavior during prolonged unconstrained standing (Freitas et al. 2005b).

In this chapter, we briefly review the control of equilibrium in humans during quiet standing and findings about prolonged unconstrained standing, and we discuss the implications of these findings for understanding the control of equilibrium in humans. But first we describe how postural sway can be evaluated. Throughout this chapter, we employ biomechanical principles to understand the control of equilibrium. The use of biomechanics to

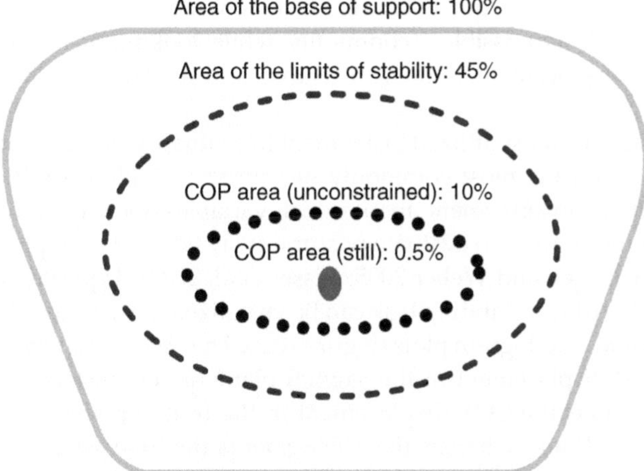

Figure 10.1 Mean values for the limits of the base of support (*solid line*), limits of stability individuals can voluntarily reach during standing (*dashed line*), center of pressure (COP) area of sway during prolonged unconstrained standing for 30 min (*dotted line*), and COP area of sway during standing still for 40 s (*filled area in the center*). Data adapted from Duarte, M., W. Harvey, and V.M. Zatsiorsky. 2000. Stabilographic analysis of unconstrained standing. *Ergonomics* 43: 1824–39; Duarte, M., and V.M. Zatsiorsky. 2002. Effects of body lean and visual information on the equilibrium maintenance during stance. *Experimental Brain Research* 146: 60–69; Freitas, S.M., J.M. Prado, and M. Duarte. 2005a. The use of a safety harness does not affect body sway during quiet standing. *Clinical Biomechanics (Bristol, Avon)* 20: 336–39; and Freitas, S.M., S.A. Wieczorek, P.H. Marchetti, and M. Duarte. 2005b. Age-related changes in human postural control of prolonged standing. *Gait & Posture* 22: 322–30, all with permission of their respective publishers.

understand the control of locomotion and the connection between motor control and biomechanics in general are addressed in the other two chapters of this section.

QUANTIFICATION OF POSTURAL SWAY DURING STANDING

Before 1950, postural sway was studied mainly by recording head oscillation, a method that is called *ataxiography*. Since then, ataxiography was almost completely forgotten and the recording of ground reaction forces and COP displacement became the prevailing approach. The quantitative evaluation of body sway via force recordings is called *posturography*, which has been divided into static posturography, when the postural control of a person is evaluated by asking that person to stand as still as possible, and dynamic posturography, when the postural responses to a perturbation applied to the person are evaluated. The most frequent measurement used in posturography is COP displacement, which can be easily measured using a force plate. The most common task used for the evaluation of postural control is the quiet standing task, in which the person is asked to stand "as still as possible," commonly while looking at a fixed target. The COP displacement is then measured and analyzed to quantify the postural sway.

Although the most utilized instrument to evaluate postural control is the force plate and the most commonly measured variable is COP displacement, there is no agreement about which variables derived from the COP signal should be used to evaluate postural sway (see, for example, Kapteyn et al. 1983; Gagey and Weber 2005; Visser et al. 2008). Typically, COP displacement during a standing task can be visualized in two ways: in statokinesigram and stabilogram plots (Figure 10.2). The *statokinesigram* is the map of the COP displacement in the sagittal plane (anteroposterior direction, COP ap) versus the COP displacement in the frontal plane (mediolateral direction, COP ml); whereas the *stabilogram* is the time series of the COP displacement in each direction. Customarily, posturographic analysis has been divided into global and structural analyses. *Global analysis* is related to the quantification of the total amount of body sway, whereas *structural analysis* quantifies particular events or components of body sway.

A large number of measures have been used to describe the amount of postural sway (Winter et al. 1990; Prieto et al. 1996; Duarte and Zatsiorsky 1999; Baratto et al. 2002; Raymakers et al. 2005; van der Kooij et al. 2005; Piirtola and Era 2006; Rougier 2008). Among them, the most common measures are COP spatial displacement (usually standard deviation in each direction or total area), mean speed or velocity, and frequency variables (usually mean or median frequency). Some of the most common variables used in the quantification of body sway in the time and frequency domains are presented in Table 10.1, and an example of the power spectral density

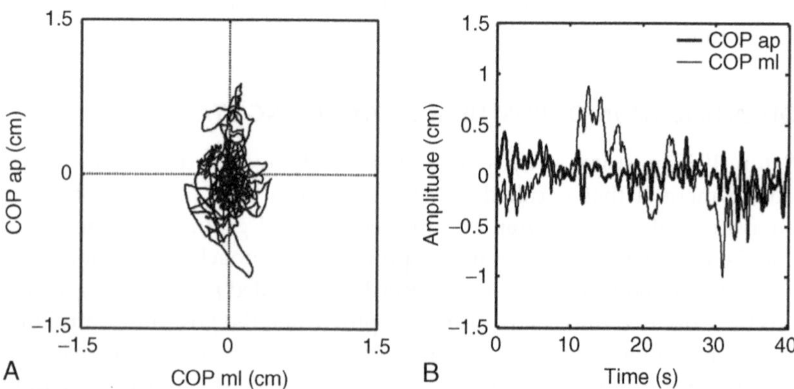

Figure 10.2 Examples of ***statokinesigram*** (A) and stabilogram (B) of center of pressure (COP) displacement during standing as still as possible on a force plate.

Table 10.1 Usual variables used in the global analysis of COP displacement and examples on how to compute these variables by using Matlab software

Variable	Matlab code
Standard deviation	std(COP)
RMS (Root Mean Square)	sqrt(sum(COP.^2)/length(COP))
Range of COP displacement	max(COP) - min(COP)
Sway path	sum(abs(COP))
Resultant sway path	sum(sqrt(COPap.^2 + COPml.^2))
Area (95% of the COP data inside)	[vec,val] = eig(cov(COPap,COPml)); Area = pi*prod(2.4478*sqrt(svd(val)))
Mean speed or velocity	sum(abs(diff(COP)))*frequency/length(COP)
Resultant mean velocity	sum(sqrt(diff(COPap).^2+diff(COPml).^2))* frequency /length(COPap)

Power spectral density
Peak (Fpeak)
Mean (Fmean)
Median (F50) frequency and the frequency band that contains up to 80% of the spectrum (F80)
	nfft = round(length(COP)/2);
	[p,f] = psd(detrend(COP),nfft, frequency,nfft,round(nfft/2));
	[m,peak] = max(p);
	area = cumtrapz(f,p);
	F50 = find(area >= .50*area(end));
	F80 = find(area >= .80*area(end));
	Fmean = trapz(f,f.*p)/trapz(f,p)
	Fpeak = f(peak)
	F50 = f(F50(1))
	F80 = f(F80(1))

estimation and its outcome variables for COP displacement during quiet standing is presented in Figure 10.3.

Baratto and collaborators (2002) examined 38 posturographic measures calculated from COP time series and examined the reliability and power of the measures to discriminate three different groups of individuals: normal individuals, parkinsonian patients, and osteoporotic patients. They concluded that only four measures were valuable for clinical practice: total sway path, frequency band, and two measures from COP decomposition called *sway-density plots*. The first two variables were derived from global analysis, whereas the other two measures were derived from structural analysis. The mean speed or velocity of the COP migration has been considered as the measure of greater consistency across repetitions (Lafond et al. 2004a; Cornilleau-Peres et al. 2005). On the other hand, Doyle and collaborators (2005) reported that peak velocity and area presented indexes of the lowest and highest reliability, respectively. Raymakers and collaborators (2005) observed that the velocity of the COP displacement was more

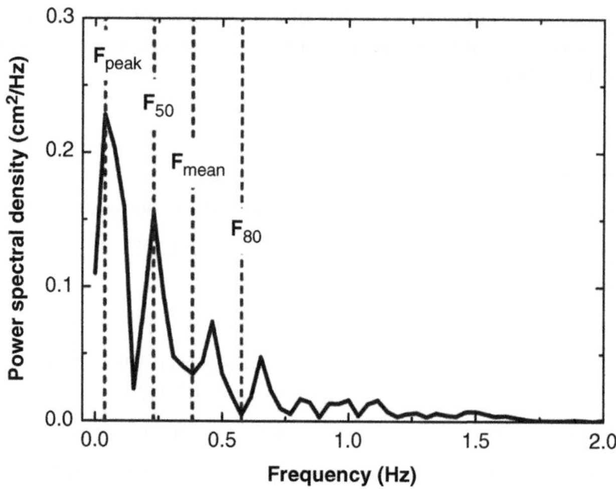

Figure 10.3 Example of the power spectral density estimation of center of pressure (COP) displacement during quiet standing. The peak (Fpeak), mean (Fmean), and median (F50) frequencies and the frequency band that contains up to 80% of the power spectrum (F80) are also shown.

reliable for comparisons between different aging groups and between groups with different health conditions. These different results can be due to the absence of standardization of the methods used to evaluate equilibrium control, such as differences in time duration (10–120 s), number of repetitions (three to nine repetitions), and frequency of data acquisition (10–100 Hz).

Center of Gravity Estimation

Typically, in posturography, instead of measuring the sway of each segment, measures of whole body sway are used; the displacements of COGv and COP are the most common measures of body sway. (However, bear in mind that the COP is not a direct measurement of postural sway of the body or its segments.) Although COP displacement can be easily measured with a force plate, the direct measurement of COGv is more complicated and typically subject to a larger error. The direct measurement of COGv is computed by recording the position of each body segment and estimating each segment mass, using an anthropometric model. More commonly, the displacement of the COGv is indirectly determined from the COP displacement, and different methods are available that produce similar results (Lafond et al. 2004b). In one of these methods, the COGv displacement is obtained by double integration of the horizontal force in combination with information from the COP displacement (King and Zatsiorsky 1997; Zatsiorsky and King 1998; Zatsiorsky and Duarte 2000). A computational algorithm implementing this method is available on the Internet (http://demotu.org/software/gline.m). A simpler method to derive the COGv displacement is to apply a low-pass filter to the COP displacement (Benda et al. 1994; Caron et al. 1997; Baratto et al. 2002). The use of a low-pass filter is motivated by modeling the mechanics of the standing-still task as an inverted pendulum, as illustrated next. Let us consider for now only the movement in the anteroposterior direction (in the sagittal plane) of a person standing still. Let us represent the human body as composed of two rigid segments articulated by a single hinge joint (feet, rest of the body, and ankle joint). Given this simplification, all the mechanical quantities important for understanding the motion of the body are represented in Figure 10.4.

Applying the second Newton-Euler equation of motion to the inverted pendulum system in this two-dimensional problem, and after a few simplifications, the following equation represents the relation between the *COGv* acceleration and the *COGv* and *COP* displacements:

$$\frac{d^2COG_v}{dt^2} \approx \frac{mgd}{I}(COG_v - COP) \qquad \text{(Eq. 1)}$$

where I is the moment of inertia of the body around the ankle.

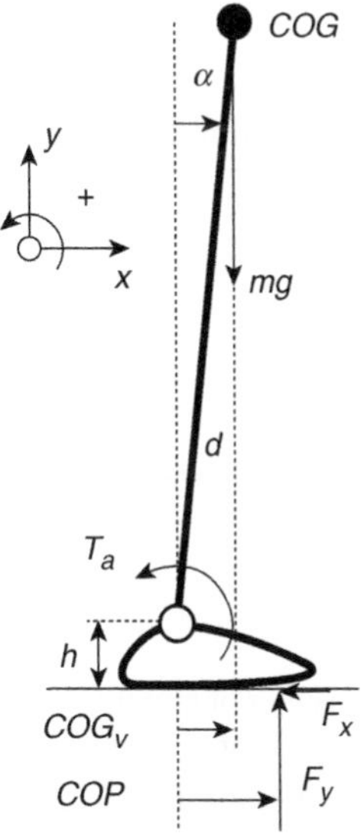

Figure 10.4 Single inverted pendulum model for the representation of a human standing. *COG*, center of gravity; COG_v, *COG* vertical projection in relation to the ankle joint; *COP*, center of pressure in relation to the ankle joint; m, g, body mass, acceleration of gravity; F_x, F_y, horizontal and vertical components of the resultant ground reaction force; T_a, torque at the ankle joint; d, distance between the *COG* and ankle joint; h, height of the ankle joint to the ground; α, angle of the body.

If we rewrite Equation 1 in the frequency domain by computing its Fourier transform, we obtain:

$$\frac{\overline{COGv}(\omega)}{\overline{COP}(\omega)} = \frac{\omega_0^2}{\omega^2 + \omega_0^2} \qquad \text{(Eq. 2)}$$

where ω is the angular frequency and $\omega_0 = \sqrt{mgd/I}$ represents the natural frequency of the pendulum.

The term on the right side of Equation 2 is always lower than 1 and indicates that COGv is indeed a filtered version of the COP in the frequency domain. For a person with 70 kg of mass and 1.70 m of height, ω_0 is equal to 3 rad/s, and the filter with this parameter will be similar to a low-pass filter with a cutoff frequency in the range of 0.4–0.5 Hz (Benda et al. 1994; Caron et al. 1997). Table 10.2 shows a Matlab code implementation of this method. A reliable estimation of the COGv based on this method depends on the assumption that the dynamics of COP and COGv can be captured by the inverted pendulum model. In addition, because of the Fourier transform, the COP data should be suitably long (at least 30 s). The mentioned above "double integration of the horizontal force" method is free from this requirement and has an additional advantage in that the COG position is determined at each instant in time and not on average over the period of observation, as in those methods based on data filtering.

Table 10.2 Matlab code for estimation of COGv from the COP displacement

```
function COGv = cogve(COP,freq,m,H)
%COGVE estimates COGv from COP using a FFT filter
%SYNTAX:
% COGv = cogve(COP,freq,m,H)
% cogve(COP,freq,m,H)
%INPUTS:
% COP: column vector of the center of pressure [m]
% freq: sampling frequency [Hz]
% m: body mass of the subject [kg]
% H: height of the subject [m]
%OUTPUT:
% COGv: column vector of the center of gravity vertical projection [m]
%cogve(COP,freq,m,H) with no output plots the COP and COGv data.

%Remove mean to decrease instabilities at the extremities:
mcop = mean(COP); COP = COP - mcop;
%Parameters:
%Height of the COG w.r.t. ankle:
h = 0.56*H - 0.039*H; %(McGinnis 2005; Winter 2005)
%Body moment of inertia around the ankle:
I = m*0.0533*H^2 + m*h^2; %(Breniere 1996)
```

(Cont'd)

Table 10.2 Matlab code for estimation of COGv from the COP displacement (*Continued*)

```
%Gravity acceleration:
g = 9.8;
%Pendulum natural frequency:
w02 = m*g*h/I;
%Make sure COP is a column vector:
if size(COP,1)==1; COP=COP'; disp('COP transformed to column vector'), end
%Number of data:
ncop = length(COP);
nfft = 2^nextpow2(ncop);
%COP fft:
COPf = fft(COP,nfft)/ncop;
%Angular frequency vector:
w = 2*pi*freq/2*linspace(0,1,nfft/2+1)';
w = [w; -w(end-1:-1:2)];
%Transfer function:
TF = w02./(w.^2 + w02);
%COGv:
COGv = real(ifft(COPf.*TF)*ncop);
COGv = COGv(1:ncop);
%Get back the mean (COP & COGv have same mean):
COP = COP + mcop; COGv = COGv + mcop;
%Plot:
t = (1:ncop)'/freq;
figure, plot(t,COP,'b',t,COGv,'r','LineWidth',2)
legend('COP','COGv','Location','best')
xlabel('Time [s]'), ylabel('Amplitude [m]')
```

This code is also available at http://demotu.org/software/cogve.m

PROLONGED UNCONSTRAINED STANDING

Under natural standing conditions, in which persons are not obliged to stand as still as possible, people usually adopt asymmetrical postures and tend to change their body position periodically while adopting relatively fixed body postures for certain periods of time. In natural standing, continuous low-amplitude and slow swaying of the body, which is normally observed during standing still, is commonly interrupted by postural changes characterized by fast and gross body movements. Hereafter, we will refer to such a task—standing for several minutes without a requirement to stay still, but with a requirement either not to change feet positions on the ground or not to step off the force plate—as prolonged unconstrained standing.

To better understand what people do during prolonged unconstrained standing, Duarte and Zatsiorsky (1999) analyzed the COP displacement of young and healthy individuals standing for 30 minutes with an upright bipedal posture on a force platform. The individuals were allowed to change their posture at any time, and there were no specific instructions on how to stand, except for the requirement to not step off the force platform. To reproduce the fact that people actually stand to do something else, the individuals were allowed to chat occasionally with another person in front of him or her. Figure 10.5 shows exemplary data for the COP displacement for one individual.

A few distinct characteristics of prolonged unconstrained standing can be noted on the COP data. First, when the COP displacement is mapped in the anteroposterior versus mediolateral plane (statokinesigram), two typical patterns can be observed: multiregion and single-region standing (Figure 10.5). In multiregion standing, the individuals tend to change the

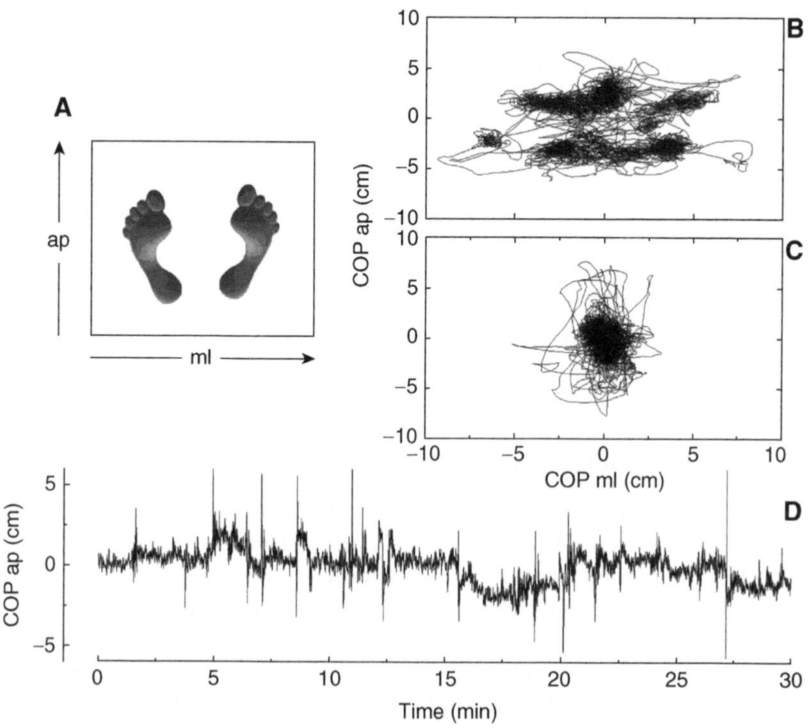

Figure 10.5 Position of the subjects on the force plate and axes convention (**A**). Two examples of statokinesigrams during prolonged unconstrained standing for 30 minutes: multiregion (**B**) and single-region standing (**C**). Exemplary center of pressure (COP) stabilogram (**D**). Data from Duarte, M., and V.M. Zatsiorsky. 2001. Long-range correlations in human standing. *Physics Letters A* 283: 124–28, with permission of the publisher.

average location of the COP several times during the trial. Second, when the COP displacement is plotted against time (stabilogram), other two characteristics can be observed (Fig. 10.5): (a) the presence of specific (localized) events of larger amplitude, which have been classified as COP migration patterns of specific types; and (b) the presence of very low frequencies in the COP displacement, a typical signature of a long-range correlation process or long-memory process. These distinct characteristics of prolonged unconstrained standing are discussed next.

The specific (localized) events in the COP data during prolonged unconstrained standing have been classified as COP migration patterns of the following types (Duarte and Zatsiorsky 1999):

- *Shifting*: a fast (step-like) displacement of the average position of the COP from one region to another;
- *Fidgeting*: a fast and large displacement and returning of the COP to approximately the same position; and
- *Drifting*: a slow continuous displacement of the average position of the COP (linear or nonlinear trend).

Figure 10.6 shows a representative example of the three patterns in a COP time series of the present study. In general, these three patterns are always observed, in varying quantities, during prolonged unconstrained standing. In fact, these patterns can be seen as different forms of shifting. Fidgeting is a shifting followed by another in the opposite direction, and drifting is a very long shifting in time.

Duarte and Zatsiorsky (1999) parameterized the COP migration patterns in terms of a few quantities, and they were able to objectively identify such parameters with computational algorithms. For recognition of shifting, any two consecutive nonoverlapping moving windows, W_1 and W_2, satisfying Equation 1 were classified as a shift:

$$\left| \frac{\overline{x}_{W1} - \overline{x}_{W2}}{\sqrt{SD_{W1}^2 + SD_{W2}^2}} \right| \geq f_{shift} \qquad \text{(Eq. 3)}$$

where $\overline{x}_{Wi}$ $(i=1,2)$ is the mean of the COP data for the windows W_1 and W_2, SD_{Wi} is the standard deviation of the COP data in the window Wi, and f_{shift} is the threshold value of the amplitude of the shift pattern (in units of $SD_{W1} + SD_{W2}$). The amplitude of the shift is defined as $|\overline{x}_{W1} - \overline{x}_{W2}|$. The estimated width of the shift (the time taken to shift the COP position) is given by the interval, W_S, separating the two consecutive windows.

For recognition of fidgeting, any peak or valley satisfying Equation 4 was classified as a fidget:

$$\left| \frac{x_F - \overline{x}_W}{SD_W} \right| \geq f_{fidget} \qquad \text{(Eq. 4)}$$

where x_F is the amplitude of the peak or valley, $\bar{x}_W$ is the mean COP data for the window W, SD_W is the standard deviation of the COP data in the window W, and f_{fidget} is the threshold value for the amplitude of the fidget pattern (in units of SD_W). The amplitude of the fidget is defined as $|x_F - \bar{x}_W|$. The width of the fidget, W_f, was estimated by the full width at half maximum of the fidget (see Fig. 10.6).

For recognition of drifting, the data between two consecutive shifts were smoothed using a low-pass filter with a variable cutoff frequency $F_C = \frac{1}{2W_D}$, where W_D was the preselected minimal drifting width. This procedure preserves only the low-frequency trend (drift) in the data. If the difference

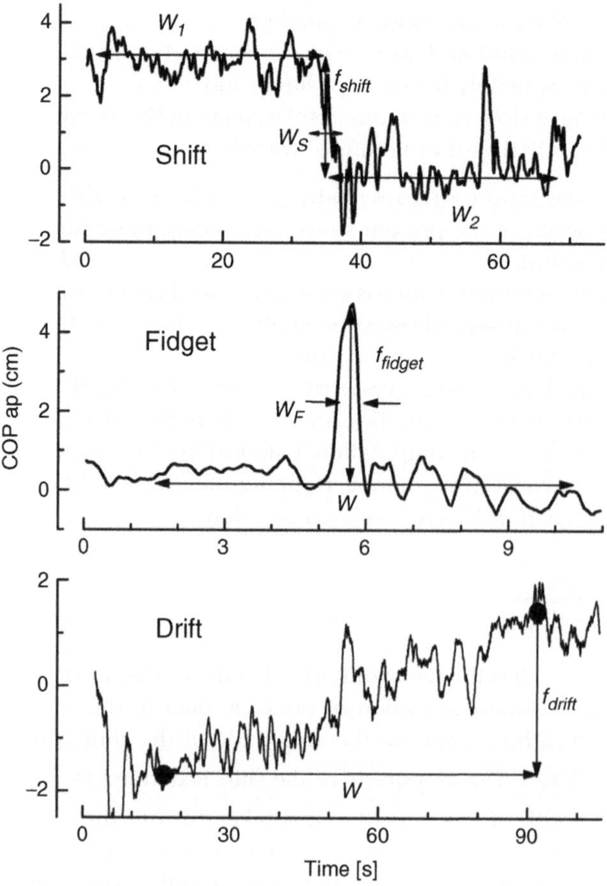

Figure 10.6 An example of shifting, fidgeting, and drifting patterns during prolonged unconstrained standing, with the corresponding parameters used for identification. Data from Duarte, M., W. Harvey, and V.M. Zatsiorsky. 2000. Stabilographic analysis of unconstrained standing. *Ergonomics* 43: 1824–39, with permission of the publisher.

between the amplitudes of two consecutive local maximum and minimum values satisfied Equation 5, the COP displacements between the consecutive maximum and minimum were classified as a drift.

$$\left|\frac{x_{\max} - x_{\min}}{SD_W}\right| \geq f_{drift} \qquad \text{(Eq. 5)}$$

where x_{max} and x_{min} are the consecutive local maximum and minimum amplitudes, SD_W is the standard deviation of the COP data in the window containing the data between the maximum and minimum values, and f_{drift} is the threshold value of the drift amplitude (in units of SD_W). The amplitude of the drift is defined as $|x_{\max} - x_{\min}|$.

Typical criterion values chosen for classifying the data as shift, fidget, or drift patterns are respectively: a minimum shift amplitude of 2 SD, a maximum shift width of 5 s, and a base window of 15 s; a minimum fidget amplitude of 3 SD, a maximum fidget width of 4 s, and a base window of 60 s; and a minimum drift amplitude of 1 SD, with a minimum drift width of 60s.

By performing the above computations, Duarte and Zatsiorsky (1999) observed that, during prolonged unconstrained standing by young healthy adults, the most common COP pattern was fidgeting, followed by shifting, and then drifting. On average, one postural change was produced every 20 s, either at the anteroposterior or at the mediolateral direction.

Why exactly postural changes are produced during prolonged unconstrained standing and how our posture is regulated by the presence of these postural changes are questions discussed next.

Basis for Postural Changes During Prolonged Unconstrained Standing

A qualitative observation of individuals during prolonged unconstrained standing reveals that the three COP patterns result from various movements of the body segments and/or the body as a whole. The most commonly observed body segments motions are arms, head, and trunk movement, as well as a redistribution of the body weight from one leg to another.

The existence of shifting and drifting fits well to the hypothesis of Lestienne and Gurfinkel (1988). These authors suggested that the motor control system responsible for balance maintenance is a hierarchical two-level system. The upper level ("conservative") determines a reference frame for an equilibrium, with respect to which the equilibrium is maintained. The low level ("operative") maintains the equilibrium around the predetermined reference position. This hypothesis was supported in studies by Gurfinkel and collaborators (1995), where the supporting surface was rotated slowly. They found that individuals maintained for some time a fixed body orientation with respect to the surface (the perceived vertical) rather than with respect to the real vertical. Lestienne and Gurfinkel (1988), as well as Gurfinkel and collaborators (1995), did not address in their studies a possible reference point migration during natural standing. The observations of shifting and drifting during prolonged unconstrained standing indeed suggest that such migration takes place.

Postural changes are most commonly viewed as a mechanism to avoid or minimize physiological fatigue and discomfort in the musculoskeletal system by decreasing venous pooling in the lower extremities, decreasing occlusion of blood flow through some regions of the sole of the foot caused by the continuous pressure in static standing, or alleviating the pressure on joints by "repumping" the cartilage fluid (Brantingham et al. 1970; Cavanagh et al. 1987; Zhang et al. 1991; Kim et al. 1994). However, at least another reason for postural changes during natural standing would be a mechanism to interact (e.g., with another person), explore, and gather information from the environment, mainly by using the visual sensory system (Riccio and Stoffregen 1988).

Duarte and collaborators (2000) tested some of these hypotheses for postural changes during prolonged unconstrained standing, employing again the analysis of COP migration patterns. They manipulated the load on the individual, under the rationale that, with the addition of an external load, the pressure on joint cartilage in the lower extremities and on the plantar sole increases. If the main reason for postural changes is to "repump" the cartilage fluid, the number of postural changes should increase when holding a load. If the reasons for postural changes are solely to decrease venous blood pooling in the lower extremities and to allow momentary blood flow through some regions of the foot sole, the number of postural changes would not vary during loaded standing. This last result would occur because the pressure on the plantar sole during normal or unloaded standing is already large enough to occlude the circulation of blood in this region (Cavanagh et al. 1987). Duarte and collaborators (2000) did not observe any increase in the number of postural changes, and so they discarded the idea of postural changes to "repump" the cartilage fluid. They also requested that participants stand with eyes closed in order to remove the visual system that is used to interact with the environment. They hypothesized that if postural changes during prolonged unconstrained standing were performed to explore the environment through the visual sensory system, then the absence of vision would lead to fewer postural changes. They also did not observe any decrease in the number of postural changes during eyes-closed standing, and so they discarded this hypothesis.

Prolonged Unconstrained Standing as a Fractal Process

The presence of fast and large fluctuations, as well as of slow and small fluctuations, in the COP displacement during prolonged unconstrained standing is a typical characteristic of a fractal process. A fractal is "a rough or fragmented geometric shape that can be split into parts, each of which is (at least approximately) a reduced-size copy of the whole" (Mandelbrot 1983). The observation of "reduced-size copy of the whole" in space is termed the *self-similarity* property; this observation in time is termed the *self-affinity* property (which can also be referred as a *long-range correlation* or *long-memory* process because the dependence of data farther apart is higher than it is expected for independent data). These two properties can be seen as scaling laws of the spatial and temporal variability of a fractal process. Duarte and Zatsiorsky (2000, 2001) analyzed the COP displacement during prolonged unconstrained standing and indeed observed that natural standing is a fractal process exhibiting these two properties, as illustrated in Figure 10.7.

The presence of long-range correlations in the COP data during natural standing is, in fact, not surprising. The branching in trees and in our lungs, the fluctuations of the waterfall sound and of our heartbeats are a few examples of the ubiquity of fractals in nature. Nevertheless, this "trivial" characteristic has important implications for the study of postural control in humans. Here are a few of them: One important issue in postural studies is the period of data acquisition (i.e., for how long should one collect data to capture essential properties of human standing?). In a frequently referenced study, Powell and Dzendolet (1984) reported low frequencies in the COP data of 130 seconds of duration. Different authors have cited this paper as a reference to justify the acquisition of data for no more than 2 minutes. Our studies suggest that, with longer acquisition time, even lower frequencies of COP could be observed. The important conclusion is that the choice of period of acquisition has to be based on which periods (frequencies) are regarded as relevant for the study in question. Another issue is whether the stabilogram can be considered a stationary process. The distinction between nonstationarity and long-range correlations in time series analysis is an ill-posed problem, and studies on stationarity in COP data have indeed shown discrepant results. Given our findings, such differences are the consequence of different periods of observation, and the investigators have tested only small portions of a longer process. Because of the presence of long-range correlations, apparent nonstationarities in short COP time series might actually represent fluctuations of a longer stationary process. Thus, the issue of stationarity cannot be adequately addressed using short time series of up to few minutes. Finally, the property of self-affinity in the COP data implies that, to properly compare COP data of different lengths (different periods of acquisition), the COP data should be scaled by the fractal exponent.

Prolonged Unconstrained Standing and Aging

It is common—but not ubiquitous—to find an increase in postural sway with aging when an individual is asked to stay as still as possible for a short

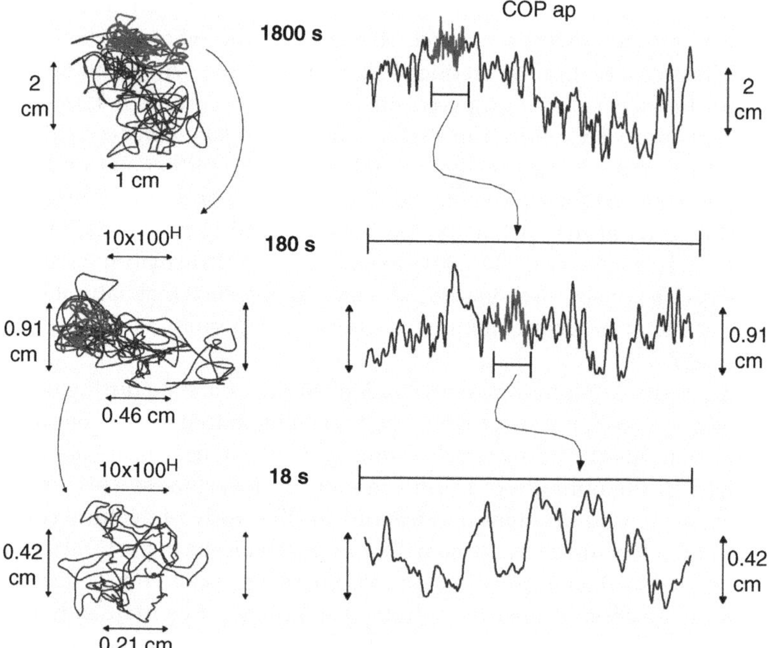

Figure 10.7 A: Statokinesigrams (*left*) and stabilograms in the anterior-posterior (ap) direction of the entire data set during natural standing (1,800 s, first row), for 1/10 of the data set (180 s, second row), and for 1/100 of the data set (18 s, third row). The *Hurst* exponent (*H*) for this example is 0.34, giving a reduction of 2.2 in the amplitude scale for each 10-fold of reduction of the time scale. Both scaled and real axes are indicated in the 180 s and the 18 s plots for illustration. Notice that after each scaling (that is related to the fractal exponent and to the period of time), the three statokinesigrams and stabilograms present roughly the same amplitudes in space. For the sake of clarity, not all points are shown for the 1,800 s and 180 s plots. The difference in the fine structure, observed for the 18 s time series compared to the other two time series, is due to the fact that center of pressure (COP) displacements for short intervals up to 1 s display a different behavior. Data from Duarte, M., and V.M. Zatsiorsky. 2000. On the fractal properties of natural human standing. *Neuroscience Letters* 283: 173–76; Duarte, M., and V.M. Zatsiorsky. 2001. Long-range correlations in human standing. *Physics Letters A* 283: 124–28, with permission of the publishers.

period of time. However, Freitas and collaborators (2005b) found that elderly individuals tend to show an opposite behavior compared to young adults during prolonged unconstrained standing. This was because elderly individuals produced fewer large-amplitude postural changes compared to young adults. Specifically, the elderly individuals produced smaller shift patterns that resulted in fewer COP multiregion patterns. Figure 10.8 shows typical examples of COP displacement in the anteroposterior direction versus the mediolateral direction during standing still and during

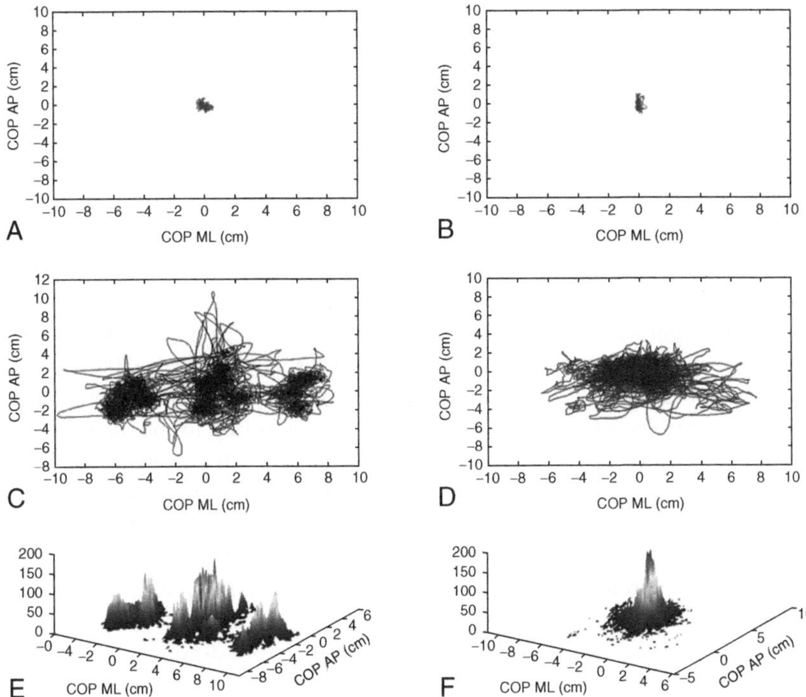

Figure 10.8 Examples of the center of pressure (COP) in the anterior-posterior (AP) direction versus the medio-lateral direction (ML) for one young adult (**A**, **C**) and one elderly individual (**B**, **D**) during standing still (**A**, **B**) and prolonged unconstrained standing (**C**, **D**). Graphs **E** and **F** show the respective COP histograms of the prolonged unconstrained standing trials.

prolonged unconstrained standing for one young adult and one elderly individual (data from Freitas et al. 2005b). The difference in the behavior of each representative participant is clear. On average, young adults ($n = 14$) exhibited six COP multiregion patterns, whereas the elderly individuals ($n = 14$) showed only one COP multiregion pattern during the 30 minutes of unconstrained standing (Freitas et al. 2005b). These results indicate that elderly individuals adopt a "freezing" strategy during prolonged standing. Because a decrease in mobility is typically observed in elderly individuals (Gunter et al. 2000; Hatch et al. 2003), Freitas and collaborators (2005b) hypothesized that the lack of mobility in elderly individuals might be responsible for the decreased numbers of postural changes of large amplitude.

More detailed examinations of the freezing strategy and the possible effect of decreased mobility on the postural changes during prolonged unconstrained standing in elderly individuals were undertaken by Prado and Duarte (2009). The hypothesis for this study was that elderly individuals produced fewer postural changes due to reduced mobility and, specifically, due to the inability to use the load/unload mechanism to transfer weight from one leg to the other. The specificity of the hypothesis is because shifts are typically a reflection of unloading and loading the body weight from one leg to the other in the mediolateral direction. As Freitas and collaborators (2005b) observed a decrease in the number of large shifts in elderly adults, this could be an indication of the inability to use such a load/unload mechanism. As early as 1913, Mosher stressed the importance of shifting the body weight from side to side for comfort (Zacharkow 1988). So, to investigate this hypothesis, Prado and Duarte (2009) used the dual force plate paradigm (one force plate under each leg) and measured the mobility of individuals. They examined 20 elderly individuals (70 ± 4 years) and 20 young adults (25 ± 4 years) without any known postural or skeletal disorders. Subjects performed two tasks: quiet standing for 60 seconds and prolonged standing for 30 minutes, standing with each leg on a force plate. In the prolonged unconstrained standing, the participants were allowed to change their posture freely at any time, and there were no specific instructions on how to stand except for the requirement not to step off the force plates. In the prolonged unconstrained standing, participants watched a television documentary displayed 3 m in front of them. The mobility of each individual was measured with the timed up-and-go test (Podsiadlo and Richardson 1991).

A change larger than 25% of the body weight in the vertical ground reaction force (Fz) on any of the force plates was counted as one transfer of weight from one leg to the other (termed shift). Different criteria for the detection of weight transfer, ranging from 0.1 to 0.5, were tested, and the comparison across groups was not affected by the criterion value. Figure 10.8 illustrates exemplary time series of the vertical ground reaction forces from the left and right legs during prolonged unconstrained standing by one young adult and one elderly adult. Again, the "freezing" behavior that elderly adults seem to adopt is evident by looking at these plots. One can observe less weight transfer from one leg to the other for the elderly adult than for the young adult, and in this particular case, the elderly adult had more weight on the left leg to begin with, with the weight share slowly increasing over time. The elderly adults significantly ($p < 0.001$) produced less weight transfers from one leg to the other and with lower amplitudes than did the young adults during prolonged unconstrained standing (Figure 10.9). For the quiet-standing task, neither group produced any weight transfer. The elderly adults may have produced less weight transfers just because they adopted a narrow base of support with their feet, and this makes it difficult to transfer weight. To investigate this possibility, Prado and Duarte (2009), using a motion capture system, also looked at the kinematics of the feet during prolonged unconstrained standing by recording the position of reflective markers placed on the participant's feet. However, they found that the base of support width of the

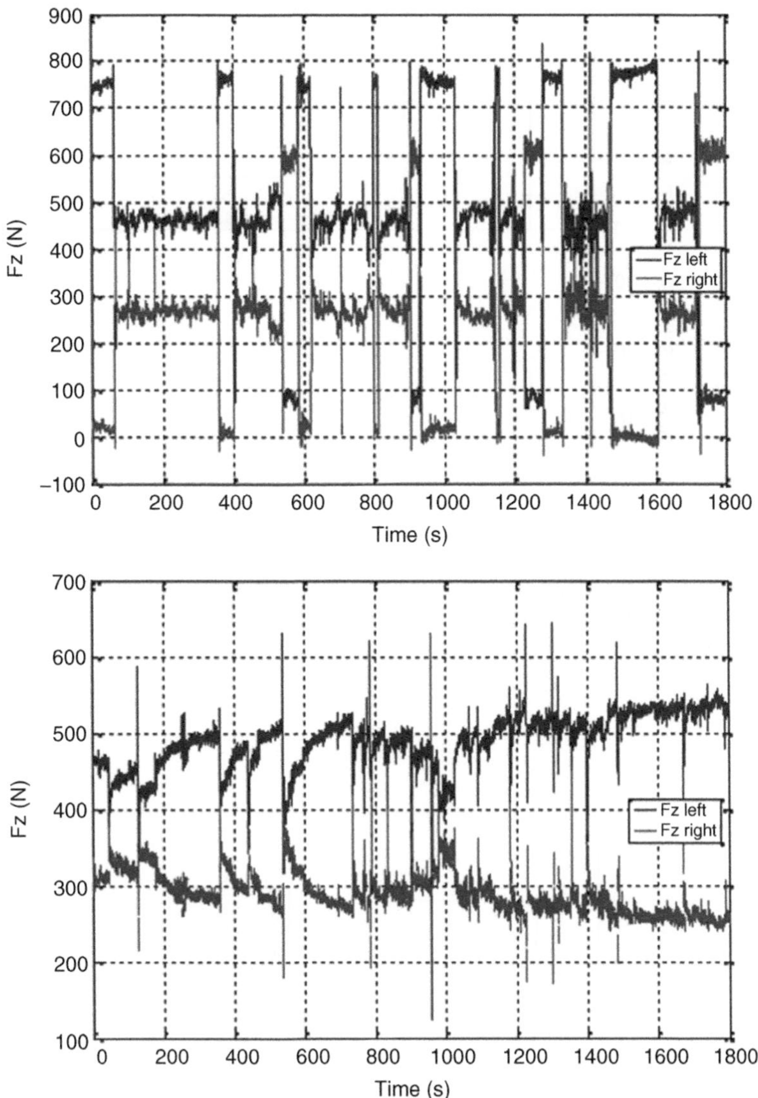

Figure 10.9 Exemplary time series of the vertical ground reaction forces from the left (Fz left, *black line*) and right (Fz right, *gray line*) legs during prolonged unconstrained standing by one young adult (*top*) and one elderly adult (*bottom*).

elderly adults was no different from that of the young adults during prolonged unconstrained standing (Figure 10.10).

Despite the decreased capacity of elderly adults to produce weight transfer, which could be viewed as a sign of decreased mobility in this group, in fact, the specific measure of mobility, the timed up-and-go

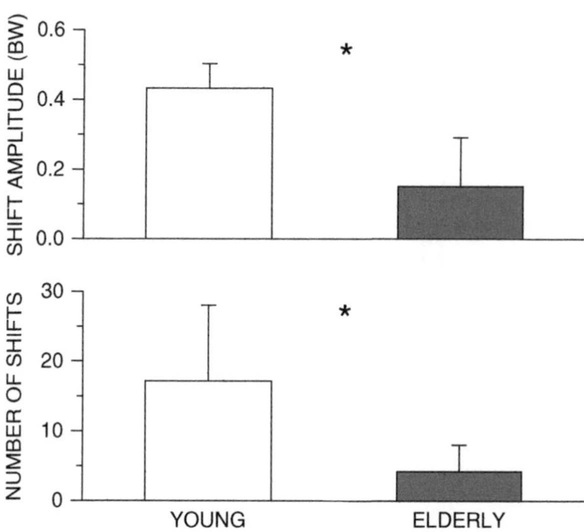

Figure 10.10 Mean and standard deviation of amplitude (*top*) and number (*bottom*) of shifts (weight transfers from one leg to the other) for young adults and elderly adults during prolonged unconstrained standing. * $p < 0.001$.

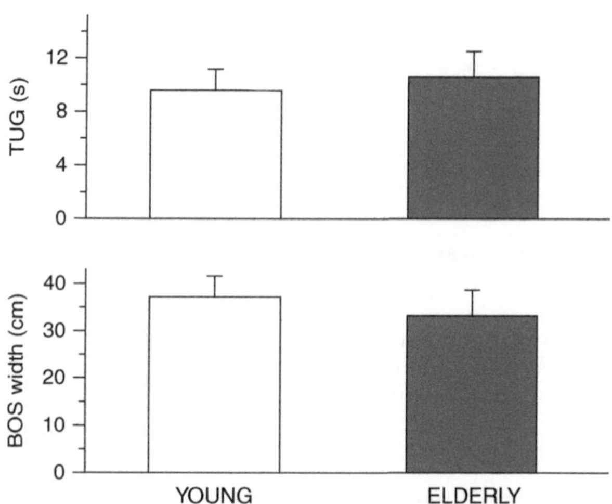

Figure 10.11 Mean and standard deviation of the base of support width for young adults and elderly adults during prolonged unconstrained standing (*left*). Mean and standard deviation of the timed up and go (TUG) test for young adults and elderly adults (*right*).

test, was not different between the young adults and the elderly adults (Figure 10.11). These results are intriguing; if the elderly adults were simply more cautious or afraid of falling, and so did not move during unconstrained standing, we should have observed a similar cautious behavior during the timed up-and-go test. But this was not the case. Therefore, we can only speculate why we observed such a difference between young and elderly individuals in producing weight transfers, but no difference in the mobility measures. If we assume that postural changes are a likely response to reduce musculoskeletal discomfort, then they are somehow initiated by proprioceptive information signaling such discomfort. It is possible that the observed decreased capacity of weight transfer by elderly adults is due to diminished somatosensory information, which is not triggering such postural changes.

Prolonged Unconstrained Standing and Musculoskeletal Problems

The observed decrease in the number and amplitude of postural changes during unconstrained standing in elderly adults may not be exclusively due to the aging factor. Rather, an immediate cause of the observed age trend could be musculoskeletal disorders associated with aging. Lafond and collaborators (2009) used the quantification of COP patterns paradigm to investigate how individuals with chronic low-back pain behave during prolonged unconstrained standing. Prolonged standing is linked with the onset of low-back pain symptoms in working populations (Macfarlane et al. 1997; Xu et al. 1997). Lafond and collaborators (2009) hypothesized that the onset of pain during prolonged standing might be due to the inability to produce postural changes during such tasks. Indeed, they found that individuals with chronic low-back pain presented fewer postural changes in the anteroposterior direction, with decreased postural sway amplitude during the prolonged standing task in comparison to the healthy group. Lafond and collaborators (2009) suggested that this deficit may contribute to low-back pain persistence or an increased risk of recurrent back pain episodes. They also linked this deficit to reduced proprioceptive information from the low back or altered sensorimotor integration in individuals with chronic low-back pain.

CONCLUDING REMARKS

Although we often refer to the postural control system as the entity responsible for the control of equilibrium during a certain body posture, this system is neither a single neuroanatomic structure in our body nor a single task that we perform. Postural control is dependent on a rich and fine integration of many sensorimotor processes in our body, the goal we are trying to accomplish, and the surrounding environment. Natural (unconstrained) standing is a good example of this complexity. The series of studies we have conducted might be useful not only for understanding how humans behave during such a task but in general how the postural control system works. The fact that during natural (unconstrained) standing humans control their posture around different reference positions with no difficulty might suggest that the postural control system in fact never specifies a fixed and unique reference position, even when standing still. When standing still, we would consciously try to avoid any postural change; however, what our postural control system adopts as an exact reference position, if it adopts one, probably is beyond our voluntary will.

ACKNOWLEDGMENTS

This work was supported by grants from Fundação de Amparo à Pesquisa do Estado de São Paulo - FAPESP/Brazil (04/10917-0 and 09/07960-4).

REFERENCES

Baratto, L., P.G. Morasso, C. Re, and G. Spada. 2002. A new look at posturographic analysis in the clinical context: Sway-density versus other parameterization techniques. *Motor Control* 6: 246–70.

Benda, B.J., P.O. Riley, and D.E. Krebs. 1994. Biomechanical relationship between center of gravity and center of pressure during standing. *Rehabilitation Engineering, IEEE Transactions* [see also *IEEE Transactions on Neural Systems and Rehabilitation*] 2: 3–10.

Bonnet, C., C. Carello, and M.T. Turvey. 2009. Diabetes and postural stability: Review and hypotheses. *Journal of Motor Behavior* 41: 172–90.

Brantingham, C.R., B.E. Beekman, C.N. Moss, and R.B. Gordon. 1970. Enhanced venous pump activity as a result of standing on a varied terrain floor surface. *Journal of Occupational Medicine* 12: 164–69.

Breniere, Y. 1996. Why we walk the way we do. *Journal of Motor Behavior* 28: 291–98.

Caron, O., B. Faure, and Y. Breniere. 1997. Estimating the centre of gravity of the body on the basis of the centre of pressure in standing posture. *Journal of Biomechanics* 30: 1169–71.

Cavanagh, P.R., M.M. Rodgers, and A. Iiboshi. 1987. Pressure distribution under symptom-free feet during barefoot standing. *Foot & Ankle* 7: 262–76.

Cornilleau-Peres, V., N. Shabana, J. Droulez, J.C. Goh, G.S. Lee, and P.T. Chew. 2005. Measurement of the visual contribution to postural steadiness from the COP movement: methodology and reliability. *Gait & Posture* 22: 96–106.

Doyle, T.L., R.U. Newton, and A.F. Burnett. 2005. Reliability of traditional and fractal dimension measures of quiet stance center of pressure in young, healthy people. *Archives of Physical Medicine and Rehabilitation* 86: 2034–40.

Duarte, M., W. Harvey, and V.M. Zatsiorsky. 2000. Stabilographic analysis of unconstrained standing. *Ergonomics* 43: 1824–39.

Duarte, M., and V.M. Zatsiorsky. 1999. Patterns of center of pressure migration during prolonged unconstrained standing. *Motor Control* 3: 12–27.

Duarte, M., and V.M. Zatsiorsky. 2000. On the fractal properties of natural human standing. *Neuroscience Letters* 283: 173–76.

Duarte, M., and V.M. Zatsiorsky. 2001. Long-range correlations in human standing. *Physics Letters A* 283: 124–28.

Duarte, M., and V.M. Zatsiorsky. 2002. Effects of body lean and visual information on the equilibrium maintenance during stance. *Experimental Brain Research* 146: 60–69.

Freitas, S.M., J.M. Prado, and M. Duarte. 2005a. The use of a safety harness does not affect body sway during quiet standing.*Clinical Biomechanics (Bristol, Avon)* 20: 336–39.

Freitas, S.M., S.A. Wieczorek, P.H. Marchetti, and M. Duarte. 2005b. Age-related changes in human postural control of prolonged standing. *Gait & Posture* 22: 322–30.

Gagey, P.-M., and B. Weber. 2005. *Posturologie: Régulation et dérèglements de la station debout*. Paris: Masson.

Gunter, K.B., K.N. White, W.C. Hayes, and C.M. Snow. 2000. Functional mobility discriminates nonfallers from one-time and frequent fallers. *Journals of Gerontology. Series A, Biological Sciences and Medical Sciences* 55: M672–76.

Gurfinkel. V.S., P. Ivanenko Yu, S. Levik Yu, and I.A. Babakova. 1995. Kinesthetic reference for human orthograde posture. *Neuroscience* 68: 229–43.

Hatch, J., K.M. Gill-Body, and L.G. Portney. 2003. Determinants of balance confidence in community-dwelling elderly people. *Physical Therapy* 83: 1072–79.

Horak, F.B., C.L. Shupert, and A. Mirka A. 1989. Components of postural dyscontrol in the elderly: a review. *Neurobiology of Aging* 10: 727–38.

Kapteyn, T.S., W. Bles, C.J. Njiokiktjien, L. Kodde, C.H. Massen, and J.M. Mol. 1983. Standardization in platform stabilometry being a part of posturography. *Agressologie* 24: 321–26.

Kim, J.Y., C. Stuart-Buttle, and W.S. Marras. 1994. The effects of mats on back and leg fatigue. *Applied Ergonomics* 25: 29–34.

King, D.L., and V.M. Zatsiorsky. 1997. Extracting gravity line displacement from stabilographic recordings. *Gait & Posture* 6: 27–38.

Lafond, D., A. Champagne, M. Descarreaux, J.D. Dubois, J.M. Prado, and M. Duarte. 2009. Postural control during prolonged standing in persons with chronic low back pain. *Gait & Posture* 29: 421–27.

Lafond, D., H. Corriveau, R. Hebert, and F. Prince. 2004a. Intrasession reliability of center of pressure measures of postural steadiness in healthy elderly people. *Archives of Physical Medicine and Rehabilitation* 85: 896–901.

Lafond, D., M. Duarte, and F. Prince. 2004b. Comparison of three methods to estimate the center of mass during balance assessment. *Journal of Biomechanics* 37: 1421–26.

Lestienne, F.G., and V.S. Gurfinkel. 1988. Posture as an organizational structure based on a dual process: A formal basis to interpret changes of posture in weightlessness. In *Vestibulospinal control of posture and locomotion*, eds., O. Pompeiano and J.H.J. Allum, vol. 76, 307–313. Amsterdam New York: Elsevier.

Macfarlane, G.J., E. Thomas, A.C. Papageorgiou, P.R. Croft, M.I.V. Jayson, and A.J. Silman. 1997. Employment and physical work activities as predictors of future low back pain. *Spine* 22: 1143–49.

Mandelbrot, B.B. 1983. *The fractal geometry of nature*. New York: W.H. Freeman.

McGinnis, P.M. 2005. *Biomechanics of sport and exercise*. Champaign, IL: Human Kinetics.

Piirtola, M., and P. Era. 2006. Force platform measurements as predictors of falls among older people: A review. *Gerontology* 52: 1–16.

Podsiadlo, D., and S. Richardson. 1991. The timed "Up & Go": A test of basic functional mobility for frail elderly persons. *Journal of the American Geriatric Society* 39: 142–48.

Powell, G.M., and E. Dzendolet. 1984. Power spectral density analysis of lateral human standing sway. *Journal of Motor Behavior* 16: 424–41.

Prado, J.M., and M. Duarte. 2009. Age-related deficit in the load/unload mechanism during prolonged standing. In *Progress in motor control VII*. Marseille, France.

Prieto, T.E., J.B. Myklebust, R.G. Hoffmann, E.G. Lovett, and B.M. Myklebust. 1996. Measures of postural steadiness: differences between healthy young and elderly adults. *IEEE Transactions in Biomedical Engineering* 43: 956–66.

Raymakers, J.A., M.M. Samson, and H.J. Verhaar. 2005. The assessment of body sway and the choice of the stability parameters. *Gait & Posture* 21: 48–58.

Riccio, G.E., E.J. Martin, and T.A. Stoffregen. 1992. The role of balance dynamics in the active perception of orientation. *Journal of Experimental Psychology. Human Perception and Performance* 18: 624–44.

Riccio, G.E., and T.A. Stoffregen. 1988. Affordances as constraints on the control of stance. *Human Movement Science* 7: 265–300.

Riley, M.A., S. Mitra, T.A. Stoffregen, and M.T. Turvey. 1997. Influences of body lean and vision on unperturbed postural sway. *Motor Control* 1: 229–46.

Riley, M.A., and M.T. Turvey. 2002. Variability of determinism in motor behavior. *Journal of Motor Behavior* 34: 99–125.

Romero, D.H., and G.E. Stelmach. 2003. Changes in postural control with aging and Parkinson's disease. *IEEE Eng Med Biol Mag* 22: 27–31.

Rougier, P.R. 2008. What insights can be gained when analysing the resultant centre of pressure trajectory? *Neurophysiology Clinics* 38: 363–73.

Slobounov, S.M., E.S. Slobounova, and K.M. Newell. 1997. Virtual time-to-collision and human postural control. *Journal of Motor Behavior* 29: 263–81.

Stoffregen, T.A., C.-M. Yang, and B.G. Bardy. 2005. Affordance judgments and non-locomotor body movement. *Ecological Psychology* 17: 75–104.

van der Kooij, H., E. van Asseldonk, and F.C. van der Helm. 2005. Comparison of different methods to identify and quantify balance control. *Journal of Neuroscience Methods* 145: 175–203.

Visser, J.E., M.G. Carpenter, H. van der Kooij, and B.R. Bloem. 2008. The clinical utility of posturography. *Clinical Neurophysiology* 119: 2424–36.

Winter, D.A. 2005. *Biomechanics and motor control of human movement*. Hoboken, NJ: John Wiley & Sons.

Winter, D.A., A.E. Patla, and J.S. Frank. 1990. Assessment of balance control in humans. *Medical Progress through Technology* 16: 31–51.

Xu, Y., E. Bach, and E. Orhede. 1997. Work environment and low back pain: the influence of occupational activities. *Occupational and Environmental Medicine* 54: 741.

Zacharkow, D. 1988. *Posture: Sitting, standing, chair design, and exercise*. Springfield, IL: Thomas.

Zatsiorsky, V.M., and M. Duarte. 2000. Rambling and trembling in quiet standing. *Motor Control* 4: 185–200.

Zatsiorsky, V.M., and D.L. King. 1998. An algorithm for determining gravity line location from posturographic recordings. *Journal of Biomechanics* 31: 161–64.

Zhang, L., C.G. Drury, and S.M. Wooley. 1991. Constrained standing: evaluating the foot/floor interface. *Ergonomics* 34: 175–92.

Part 4

Lessons from Motor Learning and Using Tools

11

Learning and Switching of Internal Models for Dexterous Tool Use

Hiroshi Imamizu

Although many animals can use simple tools, humans are unique in having remarkable abilities for the dexterous use of a wide range of tools to extend their physical capabilities. Although human faculties for tool use involve many components, Johnson-Frey (2004) reviewed neuropsychological and functional neuroimaging studies on the neural basis of tool use in humans and pointed out two major functional components. One is the semantic/conceptual knowledge about tools, representing the relationships between tools and their functions. That is, for the appropriate use of tools, humans have to understand the purpose for which an individual tool is used. It has been noted that brain damage to the left hemisphere at the intersection of the temporal-parietal-occipital cortices could selectively impair conceptual knowledge about tools (De Renzi and Lucchelli 1988). For example, it has been reported that patients with such damage attempt to brush their teeth with a comb and eat with a toothbrush. The terms "ideational" and "conceptual" apraxia have been used to refer to this type of disorder (Ochipa et al. 1992). The other major functional component is skill for tool use that helps in the production of the required actions for such tool use. Patients with damage to the left posterior parietal and/or premotor cortex retain conceptual knowledge of tools' functions and associated actions but have lost access to the representations needed to undertake the associated motor skills. This type of disorder has been named "ideomotor" apraxia, and many neuropsychological and functional neuroimaging studies have suggested that frontoparietal networks contribute to the skills (for review see Johnson-Frey 2004).

Regarding skills for tool use, however, we can consider various levels. For example, when we attempt using chopsticks for the first time, our movements are very slow and clumsy, and we make a lot of corrections based on sensory feedback. However, after gaining experience, we can manipulate them in an innate manner, as if they were parts of our own body. Several studies have suggested that the cerebellum contributes to such "expert" skills for the control of movements. In this chapter, I review studies focusing on how the cerebellum acquires skills for tool use and how the frontoparietal network and the cerebellum interact with each other for the flexible use of various types of tools. The purpose of this chapter is to delineate possible differences and interaction between skills acquired in the cerebellum and those acquired in the frontoparietal network.

INTERNAL MODELS FOR TOOL USE

Skilled manipulation of objects, including our own bodies, relies on the brain learning to control the object and predict the consequences of this control (Wolpert et al. 2001). The ability to learn the relationships between actions and resultant changes in the states of external objects is particularly important for rapid and smooth control of movements. It has been suggested that such ability is largely dependent on neural mechanisms that can model or simulate the relationships between an action and its consequences before execution. Neural mechanisms that can mimic the input-output properties of controlled objects are called internal models (Kawato et al. 1987; Wolpert et al. 1995; Kawato 1999) (see also Flanagan and Johansson, and Guigon, this volume).

In the context of arm-reaching movements, internal models transform the efference copies of a motor command into the resultant trajectory or sensorimotor feedback (Kawato et al. 1987; Miall et al. 1993; Wolpert et al. 1995) or the intended motion of the arm into the motor commands for realizing the motion (Kawato et al. 1987). Although internal models have been proposed in the context of the control of musculoskeletal systems such as limbs and eyes, it has been suggested that internal models can also contribute to predictive control of external objects such as tools. For example, skilled manipulation of a computer mouse requires the ability to predict how the mouse should be moved in order to move a cursor to a particular position on the screen and how the cursor will move on the screen if the mouse is moved in a particular direction. Using functional magnetic resonance imaging (fMRI), we have been investigating how skills for controlling a computer mouse are acquired and adaptively switched in the human brain. In the following, I summarize the results of our studies and discuss their implications for the skills needed for the use of general tools.

POSSIBLE NEURAL CORRELATES OF INTERNAL MODELS

It has been proposed that Purkinje cells in the cerebellum play an important role in representing the input-output properties of our musculoskeletal systems (Fig. 11.1; for example, Ito 1984). Purkinje cells receive major inputs

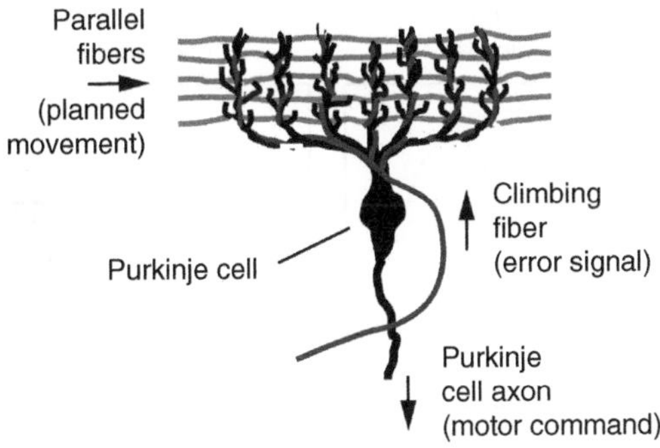

Figure 11.1 Information flow around Purkinje cells in the cerebellar cortex.

from parallel fibers and climbing fibers and send the sole output signals from the cortex. Climbing fiber inputs carry performance errors between the desired and actual movements and guide the learning acquisition of internal models by changing their synaptic efficacy. In the case of motor learning, after repetitive training, a Purkinje cell becomes capable of transforming signals representing planned movements (carried through parallel fibers) to the appropriate motor commands that realize the desired movements, as well as transforming the efference copy of motor commands to the resultant sensorimotor feedback. This learning mechanism was computationally modeled by a feedback-error-learning schema (Kawato et al. 1987; Kawato and Gomi 1992), and its biological plausibility has been investigated by neurophysiological studies in monkeys (Shidara et al. 1993; Gomi et al. 1998; Kitazawa et al. 1998; Kobayashi et al. 1998).

AN INTERNAL MODEL FOR A NOVEL TOOL IN THE CEREBELLUM

We examined whether activities reflecting an internal model and its acquisition process could be visualized in the human cerebellum by using fMRI (Imamizu et al. 2000). Subjects manipulated a computer mouse in a magnetic resonance scanner so that the corresponding cursor followed a randomly moving target on a screen (tracking task). In the test periods, the cursor appeared in a position rotated 120 degrees around the center of the screen to necessitate subject learning (novel rotated mouse; Fig. 11.2), while during baseline periods it was not rotated (normal mouse). The subjects' performance was measured by tracking errors (i.e., the distance between the cursor and the target). The errors in the test periods significantly decreased as the number of sessions increased, whereas the errors in the baseline periods were constant (Fig. 11.3A, *lower*), suggesting that learning progressed in the test periods. Activation maps obtained by subtraction of brain activity in the baseline periods, during which subjects used the

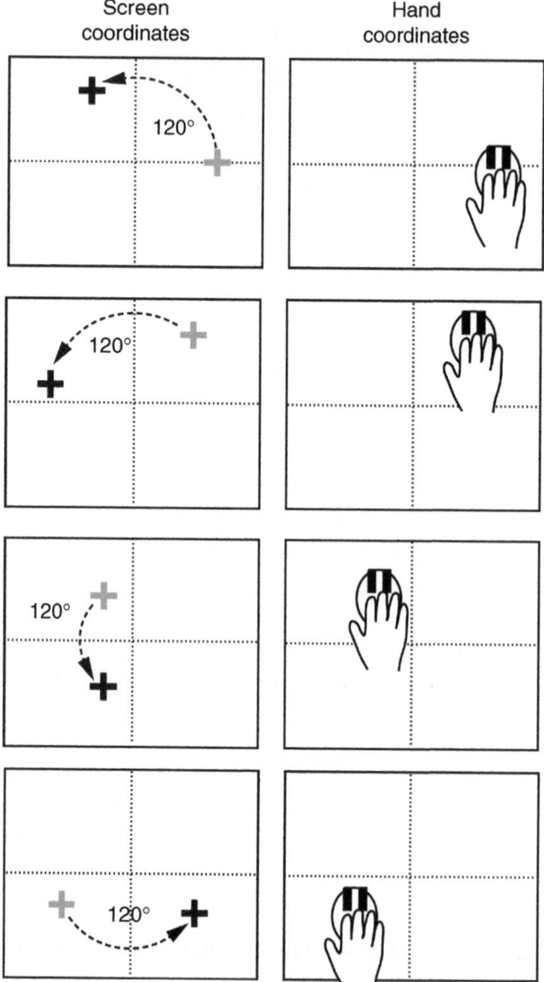

Figure 11.2 Relationship between a cursor (*left panels*) and a rotated mouse (*right panels*) at various positions. The cursor (*black cross*; +) on a computer screen appears in a position rotated 120 degrees around the screen's center. A gray cross indicates the cursor of a normal mouse.

normal mouse, from that in the test periods (Fig. 11.3A, *upper*) indicate that the activity in the lateral cerebellum decreased as learning progressed.

The decreasing activity in the lateral cerebellum might reflect performance errors that also decreased as learning proceeded. To evaluate this possibility, the subjects underwent an "error-equalized" experiment: The target velocity in the baseline periods was increased, so that the baseline error was equal to the test error (Fig. 11.3B, *lower*). There was no significant

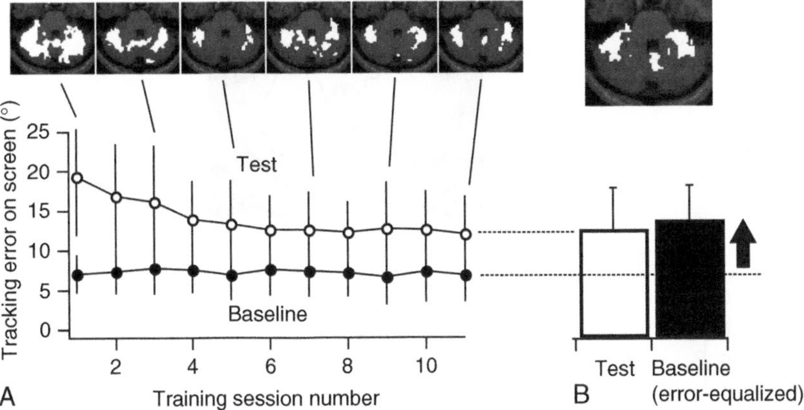

Figure 11.3 Cerebellar activity that decreased with learning progress (**A**), and the activity that remained when the tracking error was equalized (**B**). **A**: The upper panels show the activation maps of the regions significantly activated in the test periods in comparison to those in the baseline periods. The lower panel shows tracking error (mean ± SD) in the training sessions. **B**: The upper panel shows the activation map in the error-equalized session (see main text). The lower panel indicates tracking error (mean + SD) in the same session. From Imamizu, H., S. Miyauchi, T., Tamada, Y. Sasaki, R., Takino, B., Putz, et al. 2000. Human cerebellar activity reflecting an acquired internal model of a new tool. *Nature* 403: 192–95, with permission of the publisher.

difference between the test and the baseline errors, but we found cerebellar activity similar to that observed in the last stage of learning (Fig. 11.3B, *upper*). This activity cannot be related to the tracking error. The most plausible explanation is that the remaining activity reflects the acquired internal models, whereas the decrease in activity as learning progresses might largely reflect the error signals.

We examined the time courses of signal intensity during the training sessions averaged over two regions of interest. First, the error-related region was defined as voxels in the fMRI data whose signal intensities in the training sessions were significantly and positively correlated with the tracking error (white regions enclosed by solid lines in Fig. 11.4A). Second, the internal-model–related region was defined as voxels whose signal intensities were significantly higher in the test periods than in the baseline periods in the error-equalized experiments (gray hatched regions in Fig. 11.4A). The activity in the error-related region markedly decreased as the number of training sessions increased (Fig. 11.4B, *middle*). In contrast, the activity in the internal-model–related regions did not markedly decrease (Fig. 11.4B, *left*), and its correlation with the error was low ($r^2 = 0.25$) in comparison to the activity in the error-related regions ($r^2 = 0.82$). This result indicates that the activity in the internal-model–related regions might

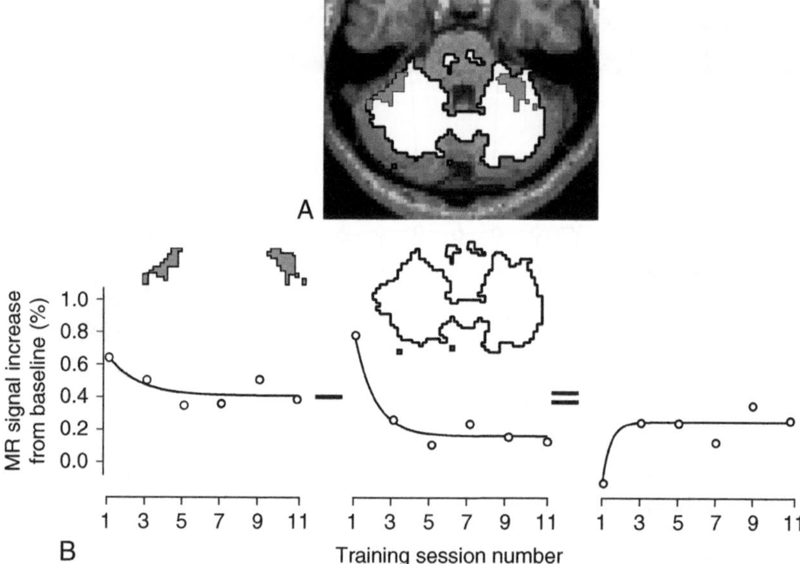

Figure 11.4 **A**: Cerebellar activity related to error signals (*white regions enclosed by solid line*) and activity related to the acquired internal model (*gray hatched regions*). **B**: Left panel shows activity change in the gray hatched regions in A. Middle panel shows activity change in the white regions in A. Right panel shows the subtraction of the activity change in the middle panel from that in the left panel. Each curve indicates the exponential function fitted to the circles. From Imamizu, H., S. Miyauchi, T. Tamada, Y. Sasaki, R. Takino, B. Putz, et al. 2000. Human cerebellar activity reflecting an acquired internal model of a new tool. *Nature* 403: 192–95, with permission of the publisher.

include components that cannot be explained solely by the error. By subtracting the activity in the error-related regions (*middle panel*) from that in the internal-model–related regions (*left panel*), we could confirm that activity reflecting the acquired internal model increased as learning progressed (Fig. 11.4B, *right*). The acquired internal model in this experiment is expected to represent the relationship between the cursor movement and mouse movement; that is, the input-output property of the novel mouse.

INTERNAL MODELS FOR TOOLS WITH DIFFERENT INPUT-OUTPUT PROPERTIES

To confirm that the described internal-model–related activity reflects the input-output properties of the novel mouse, we examined cerebellar activity after sufficiently learning another type of mouse with different input-output properties (Imamizu et al. 2003). The activity pattern in the lateral cerebellum is expected to change according to the mouse properties. In this experiment, the subjects intensively learned to manipulate two novel mice: one was the rotated mouse used in the previous experiment and the other, a velocity mouse whose cursor velocity was proportional to the mouse position (Fig. 11.5). The velocity mouse has input-output properties remarkably different from the rotated mouse, but the difficulty in manipulation, which is measured by tracking errors and the number of trials needed for learning, is almost the same as that of the rotated mouse. Thus, we could compare brain activity associated with the rotated mouse to that associated with the velocity mouse under relatively similar conditions.

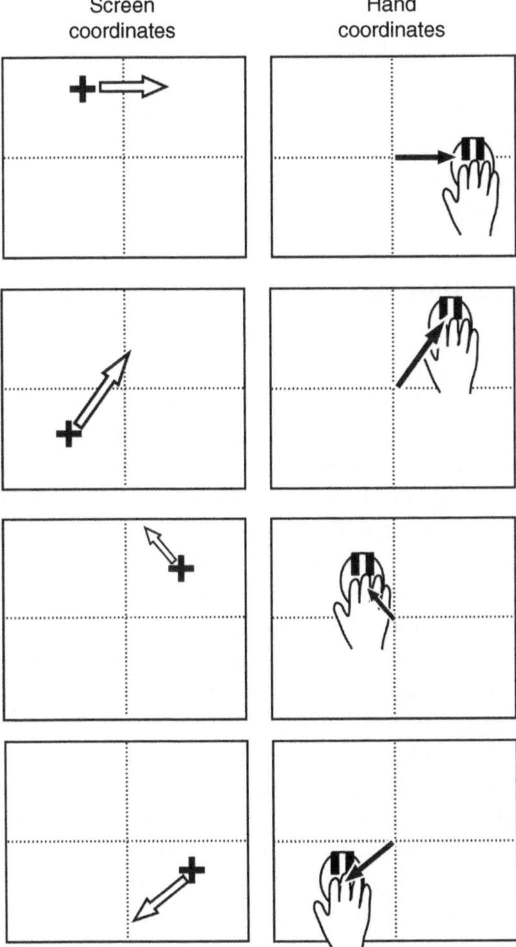

Figure 11.5 Relationship between a cursor (*left panels*) and a velocity mouse (*right panels*). The cursor's (*black cross*) velocity (*white arrow*) was proportional to the mouse displacement from the center position (*black arrow*).

There were two types of sessions when brain activity was scanned. In a rotated session, the subjects manipulated the rotated mouse during the test periods and the normal mouse during the baseline periods. In a velocity session, the same subjects manipulated the velocity mouse during the test periods and the normal mouse during the baseline periods. By increasing the target velocity during the baseline periods, the resulting errors were matched to those during the test periods according to the methods explained in the previous section (error-equalized experiment).

We subtracted the activity during the baseline period from that during test periods for each session and obtained two activation maps, each of which was related to the manipulation of the rotated mouse or the velocity mouse. Figure 11.6 shows the subtracted activity maps superimposed on horizontal sections of the cerebellum separately for two representative subjects. The white and black regions indicate activity for the rotated mouse and the velocity mouse, respectively. Mosaic regions indicate the overlap between the two types of activities. Similar regions in the lateral cerebellum were activated, but they were significantly segregated, and the rotated mouse activations tend to be located more superiorly and laterally than the velocity mouse activations.

SWITCHING MECHANISMS FOR INTERNAL MODELS

These studies indicate that the central nervous system (CNS) acquires multiple internal models. However, a question arises here as to how internal models are selected and switched appropriately for the current context. Empirically, two types of information are crucial for the switching of internal models: contextual information, such as the color or shape of the objects that can be perceived before movement execution, and information on the difference between actual and predicted sensorimotor feedback calculated during or after execution. For example, when we lift a transparent bottle, the CNS can switch between internal models for light and heavy objects in a predictive fashion since we know whether the bottle is empty or full beforehand. However, when lifting up a paper milk carton, we cannot estimate the weight, and the CNS relies on the error between the actual and predicted sensorimotor feedback (prediction error). It is probably important for anticipatory adjustment of behavior that a mechanism for predictive switching of internal models can work before movement execution, independent of a postdictive mechanism based on prediction error. The importance of prior contextual information has been suggested in other types of cognitive learning: Kole and Healy found that prior information contributes to minimizing interference in learning a large amount of information (Kole and Healy 2007).

We conducted an fMRI experiment to investigate the neural correlates for predictive and postdictive switching (Imamizu and Kawato 2008). A marker of a position recording system was attached to the subjects'

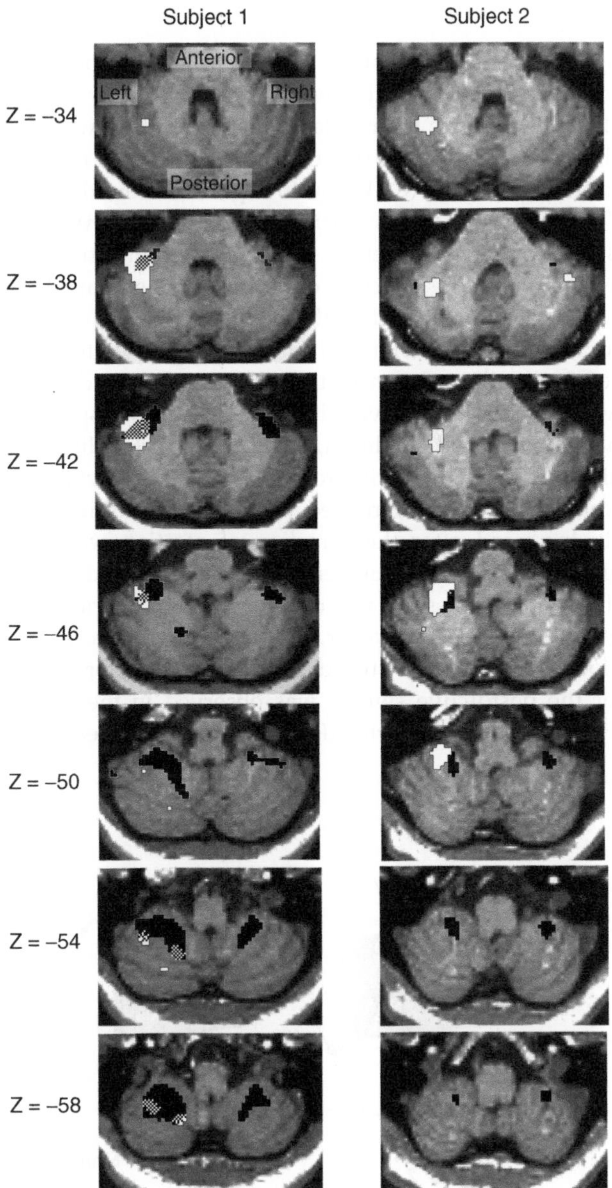

Figure 11.6 Cerebellar activity of two representative subjects in transverse sections in the order from the superior (*top panels*) to inferior (*bottom panels*) sections. White and black regions were significantly activated when subjects manipulated a rotated mouse and velocity mouse, respectively, in comparison to when subjects manipulated the normal mouse (error equalized). Z-values indicate horizontal positions in the Montreal Neurological Institute (MNI) coordinates. From Imamizu, H., T. Kuroda, S. Miyauchi, T. Yoshioka, and M. Kawato. 2003. Modular organization of internal models of tools in the human cerebellum. *Proceedings of the National Academy of Science U S A* 100: 5461–66, with permission of the publisher.

index fingers. The marker position was projected to a plane parallel to a screen, and the projected position was indicated by a cursor on the screen. Subjects learned to move their index fingers to targets while visual feedback of the finger movements (the cursor position) was rotated clockwise (CW) or counterclockwise (CCW) by 40 degrees around the initial position (Fig. 11.7). Subjects sufficiently learned the 40 degrees CW and 40 degrees CCW visuomotor rotations before scanning of brain activity, and during the fMRI experiment, the direction of rotation changed in a block-random fashion. A cue was presented at the beginning of each trial and before movement initiation. The color of the cue corresponded to the direction of rotation of the feedback in an instructed condition, and thus predictive switching was possible. However, the color did not correspond to the direction in the noninstructed condition; thus, the subjects relied on prediction errors calculated from sensorimotor feedback for switching in a noninstructed condition. Switching-related activity was identified as activity that transiently increased after the direction of rotation was changed. The switching-related activity in cue periods in the instructed condition, when a predictive switch is possible, was observed in the superior parietal lobule (SPL; Figs. 11.8A and B). However, the switching-related activity in feedback periods in the noninstructed condition, when prediction error is crucial for the postdictive switch, was observed in the inferior parietal lobule (IPL) and prefrontal cortex (PFC). These results clearly demonstrate

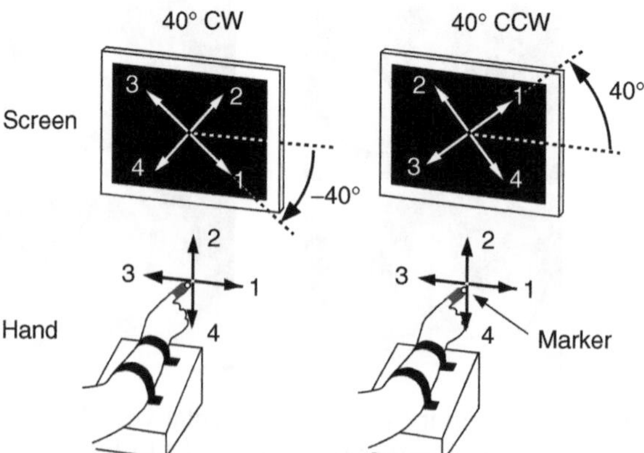

Figure 11.7 Relationship between the direction of finger movements (*black arrows*) and cursor movements (*white arrows*) under 40 degrees clockwise (*CW: left panel*) and 40 degrees counterclockwise (CCW: right panel) rotations. Numbers indicate correspondence between black and white arrows. Reproduced with permission from Imamizu, H., and M. Kawato. 2008. Neural correlates of predictive and postdictive switching mechanisms for internal models. *Journal of Neuroscience* 28: 10751–65, with permission of the publisher.

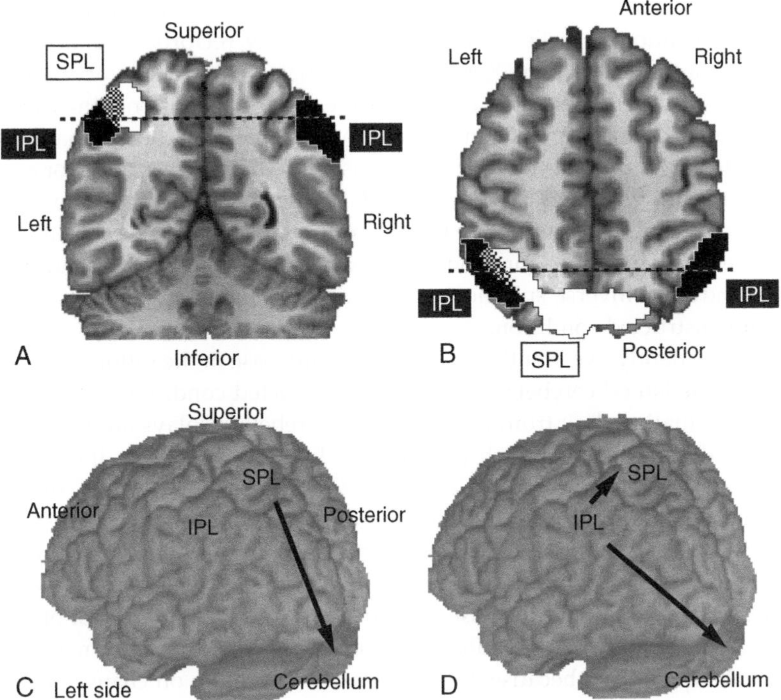

Figure 11.8 **A** and **B**: Activity in parietal regions related to predictive switch (*white*) and that related to postdictive switch (*black*) of internal models. Mosaic pattern indicates overlapped regions. Activations are superimposed on the coronal slice (**A**; y = 55 in the MNI coordinates) or the transverse (**B**; z = 50). Dashed line in each figure indicates the level of the slice in the other figure. **C** and **D**: Results of functional connectivity analysis. Influence from the superior parietal lobule (SPL) to the cerebellum was increased more during the predictive switch of internal models than during the postdictive switch (**C**). In contrast, influence from the inferior parietal lobule (IPL) to the cerebellum and to the SPL was increased more during postdictive switch than during predictive switch (**D**).

regional differences in neural substrates between the predictive and postdictive mechanisms.

We analyzed functional connectivity by using a method called dynamical causal modeling (DCM; Friston et al. 2003), which is a system identification procedure that uses Bayesian estimation to infer effective connectivity among neural systems and how it is affected by experimental conditions. Because it is impossible to investigate the connectivity among all brain regions, we made assumptions about related regions. One is that the SPL, IPL, and PFC contribute to switching, as suggested by the just described results, and the other is that the cerebellum contributes to the switching as possible neural correlates of internal models, as suggested by many of the studies mentioned earlier. We hypothesized fully reciprocal connections among these regions. Our DCM analysis estimated parameters corresponding to a modulation effect of conditions (i.e., instructed and noninstructed conditions) on each connection by using fMRI signal time courses that were extracted from the just-mentioned regions. This analysis was done for each subject, and we subtracted estimated parameter values for the noninstructed condition from those for the instructed condition across subjects to investigate increased functional connectivity in the instructed condition. We conducted inverse subtraction to investigate increased connectivity in the noninstructed condition.

Consequently, we identified a significant increase in the influence of the SPL on the lateral cerebellum during the instructed condition, suggesting that information flow from the SPL to the cerebellum plays an important role in the predictive switch (Fig. 11.8C). In contrast, during the noninstructed condition, we found an increased influence of the IPL on the lateral cerebellum, suggesting the contribution of information flow from the IPL to the cerebellum to the postdictive switch (Fig. 11.8D). We could also find increased influence from the IPL to the SPL during the noninstructed condition. This increase in influence suggests that the error of prediction for sensorimotor feedback was used as contextual information in the subsequent trial because it is important information on changes in the environment.

We observed that the accuracy of a subject's finger movements decreased immediately after changing the direction of visuomotor rotation, but the accuracy gradually improved with trials. We searched the brain regions where activity increased as subject performance improved and found that the activity increased in the supplementary motor area (SMA)/cingulate regions and in the lateral occipitotemporal cortices (LOTC), primary motor cortex (M1), middle temporal gyrus (MTG), and premotor regions (PM). We checked whether the amount of movement, which was measured by the length of the fingertip path, changed as the trial number increased but could find no significant change, suggesting that an increase in activity in these regions is related to an improvement in the subjects' performance.

Figure 11.9 illustrates a computational model of switching mechanisms (Wolpert and Kawato 1998; Haruno et al. 2001). This model hypothesizes two separate switching mechanisms for the predictive switch, based on contextual information, and for the postdictive switch, based on prediction error of sensorimotor feedback. The model also hypothesizes two types of internal models: an inverse internal model that calculates control signals from the intended motion, and a forward model that transforms control signals into predicted sensorimotor feedback. The predictive mechanism associates contextual information with an appropriate set of relative degrees of contribution of the inverse models for the current context. That is, the mechanism determines the degree of contribution of the output

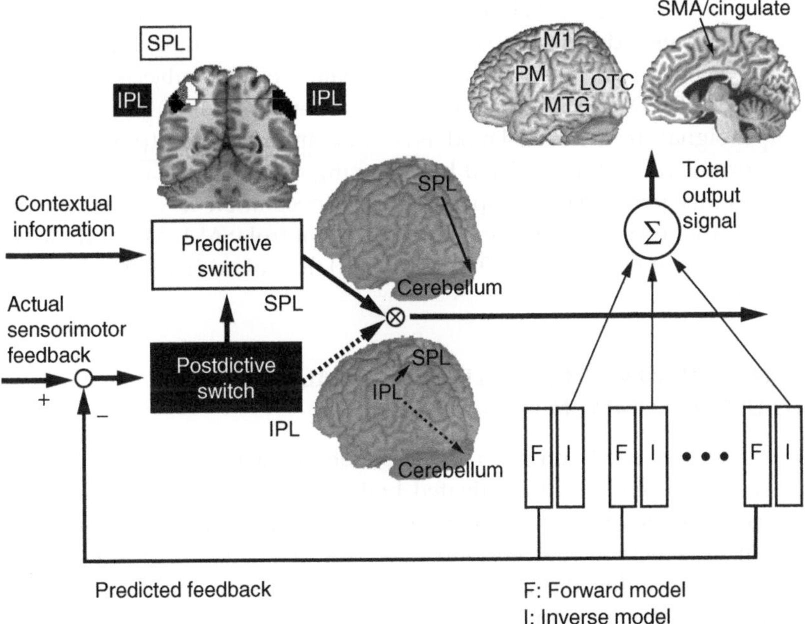

Figure 11.9 A computational model for switching of internal models with separate mechanisms for predictive and postdictive switches (Wolpert and Kawato 1998; Haruno et al. 2001). The figure also shows brain regions and functional connections that were suggested to correspond to elements and pathways in the model by an functional magnetic resonance imaging (fMRI) experiment (Imamizu and Kawato 2008). SMA: supplementary motor area, LOTC: lateral occipitotemporal cortices, M1: primary motor cortex, MTG: middle temporal gyrus, and PM: premotor region.

signal from each inverse model to the total output signal according to the contextual information. The postdictive mechanism calculates the prediction error of sensorimotor feedback by comparing actual feedback with feedback predicted by forward models. Because the smaller the error, the more likely it is that the forward model is an appropriate predictor in the current context, the postdictive mechanism increases the degree of contribution to the total output signal by the inverse model paired with the appropriate forward model.

The previously mentioned results of our fMRI study can be summarized in a computational model as follows. First, our analysis of switching-related activity suggests two separate neural substrates. The SPL and the IPL correspond to the predictive and postdictive mechanisms, respectively. Second, our connectivity analysis suggests that increased influence from the SPL to the cerebellum reflects the output signal from the predictive mechanism during the instructed condition, and that increased influence from the IPL to the cerebellum reflects the output signal from the postdictive mechanism during the noninstructed condition. Third, brain regions where activity increased as the performance of the subjects improved (SMA, LOTC, M1, MTG, and PM, see earlier discussion) might receive output signals from internal models because appropriate output signals for the current context, modulated by switching mechanisms, are believed to increase as performance improves. This speculation is consistent with notions that these regions are related to the control (SMA, M1, and PM) or observation of movement (LOTC and MTG) (Rizzolatti et al. 1996; Iacoboni et al. 2001).

CONTRIBUTION OF CEREBELLAR INTERNAL MODELS TO USE OF COMMON TOOLS

These studies used computer devices, such as a mouse and a position recording system, and investigated brain activity when humans learn a novel relationship between their hand motion and a cursor motion on a screen. This method enabled us to record the detailed motion of a subject's hand and examine the precise relationship between the change in the subject's performance and brain activity. However, these novel tools seem to be significantly different from common tools, such as scissors and a hammer. Functional imaging of activity related to the skill for use of common tools is a challenging task because it is difficult to extract activities of interest (activities related to the skills themselves) from activities related to muscle activations, as well as to proprioceptive and tactile feedback, due to complex movement of the hand and arm during manipulation of common tools.

Several studies have adopted pantomimes of tool use to reduce the tactile sensation evoked by actual interaction with tools (Moll et al. 2000; Choi et al. 2001). These studies compared activity evoked by tool-use pantomimes (gestures of tool-use without having a tool) to that evoked by a hand-movement task devoid of any tool-use connotation by matching the intrinsic properties of the movements employed in the tool-use pantomime task. The involvement of the intraparietal sulcus (IPS) was shown in tool-use skill, as well as in cognitive knowledge of tool use. However, another study pointed out that areas typically invoked by real actions may not necessarily be driven by pantomime actions, suggesting that the tool-use pantomime may not have activated skills for real tools (Kroliczak et al. 2007). Many other studies have investigated brain activity during imagining and planning the use of tools (see also Johnson-Frey, this volume) and naming tools (for review, see Lewis 2006). However, those studies focused mainly on the cerebral cortex.

We conducted an fMRI experiment to investigate the cerebellar activity while human subjects mentally imagined using 16 common tools (a pair of scissors, a hammer, chopsticks, etc.) and while they actually used them

(Higuchi et al. 2007). In an execution condition, the subjects were asked to use one of the tools along with an appropriate object with visual feedback (e.g., using scissors to cut a sheet of paper). In an imagination condition, the subjects were asked to imagine using a tool in the same way it was used in the execution condition. In this condition, the subjects were instructed not to actually manipulate the tools but to hold them while looking at the target object (e.g., paper). In a rest condition, the subjects tried not to imagine using a tool while holding a tool and looking at the object. Our hypothesis was that imagining the use of tools evokes activity related to skills (or internal models) but does not evoke activity related to muscle activation or proprioceptive and tactile feedback.

In our analysis, we calculated *t*-value–weighted centroids of activation separately for individual tools by comparing activity in the execution or the imagination condition to that in the rest condition. Consequently, centroids in the execution condition were found mainly in the anterior part of the cerebellum, consistent with the notion that the anterior part is involved in the control of limb movements, including the arm and the hand. However, most of the centroids in the imagination condition existed in the lateral part of the cerebellum (lobule VI/Crus I), where activity related to internal models for novel tools were found in our previous fMRI studies (Imamizu et al. 2000; Imamizu et al. 2003), suggesting that the lateral part also contributes to internal models for common tools. Moreover, the centroids for individual tools were not concentrated in a particular region but widely distributed over the lateral parts, indicating that different regions correspond to different tools. This suggests that internal models for common tools are stored in a modular fashion.

PREMOTOR REGION AS A TARGET OF OUTPUT FROM INTERNAL MODELS

Anatomical connectivity has been found between the ventral premotor (PMv) regions and the cerebellar output nucleus (the dentate nucleus) (Middleton and Strick 1997). Corresponding to this connection, our fMRI study suggested that the functional connectivity between the lateral cerebellum and the PMv regions increased after the acquisition of internal models (Tamada et al. 1999). This study used a novel mouse and confirmed similar change in activity to our previous study in the lateral cerebellum (Imamizu et al. 2000). Moreover, the study investigated the change in activity in cerebral regions and found a significant effect of learning on the activated volume (decrease or increase of volume) in frontal and occipital regions. The authors found that activity in the left lateral cerebellum increased after learning in comparison to the right cerebellum. In their analysis, they adopted a hypothesis suggesting that increase in activity in the right cerebral region should be observed in comparison to the left homologous region if the region has functional connectivity with the lateral cerebellum. They found that the activity in the right PMv regions increased in comparison to the left homologous regions after learning, suggesting functional connectivity between the lateral cerebellum and the PMv.

Based on these results, Higuchi and colleagues investigated the activity near the PMv regions related to imagining the use of common tools (a pencil, scissors, and chopsticks) (Higuchi et al. 2009). Such activity was found in Brodmann's area 6 and 44. Because area 44 in the left hemisphere is a part of Broca's area, which is related to language processing, they compared the activity with activity evoked when the same subjects listened to part of a story. Consequently, they found a significant overlap between the two types of activity in area 44 (a mosaic region on Fig. 11.10). These results suggest that language and tool use share common neural correlates in Broca's area. According to the authors' discussion, their tool-use task required subjects to perform hierarchical manipulation of objects and tools (e.g., moving an object while holding it with chopsticks). It has been suggested that area 44 is involved in the syntactic aspects of language (Sakai 2005) and specifically complex hierarchical processing (e.g., understanding of embedded sentences) (Friederici et al. 2006). Language understanding and the use of tools need hierarchical processing; thus, it is reasonable that both functions share neural substrates.

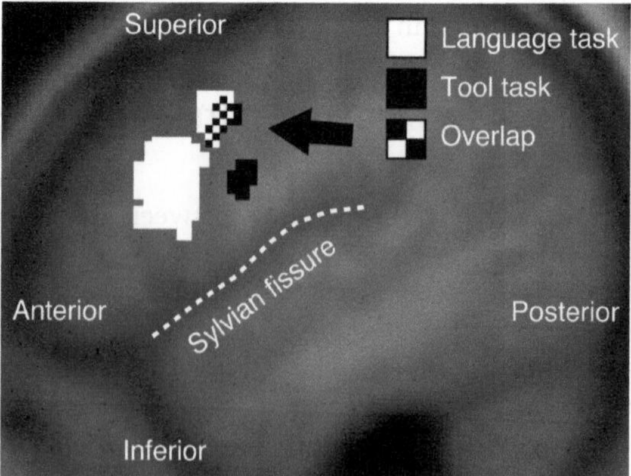

Figure 11.10 Activity near Broca's area related to language (*white*) and tool use (*black*). Activations across subjects (according to random-effect analysis) are superimposed on the sagittal section of the left hemisphere (x = – 50 in the MNI coordinates). The structural image was obtained by averaging subjects' normalized structural images. Reproduced from Higuchi, S., T. Chaminade, H. Imamizu, and M. Kawato. 2009. Shared neural correlates for language and tool use in Broca's area. *Neuroreport* 20: 1376–1381, with permission of the publisher, Wolters Kluwer Health.

DISCUSSION

In this chapter, I focused on skills for the dexterous use of tools and reviewed studies on how such skills are acquired in the lateral cerebellum, in addition to studies investigating the cerebellar-cortical loops for the flexible switching of skills depending on contextual information and sensorimotor feedback. Although these studies mainly investigated skills for novel tools (computer mice or a mouse-like device controlling a cursor by finger motion, with novel input-output properties), our recent studies on the imaginary use of common tools found activity in the lateral cerebellum that was reported in our previous studies on novel tools; it suggested that previous results could be generalized to common tools, such as the scissors and a hammer.

As mentioned at the beginning of this chapter, two major functional components have been suggested in the human faculty for tool use: semantic/conceptual knowledge about tools and sensorimotor skills for the manipulation of tools. The cerebellar internal models reviewed in this chapter are believed to contribute to the sensorimotor skills by internally representing the input-output properties of tools. However, many studies in neuropsychology and functional neuroimaging have pointed out that skills for tool use are acquired in a parietofrontal network, particularly the parietal regions (for review, see Johnson-Frey 2004; Lewis 2006). Addressed next are the differences in functions between skills acquired in the parietal regions and those acquired in the cerebellum, as well as the reasons why neuropsychological studies have drawn little attention to the cerebellum.

In engineering control theory, two major types of controllers have been proposed: a closed-loop (feedback) controller and an open-loop (feedforward) controller. The former uses feedback information, which is measured by sensors, on results caused by the body's own control signals (e.g., motor commands). The feedforward controller, on the other hand, does not rely on an external feedback loop but calculates precise control signals that can realize intended actions. This calculation of precise signals needs mechanisms that can simulate external feedback loops by representing the input-output properties of controlled objects internally. It is known that external feedback loops in biological systems are inevitably delayed by many factors, such as transmission of motor commands from the brain to the muscles, mechanical delay of muscles and external objects, and processing of visual and proprioceptive feedback information. However, humans can very rapidly and smoothly manipulate particular tools after long-term training in their use. As an extreme example, when professional carpenters use saws and cooks cut food with kitchen knives, their manipulations are often at lightning speed, and it is unlikely that they rely solely on sensorimotor feedback. Cerebellar internal models are believed to contribute to such expert skills by internally representing the input-output properties of tools. In this case, parietal regions also play key roles in sending signals representing intended motion and switching of internal models, as found by the studies reviewed in this chapter.

Figure 11.11 illustrates a hypothetical schema regarding the difference in neural networks between novice or normal use and the expert use of tools. Note that this schema supposes a situation in which a single tool is used and the switching of tools is not needed. At the novice stage (Fig. 11.11A), skills acquired in parietal (or frontal) regions play important roles in the use of tools. These skills largely depend on an external (visual and proprioceptive) feedback loop but probably can cope with many situations in which speed and precision in manipulation are not needed. However, at the expert stage, after repeated training (Fig. 11.11B), the lateral part of the cerebellum acquires internal models of tools and provides an internal simulation loop with parietal regions. At this stage, parietal regions send signals representing the intended motion to the cerebellar internal models, and the internal models then predict sensorimotor feedback and send back the predicted sensory feedback to the parietal regions (*arrows with dotted lines*). Alternatively, the internal models calculate control signals from the intended motion and send appropriate (feedforward) control signals to the frontal region (*arrows with dashed line*). Cerebellar internal models correspond to the forward model in the former route and to the inverse model in the latter route.

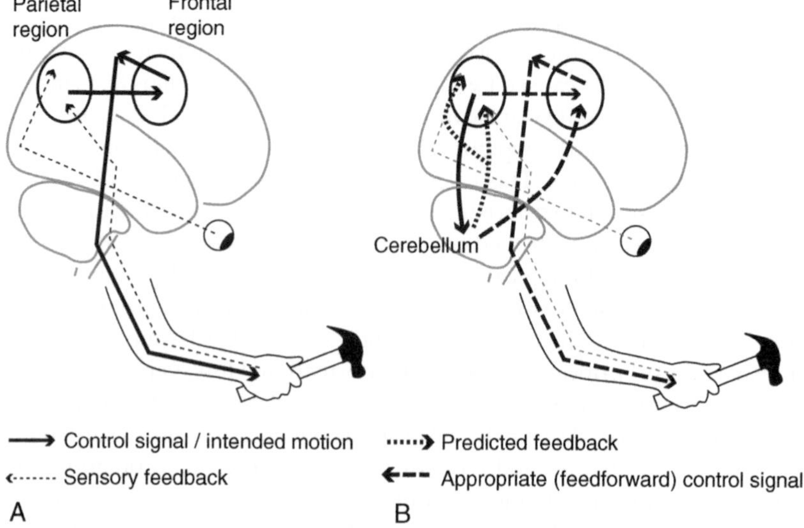

Figure 11.11 Possible major pathways of control and feedback signals during tool use (e.g., hammer) at novice (or normal) (**A**) and expert (**B**) levels.

In this schema, cerebellar internal models exist in a complementary circuit, shown by the solid and dotted lines, or a bypass route via the cerebellum for the main pathway between parietal and frontal regions. Therefore, when the cerebellum is damaged, it is unlikely that severe deficits will be observed in the manipulation of tools as long as speed and precision are not needed. This is probably the reason why deficits in the skills for tools (such as ideomotor apraxia, described earlier) have not been reported in patients with cerebellar lesions in previous neuropsychological studies. It would be expected that such patients face difficulties in using tools in a highly skillful manner, but it is often difficult to ask patients to participate in tasks requiring both speed and accuracy. In contrast, if parietal regions are damaged, problems occur in the main pathway for tool use, and patients would have severe and evident deficits in tool use. Of course, this schema is a hypothetical one and needs to be experimentally examined in future studies.

In addition to examining this schema, several hypotheses can be postulated regarding human faculty in tool use based on the studies reviewed in this chapter. First, some studies have reported that the SPL contributes to tool-use skills (Moll et al. 2000; Choi et al. 2001), whereas others have hinted at the importance of the IPL in these skills (Rumiati et al. 2004; Valyear et al. 2007). However, the functional difference in tool use between the SPL and the IPL remains unknown. Our study suggests that the SPL contributes to predictive adjustment of behaviors based on visual information, whereas the IPL contributes to postdictive or online modification of behaviors by using multisensory (proprioceptive and visual) feedback (Imamizu and Kawato 2008). Although such differences were identified in the context of switching of expert skills (internal models), it could be generalized to skills largely depending on sensory information: The SPL is involved in the manipulation of tools based on visual information, whereas the IPL plays a key role in manipulation based on multisensory feedback, not only by visual information but also by proprioceptive and tactile feedback.

Second, regarding tools, cerebellar internal models apparently contribute to skills for use, rather than the semantic/conceptual knowledge. However, our study found that activity of the MTG region increased as subject performance improved after changing the tools, suggesting that this region receives output signals from cerebellar internal models (Fig. 11.9). The MTG region has been suggested as a key region in the cortical network for the semantic/conceptual knowledge of tools (Martin et al. 1996; Johnson-Frey 2004). Input-output properties are important semantic aspects of tools; thus, internal models representing these properties may partly contribute to the identification or formation of the semantic/conceptual knowledge of tools. However, little is known about the detailed functional relationship and anatomical pathways between cerebellar internal models and the MTG regions.

Third, the parietal regions are believed to be involved in representing a body schema. An electrophysiological neuronal recording in monkeys suggested that the body schema in the parietal region is dynamically updated by training in tool use. That is, the visual response properties of bimodal (tactile and visual) neurons in the parietal regions were modified to include a hand-held tool (a rake) after monkeys were trained to use the tool to retrieve distant objects (Iriki et al. 1996). This phenomenon is considered to involve neural correlates for the perceptual assimilation of the tool and hand. It has been suggested that the anterior parts of the cerebellum contribute to the control of the body, and that homunculoid representations exist in the anterior part (Snider and Eldred 1951; Grodd et al. 2001). Consistent with this, we found that centroids of activities exist in the anterior part when subjects actually manipulate various tools with their arms and hands, but centroids were found in the lateral parts when subjects imagined the use of the tools without actual hand or arm movements (Higuchi et al. 2007). Taken together with our previous results indicating that internal models for novel tools are acquired in the lateral cerebellum (Imamizu et al. 2000; Imamizu et al. 2003), these results are believed to indicate that internal models for tools are acquired in the lateral parts. However, by analogy to the change in body schema in the parietal region, we can expect that activity related to the manipulation of a particular tool shifts from the lateral part to the anterior part when subjects gain the ability, after intensive training lasting months or years, to manipulate the tool as if it were a part of their bodies. If so, this shift would be due to the neural correlates for the sensorimotor (in contrast to perceptual) assimilation of the tool and body.

CONCLUSION

The characteristic human ability to use a wide range of tools sets us apart from other animals. This ability is based on both sensorimotor skills that are likely common to other animals and semantic/conceptual knowledge that is probably not common to them. This may be the most interesting issue in research on brain mechanisms for tool use because such ability bridges between the fundamental and higher-order functions. Thus, findings in this area are expected to provide important clues to understanding how human intelligence, such as conceptualization, emerged from fundamental functions such as sensorimotor skills, which are common to other animals.

ACKNOWLEDGMENTS

This chapter is mainly based on studies that were performed in collaboration with Drs. Satomi Higuchi, Thierry Chaminade, Tomoe Kuroda, Satoru Miyauchi, and Mitsuo Kawato. I would like to thank them for their insightful discussions and helpful comments during the collaboration.

REFERENCES

Choi, S.H., D.L. Na, E. Kang, K.M. Lee, S.W. Lee, and D.G. Na. 2001. Functional magnetic resonance imaging during pantomiming tool-use gestures. *Experimental Brain Research* 139: 311–17.

De Renzi, E., and F. Lucchelli F. 1988. Ideational apraxia. *Brain* 111: 1173–85.

Friederici, A.D., J. Bahlmann, S. Heim, R.I. Schubotz, and A. Anwander. 2006. The brain differentiates human and non-human grammars: Functional localization and structural connectivity. *Proceedings of the National Academy of Science U S A* 103: 2458–63.

Friston, K.J., L. Harrison, and W. Penny. 2003. Dynamic causal modelling. *NeuroImage* 19: 1273–1302.

Gomi, H., M. Shidara, A. Takemura, Y. Inoue, K. Kawano, and M. Kawato. 1998. Temporal firing patterns of purkinje cells in the cerebellar ventral paraflocculus during ocular following responses in monkeys I. Simple spikes [In process citation]. *Journal of Neurophysiology* 80: 818–31.

Grodd, W., E. Hulsmann, M. Lotze, D. Wildgruber, and M. Erb. 2001. Sensorimotor mapping of the human cerebellum: fMRI evidence of somatotopic organization. *Human Brain Mapping* 13: 55–73.

Haruno, M., D.M. Wolpert, and M. Kawato. 2001. Mosaic model for sensorimotor learning and control. *Neural Computation* 13: 2201–20.

Higuchi, S., T. Chaminade, H. Imamizu, and M. Kawato. 2009. Shared neural correlates for language and tool use in Broca's area. *Neuroreport* 20: 1376–1381.

Higuchi, S., H. Imamizu, and M. Kawato M. 2007. Cerebellar activity evoked by common tool-use execution and imagery tasks: an fMRI study. *Cortex* 43: 350–58.

Iacoboni, M., L.M. Koski, M. Brass, H. Bekkering, R.P. Woods, M.C. Dubeau, et al. 2001. Reafferent copies of imitated actions in the right superior temporal cortex. *Proceedings of the National Academy of Science U S A* 98: 13995–99.

Imamizu, H., and M. Kawato. 2008. Neural correlates of predictive and postdictive switching mechanisms for internal models. *Journal of Neuroscience* 28: 10751–65.

Imamizu, H., T. Kuroda, S. Miyauchi, T. Yoshioka, and M. Kawato. 2003. Modular organization of internal models of tools in the human cerebellum. *Proceedings of the National Academy of Science U S A* 100: 5461–66.

Imamizu, H., S. Miyauchi, T. Tamada, Y. Sasaki, R. Takino, B. Putz, et al. 2000. Human cerebellar activity reflecting an acquired internal model of a new tool. *Nature* 403: 192–95.

Iriki, A., M. Tanaka, and Y. Iwamura. 1996. Coding of modified body schema during tool use by macaque postcentral neurones. *NeuroReport* 7: 2325–30.

Ito, M. 1984. *The cerebellum and neural motor control.* New York: Raven Press.

Johnson-Frey, S.H. 2004. The neural bases of complex tool use in humans. *Trends in Cognitive Science* 8: 71–78.

Kawato, M. 1999. Internal models for motor control and trajectory planning. *Current Opinions in Neurobiology* 9: 718–27.

Kawato, M., K. Furukawa, and R. Suzuki. 1987. A hierarchical neural-network model for control and learning of voluntary movement. *Biological Cybernetics* 57: 169–85.

Kawato, M., and H. Gomi. 1992. A computational model of four regions of the cerebellum based on feedback-error learning. *Biological Cybernetics* 68: 95–103.

Kitazawa, S., T. Kimura, and P.B. Yin. 1998. Cerebellar complex spikes encode both destinations and errors in arm movements. *Nature* 392: 494–97.

Kobayashi, Y., K. Kawano, A. Takemura, Y. Inoue, T. Kitama, H. Gomi, and M. Kawato. 1998. Temporal firing patterns of purkinje cells in the cerebellar ventral paraflocculus during ocular following responses in monkeys II. Complex spikes [In Process Citation]. *Journal of Neurophysiology* 80: 832–48.

Kole, J.A., and A.F. Healy. 2007. Using prior knowledge to minimize interference when learning large amounts of information. *Memory & Cognition* 35: 124–37.

Kroliczak, G., C. Cavina-Pratesi, D.A. Goodman, and J.C. Culham. 2007. What does the brain do when you fake it? An FMRI study of pantomimed and real grasping. *Journal of Neurophysiology* 97: 2410–22.

Lewis, J.W. 2006. Cortical networks related to human use of tools. *Neuroscientist* 12: 211–31.

Martin, A., C.L. Wiggs, L.G. Ungerleider, and J.V. Haxby. 1996. Neural correlates of category-specific knowledge. *Nature* 379: 649–52.

Miall, R.C., D.J. Weir, D.M. Wolpert, and J.F. Stein. 1993. Is the cerebellum a Smith predictor? *Journal of Motor Behavior* 25: 203–16.

Middleton, F.A., and P.L. Strick. 1997. Dentate output channels: Motor and cognitive components. In *The cerebellum: From structure to control*, eds., C.I. de Zeeuw, P. Strata, and J. Voogd, 553–66. Amsterdam: Elsevier Science BV.

Moll, J., R. de Oliveira-Souza, L.J. Passman, F.C. Cunha, F. Souza-Lima, and P.A. Andreiuolo. 2000. Functional MRI correlates of real and imagined tool-use pantomimes. *Neurology* 54: 1331–36.

Ochipa, C., L.J. Rothi, and K.M. Heilman. 1992. Conceptual apraxia in Alzheimer's disease. *Brain* 115, Pt. 4: 1061–71.

Rizzolatti, G., L. Fadiga, M. Matelli, V. Bettinardi, E. Paulesu, D. Perani, and F. Fazio. 1996. Localization of grasp representations in humans by PET: 1. Observation versus execution. *Experimental Brain Research* 111: 246–52.

Rumiati, R.I., P.H. Weiss, T. Shallice, G. Ottoboni, J. Noth, K. Zilles, and G.R. Fink. 2004. Neural basis of pantomiming the use of visually presented objects. *NeuroImage* 21: 1224–31.

Sakai, K.L. 2005. Language acquisition and brain development. *Science* 310: 815–19.

Shidara, M., K. Kawano, H. Gomi, and M. Kawato. 1993. Inverse-dynamics model eye movement control by Purkinje cells in the cerebellum. *Nature* 365: 50–52.

Snider, R.S., and E. Eldred. 1951. Cerebro-cerebellar relationships in the monkey. *Journal of Neurophysiology* 15: 27–40.

Tamada, T., S. Miyauchi, H. Imamizu, T. Yoshioka, and M. Kawato. 1999. Cerebro-cerebellar functional connectivity revealed by the laterality index in tool-use learning. *NeuroReport* 10: 325–31.

Valyear, K.F., C. Cavina-Pratesi, A.J. Stiglick, and J.C. Culham. 2007. Does tool-related fMRI activity within the intraparietal sulcus reflect the plan to grasp? *NeuroImage* 36 Suppl 2: T94-T108.

Wolpert, D.M., Z. Ghahramani, and J.R. Flanagan. 2001. Perspectives and problems in motor learning. *Trends in Cognitive Science* 5: 487–94.

Wolpert, D.M., Z. Ghahramani, and M.I. Jordan. 1995. An internal model for sensorimotor integration. *Science* 269: 1880–82.

Wolpert, D.M., and M. Kawato. 1998. Multiple paired forward and inverse models for motor control. *Neural Networks* 11: 1317–29.

12

Variability, Noise, and Sensitivity to Error in Learning a Motor Task

DAGMAR STERNAD AND MASAKI O. ABE

When trying to understand human motor control probably the most fundamental aspect to consider is that the neuromechanical system is redundant. A task as trivial as inserting a key into a keyhole can be successfully achieved with the key approaching from a range of different orientations. Biomechanical analysis of the multisegmented arm and hand pointing the key immediately reveals that even for a single key orientation, an infinite set of joint configurations exists. Redundancy also exists at the level of muscles, such that many different muscle contractions will achieve the same joint orientation. In fact, redundancy resides across all levels of the neuromechanical system ranging from molecular, neuronal, and muscular, to behavioral processes (see also Herzog, this volume). With this multiplicity of options to achieve a given task, it is no surprise that variability at the behavioral level is ubiquitous.

Variability at the task level is also the inevitable product of multiple sources of noise in the nervous system.[1] For example, it has been shown that noise arises in signal propagation due to synaptic fluctuations that increases the irregularity of spike trains; in muscles and proprioceptors unavoidable variations are added by the transduction of a continuous signal

[1] A notational clarification on noise and variability: Although these terms are often difficult to keep apart, we distinguish between them as follows: *Variability* is the behavioral outcome of such system-intrinsic noise; capitalized *Noise* is one of the three concepts of the TCN approach and refers to the stochastic component that is assumed to be the result of intrinsic neuromotor noise; *N-Cost* is the operationalization of *Noise*. *Intrinsic (neuromotor) noise* refers to system-intrinsic fluctuations that are typically unwanted but from our perspective may also be fundamental to adaptation and control.

into discrete spike sequences (Faisal et al. 2008). Noise also occurs at all stages of the sensorimotor sequence, from the planning stage (Gordon et al. 1994; Churchland et al. 2006), the execution of movements (van Beers et al. 2004; van Beers 2009), and to the processing of sensory estimates to update motor commands (Osborne et al. 2005). This noise, or uncertainty, is also an integral element of current Bayesian approaches and has become the object of much theorizing and empirical work on perception, cognition, and motor control (van Beers et al. 2002; Körding et al. 2004; Körding and Wolpert 2004; Miyazaki et al. 2005).

Taking task redundancy and system noise together, it is no surprise that sensorimotor performance varies with every new attempt. And yet, the nervous system does not randomly vary its performance to achieve the task goal. The hypothesis of our research is that the nervous system seeks strategies that best accommodate for errors and noise; that is, it seeks solutions with stability or robustness. How is such stable coordination learned? Our research provides evidence that the central nervous system (CNS) is aware of its intrinsic noise and recognizes solutions that are robust to noise. In addition, the CNS utilizes this noise to locate the most error-tolerant solutions. Although several lines of investigation pursue similar directions, our approach is unique in postulating three conceptually different routes to performance improvement and stability.

Stability: Tolerance to Noise

Defined broadly, stable solutions are those that tolerate errors without negative effects on task performance and without requiring explicit corrections. In a continuous dynamical system, stable solutions are those that quickly recover from small perturbations (Strogatz 1994). Viewing noise as a barrage of small perturbations, more stable solutions are also more tolerant of noise. Using the frequently used image of a ball in a potential well, stability is high when the well is deep and steep (Fig. 12.1A). Stability of a system can be probed by administering small perturbations and observing how long it takes for the system to return to the stationary state (lowest point in the well). Importantly, variability is the consequence both of the steepness of the well (stability) and of the noise level. Hence, in a coordinative system, increasing stability offers a "smart" solution, as return back to steady state can happen without explicit error correction. The relevance of dynamic stability to skilled performance has been demonstrated in our previous research on rhythmically bouncing a ball (Wei et al. 2007; 2008).

A slightly different perspective on stability is required when considering a discrete system, such as a set of individual throwing actions; only discrete estimates of each throw are considered, and nothing is known about their time sequence. Unlike in continuous tasks, there is no direct

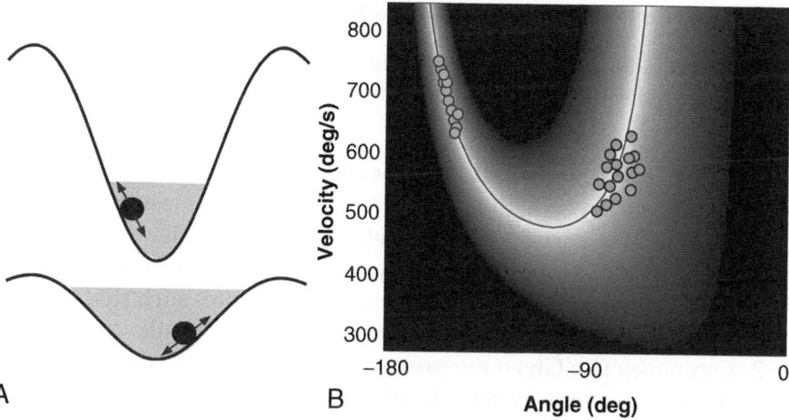

Figure 12.1 **A:** Stability and noise in a continuous dynamical system. The steepness of the well represents the stability of the system and the gray "filling" of the well represents the noise; the vertical level of the filling represents the noise level and the horizontal extent of the filling represents the effect of the variability. **B:** Discrete system with results as a function of two execution variables. The line denotes the zero-error solution manifold, darker shades denote increasing error. The two data sets exemplify how a location with shallow curvature adjacent to the solution manifold allows more noise or scatter in the data while still achieving comparable results to the data on the left.

carry-over of errors from the previous iteration and hence the concept of dynamical stability from dynamical systems theory cannot be applied "as is." Figure 12.1B schematizes such a system using our model task of target-oriented throwing: Two variables, angle α and velocity v at ball release fully determine the trajectory of the projectile and its hitting accuracy or, generally, the result: $r = f(\alpha, v)$. In the figure, every throw is characterized by one data point of (α, v) with its associated result r shown by gray shades. The task is redundant, as many combinations of α and v achieve the same outcome r (e.g., hitting accuracy or error r). The U-shaped line denotes the desired zero-error solutions, $r = 0$, that define the solution manifold. The discrete system is said to be stable when a set of performances have the same or similar results r, even though the variables α and v may vary. As in the continuous system, stability of the discrete system is assessed by considering the effect of small perturbations. In the example of Figure 12.1B, the set of data on the right is more stable or more tolerant to error as the result function is shallower around the solution manifold than on the left: small perturbations to performance on the left will lead to large increases in error.

Tolerance, Covariation, and Noise Reduction

How does the sensorimotor system deal with its intrinsic noise and perform a redundant task with stability? We propose three routes to obtain task stability (Fig. 12.2):

1. *Tolerance (T)*: The sensorimotor system seeks solutions that have low sensitivity or high tolerance to errors. In nonlinear dynamical systems this corresponds to seeking attractor states with steep wells (Fig. 12.1A); in discrete systems this implies seeking locations on the manifold with a shallow curvature, such that small deviations in α and v have minimal effect on the result.
2. *Covariation (C)*: Given the presence of intrinsic neuromotor noise, the sensorimotor system develops covariation among variables with respect to the solution manifold, such that a given amount of noise has least effect on the result.
3. *Noise (N)*: The sensorimotor system reduces the magnitude of dispersion.

Figure 12.3 illustrates these three routes with schematic data plotted in the execution space. Color shades code the result for data with different release angle and velocities; white denotes zero error, the solution manifold. Although each solution on the manifold is equivalent, different locations on the solution manifold have very different sensitivity or tolerance to errors, as illustrated by the changing width of the light gray shades adjacent to the solution manifold. The three panels contrast two data sets respectively. One data set is ideal with respect to the three components: In the left panel the two data sets have very different tolerance; the center panel illustrates how data can covary to optimize the result; the right panel illustrates how noise can be reduced.

We exemplify this three-pronged TCN approach by investigating a throwing task to demonstrate that this framework can uncover processes

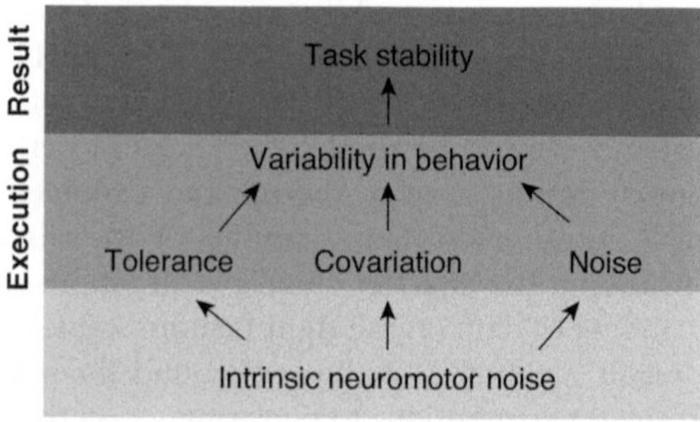

Figure 12.2 Schematic overview of the Tolerance, Covariance, Noise (TCN) approach.

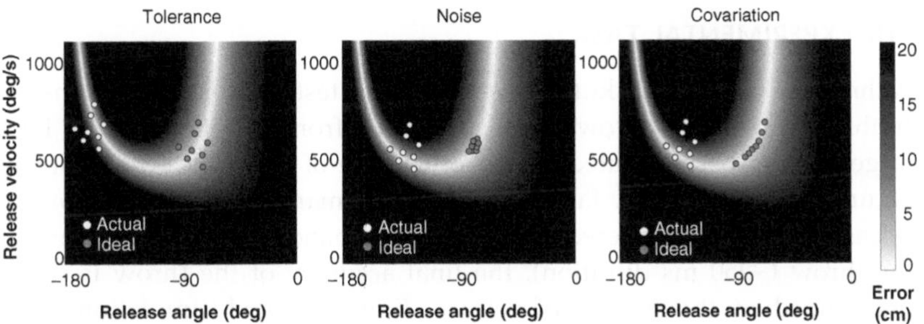

Figure 12.3 Three types of "costs" for motor variability. Actual (*white*) and ideal (*gray*) data optimized for Tolerance (*T-Cost*), Noise (*N-Cost*), and Covariation (*C-Cost*).

underlying skill improvement and learning. Specifically, we show how the three components are intertwined and how the brain uses variability to its advantage.

Related Approaches

The notion of *constraining* or *channeling* the variability such that it has little effect on the result is also a core feature in the *uncontrolled manifold* (UCM) framework (Scholz and Schöner 1999; Latash 2008; see Latash, this volume). Central to the UCM approach is the tenet that control is indicated when over-repeated performances the system's variability at the execution level shows anisotropic distribution in directions that do not affect the result (i.e., covary; Fig. 12.3). Although the notions of reducing and channeling noise are conceptually consistent with the TCN-framework, UCM uses established mathematical tools of covariance analysis to quantify the anisotropic distribution of sets of data (Craig 1986; Latash 2008). Although this affords theoretical advantages, there are also disadvantages that will be considered in the discussion (Sternad et al., 2010). A second approach that has some conceptual overlap with the TNC method is the *optimal feedback control* (OFC) framework as developed by Todorov and colleagues (Todorov 2004; Todorov 2005; see also Herzog, this volume). Extending traditional feedback control to delayed sensory estimates, OFC proposes a hierarchical control framework that applies selective control of task variables according to composite task-specific cost functions. Effectively, corrections are only applied when deviations have a devastating effect on the task goal, in the spirit of Gel'fand's minimal intervention principle (Gel'fand and Tsetlin 1962; Liu and Todorov 2007). Before elaborating on theoretical differences and possible insights derived from these different approaches, we review some recent research in our lab on the throwing task skittles.

THE EXPERIMENTAL TASK

A throwing task called skittles has served as a test bed for our hypotheses. In this task, subjects throw a ball suspended from a vertical post to hit a target skittle that is located on the other side of the post. To execute an accurate (not necessarily far) throw, subtle demands on the timing of ball release have to be mastered. While the arm/hand trajectory prepares for the throw (~250 ms duration), the final accuracy of the throw is solely determined at the instant of release. Empirical and simulation-based studies reported that the timing window for accurate throws is as short as 3–10 ms (Hore et al. 2002). This precision is astonishing, as a relatively narrow range of covarying release variables is required at the instant of release. Given these demands, the task has received considerable attention in both sports- and clinically motivated research. For example, several studies with cerebellar patients highlighted the significant involvement of the cerebellum for the coordination between the continuous trajectory and the precise timing of the release (Martin et al. 2001; Timmann et al. 2001; Hore et al. 2002).

Apparatus and Data Collection

The experimental version of our skittles task reduced the movement to a single-joint forearm rotation in the horizontal plane, where the ball release is triggered via opening a contact switch by extending the index finger during the forearm movement to simulate the throw of the ball (Fig. 12.4A). The subject grasps a ball at the tip of the lever that has the contact switch affixed. This switch can be closed by touch with the flexed index finger; opening the contact by finger extension triggers ball release. The release time determines the angular position α and angular velocity v of the arm movement from which the ball trajectory is computed. This ball traverses around the central post in an elliptic trajectory toward the skittle at the opposite side (Fig. 12.4B). The subject sees this ball trajectory online on the screen. The real arm movements with the manipulandum correspond to paddle movements on the visual display that is seen by subjects as a bar rotating around an axis. Angular displacements of the lever arm are measured by a potentiometer. The virtual task is novel to every subject, such that every learner has the same initial conditions. The task is simple enough to allow improvement within the experimental time frame, but it also provides sufficient subtleties that are only mastered with long-term practice.

The ball's elliptic trajectories are generated by a two-dimensional model, where two orthogonal springs attach the ball to the origin of the coordinate system, the center post ($x = y = 0$). Due to restoring forces proportional to the distance between ball and center post, the ball is accelerated toward the

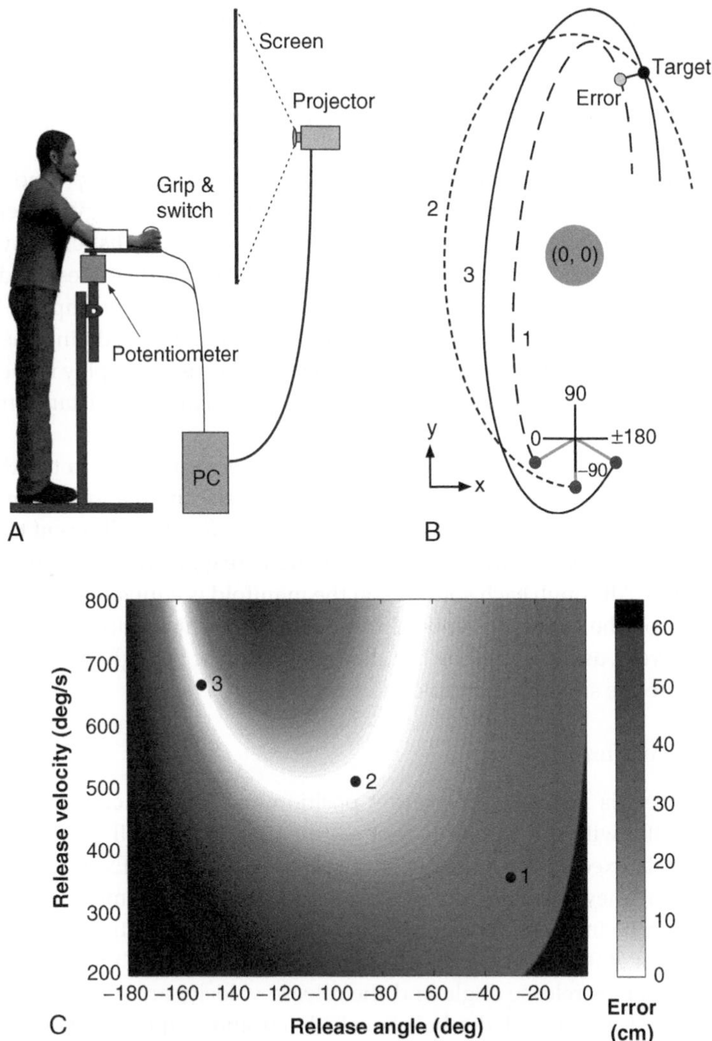

Figure 12.4 A: Experimental setup. Participants stand in front of the setup with their forearm resting on the horizontal lever arm. Rotation of the arm is recorded by a potentiometer; when the finger on the ball extends, the contact switch opens and the ball in the virtual simulation is released. Online recordings of the arm movements are displayed on the projection screen. **B**: Three exemplary throws in workspace as participants see in the experiment. The view is a top-down view onto the pendular skittles task.

center. At time t, the equations for the ball position in x- and y- direction are:

$$x(t) = A_x \sin(\omega t + \varphi_x) e^{-\frac{t}{\tau}} \qquad y(t) = A_y \sin(\omega t + \varphi_y) e^{-\frac{t}{\tau}} \qquad \text{(Eq. 1)}$$

The amplitudes A_x and A_y, as well as phase differences, φ_x and φ_y, result from the ball's release angle and velocity including energy conservation. The motions are lightly damped to approximate realistic behavior. τ denotes the relaxation time of the decay. Figure 12.4B illustrates the definitions of the Cartesian coordinates of the workspace. Three exemplary ball trajectories are displayed together with the result measure, d, defined as the minimal distance between target and trajectory. The visual display is shown to subjects on a back-projection screen that is placed at 1.2 m distance from the subject.

The execution space with three data points corresponding to the three trajectories is shown in Figure 12.4C. The result space and the solution manifold are those used for the following experiment. Note that different target locations render very different result functions (e.g., compare Figure 12.3 and 12.4C). Although each solution on the manifold is equivalent, different locations on the solution manifold have very different sensitivity or tolerance to errors, as illustrated by the changing width of the light gray shades adjacent to the solution manifold.

General Procedure

Each subject is presented the target position and is instructed to hit the target skittle with the ball in its first elliptic trajectory. In all experiments, the subjects execute their throws in a self-paced manner. Experience has shown that they can perform 300 trials within one experimental session without inducing fatigue or losing motivation and attention. The total duration for 300 trials is approximately 30 minutes. For each trial, the execution variables release angle and the release velocity are measured, and the elliptic trajectory of the ball is calculated and displayed. The result measure, d, is calculated for each trial.

TCN-Cost Analysis

Cohen and Sternad (2009) adopted an optimization perspective to quantify the three components (Cohen and Sternad 2009). Instead of calculating the difference in T, C, and N between two data sets, as developed in Müller and Sternad (2004), the new cost-based approach compares a single data set with one that is optimized in one component, keeping others constant. Note that the conceptual basis is unchanged, only the quantification is different. For a given data set, a virtual data set is numerically found that optimizes T, N, and C (see Figure 12.3 for schematic illustration): Starting with T, the actual data set is shifted across every location in execution space in a grid-like manner without changing its relative distribution; at each shift, its result is evaluated in terms of its average error; the best location in execution space is the one with the smallest error. The difference between the error of the actual and the best data set defines the cost due to nonoptimal tolerance, *T-Cost*. To determine the cost due to nonoptimal covariation, *C-Cost*, the pairing of the two execution variables of a data set is permuted to find that combination of execution variables that achieves the best possible average result. *C-Cost* is the difference between the actual and the optimal result. Last, *N-Cost* is calculated by shrinking the data set concentrically to its mean in n steps (e.g., $n = 100$). For each step, the result is evaluated and the best shrinking step is identified. Note the best result is not necessarily the single mean point, as it depends on the location. *N-Cost* is the difference in result between the initial set and the ideal one (for more details, see Cohen and Sternad 2009).

Stages of Learning: From Exploration to Increasing Covariation and Reducing Noise

What insights can this analysis yield? Are all three components decreased by the same amount with practice, or is there a component that is inaccessible to optimization? Is there a specific sequence to how the three components are optimized? What does fine-tuning of a skill imply? To address these questions, a group of 12 healthy adult subjects practiced the skittles task for six experimental sessions on 6 days. Three additional participants who had extensive previous experience with throwing continued practice for a total of 15 days; two of them were intramural Frisbee players and one was a former professional cricket player. On each day, participants completed three blocks of 60 throws, leading to a total of 1,080 throws for the normal group and 2,700 throws for the expert subjects. The goal of the long-term data collection was to examine how accurate and precise human subjects can become in this task.

A first inspection of the average error and its standard deviations per block for each participant over practice showed the expected exponential decrease of the error and also of its standard deviations (Fig. 12.5). These results are consistent with many previous reports on performance improvements with practice (Schmidt and Lee 2005) and therefore can be seen as a representative database for examining the changes in the three components *Tolerance, Covariation,* and *Noise.*

Figure 12.6 shows the data of one of the expert subjects plotted in execution space. As can be seen, on Day 1, the 60 data points of one block show a wide scatter, with most throws at larger release angles of –150 degrees. The fewer throws with a release angle around –80 degrees were later in the block, "exploring" other areas of execution space to achieve better performance with executions that are more error-*tolerant* (trial sequence in time is not visible in the figure). On Day 5, this location in execution space evidently became preferred, and the data start to cluster with some *Covariation* along the solution manifold. On Day 15 of practice, the data have become

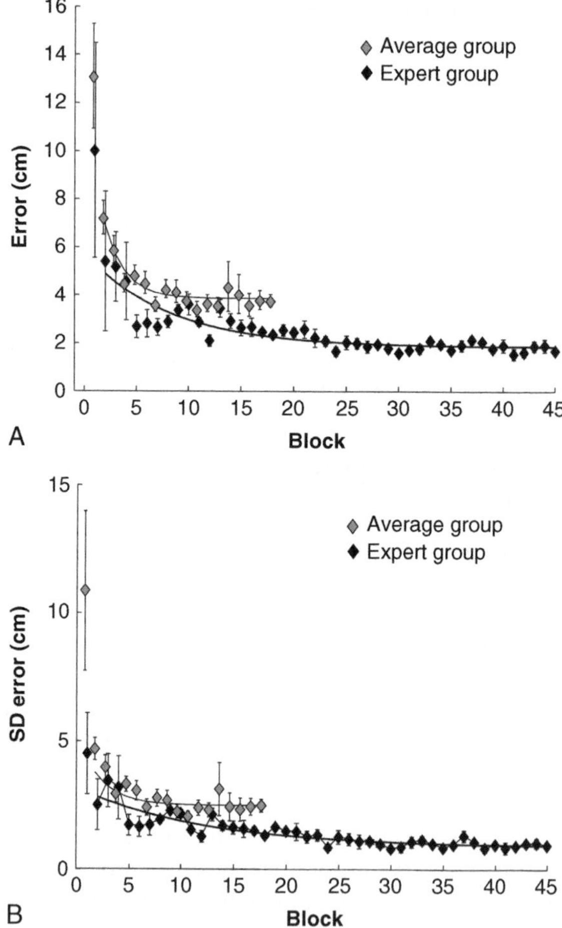

Figure 12.5 Changes in the error to the target with practice. For each block, the data of 60 trials were averaged. Participants performed three blocks of trials per day. **A:** Mean error for 12 participants over 18 blocks (6 days) of practice are shown in gray. Results for the expert participants over 45 blocks (15 days) of practice are shown in black. Error bars show standard error across participants. **B:** Standard deviations of error averaged over participants across blocks of trials. Error bars show standard error across participants.

more tightly clustered—*Noise* was reduced, and the data displayed even more pronounced *Covariation*.

Numerical estimates of the three costs were calculated for each participant for each block of 60 trials, hence rendering three estimates per day. Note the cost estimate is interpretable and expresses how much the average error could be reduced if this particular cost were minimized. The results of the three costs are therefore directly comparable. It should be

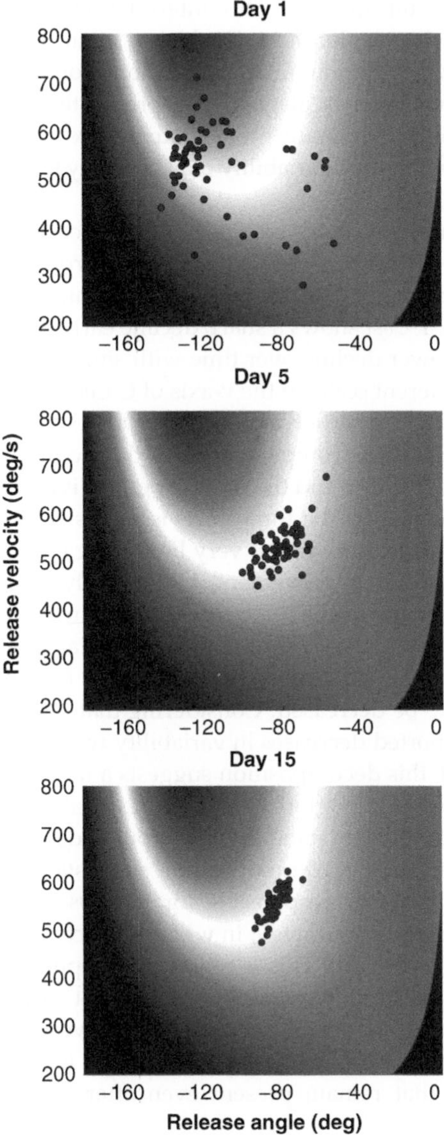

Figure 12.6 Representative example of improvement of skittles task over 15 days of practice. Data of one expert subject is plotted in execution space.

pointed out, though, that the three costs do not sum to the total error in performance. Typically, their sum is higher than the average error as the components are not exclusive and independent. Most notably, *T-Cost* of a particular data set depends on its *N-Cost*: The strategy depends on the overall dispersion of the data. Data with very little dispersion do not require a very error-tolerant strategy. This interrelation is interesting and has potential for further exploration. Could it be that, for people who have large variability, as for example due to tremor or other neurological disorders, different movement strategies are appropriate? Conversely, if people have low variability, then many more strategies are available. According to this logic, manipulation of variability may be a way to influence movement strategies.

Figure 12.7 shows the mean results of the three costs for both participant groups together with their exponential fits; the error bars denote standard error across participants. The time profiles are similar for both experts and average subjects: *T-Cost* shows a sharp decline early in practice, *C-Cost* and *N-Cost* have a slower decline over time with similar time constants; however, note the different scale on the y-axis of *C-Cost* and *N-Cost*.

Hence, plotting the fitted exponential curves in a single graph in Figure 12.8 permits better comparison of the three costs. Inspecting the profiles for the average group and the three expert individuals together reveals that the rank ordering of the three costs is consistent for all participants. *T-Cost* either drops sharply in the very beginning or is already exploited, leaving little room for improvement. Interestingly, *N-Cost* is the highest and also remains highest. The three expert individuals show that only after many days of practice does *N-Cost* approach similar levels as *C-Cost*.

These results are nontrivial, as they show that *Noise* is highest and the last component to be decreased. Considering that many studies on motor learning have reported decreases in variability with practice as the typical signature of skill, this decomposition suggests a new interpretation of this ubiquitous finding. Although the decrease of variability in error measures was typically quantified by standard deviations and interpreted as a change in random noise, the TNC-decomposition suggests that more systematic aspects of variability are responsible for the observed decrease. In the beginning are changes of strategy, in which subjects explore and find new ways of executing the task. This is followed by optimizing covariation in alignment with the solution manifold (i.e., existent variability in execution is channeled into "do-not-care-directions"). Only very late in practice does the noise component experience an improvement. It can be concluded that the fluctuations that remain present even after long practice are truly random elements.

The notion of channeling variability into do-not-care-directions is close to what the analysis approach of the UCM approach (Latash, Scholz, and Schöner, 2002) extracts from data and is also implicit in the OFC framework (Todorov and Jordan 2002; Todorov 2004). Hence, some discussion of both approaches is warranted. Before doing so, however, it should be emphasized that the present model task has redundancy in state space defined by angle and velocity at execution. As the two dimensions have different units, the space has no distance measure and does not permit the application of covariance-based analysis. The UCM and OFC approaches are

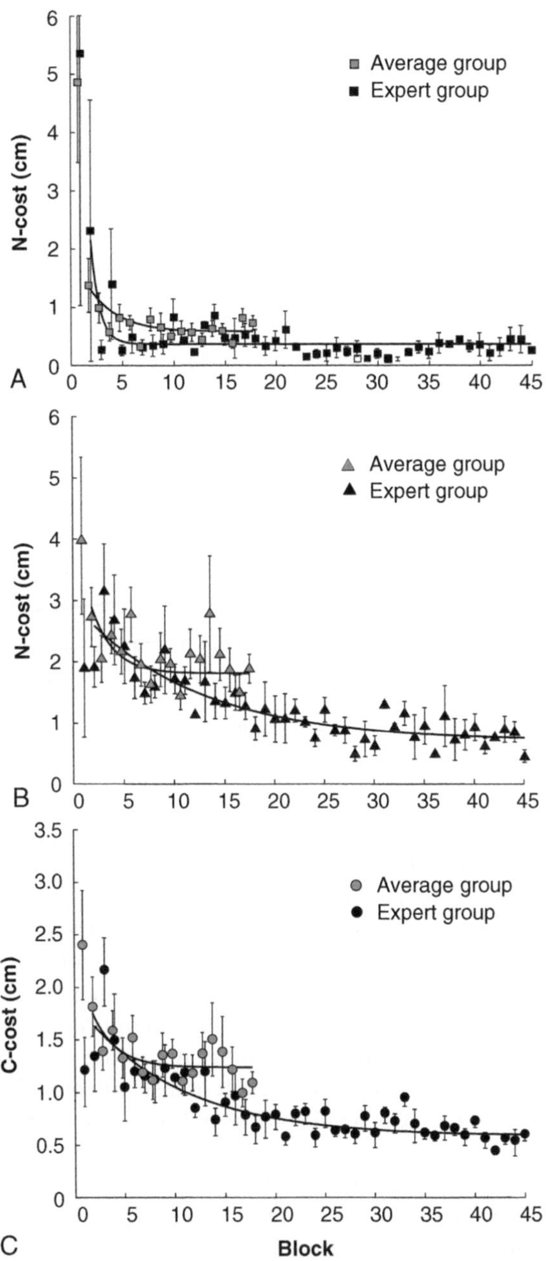

Figure 12.7 Changes in *T-Cost, N-Cost* and *C-Cost* over practice. Mean results for 12 participants over 18 blocks (6 days) of practice are shown as in gray. Results for the expert group over 45 blocks (15 days) of practice are shown in gray. Error bars show standard error across participants.

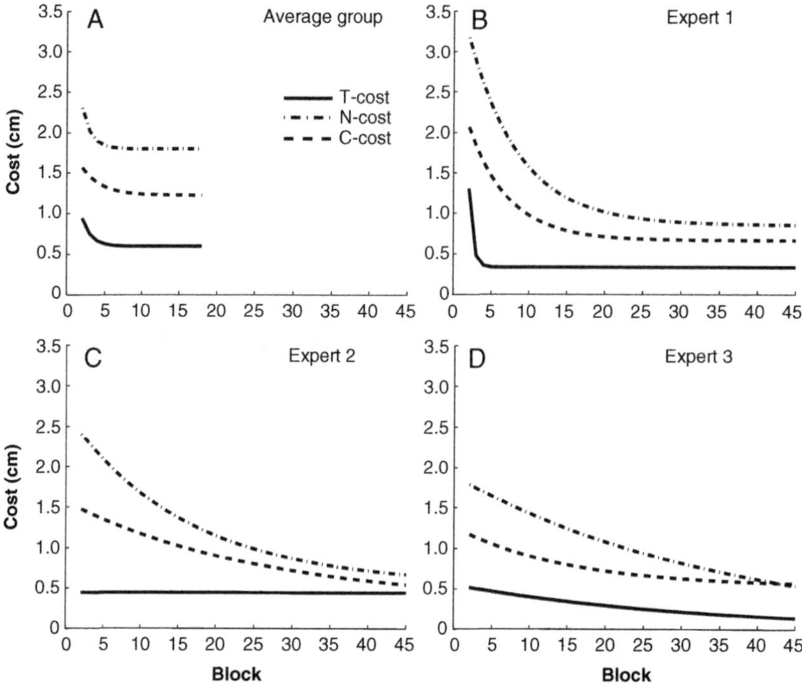

Figure 12.8 Exponential fits to *T-Cost*, *N-Cost*, and *C-Cost* for the average and the expert group data. **A**: Exponential fits to the three costs for the group. **B–D**: Exponential fits for the three expert participants.

based on the analysis of the covariance matrix, similar to many other analyses of the structure of variability, such as principal component analysis and variants of independent component analysis. Hence, orthogonality—the key concept used to apply covariance-based analyses in motor experiments—cannot be meaningfully applied to this task (Schöner and Scholz 2007; Müller and Sternad 2009; Sternad et al. 2010). A significant difference of the TCN approach is that it analyzes variability not in the space of the execution variables, but in the space of the result or task outcome. The important consequence is that the TCN analysis does not require a meaningful definition of distance in execution space.

Putting the issue of metrics aside, the distinct aspect of the TNC method is its parsing of variability into three components. In comparison, UCM distinguishes between variability parallel and orthogonal to the manifold. These correspond to covariation or the lack thereof in the TNC approach. Changes in the magnitude of the dispersion are not separated from changes in the anisotropy of the variability. That said, such an extension could be relatively straightforward. An additional conceptual difference is that the UCM analysis assumes that the system is at its best location.

In the TNC approach, the quantification of the best location that offers stability—*Tolerance*—compared to the actual location, is new and distinct. This aspect pays tribute to the fact that, in order to find the best strategy, variability is required that reveals information about where this strategy is: Variability or *Noise* presents an opportunity to learn and improve.

Sensitivity to Intrinsic Variability: Optimizing Tolerance

To what degree are subjects aware of their intrinsic noise and seek movement strategies that are tolerant to this noise? As introduced earlier in Figure 12.1, stability in both continuous and discrete dynamical systems is tightly intertwined with the noise intrinsic to the system. Hence, it is reasonable to expect that actors are aware of their inherent variability when executing a movement. However, the magnitude of this noise is not necessarily constant, and it is reasonable to assume that it is varying. One well-known determinant of the magnitude of noise is the velocity or force with which a movement is executed. The level of noise is a function of the magnitude of the signal. Such signal-dependent noise has been observed in many different motor tasks, ranging from isometric force production to rhythmic interval production, and is also conceptually consistent with Weber's Law (Worringham 1991; 1993; Ivry and Hazeltine 1995; Slifkin and Newell 1999).

Given such varying noise, how do actors plan their actions? Do they seek out the most noise-tolerant strategies as defined by the task? Or, are they aware of determinants such as velocity-dependent noise in their execution and therefore minimize their movement velocity? The costs arising from a nonoptimal movement strategy—especially *Tolerance* or *T-Cost*—can be extracted not only post hoc from the data, but can also be predicted for a given task. If the physics of the experimental task is known—as in the skittles task—stable or error-tolerant executions can be identified if a given amount of noise is assumed. Two experiments were designed to derive such predictions about tolerant solutions and to test the hypothesis that subjects seek solutions that minimize the effect of this variability on their performance result (Sternad et al. under revision).

Hypotheses and Execution Space

Three specific hypotheses were contrasted: *Hypothesis 1* states that subjects prefer those strategies that have the highest *Tolerance* or least *T-Cost.* Predictions of expected performance were calculated based on estimates of subjects' variability. The first hypothesis assumed constant levels of noise for all possible executions. If one takes into account that higher movement velocities are typically accompanied by higher variability, then it can be expected that solutions with high release velocities are avoided. Therefore, *Hypothesis 2* posits that subjects chose solutions with the lowest possible velocities. This hypothesis is also supported by the argument that lower velocities present more energy-efficient solutions. In the skittles task, these two hypotheses can make contrasting predictions when the most error-tolerant solution is not at the location with minimum velocity. Given that both criteria may compete with each other, *Hypothesis 3* posits that subjects chose solutions that trade-off between error-tolerance and low velocity-dependent noise.

To test the three hypotheses, the task was designed to create two different execution spaces by changing the location of the target skittle and the center post. Figure 12.9A illustrates the configuration of target and post in the workspace and the associated execution space and result function in Figure 12.9B for the first experiment. The locations of target and post were designed so as to achieve a result function with very different curvatures adjacent to the solution manifold (i.e., different levels of *Tolerance*). Successful solutions were relatively insensitive to release angle; that is, approximately parallel to the x-axis; the most error-tolerant location was at angle –0.7 rad and velocity 3 rad/s. Although this solution offered both error-tolerance at low velocities, solutions in this vicinity were "risky" (i.e., close to the post hits that are penalized heavily). The configuration of the second experiment, illustrated in Figure 12.9C and D, created a conflict between optimal solutions with respect to *Tolerance* and minimization of velocity. The most error-tolerant solution was at an angle of 1.5 rad, with *Tolerance* increasing only slightly, but monotonically with increasing velocity. The solution with the lowest velocity was adjacent to post hits and therefore again posed a risky strategy. If actors were aware of their intrinsic noise, a useful strategy for execution would be one that either had the lowest successful velocity or one that had slightly higher velocities but better *Tolerance*.

In the first experiment, nine subjects performed three sessions, each consisting of 180 trials, yielding a total of 540 trials; in the second experiment, nine different subjects performed five sessions, giving a total of 900 trials. In session 1 of both experiments, participants were instructed to try different release angles and release velocities to find successful strategies that achieved reliable solutions. In the subsequent sessions, participants were instructed to no longer explore but to continue with the strategy that had proven most successful. They were encouraged to fine-tune their performance and avoid hitting the center post, as they would receive a large penalty.

To quantitatively test the three hypotheses, the expected performance for each location in execution space, $E(P)$ was calculated as the average distance error d in a neighborhood around a location (α_i, v_j); the size of the neighborhood captured the subject's variability. To calculate $E(P)$, the execution space was divided into 360∗360 bins and $E(P)$ was determined for each (α_i, v_j), with $i, j = 1, 2\ldots 360$. Before these calculations, the individual

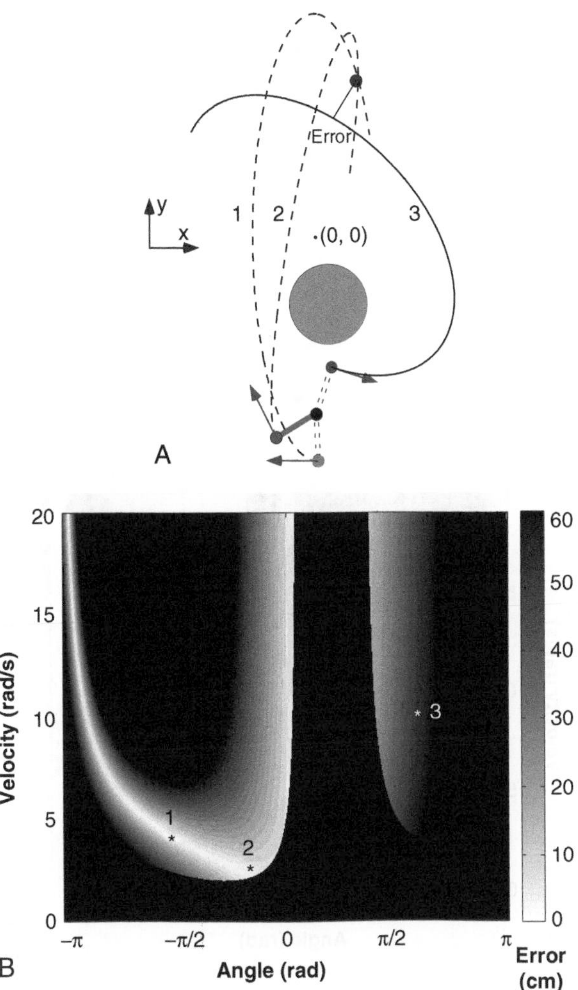

Figure 12.9 Workspace, execution space, and solution manifold. **A**: Workspace with the position of the center post and target of Experiment 1. Two ball trajectories exemplify how different release variables can lead to the same result with zero error, $d = 0$ (trajectory 1, 2, *dashed line*). Trajectory 3 shows a trajectory with non-zero error, $d = 30$ cm. **B**: Execution space and solution manifold. White denotes zero-error solutions, increasing error is shown by increasingly darker gray shades, black denotes a post hit. The release variables of trajectory 1 and 2 correspond to points 1 and 2 on the solution manifold, the variables of trajectory 3 correspond to the point 3 in a gray-shaded area.

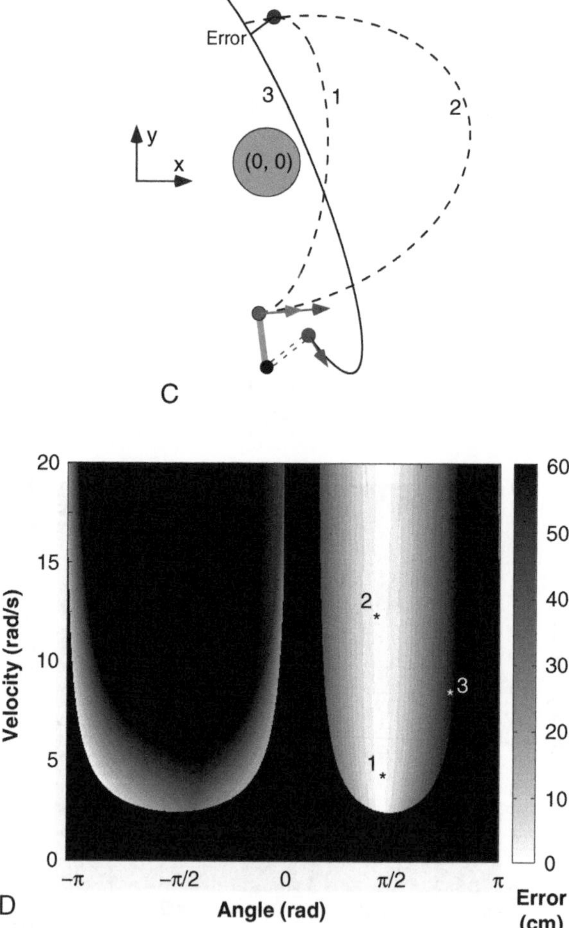

Figure 12.9 (*Continued*) **C**: Workspace with center post and target as used in Experiment 2. Three trajectories exemplify the redundancy of solutions. **D**: Corresponding execution space and solution manifold. The three points correspond to the three trajectories of panel **C**.

result or error values $d(\alpha_i, v_j)$ were transformed from a penalty function into a reward or performance function $P(\alpha_i, v_j)$:

$$P(\alpha_i, v_j) = \left| d(\alpha_i, v_j) - 60\,cm \right|$$

where 60 cm was the initially assigned post hit.

For each execution, (α_i, v_j) a matrix with Gaussian weights was defined. The size of the matrix was calculated from the actual standard deviations of angle and velocity, *SDa, SDv*, determined post hoc from all nine participants. This yielded a matrix of 15 (a, $k = -7$ to 7) × 23 (v, $n = -11$ to 11) cells with the probability distribution $p(\alpha_{i+k}, v_{j+n})$:

$$p(\alpha_{i+k}, v_{j+n}) = pdf\left(\frac{\alpha_i - \alpha_{i+k}}{SD\alpha}\right) * pdf\left(\frac{v_j - v_{j+n}}{SDv}\right), \qquad \text{(Eq. 2)}$$

where *pdf* is the probability density function of the bivariate normal distribution with mean (α_i, v_j) and standard deviations (*SDa, SDv*). The expected performance $E(P_{ij})$ at (α_i, v_j) was defined as

$$E(P_{ij}) = E(P(\alpha_i, v_j)) = \sum_{k=-7}^{7} \sum_{n=-11}^{11} p(\alpha_{i+k}, v_{j+n}) * P(\alpha_{i+k}, v_{j+n}) \qquad \text{(Eq. 3)}$$

Finally, all $E(P_{ij})$ values were normalized, dividing by the largest value to confine them to the interval between 0 and 1.

For the first experiment, the predictions for Hypothesis 1 are illustrated in Figure 12.10A: expected performance *E(P)* was highest at $\alpha = -0.7$ rad and $v = 3.0$ rad/s, defining the most error-tolerant solution. This optimum is approximately coincident with what is predicted by Hypothesis 2—where velocity is at a minimum (not shown separately). For the target constellation of the second experiment, the *E(P)* values for Hypothesis 1 are illustrated in Figure 12.10B. Importantly, the maximum *E(P)* and highest *Tolerance* was coincident with the highest velocity. In contrast, Hypothesis 2 predicted solutions at the lowest velocity at 3.1 rad/s and the invariant angle of 1.4 rad. The trade-off between maximizing error-tolerance and minimizing velocity, as posited in Hypothesis 3, was calculated with the size of the probability matrix scaled proportionally to velocity: larger sizes at higher velocities were expected from velocity-dependent noise. Hypothesis 3 is visualized in Figure 12.10C. The maximum value of *E(P)* was at $\alpha = 1.4$ rad and $v = 7.5$ rad/s.

The pooled results from all nine participants in the first experiment is shown in Figure 12.11A. The histogram pools all trials and presents the data on a grid of 36 × 36 bins. (As the focus was on solutions that participants had reached after some exploration, the first practice session was discarded from analysis.) The distribution was clearly nonuniform and clustered around a mode at −0.73 rad and 2.65 rad/s. This mode was close to the optimal *E(P)* as predicted by Hypothesis 1 (−0.70 rad, 3.0 rad/s). Note that the highest frequency of trials was also close to the locations with the high penalty; that is, executions that lead to a post hit (shown in black).

For statistical testing, these two-dimensional data were collapsed into 36 bins of the angle dimension. The same procedure was followed for the predicted *E(P)* values. Figure 12.11B shows both the data and the *E(P)* values as predicted by Hypothesis 1 and 2. The Spearman rank correlations between data and each of the two hypotheses were significant. This provided support that subjects preferred solutions with highest tolerance and lowest velocities, even though these solutions were risky.

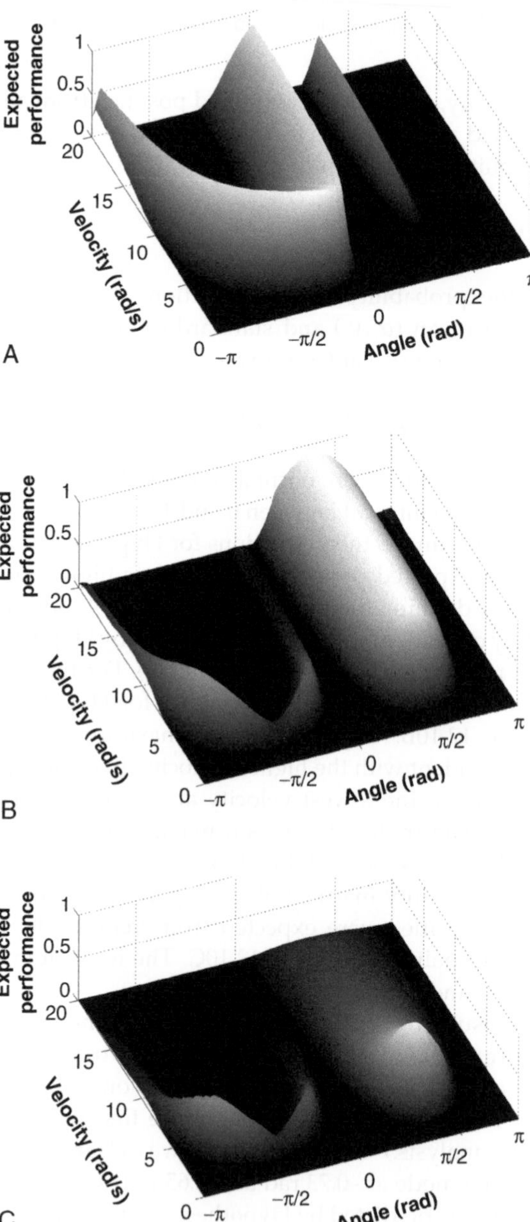

Figure 12.10 Simulation of hypotheses. **A**: Simulation of hypothesis 1 for Experiment 1: The vertical dimension represents expected performance *E(P)*, which are average values calculated from a Gaussian-weighted matrix of execution variables. The most error-tolerant solution with maximum *E(P)* is at –0.7 rad and 3 rad/s. **B**: Simulation of hypothesis 1 for Experiment 2. Expected performance *E(P)* at an angle of approximately 1.4 rad is similarly high across the entire range of velocity. **C**: Simulation of hypothesis 3 for Experiment 2. The expected performance *E(P)* decreases for higher velocity due to the simulated velocity-dependent noise. Maximum *E(P)* is at an angle of 1.4 rad with a velocity of 7.5 rad/s.

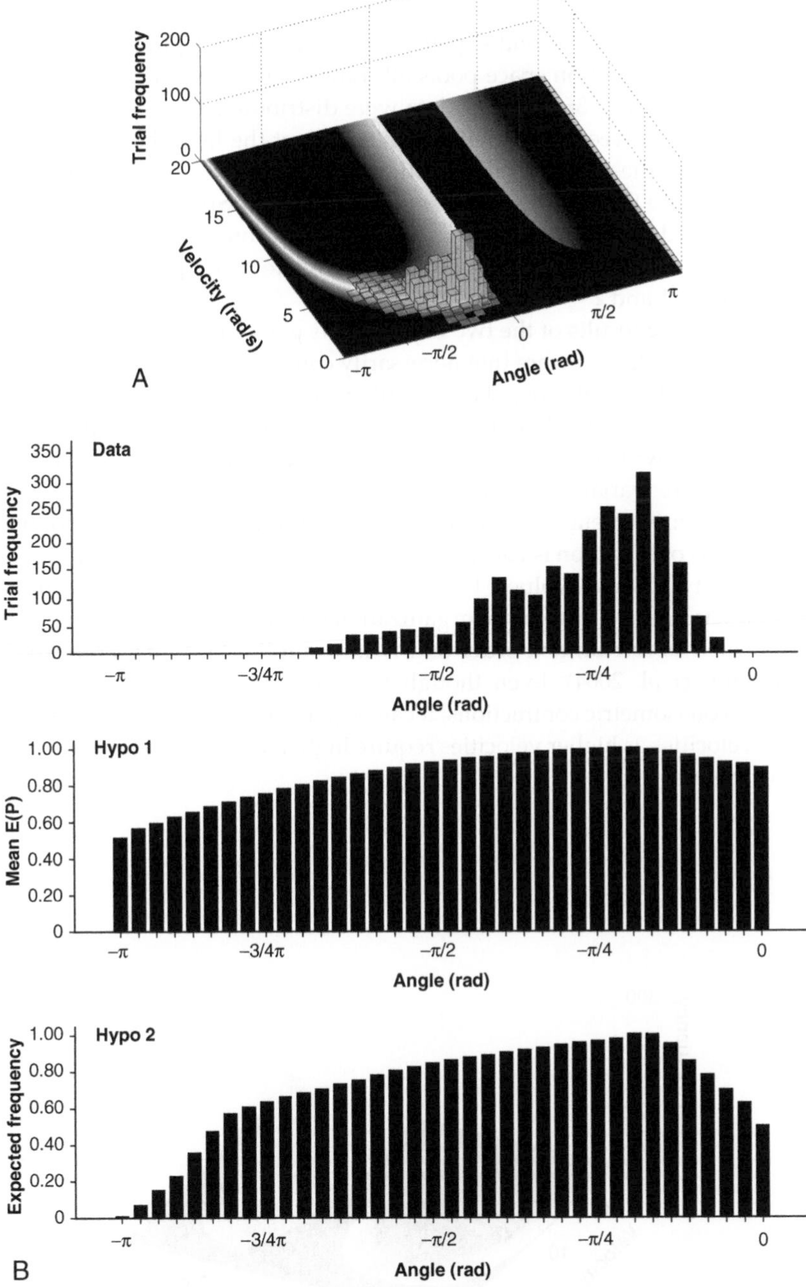

Figure 12.11 Result of Experiment 1. **A**: Histogram of all subjects' trials plotted in execution space; the mode of the two-dimensional distribution is close to the predicted location with maximum expected performance *E(P)*. **B**: Histograms in the angular dimension: Top panel shows the data distribution; middle panel shows the predicted distributions *E(P)* of Hypothesis 1; bottom panel shows the expected frequency *E(F)* of Hypothesis 2.

The results of the second experiment are shown in Figure 12.12A. The histogram in execution space pools all trials of all participants in sessions 2 to 5 onto a grid of 36 × 36. The data were distributed across a large range of velocities between 2.5 and 15.3 rad/s. To test the hypotheses, the data and the hypothesized *E(P)* distributions from the three hypotheses were collapsed onto the velocity dimensions (Fig. 12.12B). Spearman correlation tests showed that the correlation between data and Hypothesis 3 was significant, whereas the data did not correlate with predictions from Hypotheses 1 and 2.

Overall, the results of the two experiments gave support to the hypothesis that subjects are aware (not necessarily consciously) of their variability and choose those solutions that are either more tolerant to noise or have less noise associated with it. In previous work, it has been shown that variability scales with movement speed, such that performance at higher velocities is more variable (Schmidt et al. 1979; Worringham 1991; 1993). Assuming movement velocity reflects a magnitude of the motor control signal, this observation is consistent with variability increasing with signal strength (Harris and Wolpert 1998). Physiologically, this behavioral observation has been related to the organizational properties of the motor unit pool, such as recruitment order and twitch amplitudes (Jones et al. 2002; Hamilton et al. 2004). Even though these muscle–physiological studies focused on isometric contractions, it can be generalized to movements with high velocities as higher velocities require higher and faster rates of muscle contractions.

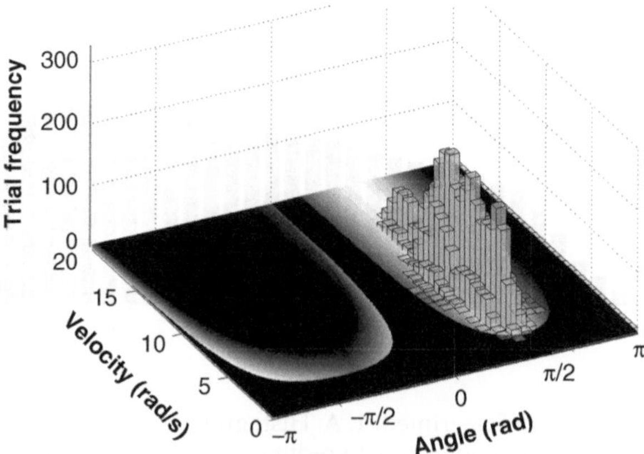

Figure 12.12 Result of Experiment 2. **A**: Histogram of all subjects' trials of four sessions plotted in execution space (720 trials per subject). The distribution is spread along a long range of velocities from 2.5 and 15.3 rad/s.

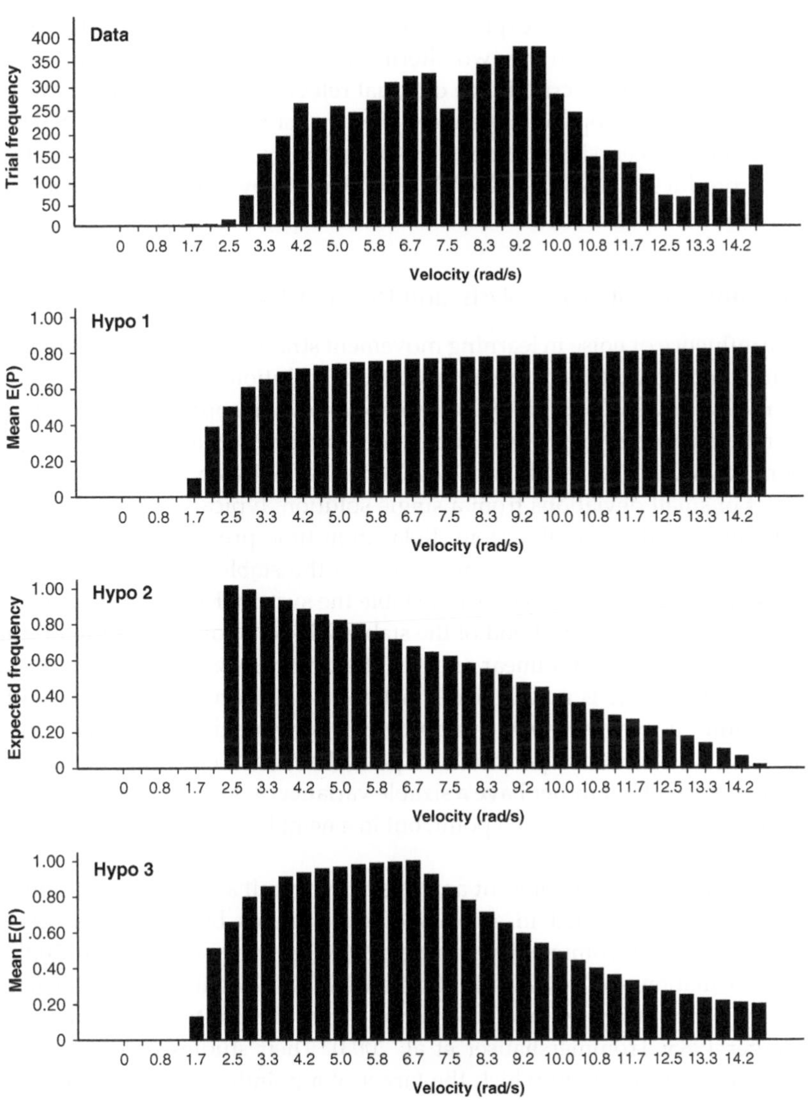

Figure 12.12 (*Continued*) **B**: Projection of the distributions to the velocity dimension. The top panel shows the data; the three panels below show the predicted distributions of Hypothesis 1, 2, and 3.

To test this alternative explanation, the second experiment was designed to distinguish between the two alternative hypotheses and test the third hypothesis that both criteria are of equal relevance. Indeed, subjects were shown to seek the optimum between the two sources of variability. Such a trade-off between signal dependent-noise and instability in an isometric force production task has recently been shown by Selen and colleagues (Selen et al. 2009).

Tolerance, Sensitivity Analysis, and Decision Theory

The influence of noise in learning movement strategies was investigated by simulations that tested the sensitivity of solutions to noise. Analysis of robustness and sensitivity is common, but our approach differs from standard sensitivity analyses as it includes variability in an extended neighborhood around each solution. Local linear stability analysis assesses the effect of small deviations from a single solution, typically, the fixed-point solution of a dynamical system. Relaxation time provides a quantitative measure for how fast a system returns to the stable solution; the faster the return, the more attractive and stable the system. Knowledge of errors in an extended neighborhood of the stable solution, however, is important when the system is nonlinear and has discontinuities. In the skittles task, the result variable is a nonlinear function of the execution variables with discontinuities; hence, such an approach is warranted. Additionally, considering that in human performance perturbations or errors are not infinitesimally small but rather have a sizable variance, it is appropriate to assess error sensitivity not only at a point, but in a neighborhood around a chosen solution.

The rationale of the present analysis is in overall accordance with decision theory as applied in a series of experiments by Trommershäuser and colleagues (Trommershäuser et al. 2003; Trommershäuser et al. 2005). The calculations for expected performance $E(P)$ are equivalent to calculating expected utility, with $P(\alpha,v)$ representing the utility or cost function (Berger 1985; Trommershäuser et al. 2003). Their studies used a speed–accuracy instruction, in which the target of a pointing task was bounded by a penalty area, and the distribution of hits was examined with respect to the relative position of target and penalty area. The gain function had an optimum defined by the weighted sum of the gain and the subject's inherent variability. The results showed systematic effects of the penalty on the data distributions and, similar to our work, supported that selection of a movement strategy was determined by the subject's inherent variability. However, the study also differed from our skittles task in that hitting success was binary (positive for the target area and negative for the penalty area). In contrast, our task permitted to estimate the continuous distance to the target, which was prerequisite to the sensitivity analysis in our study.

A Task with a Hidden Layer

The skittles task differs in one further important aspect to Trommershäuser's experiments: in the pointing task, the reward or penalty was directly visible to the subject. Hence, it is relatively straightforward in that subjects avoid the visible penalty area. In contrast, in the skittles task, the penalty or high-reward areas are sets of release parameters that are not visible. Rather, subjects have to explore the "landscape" of the task with their actions and learn the "location" of the solution manifold. This more indirect nature of the task is noticeable when we had children perform the task. Surprisingly, this "hidden layer" of the task posed severe problems to children of young age, and their typical learning patterns differed significantly from adult subjects. Children seemed to have a larger initial barrier to explore different solutions if their first attempts were not successful. Despite lack of success, they adhered more strongly to their preferred release value (Chu et al. 2009). In addition, their arm and ball trajectories were more stereotypical, even though the variability in the result error was caused by larger variance in release time along a relatively invariant trajectory. These observations indicated that, compared to adults, children were less able to use flexible search strategies and could not discover or infer the hidden nonlinear mapping between execution variables and the result. These differences highlight developmental changes in motor learning strategies (Chu et al. 2009). Hence, tasks with hidden layers pose interesting new problems for understanding processes underlying motor learning.

CONCLUSION

The reviewed findings lay the foundations for a number of new investigations. Ongoing work uses the TCN framework to assess performance of subjects with neurological impairments, such as Parkinson patients and children with cerebral palsy. The evident next step is to develop intervention techniques that influence *Tolerance, Covariation,* and *Noise* and thereby facilitate and guide skill learning and also recovery.

ACKNOWLEDGMENTS

This research was supported by grants from the National Science Foundation, BCS-0450218, the National Institutes of Health, R01-HD045639, and the Office of Naval Research, N00014-05-1-0844. We would like to express our thanks to Hermann Müller, Tjeerd Dijkstra, and Neville Hogan for many insightful discussions. We would also like to express our thanks to Virginia Chu and Terry Sanger and the members of the Action Lab, who all contributed to these experiments: Kunlin Wei, Rajal Cohen, Xiaogang Hu, and Lisa Pendt.

REFERENCES

Berger, J.O. 1985. *Statistical decision theory and Bayesian analysis*, 2nd edition. New York: Springer.

Chu, V.W.T., D. Sternad, and T.D. Sanger. 2009. Learning a redundant task in adults and children. *Society for Neuroscience Abstracts* 369–27.

Churchland, M.M., A. Afshar, and K.V. Shenoy. 2006. A central source of movement variability. *Neuron* 52:1085–96.

Cohen, R.G., and D. Sternad. 2009. Variability in motor learning: Relocating, channeling and reducing noise. *Experimental Brain Research* 193:69–83.

Craig, J.J. 1986. *Introduction to robotics*. Reading, MA: Addison-Wesley.

Faisal, A.A., L.P. Selen, and D.M. Wolpert. 2008. Noise in the nervous system. *Nature Reviews. Neuroscience* 9:292–303.

Gel'fand, I.M., and M.L. Tsetlin. 1962. Some methods of control for complex systems. *Mathematical Surveys* 17:95–116.

Gordon, J., M.F. Ghilardi, and C. Ghez. 1994. Accuracy of planar reaching movements. I. Independence of direction and extent variability. *Experimental Brain Research* 99:97–111.

Hamilton, A.F., K.E. Jones, and D.M. Wolpert. 2004. The scaling of motor noise with muscle strength and motor unit number in humans. *Experimental Brain Research* 157:417–30.

Harris, C.M., and D.M. Wolpert. 1998. Signal-dependent noise determines motor planning. *Nature* 394:780–84.

Hore, J., D. Timmann, and S. Watts. 2002. Disorders in timing and force of finger opening in overarm throws made by cerebellar subjects. *Annals of the New York Academy of Sciences* 978:1–15.

Ivry, R.B., and R.E. Hazeltine. 1995. Perception and production of temporal intervals across a range of durations: Evidence for a common timing mechanism. *Journal of Experimental Psychology. Human Perception and Performance* 21:3–18.

Jones, K.E., A.F. Hamilton, and D.M. Wolpert. 2002. Sources of signal-dependent noise during isometric force production. *Journal of Neurophysiology* 88: 1533–44.

Körding, K.P., S.P. Ku, and D.M. Wolpert. 2004. Bayesian integration in force estimation. *Journal of Neurophysiology* 92:3161–65.

Körding, K.P., and D.M. Wolpert. 2004. Bayesian integration in sensorimotor learning. *Nature* 427:244–47.

Latash, M.L. 2008. *Synergy*. Oxford: Oxford University Press.

Latash, M.L., Scholz, J.P., and G. Schöner. 2002. Motor control strategies revealed in the structure of motor variability. *Exercise and Sport Sciences Reviews* 30: 26–31.

Liu, D., and E. Todorov. 2007. Evidence for the flexible sensorimotor strategies predicted by optimal feedback control. *Journal of Neuroscience* 27:9354–68.

Martin, T.A., B.E. Greger, S.A. Norris, and W.T. Thach. 2001. Throwing accuracy in the vertical direction during prism adaptation: Not simply timing of ball release. *Journal of Neurophysiology* 85:2298–302.

Miyazaki, M., D. Nozaki, and Y. Nakajima. 2005. Testing Bayesian models of human coincidence timing. *Journal of Neurophysiology* 94:395–99.

Müller, H., and D. Sternad. 2004. Decomposition of variability in the execution of goal-oriented tasks - Three components of skill improvement. *Jonrnal of Experimental Psychology: Human Perception and Performance*, 30: 212–233.

Müller, H., and D. Sternad. 2009. Motor learning: Changes in the structure of variability in a redundant task. *Advances in Experimental Medicine and Biology* 629:439–56.

Osborne, L.C., S.G. Lisberger, and W. Bialek. 2005. A sensory source for motor variation. *Nature* 437:412–16.

Schmidt, R.A., and T. Lee. 2005. *Motor control and learning: A behavioral emphasis*, 4th edition. Champaign, IL: Human Kinetics.

Schmidt, R.A., H. Zelaznik, B. Hawkins, J.S. Frank, and J.T., Quinn Jr. 1979. Motor-output variability: A theory for the accuracy of rapid motor acts. *Psychological Review* 47:415–51.

Scholz, J.P., and G. Schöner. 1999. The uncontrolled manifold concept: Identifying control variables for a functional task. *Experimental Brain Research* 126: 289–306.

Schöner, G., and J.P. Scholz. 2007. Analyzing variance in multi-degree-of-freedom movements: Uncovering structure versus extracting correlations. *Motor Control* 11:259–75.

Selen, L.P., D.W. Franklin, and D.M. Wolpert. 2009. Impedance control reduces instability that arises from motor noise. *Journal of Neuroscience* 29:12606–16.

Slifkin, A.B., and K.M. Newell. 1999. Noise, information transmission, and force variability. *Journal of Experimental Psychology. Human Perception and Performance* 25:837–51.

Sternad, D., M.O. Abe, X. Hu, and H. Müller (under revision). Neuromotor noise, error tolerance, velocity-dependent noise in skilled performance.

Sternad, D., H. Müller, S. Park, and N. Hogan. 2010. Coordinate dependency of variability analysis. *PLoS Computational Biology* 6:e1000751.

Strogatz, S.H. 1994. *Nonlinear dynamics and chaos: With applications to physics, biology, chemistry, and engineering*. Reading, MA: Perseus Books.

Timmann, D., R. Citron, S. Watts, and J. Hore. 2001. Increased variability in finger position occurs throughout overarm throws made by cerebellar and unskilled subjects. *Journal of Neurophysiology* 86:2690–702.

Todorov, E. 2004. Optimality principles in sensorimotor control. *Nature Neuroscience* 7:907–15.

Todorov, E. 2005. Stochastic optimal control and estimation methods adapted to the noise characteristics of the sensorimotor system. *Neural Computation* 17:1084–108.

Todorov, E., and M.I. Jordan. 2002. Optimal feedback control as a theory of motor coordination. *Nature Neuroscience* 5:1226–35.

Trommershäuser, J., S. Gepshtein, L.T. Maloney, M.S. Landy, and M.S. Banks. 2005. Optimal compensation for changes in task-relevant movement variability. *Journal of Neuroscience* 25:7169–78.

Trommershäuser, J., L.T. Maloney, and M.S. Landy. 2003. Statistical decision theory and trade-offs in the control of motor response. *Spatial Vision* 16:255–75.

van Beers, R.J. 2009. Motor learning is optimally tuned to the properties of motor noise. *Neuron* 63:406–17.

van Beers, R.J., P. Baraduc, and D.M. Wolpert. 2002. Role of uncertainty in sensorimotor control. *Philosophical Transactions of the Royal Society of London. Series B, Biological Sciences* 357:1137–45.

van Beers, R.J., P. Haggard, and D.M. Wolpert. 2004. The role of execution noise in movement variability. *Journal of Neurophysiology* 91:1050–63.

Wei, K., T.M. Dijkstra, and D. Sternad. 2007. Passive stability and active control in a rhythmic task. *Journal of Neurophysiology* 98:2633–2646.

Wei, K., T.M. Dijkstra, and D. Sternad. 2008. Stability and variability: Indicators for passive stability and active control in a rhythmic task. *Journal of Neurophysiology* 99:3027–41.

Worringham, C.J. 1991. Variability effects on the internal structure of rapid aiming movements. *Journal of Motor Behavior* 23:75–85.

Worringham, C.J. 1993. *Predicting motor performance from variability measures.* Champaign, IL: Human Kinetics.

13

Forecasting the Long-range Consequences of Manual and Tool Use Actions

Neurophysiological, Behavioral, and Computational Considerations

Scott H. Frey

Healthy adults possess an easily overlooked yet remarkable ability: Without moving a muscle, we can forecast the demands of a wide variety of actions. We are, for instance, able to determine whether a stool is low enough to sit on (Warren 1984; Mark and Vogele 1987), an opening is large enough to accommodate our hand (Ishak et al. 2008), or an object is within reach (Rochat and Wraga 1997). When faced with a choice between potential actions, we are capable of selecting the least awkward alternative (Johnson 2000a). In contrast to the types of perceptual judgments that preoccupy most experimental psychologists, these tasks demand an evaluation of the relationship between external stimuli and one's own physical capabilities (Gibson 1979). Because these capabilities change as we grow, age, or experience the consequences of brain or bodily injuries, this relationship is inherently dynamic. To remain accurate, the mechanisms involved in action forecasting must therefore be capable of experience-dependent plasticity. Evidence suggests that this is the case even in response to acute manipulations, such as artificially lengthening the legs with blocks (Mark 1987), extending the arm with a tool (Witt et al. 2005), or increasing the width of the hand with a prosthesis (Ishak et al. 2008). In fact, such rapid adaptation could be fundamental to the flexible use of tools and technologies.

Although prospective estimates are often imperfect when compared to their actual movement counterparts (Fischer 2005; Rodriguez et al. 2008), the level of fidelity achieved through thought alone is nevertheless impressive. Regardless of whether one considers these tests of affordance perception or motor imagery, one thing is clear: Much more is known about the accuracy and perceptual information guiding these prospective behaviors than is understood about the neural mechanisms involved. A more complete understanding at the neurophysiological level could help to clarify the relationship between these abilities and overt motor control.

In what follows, I describe recent behavioral and functional magnetic resonance imaging (fMRI) work that focuses on identifying the brain mechanisms involved in prospectively selecting grasping actions based on use of the hands or recently mastered tool. This task appears to be solved by accurately forecasting the demands associated with the available response alternatives. Despite the complete absence of movements, we find that the parietal and premotor regions implicated in the sensorimotor control of grasping also participate in these forecasts. As a result of sensorimotor experience, these areas appear to undergo reorganizational changes that enable them to participate in accurately forecasting the demands of grasping with a formerly novel mechanical tool.

How is it possible for the same neural mechanisms to participate in both sensorimotor control and these prospective behaviors, which involve neither movement nor sensory feedback? The answer to this question has important implications both for our understanding of the functions of these brain systems and the relationship between these two classes of behaviors. I consider one possibility, that action forecasts are based on estimates of the sensory consequences that *would* be experienced if inhibited motor commands were executed. With relatively minor modifications, these long-range forecasts might be generated by the very same forward mechanisms that are hypothesized to predict the sensory consequences of ongoing movements over small increments of time.

CORTICAL MECHANISMS OF GRASPING

Manual grasping is an evolutionarily old behavior (Bloch and Boyer 2002) with well-documented neurophysiological substrates (Murata et al. 1997; Rizzolatti et al. 2002; Gardner et al. 2007a; Gardner et al. 2007b). Successfully grasping an object involves transforming sensory representations of the hand and fingers and the intrinsic spatial properties of the target object into a motor program. In macaques, this is accomplished in a network of posterior parietal and premotor regions. The anterior intraparietal area (AIP) is situated in the dorsal visual stream and projects directly to ventral premotor cortex (PMv) area F5ab (Sakata et al. 1997). In addition to cells that increase activity when macaques grasp objects in the light or dark, both AIP and F5ab contain visual neurons that respond selectively to three dimensional shapes even when no hand movements are involved. Effective stimuli are typically of a shape that is compatible with the particular cell's preferred hand configuration. Of potential relevance to prospective behaviors, these responses appear to contribute to the premovement selection of appropriate grasping and manipulation movements.

More recently, the boundaries of this parieto-premotor network have been extended by the discovery of cells that code grasp in the caudal intraparietal sulcus (V6A) (Fattori et al. 2009) and the distal forelimb field of dorsal premotor cortex (PMd or F2) (Raos et al. 2004). Of importance to the grip selection experiments discussed below that focus on selection of over- versus underhand grasps is the fact that neurons in both V6A and F2 appear to be specifically involved in coding the orientation of the wrist (i.e., hand).

Putative Parieto-premotor Homologues in the Human Brain

Two major challenges face researchers interested in determining whether a similar parieto-premotor grasp circuit exists in the human brain. First, these species last shared a common ancestor in the neighborhood of 30 million years ago, a fact that demands caution when evaluating claims of homologous brain regions. Second, comparing data from noninvasive functional neuroimaging and single-unit electrophysiology is challenging due to substantial differences in spatial and temporal resolution. Signals recorded in blood oxygen–level dependent (BOLD) fMRI are the result of hemodynamic changes tied to the activity of very large numbers of neurons and have poor temporal sensitivity, but their scope includes the entire brain. Single-unit recordings are spatially precise and have high temporal resolution, but are limited in scope.

Given these facts, it is perhaps surprising to learn that investigations of visually guided grasping consistently indicate that the functional organization of cortical networks in the human brain that are involved in grasping resemble what has been observed in macaques (Culham and Valyear 2006; Castiello and Begliomini 2008). This appears to especially be true in the parietal cortex, where significant activation within the anterior portion of the intraparietal sulcus (aIPS) is observed when objects are grasped under visual guidance (Binkofski et al. 1998; Culham et al. 2003; Frey et al. 2005; Begliomini et al. 2007; Kroliczak et al. 2007), and lesions in this region produce deficits in configuring the hand to engage objects effectively (Binkofski et al. 1998). In healthy adults, delivery of transcranial magnetic stimulation (TMS) to the contralateral aIPS interferes with the sensorimotor control of grasping (Tunik 2005; Rice et al. 2006; Rice et al. 2007). Both the aIPS and vPMC do show increased activity when subjects grasp and haptically explore objects without vision (Binkofski et al. 1999) or regulate forces applied during precision gripping (Ehrsson et al. 2001). Finally, similar to the visual neurons in macaques, the aIPS and vPMC show increased activity when participants view manipulable objects (Grafton et al. 1997; Chao and Martin 2000; Mahon et al. 2007). The approximate locations of these regions are illustrated in Figure 13.1.

Prospective Grip Selection

Earlier findings from my lab indicate that, in the absence of movement, healthy adults can evaluate the demands of grasping actions with high

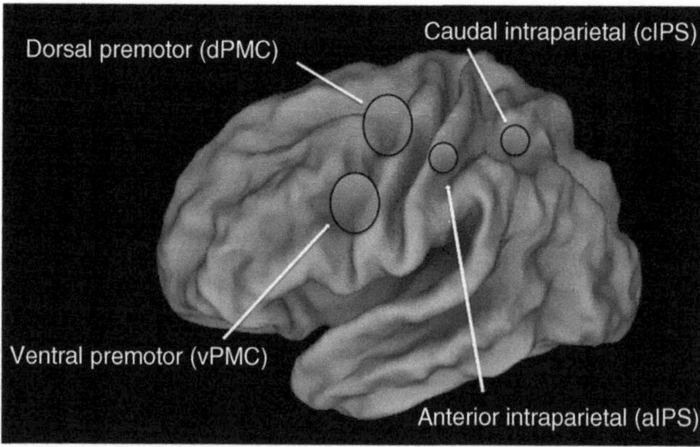

Figure 13.1 Grip preferences during overt (OGS) and prospective (PGS) grasp selection. Approximate locations of parietal and premotor areas in the human cortex that have been implicated in the representation of grasping.

fidelity and use this information to select the least awkward (most comfortable) alternative (Johnson 2000b). When asked to choose prospectively whether an under- or overhand power grip *would* be most comfortable for grasping a handle in various orientations, grip preferences are highly consistent with those expressed in a comparable reach-to-grasp task. In both conditions, participants consistently choose the grip that is experienced as least physically awkward when enacted in a separate rating task. In the *prospective grip selection* (PGS) task, the average amount of time required to select an option increases linearly as a function of the angular distance of the shortest *biomechanically plausible* path between the participants' current hand position and the preferred grip. Further, selection times are inversely related to the magnitude of the difference between ratings of the physical awkwardness of the two response alternatives. These temporal characteristics are consistent with what is expected if participants' prospective evaluations involve analog movement simulations or motor imagery. Results of subsequent fMRI work reveal that the PGS task involves a number of structures implicated in sensorimotor control of reach-to-grasp actions, including posterior parietal and premotor areas, and the lateral cerebellum (Johnson et al. 2002).

We recently returned to this issue to explore whether the same brain regions might be involved in representing grasping actions involving the hands or a mechanical tool. This involved two important changes. First, we adapted the PGS task to focus on precision gripping, because precision gripping places greater demands on configuring the hand and fingers to match the form of the object, and has been the focus of the majority of neurophysiological studies of the parietofrontal grasp circuit in monkeys and humans. Second, we manipulated the capacities of actors' limbs by requiring them to also perform the PGS task based on use of a recently mastered tool. Similar to the acute manipulations in the affordance perception literature (Mark 1987; Witt et al. 2005; Ishak et al. 2008), this novel tool mechanically altered the physical capacities of participants' hands. This allowed us to ask whether prospective estimates of grasping actions involving the tool arise from experience-dependent changes within the same brain areas implicated in manual grasping.

Use of the Hands or a Novel Tool

Prior to fMRI scanning, right-handed participants practiced an overt grip selection (OGS) task in which they used their dominant and nondominant hands and the tool (operated alternately with the left and right hands) to grasp widgets appearing in a variety of orientations. As illustrated in Figure 13.2A, the widget had two differently colored indentations that served as targets for placement of the thumb and forefinger (hand condition)

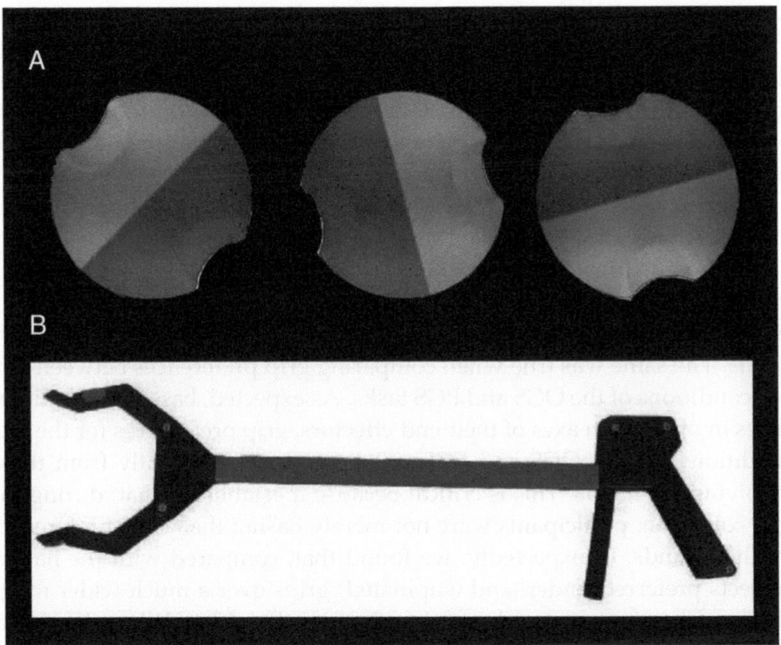

Figure 13.2 Sample stimuli (*panel A*) and the novel tool (*panel B*) from Jacobs, Danielmeier, and Frey, 2010. Note that when grasping the handle of the tool in a power grip, the opposition axis of the hand would be rotated 90 degrees relative to that of the tool's end effector. From Jacobs, S., Danielmeier, C., & Frey, S. H. (2010). Human anterior intraparietal and ventral premotor cortices support representations of grasping with the hand or a novel tool. *J Cogn Neurosci*, 22(11), 2594–2608. doi: 10.1162/jocn.2009.21372.

or the jaws of the tool (tool condition). The choice on each trial was therefore between an under- versus overhand posture. The tool was designed to mechanically transform movements of the hands in two important ways (Fig. 13.2B). While the tool was held in either hand using a power grip, synergistic extension and flexion movements of the fingers were mechanically transformed into precision gripping movements of the two jaws. Also, the opposition axis of the tool's jaws was rotated 90 degrees, relative to that of the hand operating the tool. This was expected to change the pattern of grip preferences across stimulus orientations significantly relative to those of the hands.

Next, they performed the PGS task during the acquisition of whole-brain BOLD fMRI data. Rather than actually grasping, they remained still while deciding which of the two differently colored indentations their thumb *would* be on if they grasped the widget in the most comfortable of the two precision grip postures. On trials involving the tool, they based their judgments on the placement of one of the jaws that was designated as the "thumb." During the task, they held the tool in one hand at their sides. A left- or rightward facing arrow presented at the start of each block indicated whether the upcoming series of trials should be based on use of the tool or the free hand. The tool was then switched to the opposite hand and the process was repeated. To ensure that the hands remained still, responses indicating the color of the indentation on which the "thumb" would be placed were issued using foot pedals (for additional details on this method see Jacobs et al. 2009).

As in our earlier work on power gripping, we found that participants' grip preferences in PGS (while fMRI data were acquired) were highly similar to those expressed during OGS (Fig. 13.3). This indicates that, even in the absence of sensory feedback, participants selected grips that were consistent with the respective biomechanical constraints of their left and right hands. The same was true when comparing grip preferences between tool use conditions of the OGS and PGS tasks. As expected, based on the differences in opposition axes of their end effectors, grip preferences for the tool conditions of both OGS and PGS tasks differed significantly from those involving the hands. This is critical because it establishes that, during the tool condition, participants were not merely basing their PGS preferences on their hands. Unexpectedly, we found that, compared with the hands, subjects preferred underhand (supinated) grips over a much wider range of stimulus orientations when using the tool (Fig. 13.3). When debriefed, they disclosed that in the OGS task, the underhand grip allowed them more precise control by using the palm as a platform to stabilize the tool against the forces of gravity. Remarkably, this relatively subtle compensation for the tool's dynamical properties appears to have been taken into account when selecting grips prospectively as well. Finally, the fact that participants fluidly switched between judgments based on different effectors throughout the study, with no apparent costs, would seem to indicate

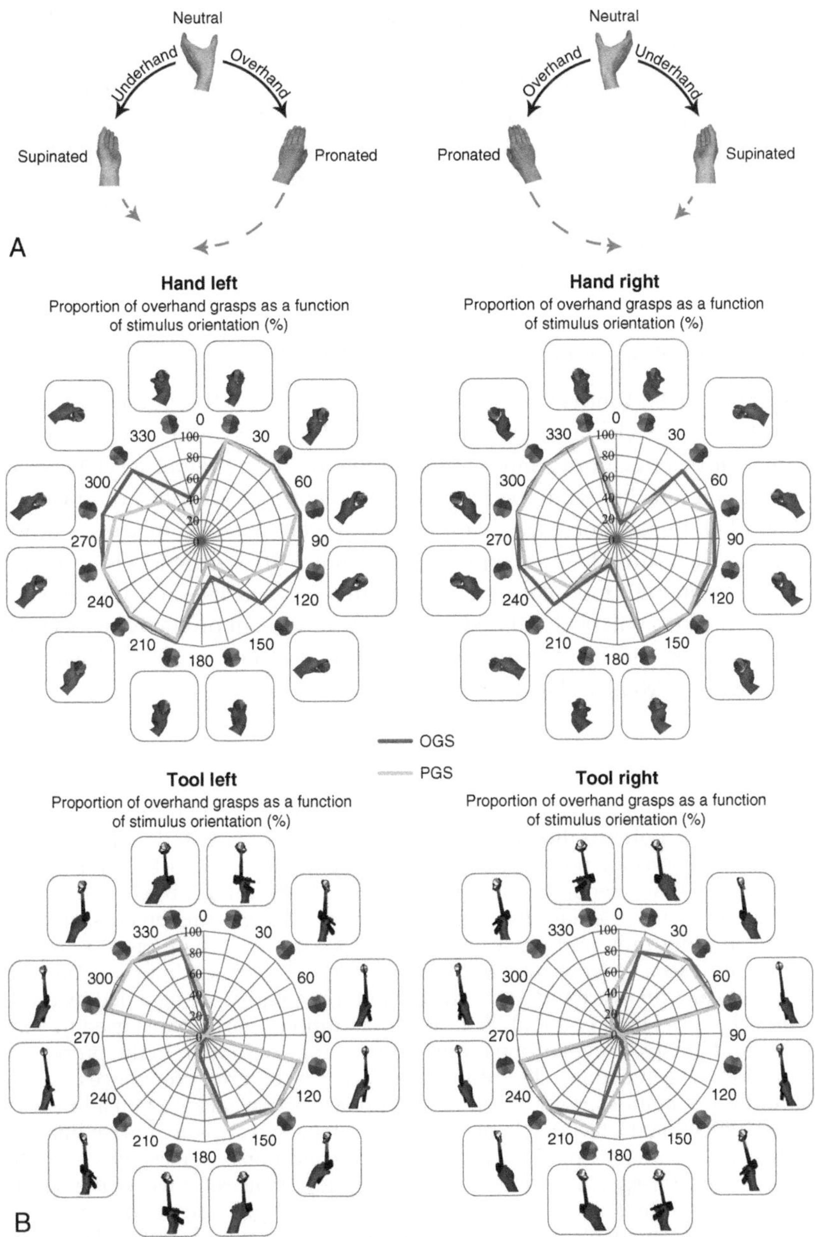

Figure 13.3 Grip preferences during overt (OGS) and prospective (PGS) grasp selection in Jacobs, Danielmeier, and Frey, 2010. **A**: Representation of the neutral, pronated and supinated postures of the left and right hand, and their relation to the definition of over- and underhand grasps. The limits of range of motion in each direction are represented by the dotted arrows. **B**: Polar plots of the average proportion of overhand grasps across subjects for each orientation

(*Continued*)

that the underlying representations of limb and tool are relatively independent.

In short, these psychophysical results are consistent with the hypothesis that participants can accurately forecast the demands of manual precision grasping while remaining still, and can use this information to select grips prospectively. Following a relatively brief period of practice (less than 1 hour), they are able to adapt these estimations to accommodate the unique mechanical and dynamical properties of a formerly novel tool. How is this possible? The results of fMRI testing provide some clues.

Neurophysiology of Prospective Grip Selection

Despite a lack of movement, fMRI data clearly show that the prospective selection of precision grips is accompanied by increased activity in the same parietal (including anterior and caudal IPs) and premotor (vPMC and dPMC) regions known to be involved in sensorimotor control of grasping (Fig. 13.4). In addition, significant increases were detected in several other regions, including the presupplementary motor area (pre-SMA)—a region that is frequently modulated in "motor imagery" tasks—and the cerebellum, which (as will be discussed later) is implicated in predictive aspects of sensorimotor control (Haruno et al. 2001; Kawato et al. 2003; Ebner and Pasalar 2008; Miall and King 2008).

Figure 13.3 (*Continued*) of the stimulus object, as observed in the OGS and PGS tasks. A data point to the periphery of the plot represents 100% of overhand grips, whereas a data point at the center of the plot means that 100% of the grips selected for that orientation were underhand. The stimulus object is shown in each of the tested orientations (15–345 degrees in 30-degree increments) and the corresponding preferred grasp (i.e., grip selected on >50% of trials) is represented next to it. A gray frame around the picture representing the preferred grip indicates an overhand grasp, while underhand grips are signaled by a red frame. In both Hand Left and Hand Right conditions, participants used mostly overhand grasps, except at the limits of their range of motion in the pronation direction. The functions describing the variation of grip preferences across stimulus orientation are 180 degrees out of phase between Hand Left and Hand Right, reflecting the fact that joint constraints of the two arms are mirror images. The same is true for Tool Left vs. Tool Right conditions. Consistent with reliance on effector-specific internal models, grip preferences for use of the hands versus tools differ substantially on both the left and right sides. In both tool use conditions, participants preferred underhand grasps for fully half of the stimulus orientations. Critically, in all four conditions, the functions describing grip preferences observed in OGS and PGS tasks were virtually identical, indicating that participants prospectively selected grips in the PGS task that were consistent with their overt behavior in the OGS task. From Jacobs, S., Danielmeier, C., & Frey, S. H. (2010). Human anterior intraparietal and ventral premotor cortices support representations of grasping with the hand or a novel tool. *J Cogn Neurosci*, 22(11), 2594–2608. doi: 10.1162/jocn.2009.21372.

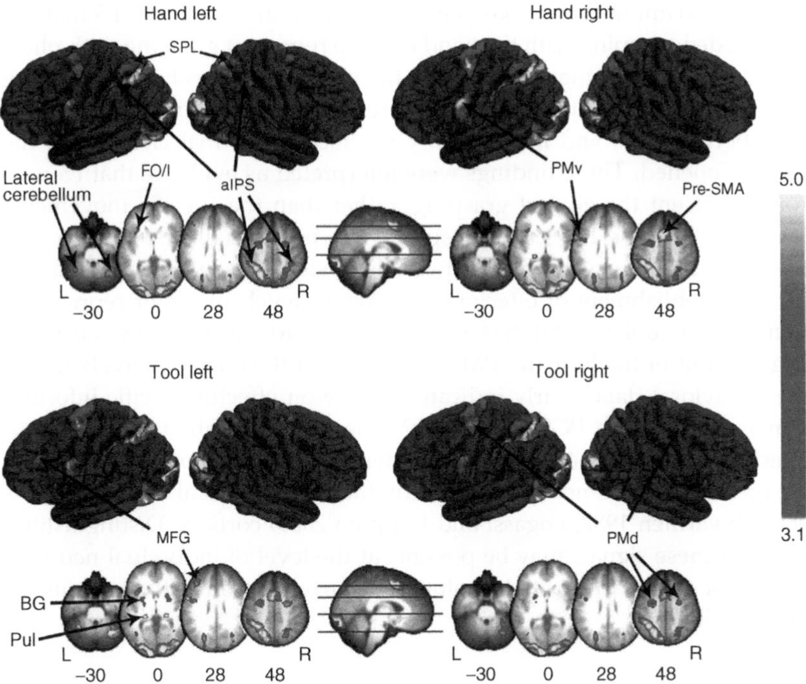

Figure 13.4 Increased neural activity associated with prospective grip selection based on use of the hands or tool. Relative to resting baseline, prospective grip selection (PGS) based on either the hands or tool was consistently associated with increased activity in parietal (anterior and caudal IPS and SPL) and premotor (PMv and PMd) areas implicated in the sensory-motor control of grasping as well as in the pre-SMA, and lateral cerebellum. Group statistical maps (Z>3.1, corrected cluster-extent significance threshold $p < 0.05$) are overlaid on the average brain of the 20 subjects. L, Left hemisphere; R, Right hemisphere.

In stark contrast to our behavioral findings, these neurophysiological responses did not differ either as a function of the side (left or right) or effector (hand or tool) involved. In fact, were it not for the clear demonstration of effector-specificity in grip preferences, it would be tempting to interpret this fMRI data as evidence for reliance on effector-independent levels of motor representation (cf. Rijntjes et al. 1999; Wing 2000). These data suggest that, as a result of experience with the tool during the OGS session, these brain regions underwent experience-dependent changes that enable them to participate subsequently in accurate prospective judgments based on either the hands or tool.

Our findings are intriguing when considered in light of experience-dependent changes related to tool use in F5 (putative vPMC) neurons of macaques (Umilta et al. 2008). Some neurons in macaque area F5 that initially coded grasping with the hand came to represent grasping with pliers after extensive training. Importantly, the movements involved in grasping do not appear to matter; comparable responses occurred when grasping with both normal and mechanically reversed pliers that close when the hand is opened. These findings were interpreted as evidence that F5 neurons represent the goal of grasping, rather than the specific movements involved. Because the goal (grasping) was not actually manipulated in these studies, however, it is also possible to view these results as evidence for the establishment of effector-independent levels of motor representation through tool use (Arbib et al. 2009). Our fMRI data do show consistent engagement of the human vPMC regardless of the effectors involved, yet the behavioral data clearly indicate reliance on effector-specific information in solving the PGS task. Why? One likely possibility is that both effector-specific and effector-independent levels of motor representation are present in the same regions of premotor (Rizzolatti et al. 1988) and parietal (Hyvarinen 1982; Fogassi and Luppino 2005) cortices. Distinguishing between these signals may be possible at the level of individual neurons, but might exceed the spatial resolution of current noninvasive neuroimaging techniques.

Alternative Explanations

One alternative possibility is that these neuroimaging findings reflect nothing more than generic processes involved in response selection, and have nothing to do with the evaluation of grasping actions. Previously, it was shown that the IPS, middle frontal gyrus, and dPMC all show increased left-lateralized activation independent of the hand used when performing a conditional versus simple response-time task (Schluter et al. 2001). Here, we do find a consistent left cerebral asymmetry for responses in the IPS, middle frontal gyrus and vPMC regardless of the side or effector involved (Fig. 13.4). Selection among candidate motor programs is inarguably a key component of the PGS task. Yet, there is a critical difference between the demands of a choice reaction-time task in which the mapping between a perceptual cue and response is fixed (Schluter et al. 2001), and the PGS task, in which the determination of which grip to select is made based on what appears to be an accurate estimation of the relationship between the stimulus and the unique physical properties of the effectors. Otherwise, there would be no reason for grip preferences in OGS and PGS to correspond. Although not detailed here, it is also worth noting that care was taken in the fMRI design to ensure that brain responses associated with the grip selection decision were not contaminated by response-button selection, which is a choice response (see details in Jacobs et al. 2009).

Another alternative is that our results are due exclusively to what has been called "motor attention." Evidence from brain-injured patients

(Rushworth et al. 1997), fMRI (Rushworth et al. 2001b), and TMS (Rushworth et al. 2001a) all implicate left inferior parietal cortex (supramarginal gyrus and aIPS), vPMc, and the adjacent inferior frontal gyrus in orienting attention to a hand for an upcoming response. There is again an important difference between these orienting tasks, in which a specific action (hand movement) is defined unambiguously by a precue, and the grip selection component of the PGS task, where participants choose a response option based on knowledge of the effectors. Motor attention, as operationalized by Rushworth and colleagues, would very likely be engaged here when the left- or rightward arrow is presented at the beginning of a block to indicate the side and effector on which the forthcoming trials will be based. Indeed, in an earlier study, we found increased left-lateralized parietal and premotor activity in association with this task component (Johnson et al. 2002). However, the current fMRI experiment was designed to enable separation of the effects related to the arrow precue from those involved in grip section (Jacobs et al. 2009), and the results presented are associated specifically with the grip selection component.

In sum, the fMRI data yielded two main findings concerning the mechanisms involved in prospective grip selection and its relationship to sensorimotor control. First, the specific parietal (anterior and caudal IPS) and premotor (vPMC and dPMC) areas involved in the sensorimotor control of manual grasping also participate in forecasting the demands of these actions. Second, as a result of practice with the formerly novel tool during the OGS task, these brain regions appear to have undergone experience-dependent changes, leading to their involvement in high-fidelity prospective judgments based on use of the tool. This complements earlier findings showing that experience with acute manipulations that modify the body's physical capabilities leads to adapting the estimates of actions afforded by perceptual stimuli (Mark 1987; Witt et al. 2005; Ishak et al. 2008).

If we accept that that our ability to accurately evaluate actions in the absence of movements does indeed arise from the very same neural mechanisms as sensorimotor control, then it is sensible to consider what shared computations are involved.

LONG-RANGE FORECASTING OF MOVEMENTS' SENSORY CONSEQUENCES

It is accepted by many that movements are controlled by both feedback and feedforward (predictive) mechanisms (for detailed reviews see Wolpert and Ghahramani 2000; Shadmehr and Krakauer 2008). These feedforward processes are believed to predict the sensory consequences that executing a motor command would have on the state of the body slightly in advance of the actual afferent signals that accompany moving. The advantage of such anticipation is that it enables rapid adjustments in behavior that would be impossible through reliance on feedback alone (see Bastian, this volume, and Flanagan, this volume). Whether or not these same forward controllers can be used to forecast sensory consequences further ahead in time, as is demanded in prospective estimation tasks, is an open question (cf. Wolpert and Flanagan 2001; Grush 2004). At the very least, this would require two modifications: inhibiting the motor command, and deweighting the contributions of actual afferent feedback to estimating the current state of one's body (cf. Grush 2004; Shadmehr and Krakauer 2008). As an illustration, consider a nontechnical sketch of what might be involved in solving the grip selection task.

As noted earlier, in both prospective and overt grip selection tasks, participants consistently prefer the response option that is perceived as least physically awkward when actually adopted (Johnson 2000b). A description of the relationship between stimulus orientations and grip preferences can therefore be thought of as a function that minimizes movements' costs. From this perspective, the question becomes how the costs associated with each response alternative can be estimated in the absence of afferent feedback. To begin, I will assume that an action has already been chosen (e.g., using the right hand to grasp the widget in an overhand precision grip). This would allow an inverse model to compute the motor command that is necessary to achieve this specific goal from a perceptual description of the stimulus and an estimate of the current state of the body (i.e., *a state estimate*). A copy of this motor command (efference copy) would be generated in parallel. During actual grasping, the motor command would make its way to the peripheral nervous system via the spinal cord, resulting in movements of the limb and the generation of afferent feedback. By contrast, in a prospective task this motor command would be inhibited somewhere along the spinocortical pathway at a point located downstream from the separation of the efference copy. In both conditions, the efference copy and the current state estimate would be input to a forward model that mimics the system whose behavior is being predicted, in this case the right upper extremity. The model then generates predictions of the motor command's sensory consequences. During actual grasping, this would occur in parallel with actual movements. However, as a result of transmission delays in peripheral and spinal systems, these centrally generated predictions would be available slightly in advance of afferent feedback. Through an iterative process that is beyond the scope of this chapter, the state estimate would be updated as the movement unfolds based on both predicted and actual sensory signals. Although accurate motor control might require a more balanced weighting of these sources, this would be detrimental to accurately forecasting the sensory consequences of motor commands in prospective tasks. The reason is that, as long as the motor command remains inhibited, one's actual state would not change. Nevertheless, the forward model would continue generating new predictions in response to the efference copy, and these could lead to misestimations of one's actual state. This difficulty might be resolved by giving no weight to predicted sensory feedback when estimating the current state of the limb (Grush 2004; Shadmehr and Krakauer 2008).

The end result of these predictive functions is an estimate of the sensory consequences that would be experienced when adopting an overhand grip of the widget with the right hand. Presumably these could be used to derive an estimate of the movement's difficultly, or costs. The same procedure would then be applied to the underhand option and a comparator mechanism could be postulated to choose the least costly of the two response alternatives. The fact that times required for prospective grip selection are inversely related to the difference between the perceived awkwardness of the two competing response alternatives seems consistent with this speculation (Johnson 2000b).

Learning

Rather than simply adapting existing models of the hands, our findings suggest that during overt practice (OGS task), participants learned a new forward model that accurately captures the mechanical and dynamical properties of the formerly novel tool (see Imamizu, this volume). The evidence for this is two-fold. First, as stressed earlier, the psychophysical results are clearly specific to the effector involved. Second, throughout the experiment, participants switched fluidly between judgments based on the hands versus tool with no apparent costs in performance. In the scheme outlined earlier, this process of model acquisition would involve a comparison of actual and predicted sensory feedback (Wolpert et al. 2001). The resulting error signal could then be used to tune the forward model, leading to more veridical predictions. By contrast, lack of afferent feedback would eliminate this error signal, and this might place severe restrictions on what aspects of a task can be learned through prospective processes alone. This could explain why participants have difficulty adapting their perceptions of affordances when the physical capabilities of the body are altered unless they are allowed to experience the sensory consequences of these manipulations directly (Mark 1987; Witt et al. 2005). The absence of an error signal during performance of prospective judgments might also explain why they are often imperfect (Fischer 2005; Rodriguez et al. 2008), as there is no opportunity to self-correct. In the present work, these imperfections are notable for stimulus orientations located at the points where actors transition between over- vs. underhand grip preferences. These transitions tend to be fuzzier (spread across more stimulus orientations) in the prospective task due to greater variability in responses.

Linkages to Neural Substrates

Finally, I briefly consider how these functions might map onto the neural substrates identified in our fMRI experiment. Previous work suggests that the cerebellum may play a key role in acquiring and supporting forward internal models (Miall 1998; Imamizu et al. 2000; Imamizu et al. 2003; Miall and King 2008). The engagement of the cerebellar hemispheres in all conditions of the PGS task could reflect the use of these models in generating long-range forecasts of the sensory consequences of grasping with hands or the tool. Moreover, there is evidence that implicates the posterior parietal cortex in computing state estimates based on both feedback and feedforward (predicted) signals (Desmurget et al. 1999; Desmurget and Grafton 2000; Mulliken et al. 2008). One possibility suggested by the present findings is that in the prospective task, the parietal cortex, along with reciprocally interconnected premotor regions, may be generating updated state estimates based exclusively on predictions arising from the forward models in the cerebellum. From this perspective, parieto-premotor circuits would participate in state estimation in both overt movement and prospective estimation tasks. The only difference would be the source(s) of information used in these computations. As introduced earlier, state estimation in sensorimotor control may be based on both feedback and feedforward signals, whereas in prospective estimation feedforward signals would be used exclusively.

Premovement Action Selection

Observations indicate that the macroscopic features of manual actions (such as over- vs. underhand) are often specified prior to movement onset (Arbib 1981; Jeannerod 1981; Keele 1981; Stelmach et al. 1994), and that predictive mechanims play an important role configuring the hand for grasping (Cesari and Newell 1999; Cesari and Newell 2000; Ansuini et al. 2006; Lukos et al. 2007). This raises an interesting question: Might these same forecasting mechanisms be used in premovement planning? Action selection is a core challenge for motor control systems because there are often a large number of possible solutions for achieving any one goal (Bernstein 1967). In the grip selection tasks described earlier, we have greatly simplified this problem by restricting the number of potential solutions for grasping the widget to two (over- or underhand). A system that simulates the details of all possible responses would certainly be untenable under more naturalistic circumstances. However, it is an empirical question whether such a mechanism could underlie the selection of the more macroscopic features of actions, with details resolved during movement execution (Johnson 2000b; Elsinger and Rosenbaum 2003).

Motor Imagery

Some authors (including myself) have claimed that action forecasting involves analog motor simulation (or motor imagery) (Rochat and Wraga

1997; Johnson 2000a; Fischer 2005). Consistent with this view is evidence that times required to perform some prospective judgments do vary in ways that are consistent with physical constraints experienced during the comparable movements (Decety et al. 1989; Johnson 2000a; Frak et al. 2001). Motor imagery tasks also are known to increase activity in the extended sensorimotor system, including many of the same regions noted in the present studies (Decety et al. 1994; Parsons et al. 1995; Grafton et al. 1996; Johnson et al. 2002). Although more work is needed to evaluate the hypothesis that motor imagery is involved in various prospective tasks, the forward processes outlined earlier could potentially yield analog movement representations (Grush 2004; Shadmehr and Krakauer 2008).

In conclusion, it may be the case that researchers from radically different theoretical perspectives have been investigating the very same processes. Whether viewed through the lens of affordance perception, motor imagery, or action selection tasks, prospective planning behaviors may all involve the same mechanisms; a hypothesis that is potentially falsifiable with current functional neuroimaging technologies.

ACKNOWLEDGMENTS AND AUTHOR NOTE

Scott H. Frey was formerly known as Scott H. Johnson and also published as Scott H. Johnson-Frey. Preparation of this chapter was supported by a grant from NIH/NINDS (#NS053962). I thank Dr. Stephane Jacobs for preparation of the original versions, from which Figures 13.2–13.4 were adapted.

REFERENCES

Ansuini, C., M. Santello, S, Massaccesi, and U. Castiello. 2006. Effects of end-goal on hand shaping. *Journal of Neurophysiology* 95:2456–65.

Arbib, M.A. 1981. Perceptual structures and distributed motor control. In *Handbook of neurophysiology: Motor control,* ed., V.B. Brooks, Part 2., Vol. 2. APA, Bethesda, MD: Am. Physiol. Assn.

Arbib, M.A., J.B. Bonaiuto, S. Jacobs, and S.H. Frey. 2009. Tool use and the distalization of the end-effector. *Psychological Research* 73:441–62.

Begliomini, C., M.B. Wall, A.T. Smith, and U. Castiello. 2007. Differential cortical activity for precision and whole-hand visually guided grasping in humans. *European Journal of Neuroscience* 25:1245–52.

Bernstein, N. 1967. *The co-ordination and regulation of movements.* Oxford: Pergamon Press.

Binkofski, F., G. Buccino, S. Posse, R.J. Seitz, G. Rizzolatti, and H. Freund. 1999. A fronto-parietal circuit for object manipulation in man: Evidence from an fMRI-study. *European Journal of Neuroscience* 11:3276–86.

Binkofski, F., C. Dohle, S. Posse, K.M. Stephan, H. Hefter, R.J. Seitz, and H.J. Freund. 1998. Human anterior intraparietal area subserves prehension: A combined lesion and functional MRI activation study. *Neurology* 50:1253–59.

Bloch, J.I., and D.M. Boyer. 2002. Grasping primate origins. *Science* 298:1606–10.

Castiello, U., and C. Begliomini. 2008. The cortical control of visually guided grasping. *Neuroscientist* 14:157–70.

Cesari, P., and K.M. Newell. 1999. The scaling of human grip configurations. *Journal of Experimental Psychology. Human Perception and Performance* 25:927–35.

Cesari, P., and K.M. Newell. 2000. Body-scaled transitions in human grip configurations. *Journal of Experimental Psychology. Human Perception and Performance* 26:1657–68.

Chao, L.L., and A. Martin. 2000. Representation of manipulable man-made objects in the dorsal stream. *Neuroimage* 12:478–84.

Culham, J.C., S.L. Danckert, J.F. DeSouza, J.S. Gati, R.S. Menon, and M.A. Goodale. 2003. Visually guided grasping produces fMRI activation in dorsal but not ventral stream brain areas. *Experimental Brain Research* 153:180–89.

Culham, J.C., and K.F. Valyear. 2006. Human parietal cortex in action. *Current Opinion in Neurobiology* 16:205–12.

Decety, J., M. Jeannerod, and C. Prablanc. 1989. The timing of mentally represented actions. *Behavioural Brain Research* 34:35–42.

Decety, J., D. Perani, M. Jeannerod, V. Bettinardi, B. Tadary, R. Woods, et al. 1994. Mapping motor representations with positron emission tomography. *Nature* 371:600–02.

Desmurget, M., C.M. Epstein, R.S. Turner, C. Prablanc, G.E. Alexander, and S.T. Grafton. 1999. Role of the posterior parietal cortex in updating reaching movements to a visual target. *Nature Neuroscience* 2:563–67.

Desmurget, M., and S. Grafton. 2000. Forward modeling allows feedback control for fast reaching movements. *Trends in Cognitive Sciences* 4:423–31.

Ebner, T.J., and S. Pasalar. 2008. Cerebellum predicts the future motor state. *Cerebellum* 7:583–88.

Ehrsson, H.H., E. Fagergren, and H. Forssberg. 2001. Differential fronto-parietal activation depending on force used in a precision grip task: An fMRI study. *Journal of Neurophysiology* 85:2613–23.

Elsinger, C.L., and D.A. Rosenbaum. 2003. End posture selection in manual positioning: Evidence for feedforward modeling based on a movement choice method. *Experimental Brain Research* 152:499–509.

Fattori, P., R. Breveglieri, N. Marzocchi, D. Filippini, A. Bosco, and C. Galletti. 2009. Hand orientation during reach-to-grasp movements modulates neuronal activity in the medial posterior parietal area V6A. *Journal of Neuroscience* 29:1928–36.

Fischer, M.H. 2005. Perceived reachability: The roles of handedness and hemifield. *Experimental Brain Research* 160:283–89.

Fogassi, L., and G. Luppino. 2005. Motor functions of the parietal lobe. *Current Opinion in Neurobiology* 15:626–31.

Frak, V., Y. Paulignan, M. Jeannerod. 2001. Orientation of the opposition axis in mentally simulated grasping. *Experimental Brain Research* 136:120–27.

Frey, S.H., D. Vinton, R. Norlund, and S.T. GraftonT. 2005. Cortical topography of human anterior intraparietal cortex active during visually guided grasping. *Brain Research. Cognitive Brain Research* 23:397–405.

Gardner, E.P., K.S. Babu, S.D. Reitzen, S. Ghosh, A.S. Brown, J. Chen, et al. 2007a. Neurophysiology of prehension. I. Posterior parietal cortex and object-oriented hand behaviors. *Journal of Neurophysiology* 97:387–406.

Gardner, E.P., J.Y. Ro, K.S. Babu, and S. Ghosh. 2007b. Neurophysiology of prehension. II. Response diversity in primary somatosensory. S-I. and motor. M-I. cortices. *Journal of Neurophysiology* 97:1656–70.

Gibson, J.J. 1979. *The ecological approach to visual perception*. Boston: Houghton Mifflin.

Grafton, S.T., M.A. Arbib, L. Fadiga, and G. Rizzolatti. 1996. Localization of grasp representations in humans by positron emission tomography. 2. Observation compared with imagination. *Experimental Brain Research* 112:103–11.

Grafton, S.T., L. Fadiga, M.A. Arbib, and G. Rizzolatti. 1997. Premotor cortex activation during observation and naming of familiar tools. *Neuroimage* 6:231–36.

Grush, R. 2004. The emulation theory of representation: Motor control, imagery, and perception. *Behavioral and Brain Sciences* 27:377–96; discussion 396–442.

Haruno, M., D.M. Wolpert, and M. Kawato. 2001. Mosaic model for sensorimotor learning and control. *Neural Computation* 13:2201–20.

Hyvarinen, J. 1982. Posterior parietal lobe of the primate brain. *Physiological Reviews* 62:1060–129.

Imamizu, H., T. Kuroda, S. Miyauchi, T. Yoshioka, and M. Kawato. 2003. Modular organization of internal models of tools in the human cerebellum. *Proceedings of the National Academy of Sciences of the USA* 100:5461–66.

Imamizu, H., S. Miyauchi, T. Tamada, Y. Sasaki, R. Takino, B. Putz, et al. 2000. Human cerebellar activity reflecting an acquired internal model of a new tool. *Nature* 403:192–95.

Ishak, S., K.E. Adolph, and G.C. Lin. 2008. Perceiving affordances for fitting through apertures. *Journal of Experimental Psychology. Human Perception and Performance* 34:1501–14.

Jacobs, S., Danielmeier, C., & Frey, S.H. (2010). Human anterior intraparietal and ventral premotor cortices support representations of grasping with the hand or a novel tool. *J Cogn Neurosci*, 22(11), 2594–2608. doi: 10.1162/jocn.2009.21372

Jeannerod, M. 1981. *The neural and behavioral organization of goal-directed movements.* New York: Oxford Science Publishers.

Johnson, S.H. 2000a. Imagining the impossible: Intact motor representations in hemiplegics. *Neuroreport* 11:729–32.

Johnson, S.H. 2000b. Thinking ahead: The case for motor imagery in prospective judgments of prehension. *Cognition* 74:33–70.

Johnson, S.H., M. Rotte, S.T. Grafton, H. Hinrichs, M.S. Gazzaniga, and H.J. Heinze. 2002. Selective activation of a parietofrontal circuit during implicitly imagined prehension. *Neuroimage* 17:1693–1704.

Kawato, M., T. Kuroda, H. Imamizu, E. Nakano, S. Miyauchi, and T. Yoshioka. 2003. Internal forward models in the cerebellum: fMRI study on grip force and load force coupling. *Progress in Brain Research* 142:171–88.

Keele, S.W. 1981. Motor control. In *Handbook in physiology, Section 1: The nervous system*, ed., W.B. Brooks, 1391–1414. Vol. 2. Baltimore: Williams & Williams.

Kroliczak, G., C. Cavina-Pratesi, D.A. Goodman, and J.C. Culham. 2007. What does the brain do when you fake it? An FMRI study of pantomimed and real grasping. *Journal of Neurophysiology* 97:2410–22.

Lukos, J., C. Ansuini, and M. Santello. 2007. Choice of contact points during multidigit grasping: Effect of predictability of object center of mass location. *Journal of Neuroscience* 27:3894–903.

Mahon, B.Z., S.C. Milleville, G.A. Negri, R.I. Rumiati, A. Caramazza, and A. Martin. 2007. Action-related properties shape object representations in the ventral stream. *Neuron* 55:507–20.

Mark, L.S. 1987. Eyeheight-scaled information about affordances: A study of sitting and stair climbing. *Journal of Experimental Psychology. Human Perception and Performance* 13:361–70.

Mark, L.S., and D. Vogele. 1987. A biodynamic basis for perceived categories of action: A study of sitting and stair climbing. *Journal of Motor Behavior* 19:367–84.

Miall, R.C. 1998. The cerebellum, predictive control and motor coordination. *Novartis Foundation Symposium* 218:272–84; discussion 284–90.

Miall, R.C., and D. King. 2008. State estimation in the cerebellum. *Cerebellum* 7: 572–76.

Mulliken, G.H., S. Musallam, and R.A. Andersen. 2008. Forward estimation of movement state in posterior parietal cortex. *Proceedings of the National Academy of Sciences of the USA* 105:8170–77.

Murata, A., L. Fadiga, L. Fogassi, V. Gallese, V. Raos, and G. Rizzolatti. 1997. Object representation in the ventral premotor cortex, area F5, of the monkey. *Journal of Neurophysiology* 78:2226–30.

Parsons, L.M., P.T. Fox, J.H. Downs, T. Glass, T.B. Hirsch, C.C. Martin, et al. 1995. Use of implicit motor imagery for visual shape discrimination as revealed by PET. *Nature* 375:54–58.

Raos, V., M.A. Umilta, V. Gallese, and L. Fogassi. 2004. Functional properties of grasping-related neurons in the dorsal premotor area F2 of the macaque monkey. *Journal of Neurophysiology* 92:1990–2002.

Rice, N.J., E. Tunik, E.S. Cross, and S.T. Grafton. 2007. On-line grasp control is mediated by the contralateral hemisphere. *Brain Research* 1175:76–84.

Rice, N.J., E. Tunik, and S.T. Grafton. 2006. The anterior intraparietal sulcus mediates grasp execution, independent of requirement to update: New insights from transcranial magnetic stimulation. *Journal of Neuroscience* 26:8176–82.

Rijntjes, M., C. Dettmers, C. Buchel, S. Kiebel, R.S. Frackowiak, and C. Weiller. 1999. A blueprint for movement: Functional and anatomical representations in the human motor system. *Journal of Neuroscience* 19:8043–48.

Rizzolatti, G., R. Camarda, L. Fogassi, M. Gentilucci, G. Luppino, and M. Matelli. 1988. Functional organization of inferior area 6 in the macaque monkey. II. Area F5 and the control of distal movements. *Experimental Brain Research* 71:491–507.

Rizzolatti, G., L. Fogassi, and V. Gallese. 2002. Motor and cognitive functions of the ventral premotor cortex. *Current Opinion in Neurobiology* 12:149–54.

Rochat, P., and M. Wraga. 1997. An account of the systematic error in judging what is reachable. *Journal of Experimental Psychology. Human Perception and Performance* 23:199–212.

Rodriguez, M., C. Llanos, S. Gonzalez, and M. Sabate. 2008. How similar are motor imagery and movement? *Behavioral Neuroscience* 122:910–16.

Rushworth, M.F., A. Ellison, and V. Walsh. 2001a. Complementary localization and lateralization of orienting and motor attention. *Nature Neuroscience* 4:656–61.

Rushworth, M.F., M. Krams, and R.E. PassinghamE. 2001b. The attentional role of the left parietal cortex: The distinct lateralization and localization of motor attention in the human brain. *Journal of Cognitive Neuroscience* 13:698–710.

Rushworth, M.F., P.D. Nixon, S. Renowden, D.T. Wade, and R.E. Passingham. 1997. The left parietal cortex and motor attention. *Neuropsychologia* 35:1261–73.

Sakata, H., M. Taira, M. Kusunoki, A. Murata, and Y. Tanaka. 1997. The TINS Lecture. The parietal association cortex in depth perception and visual control of hand action. *Trends in Neurosciences* 20:350–57.

Schluter, N.D., M. Krams, M.F. Rushworth, R.E. Passingham. 2001. Cerebral dominance for action in the human brain: The selection of actions. *Neuropsychologia* 39:105–13.

Shadmehr, R., and J.W. Krakauer. 2008. A computational neuroanatomy for motor control. *Experimental Brain Research* 185:359–81.

Stelmach, G.E., U. Castiello, and M. Jeannerod. 1994. Orienting the finger opposition space during prehension movements. *Journal of Motor Behavior* 26:178–86.

Tunik, E., S.H. Frey, and S.T. Grafton. 2005. Virtual lesions of the human anterior intraparietal area disrupt goal-dependent on-line adjustments of grasp. *Nature Neuroscience* 8:505–11.

Umilta, M.A., L. Escola, I. Intskirveli, F. Grammont, M. Rochat, F. Caruana, et al. 2008. When pliers become fingers in the monkey motor system. *Proceedings of the National Academy of Sciences of the USA* 105:2209–13.

Warren, W.H., Jr. 1984. Perceiving affordances: Visual guidance of stair climbing. *Journal of Experimental Psychology. Human Perception and Performance* 10: 683–703.

Wing, A.M. 2000. Motor control: Mechanisms of motor equivalence in handwriting. *Current Biology* 10:R245-R248.

Witt, J.K., D.R. Proffitt, and W. Epstein. 2005. Tool use affects perceived distance, but only when you intend to use it. *Journal of Experimental Psychology. Human Perception and Performance* 31:880–88.

Wolpert, D.M., and J.R. Flanagan. 2001. Motor prediction. *Current Biology* 11: R729–32.

Wolpert, D.M., and Z. Ghahramani. 2000. Computational principles of movement neuroscience. *Nature Neuroscience* 3(Suppl):1212–17.

Wolpert, D.M., Z. Ghahramani, and J.R. Flanagan. 2001. Perspectives and problems in motor learning. *Trends in Cognitive Science* 5:487–94.

14

Training Skills with Virtual Environments

Carlo A. Avizzano, Emanuele Ruffaldi, and Massimo Bergamasco

This work focuses on the concept of skills training by means of additional information being modeled within the virtual environment (VE), its control, and its interfaces. The work particularly focuses on how actuated external devices can cooperate in the control of voluntary movements to refine the quality of motor control and hence improve learning of specific abilities. The control of haptic, visual, and vibrotactile feedback in the training environment will be analyzed, and a given set of algorithms for capturing the motion, modeling the reference gestures, and rendering training feedback will be reviewed and discussed. Hence, this work introduces the information needed to model and train the motor and cognitive skills of users. A general architecture to set up a training environment that could learn from examples of experts will be presented, and it will be completed by the presentation of the "digital trainer" that uses such knowledge to drive the training feedback. Different methodologies for information representation and stimuli generation will be presented, and specific applications to haptics, audio, vision, and vibrotactile feedback will be considered. Methods for training sensorimotor coordination and procedural skills, with an analysis of the short-term memory effects, will be discussed on a specific set of test scenarios.

COMPUTERIZED TRAINING ENVIRONMENTS

The use of computers as a mean for learning began in the mid 1960s. At that time, the term *computer assisted instruction* (CAI) was coined (Carbonnell 1970) to identify programs performing tutoring based on a "question-and-answer" approach.

Computers offer a combination of low cost, programming flexibility, repeatability, accuracy in tracing user action, and precision in response that makes them the ideal instruments to create training programs. The technique of using computers for training is usually referred as *computer based training* (CBT).

The use of CBT (Lee and Owens 2004) was pioneered in late 1960s once the film-based techniques demonstrated their limitation in adapting the training material to the quality and the rhythm of students. Several factors limited the advent of CBT techniques as a broad standard adopted in education:

- In early stages of its development, the infrastructural cost, in terms of computing hardware and software development, made this resource limited to a few studies in those universities and research centers that had already gathered the hardware for different purposes.
- The weakness of standards and multimedia performance up until the 1990s, made these resources very limited, and the editing process was mostly text based. Audio and video streaming was not feasible, and only a few added interactions, mostly text-based questions/answer quizzes, were conceived.
- At that time, the digital era had not yet begun. Databases were not available, or they were not interconnected by networks, and all the information had to be brought to the program by manual inputs or scans from editors.

The use of CBT, even supported by the invention of CD-ROMs, failed to become an acceptable alternative to books and other printed material. It was only in the mid 1990s, as a side effect of the Internet boom, that people referred more and more to computers in order to find information that is not equivalently widespread and/or updated using conventional training channels.

According to Gagné (1972), the instructional areas opened by this type of technology and that are available in scientific literature can be organized into five major groups:

- Motor skills in performing physical tasks;
- Cognitive relational abilities;
- Symbolic and declarative knowledge;
- Attitudinal skills, and
- Intellectual and/or procedural skills.

In this scenario, the Internet boom gave new life to CBT, represented by two different types of realization:

- eLearning (i.e., computer- and Internet-based learning) was deeply investigated and promoted by international research plans.

eLearning faced the problem of managing distant simultaneous learning through remote student–teacher interaction, and it created a novel and completely computer-based training methodology, in which the computer replaced the teacher in guiding students to learn.

- The combination of digital libraries, advanced multimedia, and applet technologies users have begun managing learning on digital lessons deployed and personalized by computers. Webinars are now the most widespread source for this type of training.

SHORT HISTORY OF VE-BASED TRAINING

The quality, completeness, and immediacy of interaction is at the basis of VE learning capabilities. As highlighted by Barraclough and Guymer (1998), the original philosophy that motivated the investigation of VE-based training was that the more senses are stimulated, the richer is the information given to the learner and the better are the possibilities for learning. In computer-based simulation, such an approach also served to reduce the gap among the training environment and the real operational environment where the learned information should be employed.

Two elements have greatly contributed to the breakthroughs of VE in training applications: computer graphics progress in generating real-time, three-dimensional, highly immersive and interactive scenarios; and the research on and introduction into the VEs of interactive robots. Such robots, which lately have been called "force displays" (Minsky et al. 1990) or "haptic interfaces" (Klatzky 1989; Brooks 1990), enabled us to enrich those environment with fully sensory feedback, with force and tactile rendering complementing the existing audio and visual channels.

Clark and Horch (1986) already argued the possibilities offered by these kinds of devices and argued that, "Humans have remarkable ability to remember position of their limbs quite accurately and for long periods." This ability to remember motor patterns can be at the basis of motion training with haptic interfaces.

It became rapidly clear that the concept of virtual reality (VR)-based training was not limited, as it was for eLearning and CBT techniques, to mimicking the functionality of traditional training in an immersive and more expensive environment. The true application of motor training concept opened the door to a new class of interaction devices, in which users and machines share a kind of implicit knowledge (Reber 1996) of the task.

Haptic guidance was one of the first training stimuli used in combination with haptic interfaces. Training hand motion by means of haptic interfaces was investigated by several authors. In Figure 14.1, a force-feedback system to guide the hand during writing motion strokes is shown (Avizzano 2005). In these systems, haptic interfaces have a vector-based representation of all

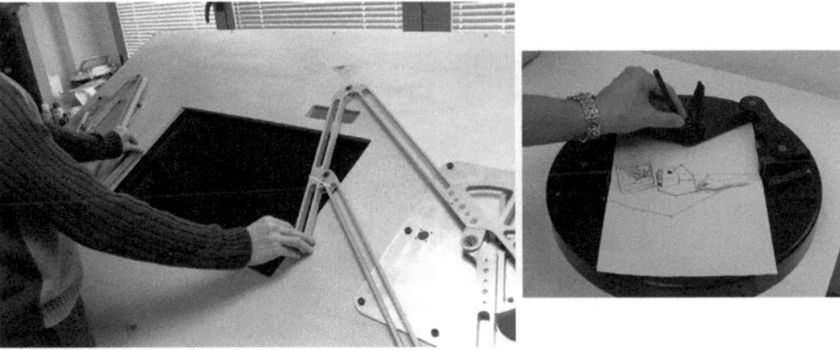

Figure 14.1 Haptic guidance by means of haptic interfaces during writing and drawing.

possible paths of motion and infer the guidance feedback using the distance to the closest path.

Haptic guidance imagines that the robot guides the user to perform motions in space, obtaining correct gestures depending on the training task. Such guidance is achieved by means of cooperation between the user and the robot. Two main types of guidance strategies were proposed and tested. In the *passive guidance approach,* the user grasps a device, which shows the user the proper trajectories and velocities to be followed. In the *active approach,* the robots only act as a "virtual" constraint that aligns the user's motion along the proper trajectory, while the user is left free to decide the velocities and energies to put in the motion.

When comparing the learning effects, both strategies have positive and negative issues that suggest, as we will show, an intermediate adaptive strategy in which the support of the computer is modulated according to the response of the learning subject.

In Figure 14.2, the intermediate strategy represents the potential offered by the combination of three-dimensional graphics with haptic interfaces (Yokokohji 1996). Yokokohji explored this paradigm by replicating an immersive ball–racket interaction in a simulated tennis exercise. He introduced the concept of the "what you see is what you feel" (WYSIWYF) interface, a system capable of generating coherent and co-located visual and haptic information that could be employed to act on virtual objects exactly as if they were real, but with added value in the fact that the physical response was completely computer controlled and therefore open to any alterations that the designer would like to introduce. The potential of this system in training applications was already addressed implicitly by Yokokohji (1996), who stated that if the "system does not provide the proper visual/haptic relationship, the training effort might not accurately reflect the real situation (no skill transfer), or even worse, the training might be counter to the real situation (negative skill transfer)."

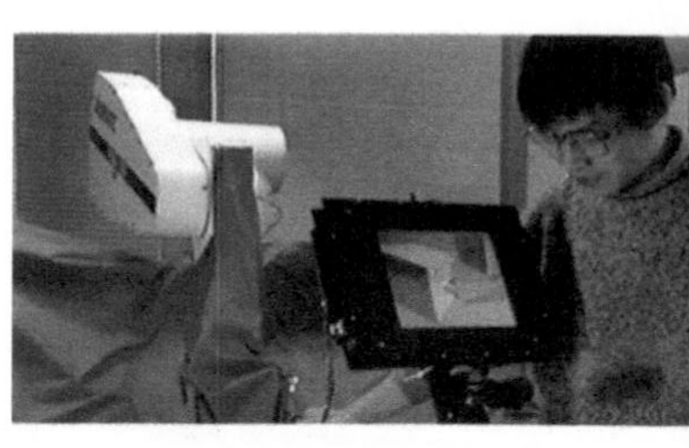

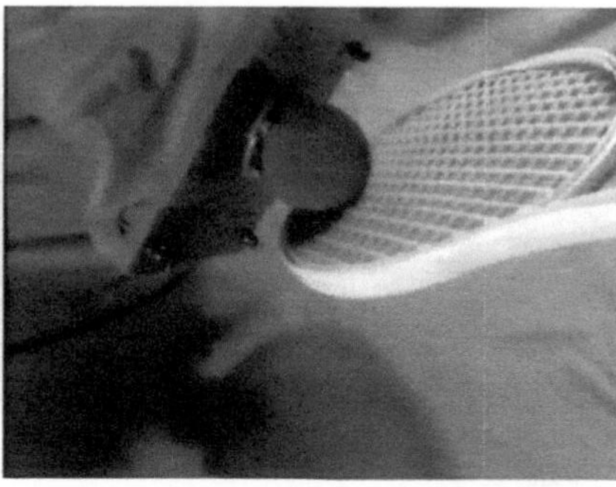

Figure 14.2 "What You See Is What You Feel" system, on the left, with a detail of the interactive virtual environment, on the right. Courtesy of the author.

In the subsequent decade, a plethora of VE-enhanced training systems were proposed. In some cases, these systems truly offered some new paradigms of training. In others, they did not provide any real benefits to what could be achieved with traditional training methodologies. At the time, it was natural that the necessity of highly costly instrumentation for VR provided a substantial benefit with respect to direct and indirect costs of training on the job. In defense of the use of haptic interfaces during training, Feygin (2002) argued that the use of this form of training was beneficial, since training occurred in body-centered (or motor) coordinates as opposed to the visuospatial coordinates that can be employed in training by shown examples (video, trainer's examples, or book). According to Feygin, this form of training "removes the need for complex sensorimotor transformation and applies to "three-or-more-dimensional motor skills that are difficult to explain and describe verbally or even visually."

Rosenberg (1993) proposed another way of formulating sensorimotor training in a VE: the concept of *virtual fixtures* (VF). Virtual fixtures were richer than the WYSIWYF concept in the sense that they also addressed the issue of what to feel when interacting with objects. This metaphor helps to identify and translate into physical structures a wide set of effects, including guiding motions, barriers, and mass properties among others. In Figure 14.3, two examples of virtual fixtures, taken from virtual assembly platforms, are shown. On the left, the internal components of a car can be mounted and assembled while the system provides force feedback related to interference and other contact properties to the user. On the right, a similar concept is extended to the maintenance and cabling of an airplane motor. Virtual fixtures in these two examples simulate interference effects during plug-and-play operation in order to verify the design optimality of maintenance operation and to train employees to proper procedural sequences.

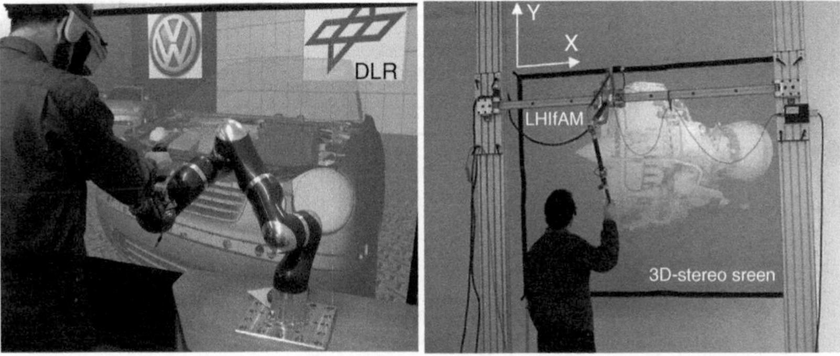

Figure 14.3 Virtual Fixtures, at Institut für Robotik und Mechatronik (*left*) and Centro de Estudios e Investigaciones Técnicas de Gipuzkoa. With permission of the authors.

The concept of VF introduced a philosophy of feedback generation that is still under investigation, both for application and behavioral training in uncommon or unfriendly environments (space or underwater operation, mission critical environments, etc.), as well as to investigate dynamic fixtures whose behavior is more complexly bound to the state of the scenario. For instance, Abbot and Okamura (2007) introduced a derivation of VF when applied strictly to robot-assisted manipulation (guided virtual fixtures, sensory substitution, cooperation and forbid region). To date, a wide amount of effects are available within this class of feedbacks. In Figure 14.4, a partial grid of the fixture set employed in our laboratory is summarized.

Virtual fixtures found their limitation in their physical bound. Fixtures were expressed as a set of object properties, which reflected the amount of knowledge that was required to properly handle a VE object using motion and guidance information. Simultaneously, Gillespie et al. (1998) and Henmi and Yoshikawa (1998) independently introduced the idea that the knowledge stored in a VE could go beyond the properties of the objects therein represented. Gillespie et al. (1998) expressly introduced the concept of the *virtual teacher*, an additional VE component represented by customized feedback and present only during specific training periods and absent during alternate performance sessions. Henmi, implemented this concept into a virtual calligraphy system (whose concept is represented in Figure 14.5) that replicated the correct drawing path showed to the system by an experienced user (the real teacher). In such a way, training systems became multistate devices, and their knowledge was not inserted a priori by experienced programmers. Such systems had at least two configurations: the learning mode (in which an instructor put his experience into the system) and a teaching mode (that transfers the previously stored experience to new users).

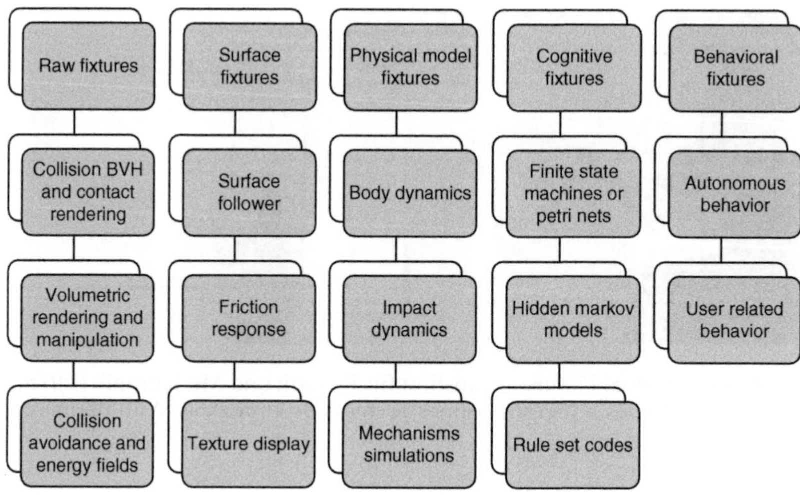

Figure 14.4 Some Virtual Fixtures represented by technological dependence.

At that time, the control issues of Henmi's proposal simply addressed a record-and-playback procedure, without taking into account the complexity factors introduced by the action repeatability. As a matter of fact, the process of handwriting only addressed proprioceptive issues of the perception action loop, with a limited impact on the process dynamics on the environment. With respect to other skills, such as tennis playing for instance, this type of ability only requires the user to control motions with respect to a given and fixed trajectory.

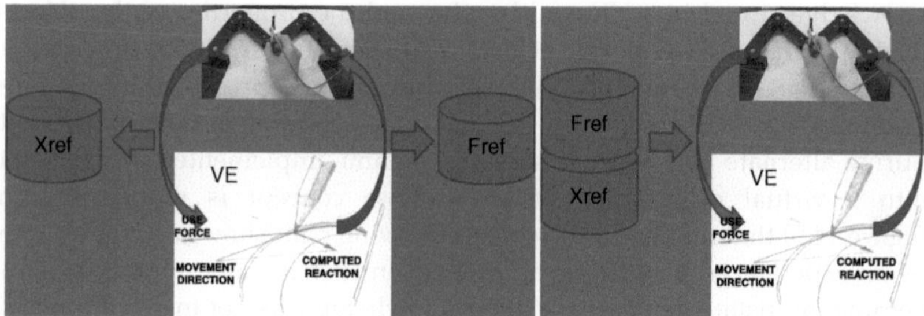

Figure 14.5 The concept of Henmi Virtual Teacher. A record (*left*) and playback (*right*) control procedure. Adapted from Henmi, K., and T. Yoshikawa T. 1998. Virtual lesson and its application to virtual calligraphy system. *Robotics and Automation Proceedings*, with permission of the publisher.

This issue was later reconsidered by several researchers who tried to employ other experts in the loop (Esen 2008) in order to improve teaching behavior or by using artificial intelligence (Sano 1999) to copy and model human control strategies.

An "extreme" application of the virtual teacher concept was achieved when cognitive training was addressed. Here, the elements suggesting to the user the proper steps to perform varied largely from blinking light elements (which represented the proper sequence) to complete agents (instructor avatars), which embedded the knowledge and describe the action to do in a simulated copy of a real plant.

Johnson et al. (2000) proposed a similar environment in which an autonomous teacher interacts with a user-controlled character and at level of speeches and environment control (see Figure 14.6).

In such an environment, it is very easy to imagine and realize systems whose utility greatly overcome their cost. The idea of using digital metrics and scoring procedures to assess the level of efficiency of such environments has been brought to light during the last few years. Ruddle and Lessels (2006) proposed a three-layer metrics to score the utility of a VR training environment. This review work was developed by taking into account learning effects of several studies all focused on a similar topic: *way finding in three-dimensional VEs*. Lessels and Ruddle concluded that at least three different levels of metrics should be taken into account:

- *Task performance during and after learning*. Task performance can be expressed with several benchmarks in the raw data and effectively represents the efficiency of the user in performing the activities in the given virtual environment.
- *Physical behavior*. Starting from the consideration that not all VEs are equivalent, it is necessary to discriminate how the design of the

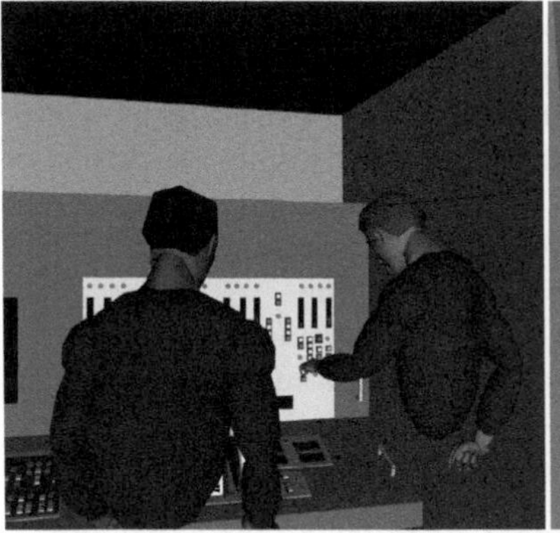
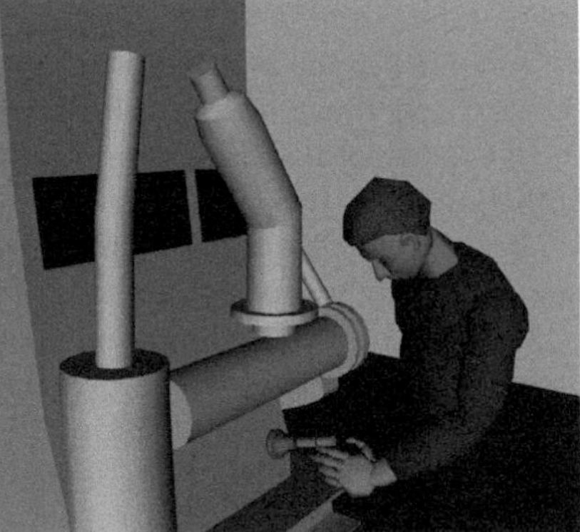

Figure 14.6 Rickel and Johnson (2000) vocational training environment.

VE affects the performance. This indirect benchmark is aimed at identifying and correlating the action performed by the user with those that he will perform in a real environment or in another VE. The physical behavior that describes how the user uses the training system is an indirect metric for at least two factors: the ergonomic aspects of the VE training system and the learning heuristics that the user develops in combination with the VT.

- *Cognitive metrics*. This metric measures the ability of the user to make use of previous knowledge and memories to optimize further action during the learning session with the VE. At least three different kinds of metrics elements could be taken into account: the memory of action patterns, the memory of required behavior, and the ability to abstract and generalize information from content.

In terms of explicit effects derived by robotic guidance, there are at least two major achievements addressed by research: the correspondence between experience and absolute, relatively simple, markers that can be identified in data recording (Moothy et al. 2003); and the ability to design and develop systems that reduce or eliminate the effect of dependence from the feedback (Li et al. 2009).

The research has so far demonstrated that even if certain type of skills can be extremely complex, their complexity can be decomposed into simpler directions, along which elementary metrics can be designed and implemented. Such metrics, once matched in training, realistically contribute to identifying if a similar level of expertise has been achieved or not. In addition, further statistical analysis has demonstrated that the modulation of the VFs during training session ("progressive shared control") helps to achieve a condition in which the same level of expertise is reached without the classical side effect of feedback dependence.

One possible conclusion of almost 20 years of research on VEs for training was presented by Sutherland (2006) in his systematic review of surgical simulators. Sutherland considered a wide database of studies (about 30) documented in the Medline and Embase databases up to April 2005, and selected only those which explicitly randomized control trials as a proof of the efficiency of the simulator. The surprising (at the time) conclusion of Sutherland was that, in contradiction to the common understanding that VE-based training was of benefit for training itself, the training results were not convincingly superior to those of standard training.

This kind of result is becoming more and more common in the scientific literature. However, such results should not compromise our judgment on the quality and usefulness of VE-based training, because additional motivations actually justify both research and use of these systems:

- In terms of applications, one cannot avoid taking the social and economic cost benefits into account. VE-based training allows learners to avoid the use of real subjects and objects, which have a high probability of being harmed by students who have not yet reached an adequate level of expertise. In addition, these tests overcome other material constraints, such as space, time, and external conditions (like weather), and they score the quality of expertise across a uniform and standardized methodology. In terms of medical and aeronautical training, the concept of transfer effectiveness ratio (TER) was introduced (Aggarwal et al. 2007) in order to quantify the effective benefits of simulators employed on operative personnel. In particular, this factor, which accounts for the time spent on the simulator in comparison to the time required to achieve the same level of practice on a real system, has high factors both when addressing airlines pilots (a TER of 0.5, which implies that each hour on the simulator reduces of 30 minutes the flight-training time required on a real airplane) and surgeons (typical TER of 2.38).

- In terms of research, the major limitations addressed by the systematic reviews seems to be solvable in a short amount of time. Most of the users employed for training so far directly coded and copied human knowledge into the training protocols, without automating the process of optimizing and refining the quality of user motion. Kimura et al. (1999) argued that the "autonomous robots must recognize human motions in real time and interact with them." In mathematical modeling, this was addressed by Rosen et al. (2001) by means of skills signatures: a specific record and modeling of human skills that will enable the machine to understand and cope with different styles.

It is therefore likely that soon a novel generation of VE-based training system will tackle the complexity of human skills and offer, if not a better quantitative feedback, at least training signals that are more contextualized and selective.

MOTION CONTROL ALGORITHMS AND PARADIGMS

At the basis of multisensory training setups, an adequate set of strategies to control user movements in coordination to what is perceived from the VE must be set. This type of control is based on three classic approaches, which have been developed during the last decade of control in haptic research. The forms in which these controls are designed strongly depend on the kind of interaction between the subject and the device. In particular, they are distinguished by:

- *Instrument replicators.* These are usually the most task-effective devices in the sense that they get the user into a training scenario that is as close as possible to the real environment. Some of the controls in such a scenario have been redesigned in order to comply and serve digital controlled loops that embed the stimuli required to train.

- *Encountered-type haptics.* This type of haptic interface can be considered a self-standing robotic system, as can all contact external devices. However, in this case, the robotic system's end-effector is not in contact with the user's hand but is tracking it at a certain distance and moves toward the contact target area only when required by the application. This type of haptic interface shows an intrinsically higher complexity, especially in control terms, with respect to external devices always in contact with the user. In the case of encountered-type systems, two additional essential characteristics should be taken into account: the tracking of the human limb's area where the contact force must be generated, and performance, in terms of the compensation of end-effector dynamics required by encountered-type haptic interfaces.
- *Contact haptic interfaces and exoskeletons.* In these system, the user grasps or is attached to the device, typically at a finite number of points, by which the force and position information necessary for training flows. These systems benefit from the fact that their control strategies can be easily taken from basic robot control, where the user is modeled as an external disturbance. Classic methods of impedance (Zilles and Salisbury 1995), admittance (Adams and Hannaford 1999), or compute torque control (Salisbury et al, 2004) can then be applied.

Most training approaches rely on the ability of the device to replicate any given (synthesis) force at the level of the user's body. The modeling of such devices is commonly addressed using the Lagrange formulation:

$$M(q)q + C(q \cdot q)q + D(q)q + G(q) = \tau_{mot} + J^T(q) F_{human} \qquad \text{(Eq. 1)}$$

Where M is the inertia matrix of the manipulator, C is the vector of Coriolis and centrifugal terms, D is the viscous friction vector, J is the Jacobian of the haptic interface, G represents gravity effect, F is the wrench applied by the operator's hand, and τ is the vector of the joint components applied by motor control. Figure 14.7 shows how these guidance motion schemas can be achieved by block constructions in control schemes. Each term of the equation can be compensated by a feedback control. This results in a map of the desired human force on motor components. In Figure 14.8, the Δ term summarizes the contribution of both viscous friction and Coriolis and centripetal terms.

In quasi-static conditions and when friction and gravity can be neglected, the mapping between the applied force/torque (wrench) and the above equation reduces to a simplified one (Marcheschi 2005), $\tau_{mot} + J^T(q) F_{human} = 0$. In this case, joint components can be derived from the principle of virtual

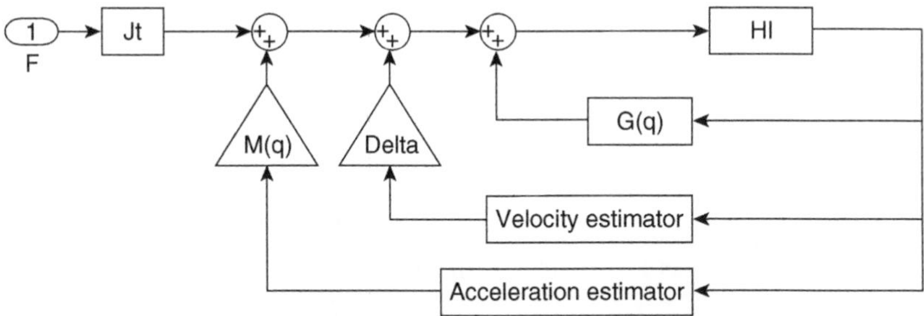

Figure 14.7 Scheme of the closed loop control procedure.

works, provided in particular by the transposition of the manipulator Jacobian: $\tau_{mot} = J^T(q)F_{des}$, where the last term represents the forces the trainer wishes to display to the user.

In more complex dynamic situations, the joint components are required to compensate for the centrifugal, inertial, viscous, and Coriolis effects that affect manipulator dynamics. If we have a good enough model of the haptic device, this compensation could be provided by cancellation. The following is the resulting torque:

$$\tau_{mot} = M^*(q)\overline{q} + C^*(q,\dot{q})\dot{q} + D^*(q)\dot{q} + G^*(q) + J^{*T}(q)F_{des} \quad \text{(Eq. 2)}$$

where the asterisk refers to model approximations of the mechanical terms. A low-level joint torque control loop is then used. Joint torque sensing allows the user to overcome the problems related to model accuracy, other friction components, and approximations in the kinematic model, and rough or no modeling at all of the device dynamics.

To identify the desired force, a contact model is usually designed. The contact model can both reproduce contact information as well as embed motion constraints and/or guidance effects. In the simplest case—contact information—the contact object is given a limited virtual stiffness that defines the apparent rigidity of the touched object.

The implementation of the virtual stiffness requires the computation of the surface normal (n) at the contact point and of the penetration vector (x, y, z) and the consequent penetration distance d:

$$d = (x\ y\ z)_{hi}\begin{pmatrix} n_x \\ n_y \\ n_z \end{pmatrix}, \quad f_{des} = \begin{cases} -\vec{n}dK_{stiff} & d > 0 \\ 0 & d \leq 0 \end{cases} \quad \text{(Eq. 3)}$$

The use of an additional digital viscosity can in some cases be added to improve stability issues when low frequency, high stiffness, and closed loops are addressed (Bergamasco 1995).

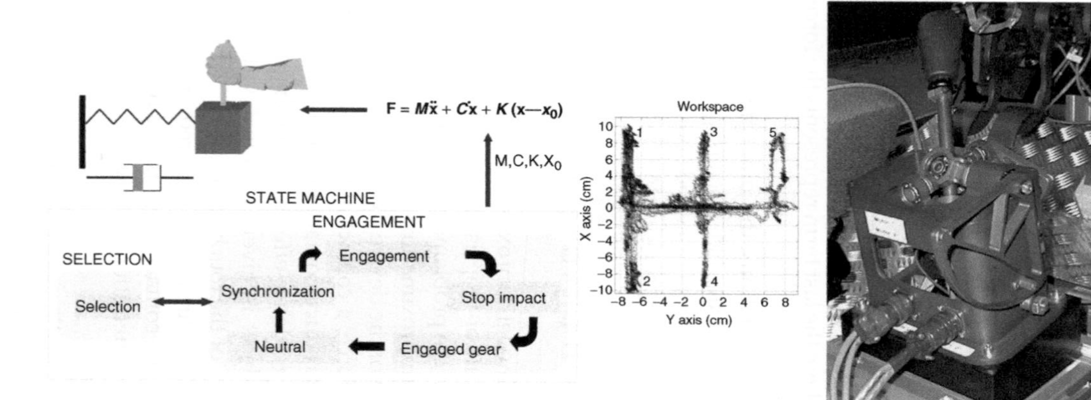

Figure 14.8 The embedded dynamics control model applied to the Gearshift interface. The figure shows the overall control scheme (*left*), simulation data (*center, x-y position*), and the employed device (*right*). From Frisoli, A., C.A. Avizzano, and M. Bergamasco. 2001. Simulation of a manual gearshift with a 2 DOF force-feedback joystick. *International Conference of Robotics & Automation*, with permission of the publisher.

When the haptic device assumes the same shape as the instrument that needs to be replicated, the control of the device can be organized as a simulation of the original instrument. If required, additional force components are added to recreate fixture and tutoring stimuli. This is generally done with a parametric closed loop that partially compensates for the interface dynamics in order to approximate the device that needs to be simulated.

Usually, in these devices, most of the mechanics are similar to those of the original device replicated, while the unseen part is different and replaced with motors. The control of these devices may be addressed in a similar way:

$$\tau_{mot} = (M^* - M_r)(q)\overline{q} + C^*(q, \dot{q})\dot{q} + (D^* - D_r)(q)\,\dot{q} + K(q - q_r) + G^*(q) \quad \text{(Eq. 4)}$$

Here, the introduction of the control law enables the user to perceive the interaction with a virtual object whose properties can be modulated by software. Once introduced in the Lagrange model and properly cancelled, the "approximated" terms of this equation lead to:

$$J^T(q)F_{human} = M_r(q)\overline{q} + D_r\dot{q} + K(q - q_r) \quad \text{(Eq. 5)}$$

or, in equivalent Cartesian coordinate systems:

$$F_{human} = \tilde{M}_r^*(x)\overline{x} + D_r^*\dot{x} + \tilde{K}_r^*(x - x_r) \quad \text{(Eq. 6)}$$

In other words, this control strategy simulates the feeling of contact between the user´s hand and a rigid object, whose properties (mass $\tilde{M}_r^{\bullet}(x)$, viscosity $\tilde{D}_r^{\bullet}$, rigidity and offset forces) are not only an element of the control strategies, but are also dynamically changeable according to the physics of the object being simulated and/or to the training strategies that need to be included in the force feedback. Different interaction behaviors can be represented through this type of control laws. This feature is achieved by programming the control feedback to compensate for component dynamics and make the mechanical response resembling that of the desired model.

The adoption of this control strategy, which only partially cancels the mass and viscous properties of the haptic interface, allows a better exploitation of the device's natural dynamics and higher thresholds in terms of effective force and dynamic ranges. An application of this control strategy was applied by Frisoli et al. (2001) in the control of a gearshift-like haptic device to be employed in a car simulator.

Figure 14.8 highlights the model of nonlinear dynamics that was implemented to simulate the effects of interacting with a real multistate object. It integrated an embedded dynamics impedance-controller with a finite state machine that changes the parameters of the model in real-time according to the state of the gear (selection, engaged, synchronizing).

Only recently have the evolution of application programming interfaces (APIs) for the simulation (PhysX 2008) and improvements in computer performance allowed the VE to simulate the entire physics of the environment to a sufficient level of detail and time granularity to allow a complete and smooth interaction using haptic devices. The combined control of what is simulated in the VE (without the notion of interactive force feedback) and of the mechanical device response is achieved by a common procedure called *virtual coupling*.

In virtual coupling, one or more parts of the user's body are in contact with an equal number of attachments to the haptic device. Those contact attachments are reflected by an equivalent set of "virtual contacts" between the manipulated objects and the interface proxies.

The virtual coupling concept is shown in Figure 14.9. The user is grasping a handle, which is virtually bound to the digital object through an elastic and damping joint that provides the feedback forces simulated in the VE to the user's hand and vice versa. Each coupling is generated on the fly, whenever the user enters into contact with a virtual object. This paradigm is particularly useful when the training VE is to teach the user the proper sensorimotor properties of an object in the environment.

Particular care should be taken with coupling properties, since poles are added for each contact and, if damping is not properly managed, an unstable condition may result. As for all digitized control systems, the use of virtual coupling adds instability to the system when the overall simulated stiffness is too high in comparison to the simulation frequency. This is true both for single contact point properties, as well as when multiple couplings interact with the same object. In such a case, the overall stiffness is the weighted series of single coupling stiffness.

LOOPS FOR TRAINING ENVIRONMENTS

To date, there have been several environments dedicated to training using VEs. Such systems can be classified into two basic categories: training environments supported by VEs, and VEs for training. Most of the systems

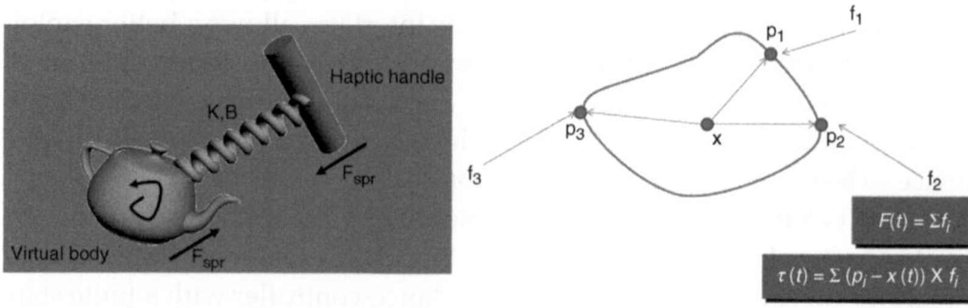

Figure 14.9 Virtual Coupling rendering approach. On the left is depicted the schema of Virtual Coupling with the Handle and the Virtual Object for the interaction. On the right is presented the schema of multiple contact points affecting a single object.

developed so far only fall into the first category since they simply use the VE as a support tool to recreate realistic conditions in which to practice skills. For the second category, we consider the presence of three basic issues that need to be addressed and implemented as an integral part of the training program:

- Bilateral interactions between the user, the real, and the digital environment, which includes a training structure to model user progress.
- A knowledge database of expert behaviors, their styles of motion, their cognitive background, and quality metrics for evaluating the achieved results.
- A training set of feedback stimuli, strictly related to user behaviors and dedicated to deliver the most effective imprint to the trainee (transfer and persistence of learning).

The proper combination of these three elements allows the design of specific training environments that may circumvent the three stages of learning as defined by Fitts and Posner (1967): cognition learning, integration learning, and automation learning.

There are several methodologies by which to approach the definition and modeling of skills. Warren (2006) inspected common approaches and identified two dominant main categories. First, the model (state space–based) approach relates to the execution of some skills primarily as a complete dynamic system, where physical bodies and muscles interact based on motor patterns commanded by the brain. Second, the embodiment and behavioral approaches decompose interactions along natural behaviors that can be shown by the actors in the environment, such as reaching, grasping, standing, etc. According to Warren (2006), both categories present positive and negative features when considering the need to explain specific elements of the interaction, such as the perception–action relationships, the emergent behaviors, optimization procedures, and the automatic learning of inverse task dynamics. Warren (2006) also highlighted the way in which different authors have explained interaction elements by referring to the properties of one or the other theoretical approach. Finally, Warren (2006) proposed a hybrid model in which both approaches were reflected.

Warren (2006) allowed three separate dynamical descriptions to identify the environment and the user's response. In addition, relationships of perception and action are modeled separately.

In Warren's approach, described in Figure 14.10, the behavior of an agent is modeled in terms of exchanges of information between the agent itself and the environment, each described as a dynamical system. The dynamics of perception and action (PA), according to Warren, can be decomposed into two basic differential equations (the ψ sensorimotor function and the χ cognitive dynamics), one environment dynamics (ϕ), and two nonlinear selection filters that map the different dynamical spaces.

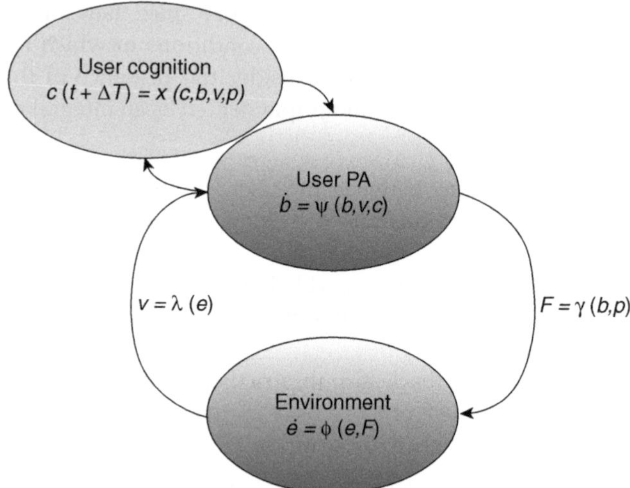

Figure 14.10 An approach to represent Perception and Action loop. Adapted Warren, W. 2006. The dynamics of perception and action. *Psychological Review* 113: 358–389, with permission of the publisher.

The environment has an internal state "e" and a descriptive function ϕ that are mapped onto the agent through an observation function λ. Similarly, the internal state of the user 'b' evolves with the ψ function and is mapped in the environment with a set of forces via the γ function. Here, two vectors of parameters guide the cognitive response (c) in performing the skill and constrain the physical limitation (p) in terms of fitness and physical abilities.

Although Warren did not describe how to introduce elements related to training, he decomposed interaction along basic, independent, and clearly defined components. We chose such a model, since it allows us to make a coherent identification of all those components required to enable digital guided training and support multiuser interaction as well.

Even if Warren did not provide any insight for modeling the internal functions: ψ, λ, χ, γ, we will show that the basic structure of his model offers the opportunity to enhance the interaction model toward a digitally mediated interaction, which handles separately the elements of style and training as discussed earlier.

The methodology described here proposes extensions to Warren's model, which applies the use of the enactive knowledge as described by Gibson (1969). This training method addresses a training process in which information connects the skill-related data to sensorimotor perception by means of immersive VEs, to allow access and acquisition of this knowledge.

Before illustrating the concept, it is useful to recall the experience of applying machine learning algorithms to robot control, as demonstrated by other research groups. Capture of style is more than capture of expert data. The preliminary experiments on point lights by Johansson (1973) more than 30 years ago demonstrated that information on gestures and walking can be encoded in a reduced set of variables. In the past decade, substantial efforts have been put into classifying and identifying human motion from observation. Troje (2008) and Gritai et al. (2004) focused on styles of walking and reduced representation for the human poses and motion. One common approach to model and classify styles is to associate them according to so-called *motion signatures* (Vasilescu 2002). Signatures identify invariant properties of the motion which can be extracted from the acquired signals through different types of data processing. Pattern simplification techniques (Davis and Gao 2003), such as principal component analysis (PCA), combined with pattern recognition, are commonly employed to determine the action style. Calinon (2006) proposed an integrated architecture that helped a robot to behave in a human-like manner in training by demonstration. The proposed system extracts relevant motion features from the observation of humans by using a probabilistic description encoded in a proper support space (determined with PCA). This behavior is created from a mixture of density function (Gaussian and Bernoulli), which defines spatiotemporal correlations across different modalities, and cognitive relationships in the observed action.

Similar concepts can be applied to robot- and VE-based training, once a proper digital model of the human skills is defined. Such a model has been designed by keeping the following factors into account:

- *The underlying components of the user–environment interaction*: For example, the amount of information to model a proper skill interaction, both in terms of observable items and controllable actions. These components are supposed to be a reduced information set of those measurable in the environment.
- *The behavioral elements that identify and classify styles*: For example, definition of the invariant and the variable elements in the constraints describing a successfully learned skill.

It is particularly relevant here that, in an approach using multimodal interfaces, we can completely or partially replace the real environment with a VE whose behavior and dynamics are defined by code and completely known to the designer. This is an essential step to digitally access measurements that are not easily caught in real environments.

The originality of our approach (Avizzano 2009) lies in the fact that the recognition is not completely performed by automated tools. Instead, it relies on a content decomposition, which has been designed in agreement with motion scientists and human factor designers (Bardy 2008). This approach has been structured by introducing the concept of subskills.

Subskills can be defined as cognitive or sensorimotor components of a task that possess specific features and metrics to be investigated with analytical tools, verified with mathematical algorithms, and stimulated with proper feedback. The subskill approach is the opposite of VFs and/or virtual teachers in the sense that it does not focus specifically on a single operation taken outside the overall task interaction. In our approach, summarized in Figure 14.11, 14 different categories of subskills have been introduced in order to measure different properties in the motor (eight categories) and cognitive (six categories) spaces. Sampling of the above-mentioned relevant points is gathered indirectly by means of *performance indicators*.

Subskills are mapped to control and training loops using a hierarchical decomposition that allows the higher semantic levels to be coordinated with the lower data content. In particular, in addition to the selected raw data and the machine learning tools described previously, the following relevant levels of information have been introduced:

Features

Features are compound logical and quantitative information that maps basic components of the motion to more relevant dimensions that characterize the style. The introduction of features in the computing process allows us to have a better targeted process, making clearer distinction between style components and focusing better on styles that are considered of primary importance by trainers. Contrary to what it seems, these

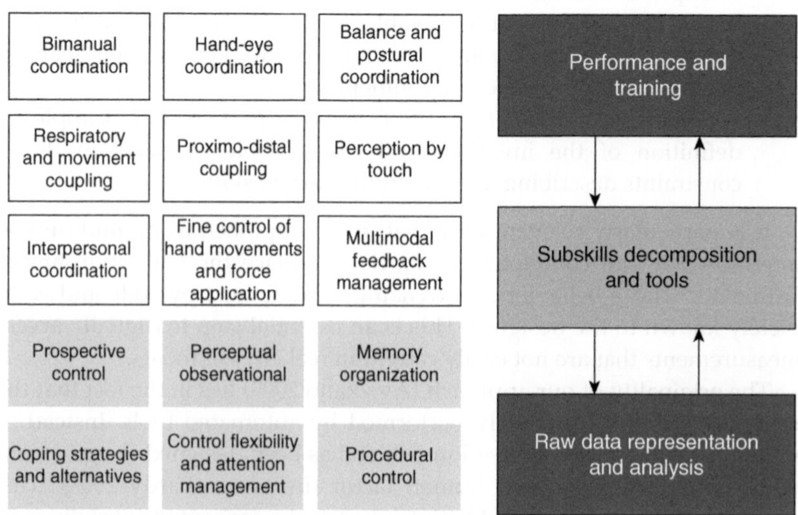

Figure 14.11 Subskill classifications (*left*) and their role in the training/learning VE (*right*).

features do not simplify the representation of the task. In fact, they increase the dimension of the representation vector and introduce more elements to be analyzed. On the other hand, features greatly simplify and improve the analysis of the performance. Each feature is designed to have a particular relationship with the performance indicators that highlight the quality of the execution of a particular phase of the skill.

Digital Subskills

Features are expected to catch a list of relevant points that could be observed in user physical and cognitive spaces (b,c) and in their characteristic evolutionary functions (ψ, χ). Hence, using features, we expect to have a methodology to qualitatively sample the hidden dynamics in those points, which the trainers consider to be of high relevance for the performing of action. The introduction of digital subskills allows immediate correlation of trainers and motion science indicators with the analytical model employed for the representation. This is performed by decomposing the user skills into the relevant subskills that are required for the specific task, then defining performance tools that measure the distance among performers. This approach allows us to redefine the digital signature of an expert style as the set of performance indicators that an expert produces when repeating a task with a given style.

Digital Training

Warren's approach has been extended to support a new model that allows training embedded in the interaction: the *digital trainer* (Fig. 14.12). The most relevant properties of the digital trainer is that it allows the user to "learn by doing," by gathering relevant task information from the direct interaction with the environment.

In the digital trainer model, the training logic and the subject interaction play a symmetric role in the hybrid virtual–real environment, within which both of them interact. The digital trainer aids the user with a set of style encodings that have been acquired from experts. With respect to traditional training, digital training can benefit from the additional power the trainer has in controlling the virtual animation of the environment.

The digital trainer has additional capabilities with respect to those at the disposal of a real trainer acting in the same situation. In particular, the observation of the subject is not limited to the external observation of actions but is enhanced with real-time biometric measurements (electroencephalograph [EEG], electromyelograph [EMG], electrocardiograph [ECG], oxygen consumption, eye tracking, etc.). These measures provide a more accurate discrimination of conditions that determine a user's responses and actions. In addition, the feedback from the trainer to the environment can bypass the need for physical interaction and directly affect the behavior

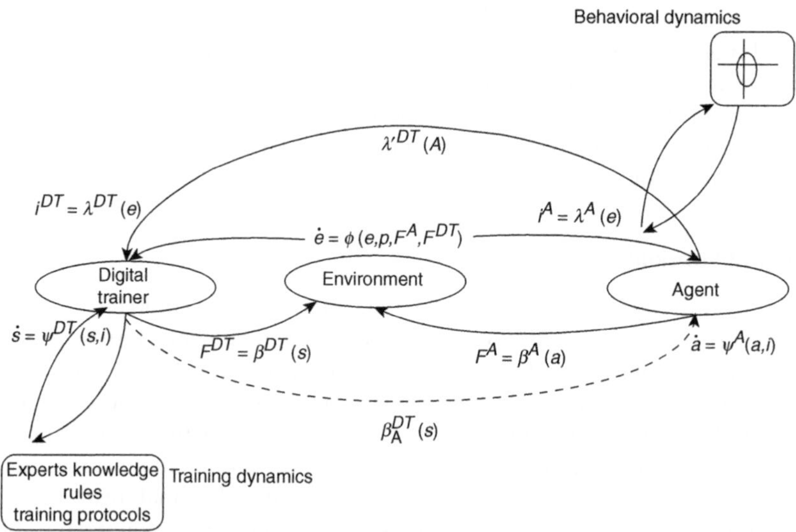

Figure 14.12 The Digital Trainer model. The Digital Trainer model extends Warren's approach (*right side*) to include the dynamics of the interactive VE and the train controller (*left side*). From Avizzano et al. 2009.

of the environment. Finally, the digital trainer feedback can completely bypass the environment and communicate directly to the user by means of real-time rendering for the purpose of driving actions or correcting errors (e.g., by means of vibrotactile stimuli, haptics, or sound).

IMPLEMENTATION

The implementation of a control framework to support digital training requires a complex integration between the architecture of the VE and the architecture of the learning control. The initial step is to model and maintain user- and expert-related knowledge with a stable source of information. In our work, this has been achieved by interconnecting the information related to user skills into a portable database. Such a repository system is based on SQlite (Owens 2006). The choice of SQlite as a reference database was explicitly done in order to embed the data capture and to maintain the data collection in a unique structure. SQlite has some unique features in terms of performance, portability, supported languages, and manipulation tools that currently make it the most suitable platform.

Additionally, in order to maintain a clear organization of the information archived into the database, a systematic tool to describe, organize, store, and recall the information has been developed. The information stored at this level exactly mirrors the hierarchy of information described earlier, which spans raw data up to digital subskills. Raw variables are the starting point of the services offered by the database. They store the data gathered from the experimental sessions, but do not highlight the semantic knowledge that is encoded in them.

An overall structure of the repository system architecture is represented in Figure 14.13. The VE has been decomposed into its different functions (i.e., interconnection, capturing, and rendering of information). In such a way, it is possible for the digital trainer to connect to and interact with real-time control processes of the environment's interaction with knowledge stored into databases.

Therefore, the repository systems also offer an additional level of information storage in order to embed a more complex organization of information in the data values and their semantic content. This is achieved by tools that process data inside of the repository and create higher levels of abstraction, which can be employed by the digital trainer in further training. Three kinds of operation are possible: outer processing, inner processing, and fruition. In *outer processing mode,* an external program will provide handles to the data in order to create higher levels of representation. *Inner processing mode* is similar but exploits functions encoded into the database to execute mathematical algorithms stored inside embedded python code. Finally, *fruition* operations retrieve information for analyzing and comparing the progress of training with respect to the signatures left by experts during their sessions.

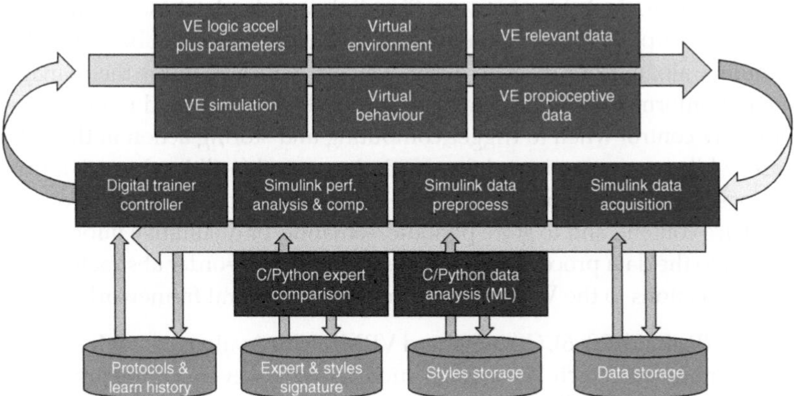

Figure 14.13 Integrated structures adopted for the digital trainer implementation. From Avizzano, C.A., E. Ruffaldi E., and V. Lippi. 2009. *Skills Digital Representation and Storage*, SKILLS09 International Conference on Multimodal Interfaces for Skills Transfer, Bilbao, Spain, with permission.

The data processing of information makes use of several types of algorithms. Principal component analysis, dynamic time warping (DTW), K-means, and other similar techniques are used to filter and classify expert motions, while trained hidden Markov models (HMM), probabilistic neural networks, and similar tools are employed to deliver computational results in real time. The information related to training and to expert references is derived by preprocessing the samples from experts into a properly encoded form for interactive use.

The bridge among the processing frameworks, the VE, and the expert knowledge is provided using a commercial tool for control simulation and hardware in the loop control, Matlab/Simulink®. Such a tool implements most of the basic building blocks to perform continuous signal handling, basic neural networks, and the like, while more complex computation can easily be introduced into the environment by means of C-based S-functions plugged into the system.

This has been achieved by developing a full set of Simulink toolboxes that handle the archiving and retrieval functions by using Simulink components, which can manipulate data in real time and embed the results in interactive VE trainers. Specific scripting modules and online filters allow the user to implement any sort of training data, performance indicators, and expert models.

The Matlab/Simulink environment also provides a bridge toward information stored in the database. Such a choice brings the following benefits: First, it completely decouples information processing from the interaction data managed within the VE algorithms, and second, it allows processing information in a unique, coherent, and graphical approach that can be clearly understood and reusable by exploiting the graphical expression of the Simulink schematics.

In addition, the bridge between Simulink and the database organization allows decoupling of the continuous time control, which can be handled in Simulink alone, from discrete event systems, which requires the management of information in the database. Specific blocks provided in the library precisely control when to trigger computing and storing action in the database, while interacting in real time with the control facilities. In such a way, it is possible to simultaneously retrieve behavioral data information from the database content, and to store periodic, semantic, or qualitative information related to the data processing, such as styles and high-order abstraction.

Connections to the VE have been created for several frameworks:

XVR (Ruffaldi 2006), OpenSG, and VRML with Avalon Instant Reality (Behr and Froehlich 1998). In all such cases, however, VE integration requires that the VE exports the basic interaction elements described in Figure 14.13, in order for the digital trainer to control the learning approach. Using such a framework, it is thus possible to implement performance indicators, style identifiers, training protocols, and

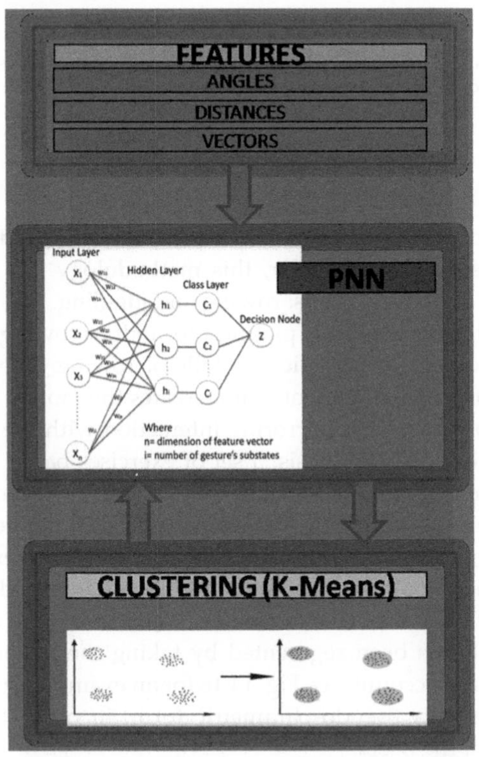

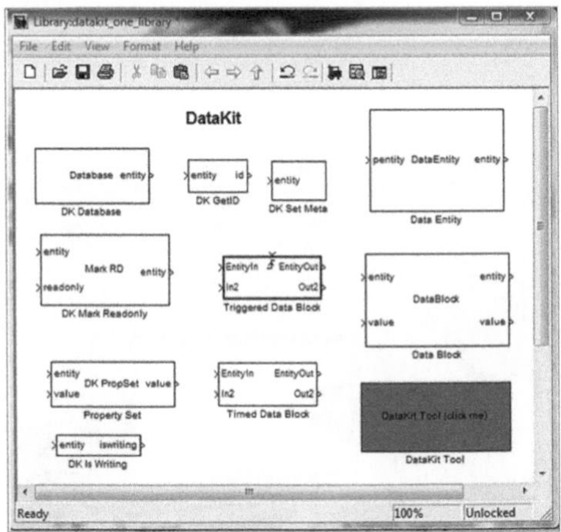

Figure 14.14 Example of data processing (*left*; from Portillo-Rodriguez et al. [2008]) and graphical user interface in Simulink (*right*; from Avizzano [2009]). From Portillo-Rodriguez, O., C. Sandoval-Gonzalez; A. Avizzano, E. Ruffaldi, D. Vercelli, and M. Bergamasco. 2008. *Development of a 3D real time gesture recognition methodology for virtual environment control.* In the 17th IEEE International Symposium on Robot and Human Interactive Communication RO-MAN, 279–84; and Avizzano, C.A., E. Ruffaldi, and V. Lippi. 2009. *Skills Digital Representation and Storage,* SKILLS09 International Conference on Multimodal Interfaces for Skills Transfer, Bilbao, Spain, with permission of the publishers.

learning accelerators according to the theories of sensorimotor learning by Schoner and Kelso (1988).

EXPERIMENTAL CASE STUDIES

Several types of demonstrators that exploit such a paradigm have been developed recently. In particular, this methodology has presently been applied to two specific domains: rowing and juggling. The *SPRINT rowing system* (Ruffaldi et al. 2009) is a platform for indoor rowing training that is aimed at improving the specific subskills of rowing. The system has as its basis a simulation component that recreates the motion of the user and provides a haptic feedback mirroring interaction with the water (see Fig. 14.15). Over the simulation basis, a set of exercises based on multimodal feedback for training specific subskills is built: technique procedure, energy management, and coordination. Relevant expert data has been collected by tracking the angles of the oars, the trolley position, the exerted forces, and the head position. Data segmentation and clustering made it possible to identify the path that is most efficient for both boat motion and user physiology. The path has been segmented by taking the major elements of a rowing stroke into account (see Fig. 14.16 for an example), and successively modeling these in a pseudo-parametric form, in order to adapt to the different sizes of the users.

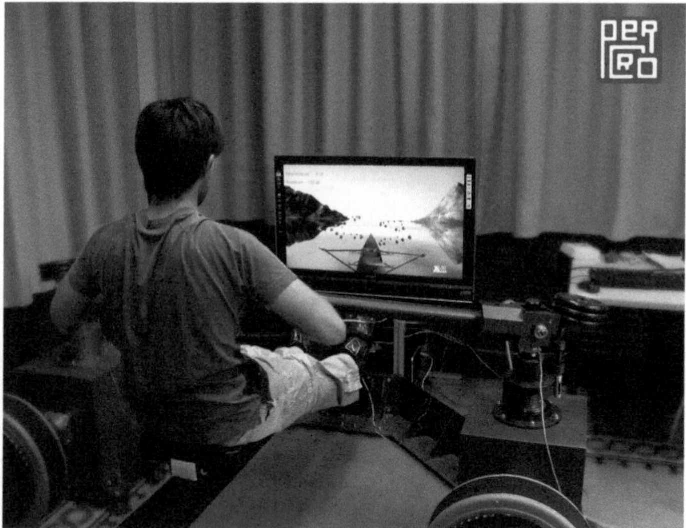

Figure 14.15 Photography of the rowing training system SPRINT.

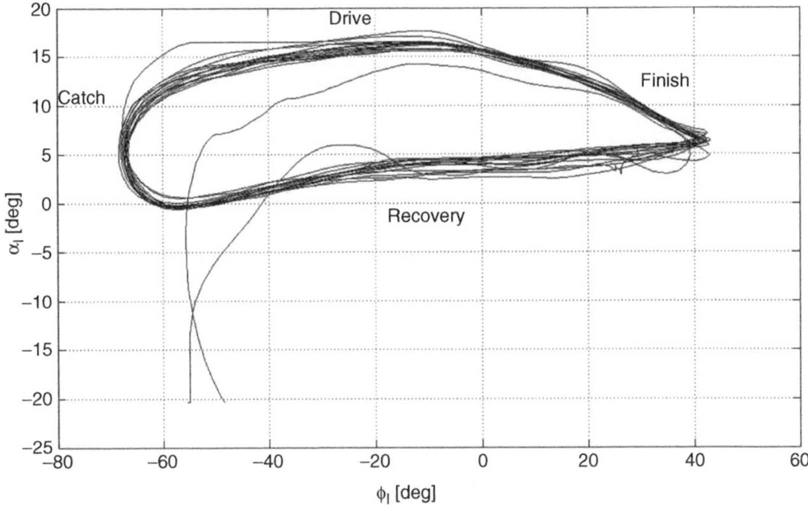

Figure 14.16 Sample trajectory of a rowing cycle shown in the space of the fundamental oars angles (tilt vs. swing).

This model is then used for training purposes. Two types of feedback, one based on the visual presentation of the trajectory (both in real-time and after the task) and the other in the form of vibrotactile feedback, show the user his or her motion errors.

In the *juggling trainer*, a VE has been designed to improve the technique of the juggler in performing specific tricks. The training elements considered as relevant for training were spatial coordination properties, as well as timing synchronization. The trainer provides two types of platform: a purely visual guidance that uses Polhemus sensors and VR-based animation to represent hands, balls, motion, and training stimuli, and a haptic training platform based on encountered-type haptic interfaces (Tripicchio et al. 2009; shown in Fig. 14.17. Here, a couple of symmetric haptic devices serve to present the relevant stimuli to left and right hands as they catch balls. The training system simulates ball trajectories and coordinates the robotic devices to improve the control of sensorimotor coordination.

CONCLUSION

Novel multimodal interactive systems enable researchers to develop integrated systems that handle sophisticated interaction protocols within the interaction loops. In the case of training systems, this is achieved by integrating the existing knowledge on required motions and experts' samples

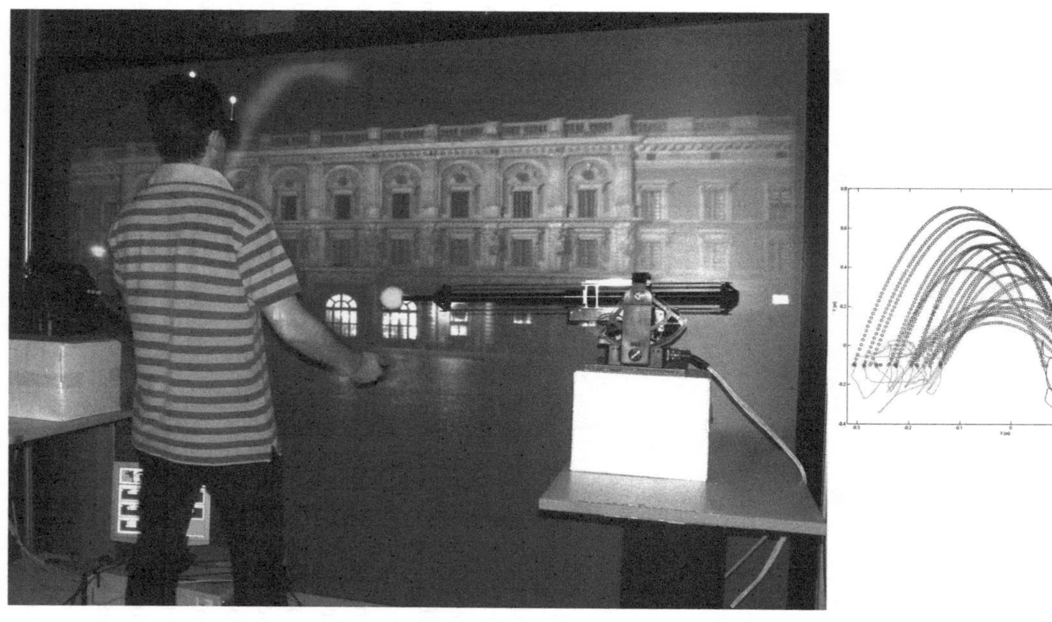

Figure 14.17 Juggling virtual trainer. An integrated visuo-haptic platform, on the left, interacts to show the user correct motion sequences. Raw data plot of hands and balls tracking are reported on the right. From Bardy, B.G., C.A. Avizzano C.A., et al. 2008. Introduction to the Skills project and its theoretical framework. *IDMME-Virtual Concept*, Berlin: Springer-Verlag.

with a proper feedback that stimulates user perception without disturbing the main components of the perception action loop. Here, we presented an integrated architecture to merge present VE systems with known learning and interaction models. In particular, the proposed architecture highlights the presence and the core role of a digital trainer, a software tutor that senses user actions and controls the configuration parameters of a VE to facilitate and accelerate learning.

The methodology to design the digital trainer has been discussed by correlating the technical constraints to the human factors considered relevant. The resulting process has shown the necessity of introducing a new concept into the control design: the digital skill, a mathematical entity that links the data required for the technical implementation and the information handled by trainers, experts, and researchers on human factors. The current work has also shown how the information required for the digital skill can be extracted from experts' examples by the adoption of existing machine learning and control tools. The implementation of these concepts on two platforms developed in the context of the EU-SKILLS integrated project have also been shown.

REFERENCES

Abbott, J., and A. Okamura. 2007. Pseudo-admittance bilateral telemanipulation with guidance virtual fixtures. *International Journal of Robotics Research* 26: 865–71.

Adams, R., and B. Hannaford. 1999. Stable haptic interaction with virtual environments. *IEEE Transactions on Robotics and Automation* 15:465–74.

Aggarwal, R., J. Ward, I. Balasundaram, P. Sains, T. Athanasiou, and A. Darzi. 2007. Proving the effectiveness of virtual reality simulation for training in laparoscopic surgery. *Annals of Surgery* 246:771–76.

Avizzano, C.A., E. Ruffaldi, and V. Lippi. 2009. *Skills Digital Representation and Storage*, In Proceedings of SKILLS09 International Conference on Multimodal Interfaces for Skills Transfer, Bilbao, Spain. ISBN:978-84-613-5456-5.

Avizzano, C.A., M. Raspolli, S. Marcheschi, and M. Bergamasco. 2005. Haptic desktop for office automation and assisted design. In Proceedings of *IEEE International Conference on Robotics and Automation* 4086–91, Barcelona.

Barraclough, A., I. Guymer. Virtual Reality 1998. -A Role In Environmental Engineering Education?. Wien: Water Science & Technology, Vol. 38(11): 303–310.

Bardy, B.G., C.A. Avizzano. et al. 2008. Introduction to the Skills Project and its theoretical framework. *IDMME-Virtual Concept*, Berlin: Springer.

Behr, J., and A. Froehlich. 1998. AVALON, an open VRML VR/AR system for dynamic application. *Computer Graphics Topics* 10:28–30.

Bergamasco, M. 1995. Force replication to the human operator: The development of arm and hand exoskeletons as haptic interfaces. In *Robotics Research*, eds., G. Giralt and H. Hirzinger. Berlin: Springer.

Brooks, F.P., M. Ouh-Young, J.J. Batter, and P.J. Kilpatrick. 1990. Project GROPE - haptic displays for scientific visualization. *Computer Graphics* 24:177–85.

Calinon, S., F. Guenter, and A. Billard. 2006. On learning, representing and generalizing a task in a humanoid robot. *IEEE Transactions on Systems, Man and Cybernetics* 37:286–98.

Carbonell, J. 1970. AI in CAI: An artificial-intelligence approach to computer-assisted instruction. *IEEE Transactions on Man-machine Systems* 11:190–202.

Clark, F.J., K.W. Horch. 1986. Kinesthesia. In *Handbook of human perception and performance*, Vol. I, eds., B.F. Boff, L.L. Kaufman and J.P. Thomas. New York: John Wiley & Sons.

Davis, J., and H. Gao. 2003. Recognizing human action efforts: An adaptive three-mode PCA framework. *Computer Vision Proceedings* 1463–69.

Esen, H., K. Yano, and M. Buss. 2008. Force skill training with hybrid trainer model. In Proceedings of *IEEE International Workshop on Robot and Human Interactive Communication Proceedings* 9–14. ISBN: 978-1-4244-2212-8.

Feygin, D., M. Keehner, and R. Tendick. 2002. Haptic guidance: Experimental evaluation of a haptic training method for a perceptual motor skill. Haptic Interfaces for Virtual Environment and Teleoperator Systems Proceedings 40–47, ISBN: 0-7695-1489-8.

Fitts, P., and M. Posner. 1967. *Human performance.* Brooks/Cole Publishing Co.

Frisoli, A., C.A. Avizzano, E. Ruffaldi, A. Filippeschi, and M. Bergamasco. 2008. Preliminary design of rowing simulator for in-door skill training. In Proceedings of *Ambient Media and Systems.*, ICST Brussels.

Frisoli, A., C.A. Avizzano, and M. Bergamasco. 2001. Simulation of a manual gear-shift with a 2 DOF force-feedback joystick. In Proceedings of *International Conference of Robotics and Automation.* 2:1364–1369. Seoul, Korea.

Gagné, R. 1972. *Interchange, in domains of learning* 87–105. Berlin: Springer.

Gibson, E. 1969. *Principles of perceptual learning and development.* New York: Prentice Hall.

Gillespie, R., S. O'Modhrain, P. Tang, D. Zaretzky, and C. Pham. 1998. The virtual teacher. In Proceedings of *ASME International Mechanical Engineering Conference and Exposition, Dynamic Systems and Control* 171–178.

Gritai, A., Y. Sheikh, and M. Shah. 2004. On the use of anthropometry in the invariant analysis of human actions. *International Conference on Pattern Recognition Proceedings* 2:923–26. ISBN: 0-7695-2128-2.

Henmi, K., and T. Yoshikawa. 1998. Virtual lesson and its application to virtual calligraphy system. In Proceedings of *IEEE International Conference on Robotics and Automation,* Leuven, Belgium. 2:1275–1280

Johansson, G. 1973. -Visual perception of biological motion and a model for its analysis. *Perception & Psycholophysics, 14,* 201–211. Lawrence Erlbaum

Johnson, W., J. Rickel, and J. Lester. 2000. Animated pedagogical agents: Face-to-face interaction in interactive learning environments. *International Journal of Artificial Intelligence in Education* 11:47–78.

Kimura, H., T. Horiuchi, and K. Ikeuchi. 1999. Task-model based human robot cooperation using vision. In Proceedings of *IEEE International Conference on Intelligent Robots and Systems Proceedings* 2:701–706. ISBN: 0-7803-5184-3

Klatzky, R., S. Lederman, and C. Reed. 1989. Haptic integration of object properties: Texture, hardness, and planar contour. *Journal of Experimental Psychology: Human Perception and Performance* 15:45–57.

Lee, W., and D. Owens. 2004. *Multimedia-based instructional design: Computer-based training, web-based training, distance broadcast training, performance-based solutions.* New York: John Wiley and Sons.

Li, Y., J. Huegel, V. Patoglu, and M. O'Malley. 2009. Progressive shared control for training in virtual environments. *World Haptics Proceedings,* IEEE Computer Society: 332–37, Salt Lake City. ISBN: 978-1-4244-3858-7.

Marcheschi, S., A. Frisoli, C.A. Avizzano, and M. Bergamasco. 2005. A method for modeling and control complex tendon transmissions in haptic interfaces. In Proceedings of *IEEE International Conference on Robotics and Automation Proceedings* 1773–78, Barcelona. ISBN: 0-7803-8914-X.

Minsky, M., M. Ouh-Young, O. Steele, F.P. Brooks, and M. Behensky. 1990. Feeling and seeing: Issues in force display. *Computer Graphics* 24:235–43.

Moorthy, K., Y. Munz, S. Sarker, and A. Darzi. 2003. Objective assessment of technical skills in surgery. *British Medical Journal* 327:1032–37.

Owens, M. 2006. *The definitive guide to SQLite.* Berkeley, CA: Apress. doi: 10.1007/978-1-4302-0172-4.

PhysX. 2008. AGEIA.

Reber, A. 1996. *Implicit learning and tacit knowledge: An essay on the cognitive unconscious.* New York: Oxford University Press.

Rosen, J., B. Hannaford, C. Richards, and M. Sinanan. 2001. Markov modeling of minimally invasive surgery based on tool/tissue interaction and force/torque signatures for evaluating surgical skills. *IEEE transactions on Biomedical Engineering* 48:579–91.

Rosenberg, L.B. 1993. Virtual fixtures: Perceptual tools for telerobotic manipulation. In Proceedings of *Virtual Reality Annual Symposium* 76–82, ISBN: 0-7803-1363-1.

Ruddle, R., and S. Lessels. 2006. Three levels of metric for evaluating wayfinding. *Presence: Teleoperators and Virtual Environments* 15:637–54.

Ruffaldi, E. 2006. Haptic web: Haptic rendering and interaction with XVR. In *Proceedings of XVR Workshop*. Pisa: VRmedia.

Ruffaldi, E., A. Filippeschi, A. Frisoli, O. Sandoval, C.A. Avizzano, and M. Bergamasco. 2009. Vibrotactile perception assessment for a rowing training system. *World Haptics Proceedings,* IEEE Computer Society: 350–355, ISBN: 978-1-4244-3858-7.

Salisbury, K., F. Conti, and F. Barbagli. 2004. Haptic rendering: Introductory concepts. *IEEE Computer Graphics and Applications 24(2):* 24–32.

Sano, A., H. Fujimoto, and K. Matsushita. 1999. Machine mediated training based on coaching. *IEEE System, Man, and Cybernetics Proceedings* 2:1070–75.

Schoner, G., and J. Kelso. 1988. Dynamic pattern generation in behavioral and neural systems. *Science* 239:1513.

Sutherland, L., P. Middleton, A. Anthony, J. Hamdorf, P. Cregan, D. Scott, and G. Maddern. 2006. Surgical simulation: A systematic review. *Annals of Surgery* 243:291–99.

Tripicchio, P., E. Ruffaldi, C.A. Avizzano, and M. Bergamasco. 2008. Virtual laboratory: A virtual distributed platform to share and perform experiments. *Haptic Interfaces for Virtual Environment and Teleoperator Systems* 311–18, ISBN: 978-1-4244-2005-6.

Tripicchio, P., E. Ruffaldi, C.A. Avizzano, and M. Bergamasco. 2009. Control strategies and perception effects in co-located and large workspace dynamical encountered haptics. *World Haptics Proc.* IEEE Computer Society 63–68.

Troje, N. 2008. *Retrieving information from human movement patterns.* New York: Oxford University Press.

Vasilescu, M. 2002. Human motion signatures: Analysis, synthesis, recognition. In Proceedings of *International Conference on Pattern Recognition* 3:456–60, ISBN: 0-7695-1695-X.

Warren, W. 2006. The dynamics of perception and action. *Psychological Review* 113:358–89.

Yokokohji, Y., R. Hollis, T. Kanade, K. Henmi, and T. Yoshikawa. 1996. Toward machine mediated training of motor skills. Skill transfer from human to human via virtual environment. In Proceedings of *IEEE International Workshop on Robot and Human Communication Proceedings* 5:32–37, ISBN: 0-7803-3253-9.

Zilles, C., and J. Salisbury. 1995. A Constraint-based God-object method for haptic display. In Proceedings of *International Conference on Intelligent Robots and Systems Proceedings* 3(3):3146–52, ISBN:0-8186-7108-4.

Part 5

Lessons from Studies of Aging and Motor Disorders

15

Brain and Behavior Deficits in De Novo Parkinson Disease

David E. Vaillancourt and Janey Prodoehl

BRIEF TUTORIAL: BASAL GANGLIA FUNCTION IN PARKINSON DISEASE

Parkinson disease (PD) is an insidious disease that affects motor, cognitive, and emotional brain systems. The prevalence of PD varies from study to study based on differences in methodology, but most estimates suggest an overall prevalence ranging from 100 to 200 per 100,000 (Marras and Tanner 2004). Some estimates suggest that over the next 25 years, the number of individuals over the age of 50 who are diagnosed with PD will exceed 8.5 million worldwide (Dorsey et al. 2007). Comparing healthy age-matched individuals to individuals with PD, the mortality rate is two to five times higher for individuals with PD (Bennett et al. 1996; Morens et al. 1996; Louis et al. 1997), which means that PD patients have a shorter life expectancy (Morens et al. 1996; Morgante et al. 2000). The cost of treating PD will likely increase unless preventative measures can be put in place that either slow or stop its progression (Weintraub et al. 2008).

The classic motor symptoms of PD include bradykinesia, tremor, and rigidity, and it is hypothesized that these symptoms are due to abnormal functioning of the basal ganglia-thalamo-cortical circuit. Within the basal ganglia lies the substantia nigra pars compacta, which provides massive dopaminergic input into the striatum (putamen and caudate). In PD, the dopaminergic neurons in the substantia nigra pars compacta are progressively lost, and it is estimated that at least 50% of the cells die before the motor symptoms become apparent (Braak et al. 2003; Hodaie et al. 2007). The death of dopaminergic cells leads to reduced levels of dopamine in the striatum, and it is estimated that, upon clinical expression of PD, at least 80% of the striatal dopamine has already been depleted (Hodaie et al. 2007). Although the exact mechanisms underlying dopaminergic cell death are unknown, many scientists believe that nigral neuronal death is initiated by the interaction of environmental neurotoxins and a genetic predisposition that could induce mitochondrial dysfunction and oxidative damage in nigra neurons, which are thought to die from apoptosis (Anglade et al. 1997; Olanow and Tatton 1999; Mizuno et al. 2004).

The consequences of dopaminergic cell death in the pars compacta of the substantia nigra is a disturbance of activity in the basal ganglia circuitry that manifests behaviorally as motor deficits. The basal ganglia circuitry is a collection of interconnected nuclei—substantia nigra pars reticulate (SNr), substantia nigra pars compacta (SNc), caudate, putamen, internal globus pallidus (GPi), external globus pallidus (GPe), and subthalamic nucleus (STN)—which have an indirect but important influence on motor function. In the basal ganglia circuitry, the striatum (caudate and putamen) receives excitatory input from the cortex, and it, in turn, inhibits the output from GPi and SNr. This is termed the *direct pathway*, and activity here results in reduced inhibitory output from GPi and SNr onto the thalamocortical circuitry, thereby increasing the thalamocortical drive (Albin et al. 1989; DeLong 1990; DeLong and Wichmann 2007). In contrast, the *indirect pathway* inhibits voluntary movement by reducing the thalamocortical drive. In this pathway, the striatum inhibits GPe, which results in reduced inhibition of STN. The STN makes an excitatory projection and contacts GPi and SNr (DeLong and Wichmann 2007). Increased excitation of GPi and SNr results in increased inhibitory output from these nuclei to the thalamus, thereby reducing the thalamocortical drive.

Dopamine, a neurotransmitter, is required to preserve the balance in neuronal output from the direct and indirect basal ganglia pathways. In the basal ganglia circuitry, two types of receptors at the striatum are integral binding sites for dopamine—the D_1 and D_2 receptors. Release of dopamine that influences the direct pathway occurs via activation of the D_1 receptors, whereas activation of the D_2 receptors tends to inhibit the indirect pathway. Both D_1 and D_2 receptors are located in the dendritic spines of striatal output neurons, thereby allowing dopamine to modulate corticostriatal signals. Since dopamine has a differential effect on these two types of receptors (i.e., it exerts an excitatory influence on D_1 receptors and an inhibitory influence on D_2 receptors), a lack of dopamine will cause corticostriatal signals to be abnormal. The end result of a dopaminergic deficit is an abnormal balance of inhibition and excitation between the direct and indirect striatopallidal circuit, which results in abnormal motor control. This theoretical perspective has led to the development of new pharmacological agents that increase dopamine activity in the nigrostriatal pathway (Poewe et al. 2004), and has also led to new surgical interventions, such as deep brain stimulation, which aim to modify brain activity in these pathways (Perlmutter and Mink 2006). Next, we discuss the animal models of PD that have been developed and that underlie this theoretical model, and present a major problem confronting future PD research for both animal and human studies.

PROBLEM: RELATING ANIMAL MODELS OF THE BASAL GANGLIA TO HUMANS WITH PD

A little over half a century has passed since dopamine was identified as a neurotransmitter, and it was recognized that depleting monoamines in the brain via administration of reserpine caused hunched immobility in rodents (Carlsson et al. 1957). It was also shown that levodopa, a precursor to the neurotransmitter dopamine, could reverse some of the effects that reserpine induced in the rodents (Carlsson 1959). The use of reserpine as a rodent model of PD, however, is transient, and does not induce the pathological features typically seen in humans with PD. Another rodent model of PD has also proven very useful. When 6-hydroxydopamine (6-OHDA), a neurotoxin, is injected into the substantia nigra, medial forebrain, or striatum, degeneration occurs in the nigrostriatal pathway and striatal dopamine is reduced (Ungerstedt 1968; Ungerstedt and Arbuthnott 1970). Although the symptoms of the 6-OHDA rodent model of PD do not reflect those of humans with PD, and it can actually induce circling behaviors not seen in humans, the model has allowed significant advances in drug development (Jenner 2008). In fact, the 6-OHDA rodent model is highly predictive of the effects of dopaminergic drugs in humans, and has been suggested as a model for studying dyskinesias, an unfortunate side effect of levodopa therapy consisting of involuntary and uncontrolled jerky body and limb movements (Papa et al. 1994; Lindgren et al. 2007).

A more influential experimental model of PD has been the 1-methyl-4-phenyl-1,2,3,6-tetrahydropyridine (MPTP) model in nonhuman primates (Davis et al. 1979; Langston et al. 1983). The original discovery of MPTP came surprisingly in humans, when seven young adults took experimental drugs that were contaminated with MPTP. These seven adults subsequently developed parkinsonism, and the discovery that MPTP was the culprit led to the development of the MPTP model of PD in nonhuman primates that is commonly used today (Langston et al. 1983; Kordower et al. 2000). Injecting MPTP into the carotid artery of a nonhuman primate will cause significant death of dopaminergic neurons in the substantia nigra and cause the animal to develop most symptoms that mimic PD. In addition, the drugs used to treat humans with PD also have positive effects for treating symptoms in the nonhuman primate rendered parkinsonian by MPTP. Although initial studies using MPTP in rodents were not successful, in recent years, a rodent model of PD using MPTP has been further developed and refined (Jackson-Lewis and Przedborski 2007).

Despite the fact that animal models of PD have led to the development of symptomatic therapies for treating PD, these models have been far less successful for developing neuroprotective drugs for PD. A neuroprotective drug is one designed to prevent the disease from occurring or progressing. There may be several reasons for this lack of progress. First, although useful for drug development, the 6-OHDA rodent model of PD does not produce symptoms of PD, and the MPTP model in nonhuman primates does not typically induce tremor in the animals. Although tremor does not occur in all patients with PD, it does occur in the majority of patients with PD, and tremor can be a disabling symptom (Elble and Koller 1990). Second, most animal models produce a sudden loss of dopaminergic neurons selectively in the substantia nigra, whereas developing PD occurs over many years through progressive and gradual loss of dopaminergic neurons in the substantia nigra and other brainstem areas (Braak et al. 2003). Third, humans with PD have degeneration in areas of the cortex and brainstem that are not always mimicked through the 6-OHDA and MPTP animal models of PD. Fourth, following the diagnosis of PD, the symptoms of a patient will progress over time, whereas most animal models of PD are not progressive. As such, there is a need for new animal models of PD that mimic the progression of PD in humans. At the same time, it is important to study PD in humans to understand how PD develops in the early stages of the disease before drug therapy has begun—so called de novo PD. Although a few studies have compared de novo PD to levodopa-treated PD, it is not always clear what changes are due to disease progression in these disparate groups and what changes are due to chronic exposure to levodopa (Marsden 1994; Ellis et al. 1997; Hershey et al. 2003). In addition, there is a need to understand how PD progresses from the de novo state to moderate and advanced PD.

Although there have been a substantial number of behavioral motor control and brain imaging studies in humans with PD (Grafton 2004; van Eimeren and Siebner 2006), the vast majority of these studies have focused on patients already treated by dopaminergic therapy who have advanced symptoms. Far less is known about how motor control is affected in de novo PD, and how brain structure and function is affected in de novo PD. As such, the problem addressed in this chapter examines what is currently known about behavioral deficits, brain structure, and brain function in de novo PD. The following sections examine how both nonmotor and motor behavior are affected in de novo PD, and how various electrophysiological and neuroimaging techniques have shed light on how PD affects the basal ganglia and cortex prior to patients beginning drug treatment.

REVIEW: STUDIES OF DE NOVO PD USING BEHAVIORAL, ELECTROPHYSIOLOGICAL, AND BRAIN IMAGING METHODS

Behavioral Nonmotor Studies in De Novo PD

Although PD has classically been described as a motor disorder, many studies have clearly shown that nonmotor symptoms are also present

(Chaudhuri et al. 2006; Chaudhuri and Naidu 2008). The nonmotor symptoms include neuropsychiatric symptoms (depression, cognitive dysfunction, hallucinations, dementia, confusion), sleep disorders (restless leg syndrome, rapid eye movement sleep disorders, insomnia), autonomic symptoms (bladder disturbances, sweating, orthostatic hypotension, erectile impotence), gastrointestinal symptoms (dribbling of saliva, dysphagia, constipation, nausea), fatigue, and sensory symptoms (pain, paraesthesia, visual dysfunction, olfactory disturbances) (Chaudhuri and Schapira 2009). These nonmotor symptoms may be a consequence of dopaminergic and other pharmacological treatments that PD patients receive. Alternatively, these nonmotor symptoms may be related to dopaminergic dysfunction inherent to PD in areas such as the ventral tegmental area and hypothalamus. For instance, a recent study using positron emission tomography showed that PD patients had reduced binding of ^{11} C-raclopride in the hypothalamus (Politis et al. 2008). Such findings point to the potential that some nonmotor features of PD may be due to the inherent degeneration of subcortical regions that occur with the natural course of PD. Several recent studies have investigated some of these nonmotor features in de novo PD.

Aarsland and colleagues (2009) studied neuropsychiatric issues in recently diagnosed PD patients who were untreated in four counties spanning western and southern Norway. The Neuropsychiatric Inventory (NPI) was administered to 175 PD patients and 166 healthy control subjects with a similar age and sex. The overall proportion of individuals with NPI symptoms was significantly higher in patients with PD (56%) compared with control subjects (22%). In the patients with PD, depression (37%), apathy (27%), sleep disturbances (18%), and anxiety (17%) were the most common nonmotor symptoms. What seems most important was that, when thresholds were used to identify clinically significant symptoms, 22% of PD patients had clinically significant symptoms versus only 3% of healthy control subjects.

Olfaction has been one of the most widely studied nonmotor features of PD. In studies that focus on treated PD patients at differing stages of disease progression, it has been shown that up to 90% of PD patients have some form of olfactory impairment (Katzenschlager and Lees 2004). Also, population-based studies have identified that olfactory dysfunction seems to occur in patients not yet diagnosed as having PD. For instance, olfaction was assessed in 2,267 elderly subjects without PD and dementia in the Honolulu Heart Program (Ross et al. 2008). After 8 years, 35 of the subjects developed PD, and these individuals scored in the lower quartile range of the odor identification test. In addition, there were 164 patients who later died without being diagnosed as having PD and these patients underwent postmortem examination. Of these individuals, 17 had incidental Lewy bodies in the substantia nigra and locus coeruleus, and these patients had a mean odor detection score that was significantly lower than the subjects without incidental Lewy bodies at autopsy (Ross et al. 2006). Along with the loss of dopaminergic neurons, the presence of Lewy bodies is the main pathological hallmark of clinical PD (Hughes et al. 2002). In a study of both de novo PD and treated PD, olfaction was tested and compared with a healthy control group (Tissingh et al. 2001). The authors found that both de novo and treated PD patients scored significantly lower on all olfactory tests. In addition, within the PD group, there was a significant relation between odor discrimination and measures of disease severity.

In a study of reward learning and novelty-seeking personality, newly diagnosed de novo patients with PD were studied (Bodi et al. 2009). Patients recently treated with a dopamine agonist (a medication that directly stimulates the receptors in nerves in the brain that normally would be stimulated by dopamine) and healthy control subjects were studied (Bodi et al. 2009). The task used in the study was a feedback-based probabilistic classification task. The de novo patients were also evaluated after 12 weeks of treatment with dopamine agonists. The authors found that de novo PD patients had selective deficits on reward-processing and novelty-seeking aspects of the task. In addition, dopamine agonists increased novelty seeking, enhanced reward processing, and decreased punishment-processing behaviors.

In summary, the nonmotor features of PD are becoming more apparent to movement disorders specialists (Chaudhuri and Schapira 2009). Despite the heightened awareness among movement disorders specialists however, this level of awareness has not reached the general public or health-care professionals. For instance, a recent survey showed that up to 62% of nonmotor symptoms of PD may go unreported because patients are either embarrassed or because they are unaware that these symptoms may be related to PD (Chaudhuri and Schapira 2009). It remains to be determined to what extent the motor and nonmotor features of PD have a common or separate underlying pathophysiology.

Behavioral Motor Control Studies in De Novo PD

A limited number of behavioral studies have shown that de novo PD patients have significant motor deficits compared to controls even in the very early stages of disease. One study found that PD patients are impaired relative to controls when performing complex unimanual upper limb motor tasks such as hand writing, pointing, and aiming (Ponsen et al. 2008). During the writing task, for example, PD patients had a reduced sentence length, writing velocity, and letter height compared to controls. Unlike controls, PD patients performed the aiming task more slowly when moving to a target than when moving beyond a target, and patients were less accurate than controls during the pointing task (Ponsen et al. 2008). The authors have also studied complex upper limb movements and found that de novo PD patients had impaired coordination relative to controls during a bimanual circle-drawing task (Ponsen et al. 2006). Specifically, PD patients had a significantly higher percentage of unsuccessful trials compared to controls and were less accurate with their nondominant hand. Also, when subjects were required to perform antiphase movements at low frequency (i.e., 1 Hz), PD patients had greater difficulty in keeping both hands in the antiphase coordination pattern (Ponsen et al. 2006).

Other work has found that, compared to controls, de novo PD patients exhibit kinematic deficits and abnormalities in muscle activation during a simpler task, such as rapid elbow flexion movements of different distances (Pfann et al. 2001). This study found that the elbow movements of PD patients had lower peak velocity than controls, and that PD patients showed a reduced ability to scale movement velocity as movement distance increased. Analysis of electromyographic (EMG) data revealed that de novo PD patients have specific deficits in modulating the first agonist burst in response to task demands, and that the timing of the antagonist burst becomes impaired in patients with greater disease severity (Pfann et al. 2001).

Figure 15.1 shows a schematic representing the hypothesized EMG modulation for the control of movement distance with the onset of PD and

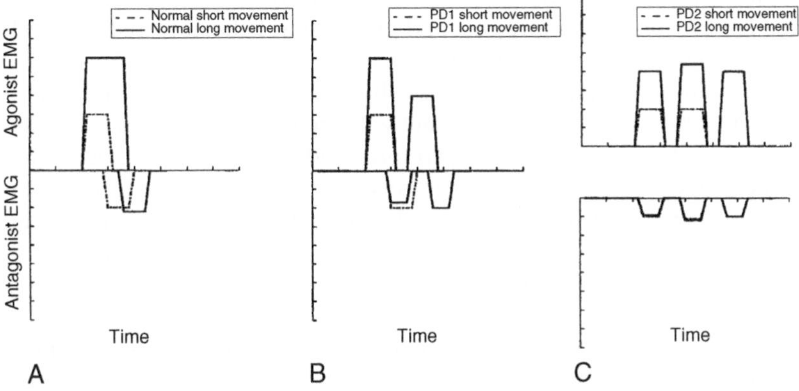

Figure 15.1 Schematic of changes in electromyographic (EMG) modulation with disease progression. Each plot shows a schematic of agonist and antagonist EMG for a short (*dot-dash line*) and long (*solid line*) movement. **A**: EMG modulation typical of healthy subjects: an increase in magnitude and duration of the agonist burst and a delay in the antagonist burst for the longer movement. **B**: Changes that occur relatively early in PD: a loss of duration modulation and an increase in the number of EMG bursts. **C**: Changes that occur later in PD: a decrease in agonist magnitude, a possible further increase in the number of bursts, a decrease in antagonist EMG magnitude, and a shift in the timing of the antagonist activity relative to the timing of the agonist activity. The agonist and antagonist EMGs are separated in plot 3 to suggest that we do not know whether or not these changes all emerge at the same time or at different times in terms of disease progression. Adapted from Pfann, K.D., A.S. Buchman, C.L. Comella, and D.M. Corcos. 2001. Control of movement distance in Parkinson's disease. *Movement Disorders* 16: 1048–65, with permission of the publisher.

increased severity of PD. The left panel shows the typical EMG modulation for a short and long movement distance in the agonist and antagonist muscle of a healthy individual. What is evident is that healthy subjects should be able to increase the duration of the EMG agonist burst and amplitude of the EMG agonist burst for a long distance compared with a short distance. In patients with early PD (Fig. 15.1B), the model predicts that duration modulation is impaired, and that PD patients are only able to scale the amplitude of the EMG burst. In addition, multiple EMG bursts may become present in early-stage de novo PD. Additional EMG bursts create additional muscle force, which can help the patient move the limb to the target. In advanced PD, several changes in the EMG are hypothesized. Figure 15.1C predicts that the agonist amplitude would be decreased, there would be an additional increase in the number of agonist bursts, a decrease in the amplitude of the antagonist EMG signal, and an increase in the overlap of the agonist and antagonist burst. Interestingly, it has been shown that all of the features of advanced PD predicted in Figure 15.1C are modified by both deep brain stimulation of the STN and levodopa therapy (Vaillancourt et al. 2004).

In addition to limb movement deficits, recent models of the basal ganglia have incorporated gripping and grasping as behaviors that are modified by the basal ganglia (Prodoehl et al. 2009). In a study of de novo PD, Fellows and colleagues (2004) have shown that grip force abnormalities exist in patients who did not present with tremor. The authors found that the time between the onset of grip force and the lift-off of an object was greater for de novo PD than for controls. PD patients also produced higher grip force amplitude than did controls during both the lifting and holding phases of the task. The authors concluded that the grip force abnormalities are intrinsic features of PD and are not the consequence of dyskinesias or tremor.

A diagnostic test battery has been developed that includes tests of motor function, olfaction, and mood (Montgomery et al. 2000a). Using the test battery, Montgomery and colleagues (2000b) have studied patients with mild symptoms who did not yet meet diagnostic criteria for PD. For the motor function tests, patients performed wrist flexion and extension movements to different targets, and movement velocity was recorded. Olfaction was measured using the University of Pennsylvania Smell Identification Test. Mood was assessed using the Beck Depression Inventory. The authors studied 194 patients for 1 year. Of these patients, 59 were subsequently diagnosed with PD, 40 as neurologically normal, and the remaining 106 were deemed to have a neurological condition other than PD. In total, the test battery was 92% specific and 68% sensitive for PD, and the area under the receiver operator characteristics (ROC) curve was 0.88 for predicting the development of PD. It seems likely therefore that diagnostically, success may come from consideration of both the nonmotor and motor features of the disease.

In summary, previous work demonstrates that de novo PD patients exhibit both motor and nonmotor deficits. The nonmotor deficits can range from depression, apathy, sleep disturbances, anxiety, olfactory disturbances, and deficits in reward-learning and novelty-seeking behaviors. The motor deficits in de novo PD have been shown during a variety of motor tasks that include handwriting, bimanual coordination, elbow flexion and extension, wrist flexion and extension, and grip force control. The fact that the patients in these studies have never been exposed to antiparkinsonian medication confirms that the deficits in motor control are intrinsic features of PD and are not due to medication exposure. Moreover, as shown in Figure 15.1, the presence of abnormalities in the EMG of de novo patients suggests that the neural control of muscle activation is deficient in de novo PD. This raises questions about whether changes in brain structure and function also occur in the early stages of PD, before patients begin a medication regimen. The next section reviews the current understanding of brain abnormalities in de novo PD from electrophysiological studies of brain activity.

ELECTROPHYSIOLOGICAL STUDIES IN DE NOVO PD

Electroencephalography (EEG) and transcranial magnetic stimulation (TMS) are two electrophysiological techniques that have been used to examine cortical function in de novo PD. One EEG experiment used a "flanker task" to investigate event-related potentials related to error-processing mechanisms in de novo PD patients and healthy controls (Beste et al. 2009). Beste and colleagues (2009) found that the amplitude of the error-related negativity of the event-related potential was significantly reduced in PD patients compared to controls. Using TMS, Pierantozzi and colleagues (2001) showed that, compared to healthy control subjects, de novo PD patients had significantly reduced early and late cortical inhibition. This abnormal inhibition could be reversed by acute administration of apomorphine, a dopamine receptor agonist, thus suggesting that abnormal cortical inhibitory mechanisms in early PD may be associated with altered cortical and/or subcortical dopaminergic transmission. Also using TMS, Cantello and colleagues (2007) showed that, compared to controls, de novo PD patients exhibited a late long-latency cortical inhibition peak that was absent among controls. This pathological enhancement of late long-latency cortical inhibition is also found in patients with more advanced PD and has been suggested to have a pathological role in the impairment of rapid, sequential voluntary movements in PD (Berardelli et al. 1996). In addition, abnormal cortical inhibitory mechanisms have been suggested as underlying abnormal voluntary muscle relaxation in de novo PD (Labyt et al. 2005).

Repetitive TMS (rTMS) has been used to examine cortical excitability in de novo PD. Buhman and others (2004) used rTMS to examine cortical excitability in de novo PD and found that, at an intermediate interstimulus interval of 5 ms, rTMS over the premotor cortex led to reduced excitability in the primary motor cortex in de novo PD. In contrast, healthy control subjects showed increased cortical excitability following rTMS. These results suggest an abnormal modifiability in the premotor–motor connections in early stage PD. Taken together, these findings from electrophysiological studies in de novo PD suggest changes in cortical excitability and inhibition early on in the disease. However, these techniques do not allow examination of deeper subcortical structures. To that end, various brain imaging techniques have been developed and utilized in the examination of brain structure and function in de novo PD.

BRAIN IMAGING STUDIES IN DE NOVO PD

Numerous techniques have been developed to investigate brain function over the past several decades. Studies have begun to utilize many of these different brain imaging techniques to characterize the changes in brain structure and function in de novo PD, particularly in the deeper subcortical regions where PD is thought to originate. These techniques include magnetic resonance spectroscopy, positron emission tomography (PET), single-photon emission computerized tomography (SPECT), voxel-based morphometry, functional magnetic resonance imaging (fMRI), and diffusion tensor imaging (DTI). Findings from de novo PD studies utilizing each of these techniques are discussed below.

Within the basal ganglia, Ellis and colleagues (1997) used magnetic resonance spectroscopy to investigate whether significant metabolic changes occurred in the putamen of de novo PD compared to more advanced patients chronically exposed to levodopa and compared to healthy controls. They found a significant reduction in the N-acetylaspartate-to-choline ratio from the putamen contralateral to the most affected side in the de novo group but not in the levodopa-treated group or the control group. This altered ratio may reflect loss of nigrostriatal dopamine terminals or a functional abnormality of striatal putaminal neurons in the de novo group.

A number of PET and SPECT experiments have shown that several characteristic changes occur in the basal ganglia of de novo PD. One PET study found that de novo PD patients have increased microglial activation in the striatum relative to controls, and that this increase is correlated with reduced presynaptic dopamine transporter density in the putamen (Ouchi et al. 2005). Ouchi and colleagues (2005) interpreted this finding to suggest that neuroinflammatory processes mediated by microglia within the striatum contribute to the degeneration of dopaminergic function in the striatum. Several other PET and SPECT studies using a variety of ligands have extended this finding to reveal several general characteristics of nigrostriatal degeneration in de novo PD. For instance, these studies demonstrate that the putamen and caudate are differentially affected in de novo PD

(Tissingh et al. 1998b; Ouchi et al. 1999; Nurmi et al. 2000; Nurmi et al. 2001; Rinne et al. 2001; Nurmi et al. 2003; Bruck et al. 2005; Ouchi et al. 2005; Bruck et al. 2006; Isaias et al. 2007). Specifically, the posterior portion of the putamen is more affected than the anterior portion of the putamen, and the caudate is the least affected region of the striatum. Moreover, the striatum contralateral to the most symptomatically affected side is more affected than the ipsilateral striatum (Rinne et al. 1997; Tissingh et al. 1998b; Ouchi et al. 1999; Nurmi et al. 2003; Ouchi et al. 2005; Bruck et al. 2006; Isaias et al. 2007). Although the primary goal of many of these neuroimaging studies has been to discriminate de novo PD patients from healthy controls, other work has identified significant relations between measures of degeneration in the basal ganglia and measures of disease severity. Ouchi and colleagues (2005) found that the level of microglial activation is positively correlated with the motor severity of de novo PD, as evaluated by the Unified Parkinson's Disease Rating Scale (UPDRS). Other work found a negative correlation between dopamine transporter activity and the Hoehn and Yahr stage in both the putamen and caudate nucleus of de novo PD (Rinne et al. 1997) and between putamen and caudate dopamine transporter activity and disease severity as measured by the UPDRS (Tissingh et al. 1998a). Tissingh and colleagues also clearly showed that there is a bilateral loss of striatal dopamine transporters, particularly in the putamen, in patients early on in the disease process who manifest only unilateral symptoms.

Human neuroimaging studies have also identified significant pharmacological and metabolic changes in the cortex of de novo PD. Voxel-based morphometry in de novo PD has shown no changes in intracranial volume, whole-brain gray matter, or whole-brain white matter between patients and controls after controlling for sex and age (Martin et al. 2009). However, decreased white matter volume in the anterior right fusiform gyrus and superior temporal gyrus has been found with the earliest changes in a de novo PD group, likely occurring in subcortical white matter rather than in the temporal cortex itself. These areas are beyond the classic basal ganglia-thalamo-cortical loop. This finding needs replication because it suggests that areas may be affected in PD that are not classically associated with motor symptoms. Two studies using magnetic resonance spectroscopy have investigated whether there are significant metabolic changes in motor cortex associated with de novo PD. One of these studies investigated the motor cortex of de novo PD and found that metabolite ratios (i.e., choline-to-creatine and N-acetylaspartate-to-creatine) are abnormally low compared to healthy controls (Lucetti et al. 2007). Another study used similar methods and found that these metabolite ratios were similar in the pre-supplementary motor cortex of de novo PD patients and control subjects (Martin et al. 2008b). Additionally, a previous PET study found that dopamine uptake is significantly increased for de novo PD compared to controls in other cortical areas, including the premotor, parietal, medial and lateral frontal, and cingulate cortices (Bruck et al. 2006).

Very few human studies have been performed comparing neural activation in patients with de novo PD and healthy controls performing behavioral tasks using BOLD fMRI. Marklund et al. (2009) used fMRI to investigate the tonic and phasic components of the BOLD response in the basal ganglia of de novo PD patients performing a working memory task. The tonic and phasic components represent different time scales of change for the BOLD response. The authors found that phasic BOLD responses were greatly reduced in the caudate, putamen, and globus pallidus of PD patients relative to controls. Conversely, tonic BOLD responses were similar for PD patients and controls in all areas of the basal ganglia except the anterior portion of the putamen (Marklund et al. 2009). Another fMRI study compared BOLD activation in drug-naïve PD and healthy controls performing a motor task. This study found that, relative to controls, PD patients had reduced activation volume in the bilateral SMA and primary motor cortex (M1) contralateral to the most symptomatically affected side during a simple finger opposition task (Buhmann et al. 2003). Patients were scanned again after an intake of dopamine and the BOLD signal in M1 and SMA increased. Moreover, the intake of dopamine improved the motor performance of the PD patients, and there was a strong correlation between motor performance and BOLD activation in contralateral M1 for all patients and in SMA for most patients (Buhmann et al. 2003). This finding of reduced BOLD activation is contradictory to other fMRI studies that have observed increased BOLD activation in PD patients relative to controls performing simple motor tasks, such as finger tapping (Yu et al. 2007), sequential finger tapping/fist clenching (Sabatini et al. 2000), or joystick movements (Haslinger et al. 2001). Haslinger and colleagues (2001) hypothesized that the BOLD hyperactivity associated with PD is caused by reorganization of motor cortex to compensate for impairments of the motor system. The findings of Buhmann and colleagues (2003) support this hypothesis by demonstrating that reorganization has yet to occur in early-stage de novo PD patients, and that BOLD hypoactivation in M1 and SMA may reflect decreased input from the basal ganglia and thalamus. However, since the fMRI data collected by Buhmann and colleagues (2003) only included the frontal, parietal, and temporal cortices, it remains unclear how the pathophysiology of early-stage, de novo PD alters BOLD activation in subcortical structures such as the BG during motor tasks.

Our laboratory conducted a study to determine which subcortical structures are affected during the performance of a force control task in de novo PD. In particular, the study determined if only selected basal ganglia nuclei, or if all basal ganglia nuclei are affected in de novo PD (Spraker et al. manuscript under review). Since the cerebellum is hyperactive in moderate to advanced PD, the study also determined if cerebellar hyperactivity is found early in the course of de novo PD. BOLD fMRI was compared between 14 early-stage de novo PD patients and 14 controls performing two precision grip force tasks. The grip tasks used in the study were chosen because both tasks are known to provide robust activation in BG nuclei (Spraker et al. 2007; Vaillancourt et al. 2007), and the two tasks were similar except that the 2-second task required more switching between contraction and relaxation than the 4-second task. The 4-second task revealed that PD patients were hypoactive relative to controls only in putamen and external globus pallidus, and thalamus. In the 2-second task, PD patients were hypoactive throughout all the BG nuclei, thalamus, M1, and SMA. There were no differences in cerebellar activation between groups during either task. Regions-of-interest analysis revealed that the hypoactivity observed in PD patients during the 2-second task became more pronounced over time as patients performed the task. This suggests that a motor task that requires increased switching can accentuate abnormal activity throughout all BG nuclei in early-stage de novo PD, and that the abnormal activity becomes more pronounced with repeated task performance in these patients. The results are also consistent with the hypothesis that cerebellar compensation has not yet occurred in early-stage de novo PD. For similar arguments on compensation during aging, the readers should see the chapter by Swinnen and colleagues, this volume.

Both PET (Eidelberg et al. 1997; Eckert et al. 2007; Ma et al. 2007) and SPECT (Feigin et al. 2007) studies have shown that, when at rest, PD patients off medication have increased perfusion and glucose metabolism in the putamen and globus pallidus, relative to controls. This increased metabolism at rest could result in a reduced BOLD response during force production. As such, the two basal ganglia areas (putamen and globus pallidus) that were hypoactive in the 4-second force task could have been caused by altered metabolism at rest. However, since the study found additional areas with hypoactive BOLD in the de novo PD group during the 2-second task, it seems unlikely that hypermetabolism at rest explains the findings in caudate, STN, and substantia nigra. In addition, the fact that the hypoactivity became more pronounced with repeated performance of the 2-second task suggests that mechanisms related to the force task may explain the dynamics of the BOLD signal in the basal ganglia rather than increased resting metabolism. Further studies are required to explain the relationship between resting metabolic changes in PD and the BOLD response underlying movement tasks in different basal ganglia nuclei.

Another technique that has recently received considerable interest in the study of de novo PD is diffusion tensor imaging (DTI). Although DTI has typically been used to study white matter tracts (Mori and Zhang 2006; Kraus et al. 2007), it also holds promise for studying abnormalities in gray matter areas. As a method, DTI is based upon the diffusivity of water molecules, which exhibit a varying degree of tissue-dependent anisotropy. In white matter, water molecules are limited in the directions of diffusion, resulting in a high value of fractional anisotropy (FA) (Basser et al. 1994). However, in gray matter and in cerebrospinal fluid, water molecular diffusion exhibits significantly less directional dependence, causing low FA values relative to white matter. Tessa and colleagues (2008) studied 27 de novo PD patients using whole-brain DTI and T1-weighted MRI. The authors found that total brain volume, gray matter volume, and white matter were not different in de novo PD compared with control subjects. The de novo PD patients had an increase of the 25th percentile of the FA histogram relative to control subjects. The authors suggested that these changes reflected subtle loss of gray matter, consistent with the hypothesis that widespread neurodegeneration has occurred in de novo PD at the time of clinical diagnosis. This conclusion is consistent with two other DTI studies of patients with PD (Karagulle Kendi et al. 2008; Gattellaro et al. 2009).

Although whole-brain DTI approaches have revealed that de novo PD shows changes in the cortex beyond the basal ganglia, degeneration is thought to initially occur in the brainstem, and one critical area is the substantia nigra region of the BG. Our laboratory has recently used DTI to study the substantia nigra using hand-drawn regions of interest that were anatomically defined according to known patterns of degeneration in the substantia nigra (Vaillancourt et al. 2009). The rationale for studying the substantia nigra is that DTI performed in the MPTP mouse model of PD suggests that the measures extracted from DTI relate to the number of dopaminergic cells in the substantia nigra (Boska et al. 2007). The authors suggested that DTI can provide an indirect measure of dopaminergic degeneration within the substantia nigra, presumably because cell loss in the substantia nigra alters the microstructural integrity and diffusivity of water molecules. We studied 28 subjects (14 with early-stage, untreated PD and 14 age- and gender-matched controls) with a high-resolution DTI protocol at 3 Tesla using an eight-channel phase-array coil and parallel imaging to study specific segments of degeneration in the substantia nigra (Vaillancourt et al. 2009). Regions of interest were hand-drawn in the rostral, middle, and caudal substantia nigra by two blinded and independent raters. Figure 15.2A shows data from one of the raters indicating the degeneration pattern observed from rostral to caudal. In the rostral substantia nigra, there was no difference between groups for FA. However, in the middle and caudal substantia nigra, FA was reduced in PD compared with healthy control subjects. In addition, radial diffusivity was increased in the PD subjects compared with healthy control subjects. Figure 15.2B shows the results for FA in the caudal substantia nigra for each of the 14 patients (*gray*) and 14 control subjects (*black*). The finding that FA was reduced for PD patients caudally but not rostrally was consistent with other studies of iron content using a multiple gradient echo sequence of the proton transverse relaxation rate (Martin et al. 2008a). A receiver operator characteristic analysis confirmed the observations in Figure 15.2B that, in the caudal substantia nigra, the sensitivity and specificity were 100% for distinguishing PD patients from healthy subjects. Findings were consistent across both raters, who were blinded to the status of each patient group. As such, these

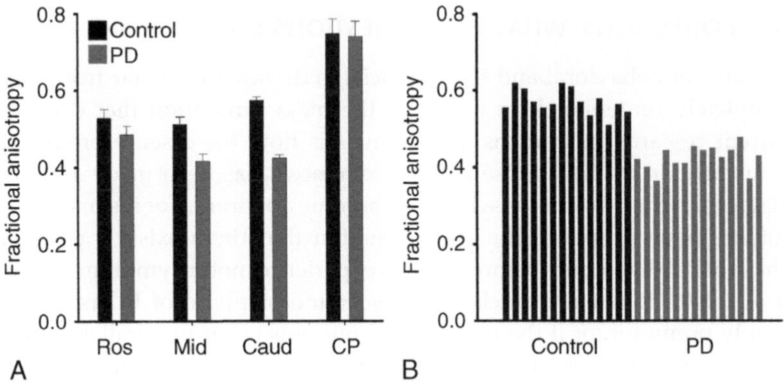

Figure 15.2 Changes in fractional anisotropy (FA) in different segments of the substantia nigra in de novo PD. **A**: FA averaged across 14 PD patients (*gray bars*) and 14 healthy control subjects (*black bars*) in the rostral, middle, and caudal region of the substantia nigra. The FA values for the cerebral peduncle (CP) are also shown for comparison, and there was no difference in FA in the CP. Error bars represent ± 1 SD. **B**: The FA values from one of the blinded raters from the study for all 14 PD patients (*gray bars*) and all 14 healthy controls (*black bars*) from the caudal region of interest. The caudal region had the greatest sensitivity and specificity. Adapted from Vaillancourt, D.E., M.B. Spraker, J. Prodoehl, I. Abraham, D.M. Corcos, X.J. Zhou, et al. 2009. High-resolution diffusion tensor imaging in the substantia nigra of de novo Parkinson disease. *Neurology* 72: 1378–84, with permission of the publisher.

findings provide evidence that high-resolution diffusion tensor imaging in the substantia nigra can distinguish early-stage, de novo patients with PD from healthy individuals on a patient-by-patient basis and has the potential to serve as a noninvasive early biomarker for PD.

In summary, a relatively small number of studies have investigated the structural and functional changes in the brain that are present in the very early stages of PD, before patients have been exposed to antiparkinsonian medication. Numerous techniques, including EEG, TMS, PET, SPECT, fMRI, DTI, and MRI, have been used. The general observation that can be gleaned from the literature thus far is that all BG nuclei are functioning abnormally in early-stage, de novo PD, but that only specific tasks elicit the differences between groups in all nuclei. Early on in the disease, adaptive changes in the cerebellum and cortex have not yet occurred. In addition, a consistent finding has been that the striatum is hypermetabolic at rest, with limited morphological changes in the cortex. Diffusion tensor imaging in the cortex has been able to detect microstructural changes in de novo PD, but these effects are not as reliable as those identified for the substantia nigra using DTI.

OPEN QUESTIONS: WHAT OPEN QUESTIONS STILL REMAIN?

The area of behavioral and brain deficits in de novo PD is far from being completely understood. In addition, the major limitation that confronts current research in humans and animals is how the disease progresses, both early on in the disease before a diagnosis has been made and after diagnosis, when the motor symptoms become apparent. For instance, some authors have proposed the general notion that there exists a premotor phase of PD that occurs before patients experience motor symptoms (Tolosa et al. 2009). It remains unclear if this premotor phase of PD is actually simply premotor, or if the nonmotor symptoms occur in parallel with the motor symptoms. The reason that a premotor phase is suspected is that large-scale studies have been conducted when other symptoms are experienced by a patient before the patient notices obvious motor symptoms (Tolosa et al. 2009). Also, studies such as the Honolulu Heart Program have found that patients who had an abnormal odor identification test were more susceptible to developing PD (Ross et al. 2008). It is unclear, however, how long the premotor phase is, and whether these large-scale studies could have detected motor symptoms had they used motor measures that were sensitive enough to detect PD. Potentially sensitive motor measures include measures of tremor and the use of the variability of the EMG bursting pattern in patients with PD. When assessing tremor in the clinic, most

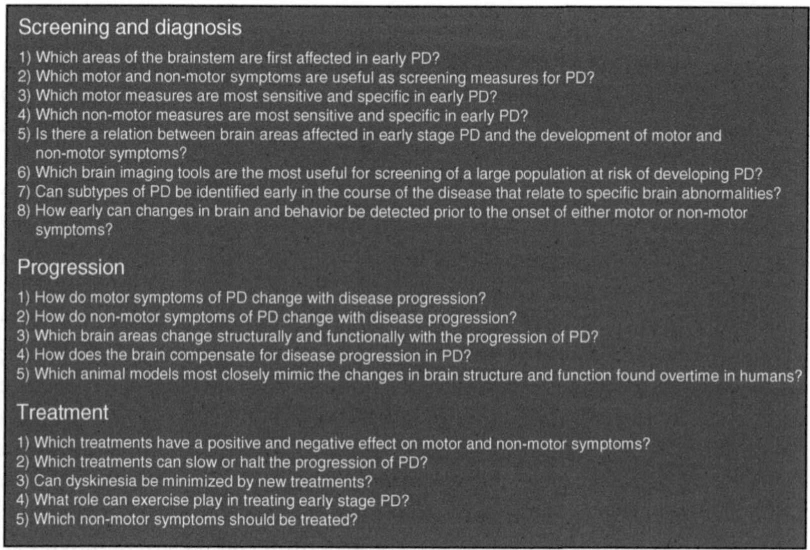

Figure 15.3 Some of the central questions that may drive future research studies into the screening and diagnosis, progression, and treatment of Parkinson disease.

neurologists rely upon the amplitude of tremor. In a study of patients with PD who did not experience tremor, it was shown that, although the amplitude of tremor was not different between PD patients and control subjects, the structure of tremor assessed using the measure of approximate entropy was reduced in patients with PD (Vaillancourt and Newell 2000). In addition, during a single-joint flexion movement task, the variability of the EMG bursting pattern was highly sensitive (90% sensitivity) at differentiating 30 patients with PD from ten healthy control subjects (Robichaud et al. 2009). Moreover, one of the healthy subjects had values of EMG variability that were abnormal, and 30 months after her initial testing she was subsequently diagnosed with PD. As such, using more sensitive motor measures in large-scale population-based studies could reveal that the premotor phase of PD is actually occurring in parallel with the motor phase of PD.

The preclinical phase of PD is an area that deserves future research. In Figure 15.3, we list several unresolved questions that may help guide future work in behavioral and brain deficits in PD. We have categorized these questions into themes that include screening and diagnosis, progression, and treatment. These questions are not meant to be fully inclusive, but they reflect central questions that may guide future studies.

CONCLUSION

Understanding the pathophysiology of PD is an important goal, given the prevalence of the disease and its morbidity and mortality. Although the development of animal models of PD has proved useful for the development of symptomatic therapies for the disease, these models do not capture all features of the disease, nor do they allow us to examine how the disease develops across time. Much of the literature in humans to date has focused on PD patients with more advanced stages of the disease who have already been exposed to symptomatic treatments. It is well established that chronic exposure to antiparkinsonian medication changes brain function. Much less is known about the motor and nonmotor deficits and brain structure and function in early-stage PD patients who are naïve to the effects of antiparkinsonian medication.

Examination of behavior and brain structure and function in PD patients who have not yet been exposed to symptomatic treatments offers the promise of helping to understand how the brain is altered by the disease, independent of the effects of symptomatic treatment. Advances in neuroimaging techniques such as PET, SPECT, fMRI, and DTI hold promise for the development of measures with which to help confirm diagnosis and track disease progression in PD. However, large-scale studies that examine the preclinical phase of PD are needed to help develop diagnostic tests that are practical and feasible to perform on a large, multisite scale. It is estimated that at least 50% of the dopaminergic neurons in the substantia nigra pars compacta die before motor symptoms appear in PD. Developing sensitive and specific measures of PD prior to symptom onset is needed. Only then can neuroprotective agents that slow or halt the progression of the disease be fully utilized.

ACKNOWLEDGMENTS

This research was supported in part by grants from the National Institutes of Health (R01-NS-52318, R01-NS58487) and the Michael J. Fox Foundation.

REFERENCES

Aarsland, D., K. Bronnick, G. Alves, O.B. Tysnes, K.F. Pedersen, U. Ehrt, and J.P. Larsen. 2009. The spectrum of neuropsychiatric symptoms in patients with early untreated Parkinson's disease. *Journal of Neurology, Neurosurgery, & Psychiatry* 80: 928–30.

Albin, R.L., A.B. Young, and J.B. Penney. 1989. The functional anatomy of basal ganglia disorders. *Trends in Neuroscience* 12: 366–75.

Anglade, P., S. Vyas, F. Javoy-Agid, M.T. Herrero, P.P. Michel, J. Marquez, et al. 1997. Apoptosis and autophagy in nigral neurons of patients with Parkinson's disease. *Histology & Histopathology* 12: 25–31.

Basser, P.J., J. Mattiello, and D. LeBihan. 1994. MR diffusion tensor spectroscopy and imaging. *Biophysics Journal* 66: 259–67.

Bennett, D.A., L.A. Beckett, A.M. Murray, K.M. Shannon, C.G. Goetz, D.M. Pilgrim, and D.A. Evans. 1996. Prevalence of parkinsonian signs and associated mortality in a community population of older people. *New England Journal of Medicine* 334: 71–76.

Berardelli, A., S. Rone, M. Inghilleri, and M. Manfredi. 1996. Cortical inhibition in Parkinson's disease. A study with paired magnetic stimulation. *Brain* 119: 71–77.

Beste, C., R. Willemssen, C. Saft, and M. Falkenstein. 2009. Error processing in normal aging and in basal ganglia disorders. *Neuroscience* 159: 143–49.

Bodi, N., S. Keri, H. Nagy, A. Moustafa, C.E. Myers, N. Daw, et al. 2009. Reward-learning and the novelty-seeking personality: A between- and within-subjects study of the effects of dopamine agonists on young Parkinson's patients. *Brain* 132: 2385–2395.

Boska, M.D., K.M. Hasan, D. Kibuule, R. Banerjee, E. McIntyre, J.A. Nelson, et al. 2007. Quantitative diffusion tensor imaging detects dopaminergic neuronal degeneration in a murine model of Parkinson's disease. *Neurobiology of Disease* 26: 590–96.

Braak, H., K. Del Tredici, U. Rub, R.A. de Vos, E.N. Jansen Steur, and E. Braak. 2003. Staging of brain pathology related to sporadic Parkinson's disease. *Neurobiology of Aging* 24: 197–211.

Bruck, A., S. Aalto, E. Nurmi, J. Bergman, and J.O. Rinne. 2005. Cortical 6-[18F]fluoro-L-dopa uptake and frontal cognitive functions in early Parkinson's disease. *Neurobiology of Aging* 26: 891–98.

Bruck, A., S. Aalto, E. Nurmi, T. Vahlberg, J. Bergman, and J.O. Rinne. 2006. Striatal subregional 6-[18F]fluoro-L-dopa uptake in early Parkinson's disease: A two-year follow-up study. *Movement Disorders* 21: 958–63.

Buhmann, C., V. Glauche, H.J. Sturenburg, M. Oechsner, C. Weiller, and C. Buchel. 2003. Pharmacologically modulated fMRI–cortical responsiveness to levodopa in drug-naive hemiparkinsonian patients. *Brain* 126: 451–61.

Buhmann, C., A. Gorsler, T. Baumer, U. Hidding, C. Demiralay, K. Hinkelmann, et al. 2004. Abnormal excitability of premotor-motor connections in de novo Parkinson's disease. *Brain* 127: 2732–46.

Cantello, R., R. Tarletti, C. Varrasi, M. Cecchin, and F. Monaco. 2007. Cortical inhibition in Parkinson's disease: New insights from early, untreated patients. *Neuroscience* 150: 64–71.

Carlsson, A. 1959. The occurrence, distribution and physiological role of catecholamines in the nervous system. *Pharmacology Review* 11: 490–93.

Carlsson, A., M. Lindqvist, and T. Magnusson. 1957. 3,4-Dihydroxyphenylalanine and 5-hydroxytryptophan as reserpine antagonists. *Nature* 180: 1200.

Chaudhuri, K.R., D.G. Healy, and A.H. Schapira. 2006. Non-motor symptoms of Parkinson's disease: Diagnosis and management. *Lancet Neurologyogy* 5: 235–45.

Chaudhuri, K.R., and Y. Naidu. 2008. Early Parkinson's disease and non-motor issues. *Journal of Neurology* 255 (Suppl 5): 33–38.

Chaudhuri, K.R., and A.H. Schapira. 2009. Non-motor symptoms of Parkinson's disease: Dopaminergic pathophysiology and treatment. *Lancet Neurology* 8: 464–74.

Davis, G.C., A.C. Williams, S.P. Markey, M.H. Ebert, E.D. Caine, C.M. Reichert, and I.J. Kopin. 1979. Chronic Parkinsonism secondary to intravenous injection of meperidine analogues. *Psychiatry Research* 1: 249–54.

DeLong, M.R. 1990. Primate models of movement disorders of basal ganglia origin. *Trends in Neuroscience* 13: 281–85.

DeLong, M.R., and Wichmann T. 2007. Circuits and circuit disorders of the basal ganglia. *Archives of Neurology* 64: 20–24.

Dorsey, E.R., R. Constantinescu, J.P. Thompson, K.M. Biglan, R.G. Holloway, K. Kieburtz, et al. 2007. Projected number of people with Parkinson disease in the most populous nations, 2005 through 2030. *Neurology* 68: 384–86.

Eckert, T., C. Tang, and D. Eidelberg. 2007. Assessment of the progression of Parkinson's disease: A metabolic network approach. *Lancet Neurology* 6: 926–32.

Eidelberg, D., J.R. Moeller, K. Kazumata, A. Antonini, D. Sterio, V. Dhawan, et al. 1997. Metabolic correlates of pallidal neuronal activity in Parkinson's disease. *Brain* 120 (Pt 8): 1315–24.

Elble, R.J., and W.C. Koller. 1990. *Tremor*. Baltimore: The John Hopkins University Press.

Ellis, C.M., G. Lemmens, S.C. Williams, A. Simmons, J. Dawson, P.N. Leigh, and K.R. Chaudhuri. 1997. Changes in putamen N-acetylaspartate and choline ratios in untreated and levodopa-treated Parkinson's disease: A proton magnetic resonance spectroscopy study. *Neurology* 49: 438–44.

Feigin, A., M.G. Kaplitt, C. Tang, T. Lin, P. Mattis, V. Dhawan, M.J. During, and D. Eidelberg. 2007. Modulation of metabolic brain networks after subthalamic gene therapy for Parkinson's disease. *Proceedings of the National Academy of Science U S A* 104: 19559–64.

Fellows, S.J., and J. Noth. 2004. Grip force abnormalities in de novo Parkinson's disease. *Movement Disorders* 19: 560–65.

Gattellaro, G., L. Minati, M. Grisoli, C. Mariani, F. Carella, M. Osio, et al. 2009. White matter involvement in idiopathic Parkinson disease: A diffusion tensor imaging study. *AJNR American Journal of Neuroradiology* 30: 1222–26.

Grafton, S.T. 2004. Contributions of functional imaging to understanding parkinsonian symptoms. *Current Opinions in Neurobiology* 14: 715–19.

Haslinger, B., P. Erhard, N. Kampfe, H. Boecker, E. Rummeny, M. Schwaiger, et al. 2001. Event-related functional magnetic resonance imaging in Parkinson's disease before and after levodopa. *Brain* 124: 558–70.

Hershey, T., K.J. Black, J.L. Carl, L. McGee-Minnich, A.Z. Snyder, and J.S. Perlmutter. 2003. Long term treatment and disease severity change brain responses to levodopa in Parkinson's disease. *Journal of Neurology, Neurosurgery, & Psychiatry* 74: 844–51.

Hodaie, M., J.S. Neimat, and A.M. Lozano. 2007. The dopaminergic nigrostriatal system and Parkinson's disease: Molecular events in development, disease, and cell death, and new therapeutic strategies. *Neurosurgery* 60: 17–28; discussion 28–30.

Hughes, A.J., S.E. Daniel, Y. Ben-Shlomo, and A.J. Lees. 2002. The accuracy of diagnosis of parkinsonian syndromes in a specialist movement disorder service. *Brain* 125: 861–70.

Isaias, I.U., R. Benti, R. Cilia, M. Canesi, G. Marotta, P. Gerundini, et al. 2007. [123I] FP-CIT striatal binding in early Parkinson's disease patients with tremor vs. akinetic-rigid onset. *Neuroreport* 18: 1499–1502.

Jackson-Lewis, V., and S. Przedborski. 2007. Protocol for the MPTP mouse model of Parkinson's disease. *Nat Protoc* 2: 141–51.

Jenner, P. 2008. Functional models of Parkinson's disease: A valuable tool in the development of novel therapies. *Annals of Neurology* 64 (Suppl 2): S16–29.

Karagulle Kendi, A.T., S. Lehericy, M. Luciana, K. Ugurbil, and P. Tuite. 2008. Altered diffusion in the frontal lobe in Parkinson disease. *AJNR American Journal of Neuroradiology* 29: 501–505.

Katzenschlager, R., and A.J. Lees. 2004. Olfaction and Parkinson's syndromes: Its role in differential diagnosis. *Current Opinions in Neurology* 17: 417–23.

Kordower, J.H., M.E. Emborg, J. Bloch, S.Y. Ma, Y. Chu, L. Leventhal, et al. 2000. Neurodegeneration prevented by lentiviral vector delivery of GDNF in primate models of Parkinson's disease. *Science* 290: 767–73.

Kraus, M.F., T. Susmaras, B.P. Caughlin, C.J. Walker, J.A. Sweeney, and D.M. Little. 2007. White matter integrity and cognition in chronic traumatic brain injury: A diffusion tensor imaging study. *Brain* 130: 2508–19.

Labyt, E., F. Cassim, D. Devos, J.L. Bourriez, A. Destee, J.D. Guieu, et al. 2005. Abnormal cortical mechanisms in voluntary muscle relaxation in de novo parkinsonian patients. *Journal of Clinical Neurophysiology* 22: 192–203.

Langston, J.W., P. Ballard, J.W. Tetrud, and I. Irwin. 1983. Chronic Parkinsonism in humans due to a product of meperidine-analog synthesis. *Science* 219: 979–80.

Lindgren, H.S., D. Rylander, K.E. Ohlin, M. Lundblad, and M.A. Cenci. 2007. The "motor complication syndrome" in rats with 6-OHDA lesions treated chronically with L-DOPA: Relation to dose and route of administration. *Behavior Brain Research* 177: 150–59.

Louis, E.D., K. Marder, L. Cote, M. Tang, and R. Mayeux. 1997. Mortality from Parkinson disease. *Archives of Neurology* 54: 260–64.

Lucetti, C., P. Del Dotto, G. Gambaccini, R. Ceravolo, C. Logi, C. Berti, et al. 2007. Influences of dopaminergic treatment on motor cortex in Parkinson disease: A MRI/MRS study. *Movement Disorders* 22: 2170–75.

Ma, Y., C. Tang, P.G. Spetsieris, V. Dhawan, and D. Eidelberg. 2007. Abnormal metabolic network activity in Parkinson's disease: Test-retest reproducibility. *Journal of Cerebral Blood Flow & Metabolism* 27: 597–605.

Marklund, P., A. Larsson, E. Elgh, J. Linder, K.A. Riklund, L. Forsgren, and L. Nyberg. 2009. Temporal dynamics of basal ganglia under-recruitment in Parkinson's disease: Transient caudate abnormalities during updating of working memory. *Brain* 132: 336–46.

Marras, C., and C.M. Tanner. 2004. Epidemiology of Parkinson's disease. In *Movement disorders: Neurologic principles and practice*, vol. 2, eds., R. L. Watts and W.C. Koller, 177–95. New York: McGraw-Hill.

Marsden, C.D. 1994. Parkinson's disease. *Journal of Neurology, Neurosurgery, & Psychiatry* 57: 672–81.

Martin, W.R., M. Wieler, and M. Gee M. 2008a. Midbrain iron content in early Parkinson disease: A potential biomarker of disease status. *Neurology* 70: 1411–17.

Martin, W.R., M. Wieler, M. Gee, and R. Camicioli. 2009. Temporal lobe changes in early, untreated Parkinson's disease. *Movement Disorders* 24(13): 1949–54.

Martin, W.R., M. Wieler, M. Gee, C.C. Hanstock, and R.M. Camicioli. 2008b. Intact presupplementary motor area function in early, untreated Parkinson's disease. *Movement Disorders* 23: 1756–59.

Mizuno, Y., N. Hattori, and H. Mochizuki. 2004. Etiology of Parkinson's disease. In *Movement disorders: Neurologic principles and practice*, vol. 2, eds., R.L. Watts and W.C. Koller WC, 209–32. New York: McGraw-Hill.

Montgomery, E.B., Jr., W.C. Koller, T.J. LaMantia, M.C. Newman, E. Swanson-Hyland, A.W. Kaszniak, and K. Lyons. 2000a. Early detection of probable idiopathic Parkinson's disease: I. Development of a diagnostic test battery. *Movement Disorders* 15: 467–73.

Montgomery, E.B., Jr., K. Lyons, and W.C. Koller. 2000b. Early detection of probable idiopathic Parkinson's disease: II. A prospective application of a diagnostic test battery. *Movement Disorders* 15: 474–78.

Morens, D.M., J.W. Davis, A. Grandinetti, G.W. Ross, J.S. Popper, and L.R. White. 1996. Epidemiologic observations on Parkinson's disease: Incidence and mortality in a prospective study of middle-aged men. *Neurology* 46: 1044–50.

Morgante, L., G. Salemi, F. Meneghini, A.E. Di Rosa, A. Epifanio, F. Grigoletto, et al. 2000. Parkinson disease survival: A population-based study. *Archives of Neurology* 57: 507–12.

Mori, S., and J. Zhang. 2006. Principles of diffusion tensor imaging and its applications to basic neuroscience research. *Neuron* 51: 527–39.

Nurmi, E., J. Bergman, O. Eskola, O. Solin, S.M. Hinkka, P. Sonninen, and J.O. Rinne. 2000. Reproducibility and effect of levodopa on dopamine transporter function measurements: A [18F]CFT PET study. *Journal of Cerebral Blood Flow & Metabolism* 20: 1604–09.

Nurmi, E., J. Bergman, O. Eskola, O. Solin, T. Vahlberg, P. Sonninen, and J.O. Rinne JO. 2003. Progression of dopaminergic hypofunction in striatal subregions in Parkinson's disease using [18F]CFT PET. *Synapse* 48: 109–15.

Nurmi, E., H.M. Ruottinen, J. Bergman, M. Haaparanta, O. Solin, P. Sonninen, and J.O. Rinne. 2001. Rate of progression in Parkinson's disease: A 6-[18F]fluoro-L-dopa PET study. *Movement Disorders* 16: 608–15.

Olanow, C.W., and W.G. Tatton. 1999. Etiology and pathogenesis of Parkinson's disease. *Annual Review of Neuroscience* 22: 123–44.

Ouchi, Y., T. Kanno, H. Okada, E. Yoshikawa, M. Futatsubashi, S. Nobezawa, T. Torizuka, and M. Sakamoto. 1999. Presynaptic and postsynaptic dopaminergic binding densities in the nigrostriatal and mesocortical systems in early Parkinson's disease: A double-tracer positron emission tomography study. *Annals of Neurology* 46: 723–31.

Ouchi, Y., E. Yoshikawa, Y. Sekine, K. Futatsubashi, T. Kanno, T. Ogusu, and T. Torizuka. 2005. Microglial activation and dopamine terminal loss in early Parkinson's disease. *Annals of Neurology* 57: 168–75.

Papa, S.M., T.M. Engber, A.M. Kask, and T.N. Chase. 1994. Motor fluctuations in levodopa treated parkinsonian rats: Relation to lesion extent and treatment duration. *Brain Research* 662: 69–74.

Perlmutter, J.S., and J.W. Mink. 2006. Deep brain stimulation. *Annual Reviews of Neuroscience* 29: 229–57.

Pfann, K.D., A.S. Buchman, C.L. Comella, and D.M. Corcos. 2001. Control of movement distance in Parkinson's disease. *Movement Disorders* 16: 1048–65.

Pierantozzi, M., M.G. Palmieri, M.G. Marciani, G. Bernardi, P. Giacomini, and P. Stanzione. 2001. Effect of apomorphine on cortical inhibition in Parkinson's disease patients: A transcranial magnetic stimulation study. *Experimental Brain Research* 141: 52–62.

Poewe, W., R. Granata, and F. Geser. 2004. Pharmacologic treatment of Parkinson's disease. In *Movement disorders: Neurologic principles and practice*, vol. 2, eds. R.L. Watts and W.C. Koller, 247–71. New York: McGraw-Hill.

Politis, M., P. Piccini, N. Pavese, S.B. Koh, and D.J. Brooks. 2008. Evidence of dopamine dysfunction in the hypothalamus of patients with Parkinson's disease: An in vivo (11. C-raclopride PET study. *Experimental Neurology*. Epub ahead of print.

Ponsen, M.M., A. Daffertshofer, E. van den Heuvel, E. Wolters, P.J. Beek, and H.W. Berendse. 2006. Bimanual coordination dysfunction in early, untreated Parkinson's disease. *Parkinsonism & Related Disorders* 12: 246–52.

Ponsen, M.M., A. Daffertshofer, E. Wolters, P.J. Beek, and H.W. Berendse. 2008. Impairment of complex upper limb motor function in de novo Parkinson's disease. *Parkinsonism & Related Disorders* 14: 199–204.

Prodoehl, J., D.M. Corcos, and D.E. Vaillancourt. 2009. Basal ganglia mechanisms underlying precision grip force control. *Neuroscience & Biobehavioral Reviews* 33: 900–908.

Rinne, J.O., J.T. Kuikka, K.A. Bergstrom, J. Hiltunen, and H. Kilpelainen. 1997. Striatal Dopamine transporter in Parkinson's disease: A study with a new radioligand, [(123. I]B-CIT-FP. *Parkinsonism & Related Disorders* 3: 77–81.

Rinne, O.J., E. Nurmi, H.M. Ruottinen, J. Bergman, O. Eskola, and O. Solin. 2001. [(18. F]FDOPA and [(18. F]CFT are both sensitive PET markers to detect presynaptic dopaminergic hypofunction in early Parkinson's disease. *Synapse* 40: 193–200.

Robichaud, J.A., K.D. Pfann, S. Leurgans, D.E. Vaillancourt, C.L. Comella, and D.M. Corcos. 2009. Variability of EMG patterns: A potential neurophysiological marker of Parkinson's disease? *Clinical Neurophysiology* 120: 390–97.

Ross, G.W., R.D. Abbott, H. Petrovitch, C.M. Tanner, D.G. Davis, J. Nelson, et al. 2006. Association of olfactory dysfunction with incidental Lewy bodies. *Movement Disorders* 21: 2062–67.

Ross, G.W., H. Petrovitch, R.D. Abbott, C.M. Tanner, J. Popper, K. Masaki, et al. 2008. Association of olfactory dysfunction with risk for future Parkinson's disease. *Annals of Neurology* 63: 167–73.

Sabatini, U., K. Boulanouar, N. Fabre, F. Martin, C. Carel, C. Colonnese, et al. 2000. Cortical motor reorganization in akinetic patients with Parkinson's disease: A functional MRI study. *Brain* 123 (Pt 2): 394–403.

Spraker, M.B., J. Prodoehl, D.M. Corcos, C.L. Comella, and D.E. Vaillancourt. 2010. Basal ganglia hypoactivity during grip force in drug naive Parkinson's disease. *Human Brain Mapping* Epub Ahead of Print.

Spraker, M.B., H. Yu, D.M. Corcos, and D.E. Vaillancourt. 2007. Role of individual basal ganglia nuclei in force amplitude generation. *Journal of Neurophysiology* 98: 821–34.

Tessa, C., M. Giannelli, R. Della Nave, C. Lucetti, C. Berti, A. Ginestroni, et al. 2008. A whole-brain analysis in de novo Parkinson disease. *AJNR American Journal of Neuroradiology* 29: 674–80.

Tissingh, G., H.W. Berendse, P. Bergmans, R. DeWaard, B. Drukarch, J.C. Stoof, and E.C. Wolters. 2001. Loss of olfaction in de novo and treated Parkinson's disease: Possible implications for early diagnosis. *Movement Disorders* 16: 41–46.

Tissingh, G., P. Bergmans, J. Booij, A. Winogrodzka, E.A. van Royen, J.C. Stoof, and E.C. Wolters. 1998a. Drug-naive patients with Parkinson's disease in Hoehn and Yahr stages I and II show a bilateral decrease in striatal dopamine transporters as revealed by [123I]beta-CIT SPECT. *Journal of Neurology* 245: 14–20.

Tissingh, G., J. Booij, P. Bergmans, A. Winogrodzka, A.G. Janssen, E. A. van Royen, J.C. Stoof, and E.C. Wolters. 1998b. Iodine-123-N-omega-fluoropropyl-2beta-carbomethoxy-3beta-(4-iod ophenyl) tropane SPECT in healthy controls and early-stage, drug-naive Parkinson's disease. *Journal of Nuclear Medicine* 39: 1143–48.

Tolosa, E., C. Gaig, J. Santamaria, and Y. Compta. 2009. Diagnosis and the premotor phase of Parkinson disease. *Neurology* 72: S12–20.

Ungerstedt, U. 1968. 6-Hydroxy-dopamine induced degeneration of central monoamine neurons. *European Journal of Pharmacology* 5: 107–10.

Ungerstedt, U., and G.W. Arbuthnott. 1970. Quantitative recording of rotational behavior in rats after 6-hydroxy-dopamine lesions of the nigrostriatal dopamine system. *Brain Research* 24: 485–93.

Vaillancourt, D.E., and K.M. Newell. 2000. The dynamics of resting and postural tremor in Parkinson's disease. *Clinical Neurophysiology* 111: 2046–56.

Vaillancourt, D.E., J. Prodoehl, L. Verhagen Metman, R.A. Bakay, and D.M. Corcos. 2004. Effects of deep brain stimulation and medication on bradykinesia and muscle activation in Parkinson's disease. *Brain* 127: 491–504.

Vaillancourt, D.E., M.B. Spraker, J. Prodoehl, I. Abraham, D.M. Corcos, X.J. Zhou, et al. 2009. High-resolution diffusion tensor imaging in the substantia nigra of de novo Parkinson disease. *Neurology* 72: 1378–84.

Vaillancourt, D.E., H. Yu, M.A. Mayka, and D.M. Corcos. 2007. Role of the basal ganglia and frontal cortex in selecting and producing internally guided force pulses. *Neuroimage* 36: 793–803.

van Eimeren, T., and H.R. Siebner. 2006. An update on functional neuroimaging of parkinsonism and dystonia. *Current Opinions in Neurology* 19: 412–19.

Weintraub, D., C.L. Comella, and S. Horn. 2008. Parkinson's disease—Part 1: Pathophysiology, symptoms, burden, diagnosis, and assessment. *American Journal of Managed Care* 14: S40–48.

Yu, H., D. Sternad, D.M. Corcos, and D.E. Vaillancourt. 2007. Role of hyperactive cerebellum and motor cortex in Parkinson's disease. *Neuroimage* 35: 222–33.

16

Emerging Principles in the Learning and Generalization of New Walking Patterns

Erin V. L. Vasudevan, Amy J. Bastian, and Gelsy Torres-Oviedo

Locomotion is one of the most fundamental animal behaviors. An essential feature of locomotion is that it is done effortlessly—we don't pay attention to the patterns of our leg motions, but instead focus on things like our destination or the person walking with us. Yet, locomotion is not just a rote motor pattern. It must constantly be adjusted to deal with changes in the environment (e.g., mud versus snow), body (e.g., fatigue, weight gain), or other conditions (e.g., high-heeled shoes). Some gait modifications can occur almost instantly in response to sensory feedback, such as tripping over a root while hiking, and are thought to be coordinated primarily by spinal pattern-generating networks that allow automatic, self-sustaining control of the gait cycle across many species (see Knuesel et al., see Chapter 18 in this volume). However, when changes in the body or environment are sustained and predictable, the nervous system can adapt, or learn to account for them via supraspinal mechanisms. Here, we define adaptation as a form of short-time scale learning. It is the trial-and-error process of changing a movement pattern in response to predictable circumstances. Adaptation requires error feedback: the motor pattern is adjusted in response to errors on a time scale of minutes to hours. An important feature of adaptation is that the new pattern is stored and expressed as an aftereffect when the predictable perturbation is removed. This aftereffect has to actively be "unlearned" or washed out.

We have focused on a form of locomotor adaptation that occurs when people walk on a split-belt treadmill (Reisman et al. 2005, also shown in Figure 16.1). In our paradigm, subjects are asked to walk in a baseline condition with the belts "tied" at the same speed. They then adapt their locomotor pattern to a split-belt condition, in which one belt moves faster than the other. This initially disrupts the normal antiphase motion of the two

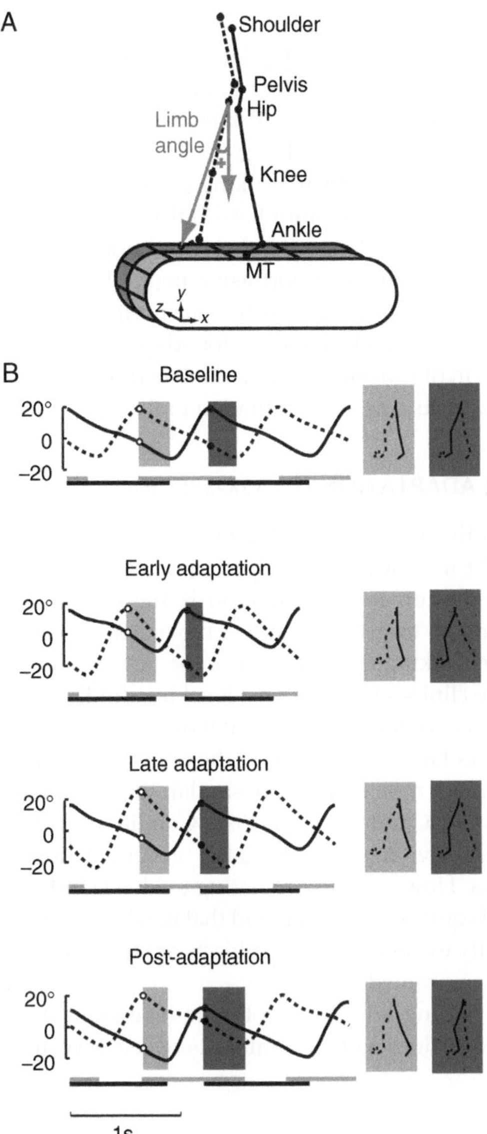

Figure 16.1 Example data showing split-belt adaptation. **A**: Stick figure illustrates placement of infrared markers for movement analysis and limb angle, which is defined as the angle between a vertical line and a vector drawn from the hip to the toe (metatarsal or MT). Positive limb angles occurred when the limb was forward of the vertical line. **B**: Example limb angle trajectories during forward walking at baseline (tied belts), early and late adaptation (split belts), and early post-adaptation (tied belts). The leg trained on the fast and slow belts during adaptation are referred to as the fast leg (*dotted*) and slow leg (*solid*), respectively. Horizontal bars below represent stance phases for the fast (*gray*) and slow leg (*black*). Gray-shaded boxes represent the double support periods,

(*Continued*)

legs, and causes asymmetry in step length and double-support times. It is possible that biomechanical factors important for gait, such as stability, energy, and mechanical stress (see Prilutsky and Klishko, Chapter 9 in this volume), are perturbed by this change in the environment, leading to inefficient gait. Subjects adapt their walking patterns over the course of minutes to reestablish symmetric, antiphase limb movements. After adaptation, when the subjects return to the tied-belt condition, they show after effects in step length and double-support asymmetry. These aftereffects require more walking to wash out and return to the normal pattern. In this review, we highlight our new work on locomotor adaptation, focusing on the specificity of this form of learning, the potential neural substrates involved, and the potential for its use as a rehabilitation tool.

LOCOMOTOR ADAPTATION IS TASK-SPECIFIC

Studies of adaptive processes, including split-belt adaptation, can provide valuable insight into how people learn new movements. For example, a fundamental question in rehabilitation is the extent to which a newly learned movement transfers to other movements. This is of particular importance for walking therapies, since the task that is often trained and practiced in the clinic— walking on a level treadmill at constant speed—is rarely, if ever, encountered in the "real world." Although many studies of upper limb tasks have demonstrated the ability of the nervous system to generalize learned motor skills to similar movements (Shadmehr and Mussa-Ivaldi 1994; Gandolfo et al. 1996; Conditt et al. 1997; Malfait et al. 2002), relatively few have investigated generalization across different locomotor tasks. However, accumulating evidence indicates that locomotor adaptation is quite task-specific and that newly learned walking patterns are preferentially expressed when subjects are tested on tasks very similar to those that were trained.

One robust finding arising from two independent studies is that locomotor adaptation does not generalize between forward and backward

Figure 16.1 (*Continued*) when both legs were in stance—light-gray corresponds to when the fast leg was leading; dark-gray corresponds to when the slow leg was leading. Stick figures on the right illustrate limb configurations corresponding to the beginning of stance phase (also shown by open and closed circles in the limb angle plots, representing limb angle at heel strike of the fast and slow legs, respectively). Note the development of asymmetries in double-support (width of gray boxes) and the step lengths (distance between ankle markers in stick figures) during early adaptation. The asymmetries are reduced by late adaptation and reversed during postadaptation. Adapted from Choi, J.T., and A.J. Bastian. 2007. Adaptation reveals independent control networks for human walking. *Nature Neuroscience* 10:1055–62, with permission of the publisher, Macmillan Publishers Ltd.

walking (Choi and Bastian 2007; Reynolds and Bronstein 2004). In one, subjects adapted to walking onto a moving platform: an experience similar to stepping onto a moving sidewalk in an airport (Reynolds and Bronstein 2004). Subsequently, aftereffects (i.e., postural sway) were measured when the platform was adjusted to be stationary. The authors found that when subjects practiced stepping onto the moving platform during forward walking, aftereffects did not carry over to backward walking. Moreover, aftereffects reemerged when subjects went back to forward walking on the stationary platform, indicating that they had been stored for subsequent release. We found similar results using a split-belt adaptation paradigm (Choi and Bastian 2007): aftereffects of split-belt adaptation did not carry over to backward walking if forward walking was trained, and vice versa (Fig. 16.2). Of particular interest was the finding that subjects who practiced split-belt walking with the belts running in different directions ("hybrid" walking) expressed aftereffects during both forward and backward walking, even when aftereffects in one direction were completely washed out before testing the other. Therefore, not only are functional networks for forward and backward walking adapted separately in humans, but the circuits controlling each leg can be trained individually.

Although it has been established that there is no transfer of learning between different directions of walking, it is less clear to what extent locomotor tasks must resemble one another for transfer to occur. Lam and Dietz (2004) showed that subjects who learned an obstacle-avoidance strategy could transfer the acquired performance to other forms of treadmill walking, like walking downhill or with additional weight attached to the leg. However, this task likely involves more explicit (i.e., conscious) learning processes than other adaptation tasks, which are largely implicit (i.e., unconscious), thus it is not known if this result could be replicated using a split-belt treadmill paradigm. Recently, we have begun to characterize the dynamic range of split-belt adaptation by testing transfer to different speeds of walking (Vasudevan and Bastian 2010). We found that this range was narrower than we anticipated: the largest aftereffects occurred when belts were tied at the same speed as the slow belt during adaptation and, in some cases, a speed difference of only 0.175 m/s was sufficient to see significant reductions in aftereffect size. We also found that washing out aftereffects at a fast speed (e.g., 1.4 m/s) did not abolish the aftereffects at a slow speed (e.g., 0.7 m/s), thus demonstrating that there is only partial overlap in the functional networks coordinating different walking speeds. This is supported by recent findings in other vertebrates showing that different classes of neurons are specifically recruited for the generation of fast and slow locomotion (McLean et al. 2008; McLean and Fetcho 2009). Taken together, these results reveal the importance of carefully selecting the training task to resemble the task, or range of tasks, that one aims to improve.

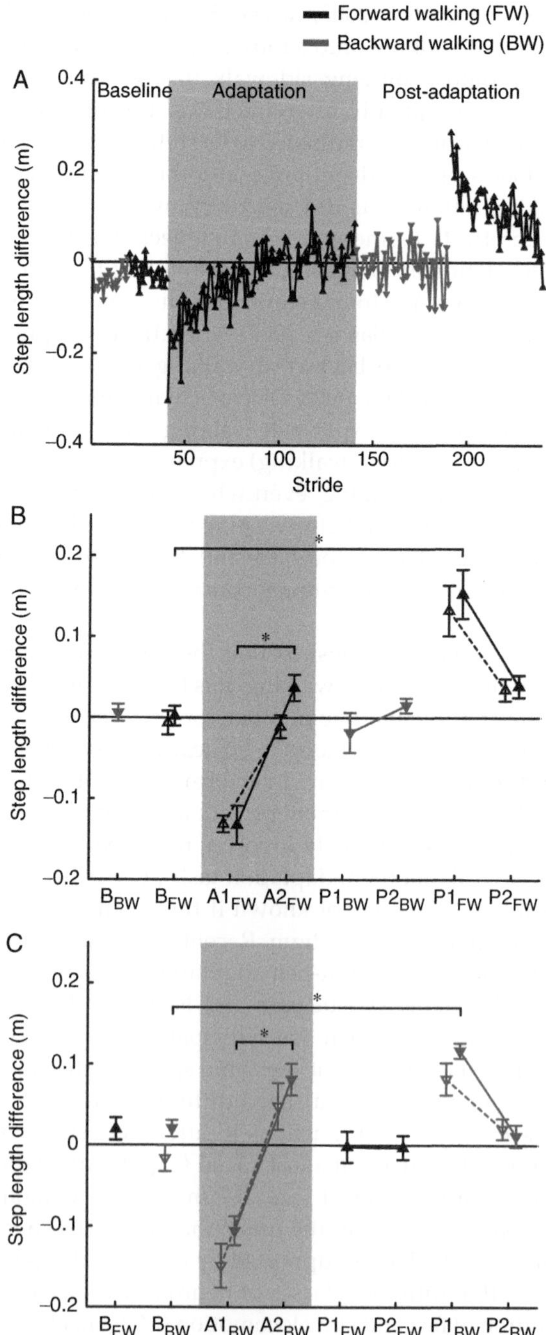

Figure 16.2 Transfer of split-belt adaptation between forward walking (FW) and backward walking (BW). **A**: Changes in step length (anterior-posterior

LOCOMOTOR ADAPTATION IS CONTEXT-SPECIFIC

Another critical issue for rehabilitation is the extent to which movements learned on a device generalize to free-space movements. Several studies of device-induced learning in upper limb movements have noted limited generalization to the behavior when off the device. For example, reaching movements can be adapted by using a robot that applies forces to the hand when reaching toward a target (Shadmehr and Mussa-Ivaldi 1994). Aftereffects induced are, however, significantly smaller when subjects reached without holding the device handle (Cothros et al. 2006) or when holding the handle in the absence of the device, so that the contextual cues related to hand grasp are conserved (Kluzik et al. 2008). Therefore, the learning in reaching adaptation seems to be specific to the training device. Not surprisingly, split-belt adaptation also shows limited generalization to free-space movements, as evidenced by small aftereffects resulting from this training when walking off of the treadmill (e.g., over-ground walking; Reisman et al. 2009). These findings suggest that, during training, subjects acquire or update an internal model of the body interacting with the device and not of the body alone (see Imamizu, Chapter 11 this volume).

Figure 16.2 (*Continued*) distance between ankle markers at heel strike) in a typical subject. Step length difference is equal to the fast leg's step length minus the slow leg's step length; a value of 0 indicates perfect symmetry. During baseline BW and FW, steps were the same size on both sides. During split-belt FW adaptation, the fast leg initially took a shorter step than the slow leg, and the step lengths gradually became more symmetric. When normal walking conditions were restored in post-adaptation (tied belts), step lengths were symmetric in BW indicating a lack of adaptation transfer. Despite 5 minutes of BW washout, FW showed strong after-effects in step length symmetry on tied-belts. **B**: Average step length difference for all subjects who were adapted during FW ($n = 7$; *solid line*). Differences were calculated for baseline BW and FW, early and late FW adaptation, early and late BW post-adaptation, and early and late FW post-adaptation. A repeated-measures ANOVA indicated significant changes in step length from early to late FW adaptation and from FW baseline to early FW post-adaptation ($p < 0.001$). There was no difference between BW baseline and early BW post-adaptation ($p \geq 0.5$) and there was no difference between the two groups that did the experiment with (*solid line*) and without (*dashed line*) BW washout (group effect, $p = 0.3$). **C**: Average step length differences for subjects who were adapted during BW ($n = 7$; *solid line*). A repeated-measures ANOVA showed significant changes in step length from early to late BW adaptation and from BW baseline to early BW post-adaptation on tied-belts ($p < 0.001$). Step length was not significantly different between FW baseline and FW early post-adaptation on tied-belts ($p \geq 0.5$). There was no difference between two groups with (*solid line*) and without (*dashed line*) FW washout (group effect, $p = 0.1$). Adapted from Choi, J.T., and A.J. Bastian. 2007. Adaptation reveals independent control networks for human walking. *Nature Neuroscience* 10:1055–62, with permission of the publisher, Macmillan Publishers Ltd.

Consequently, the motor memory acquired on devices can only be accessed and updated on the same device.

A promising study in human reaching has, however, demonstrated that device-induced learning can be manipulated to increase the transfer of learning to the behavior off of the device (Kluzik et al. 2008). More generalization was observed when subjects adapted their reaching to gradual as opposed to abrupt perturbations. During gradual adaptation, subjects experienced small perturbations that gradually increased during adaptation, whereas during abrupt adaptation, they experienced a single large perturbation that was abruptly introduced and maintained during adaptation. It has been suggested that small errors, like those resulting from gradual perturbations, can more easily be attributed to the individual's own motor commands, as opposed to the device (Diedrichsen et al. 2005), resulting in larger generalization. Credit assignment, defined as the ability of the nervous system to assign errors to the body or the environment, may therefore underlie the generalization of learning to the behavior off of the device. Theoretical work proposes that subjects form an estimate of the source of error during adaptation (Berniker and Kording 2008). This suggests that, when the estimate of the source of error is the body, people will generalize the learned behavior more than when they attribute the error to a device. Whether credit assignment can be manipulated for split-belt adaptation is yet to be investigated.

NEURAL SUBSTRATES FOR ADAPTATION

In a number of different experimental paradigms, the cerebellum has been shown to be essential for making the feedforward predictions that are the basis of adaptation (Horak and Diener 1994; Lang and Bastian 1999; Martin et al. 1996; Maschke et al. 2004; Smith and Shadmehr 2005; Xu-Wilson et al. 2009). We found that the cerebellum was required for locomotor adaptation as well, since people with damage to the cerebellum were impaired in adapting to the split-belt treadmill (Morton and Bastian 2006; see Figure 16.3A and B). Specifically, the most impaired subjects presented with high levels of gait ataxia in relation to limb ataxia, indicating that the cerebellar regions controlling posture and gait (i.e., the vermis and fastigial nuclei; Sprague and Chambers 1953; Chambers and Sprague 1955a; Chambers and Sprague 1955b; Thach et al. 1992) may play a particularly important role in the control of predictive gait adaptations. In contrast, adults and children with cerebral damage due to stroke (cortical or subcortical) or hemispherectomy were capable of adapting and storing aftereffects (Reisman et al. 2007; Choi et al. 2009; see Fig. 16.3C and D), thus demonstrating that the cerebrum is not essential for locomotor adaptation (also see Yanagihara et al. 1993).

It is thought that the cerebellum is ideally suited to recalibrate the predictive feedforward control of stepping since it receives inputs that allow

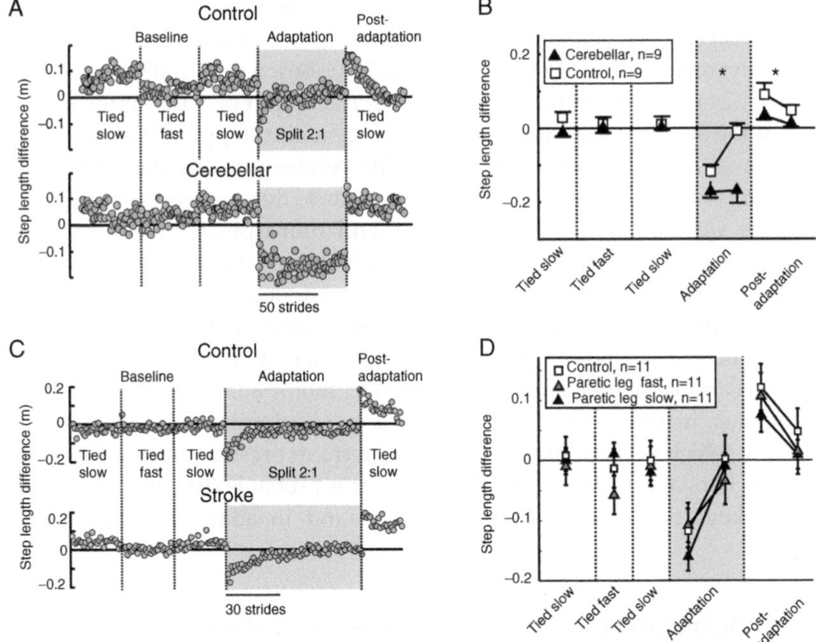

Figure 16.3 Split-belt adaptation in people with cerebellar (**A,B**) or cerebral (**C,D**) damage. **A**: Step length differences for a typical control subject (*top row*) and from a subject with cerebellar damage (*bottom row*). Note that both subjects were initially perturbed (i.e., made asymmetric) by the introduction of split-belts at the beginning of adaptation; however, while the control subject was able to gradually make step lengths equal, the subject with cerebellar damage was unable to make these adjustments. Significant aftereffects were only observed in the control subject, and not in the subject with cerebellar damage. **B**: Average step length differences for control and cerebellar groups. Each data point represents values averaged over the early or late portions of each testing period (± SEM). Asterisks indicate significant differences between cerebellar and control groups ($p < 0.05$). **C**: Step length differences for a typical control (*top row*) and a stroke (*bottom row*) subject. Note that, in contrast to the cerebellar subject shown in A, both the control and stroke subjects gradually adapted to the split-belts and both showed significant aftereffects in the post-adaptation period. **D**: Average step length differences shown as in B. Data from experiments when stroke subjects were adapted to split-belts with their paretic leg on the fast belt are shown in gray triangles; data from when subjects were adapted with the paretic leg on the slow belt are shown in black triangles. Regardless of which belt the paretic leg was on, stroke subjects were capable of adapting and storing aftereffects. **A, B** are adapted from Morton, S.M., and A.J. Bastian. 2006. Cerebellar contributions to locomotor adaptations during split-belt treadmill walking. *Journal of Neuroscience* 26:9107–16, with permission of the publisher, Society for Neuroscience. **C, D** are adapted from Reisman, D.S., R. Wityk, K. Silver, and A.J. Bastian. 2007. Locomotor adaptation on a split-belt treadmill can improve walking symmetry post-stroke. *Brain* 130:1861–72, with permission of the publisher, Oxford University Press.

comparisons of the anticipated and actual movement. Afferent signals from the dorsal spinocerebellar pathways inform the cerebellum about the ongoing movement of the legs (Poppele et al. 2003; Bosco et al. 2005; Bosco et al. 2006), whereas the ventral spinocerebellar tract input provides information about the activity of spinal networks that generate stepping (i.e., intended movement) (Arshavsky et al. 1978). The cerebellum can then influence walking patterns through efferent projections to descending tracts, including the vestibulospinal, reticulospinal, and rubrospinal tracts (Orlovsky 1972a; Orlovsky 1972b). Indeed, in decerebrate cats, Purkinje cell complex spikes increase in firing rate during the initial period of walking on a split-belt treadmill (Yanagihara and Udo 1994). These complex spikes likely represent error signals in the control of movement (Gilbert and Thach 1977; Medina and Lisberger 2008). Moreover, locomotor adaptation is abolished altogether in these cats following nitric oxide deprivation in cerebellar tissues, which is thought to reduce long-term depression in Purkinje cells (Yanagihara and Kondo 1996). Therefore, it is probable that the cerebellum has a key role in locomotor adaptation and in adaptive processes in general.

CAN LOCOMOTOR ADAPTATION BE USED FOR REHABILITATION?

Since cerebral damage does not impair a person's ability to make adaptations and store aftereffects during split-belt treadmill walking (Reisman et al. 2007; Choi et al. 2009), this raises the exciting possibility that adaptive strategies may be used to correct walking deficits following stroke or other brain lesions (e.g., hemispherectomy). Supporting this is the finding from Reisman and colleagues (2007) that adult stroke survivors with a hemiparesis (i.e., gait asymmetry or "limp") could temporarily improve their walking pattern following a single training session on a split-belt treadmill. Adaptive strategies can also be used to correct upper limb movements: practicing reaching in a force field applied by a robot can cause aftereffects that reduce baseline errors (Patton et al. 2006). Importantly, in both cases, the perturbations imposed by the treadmill or robot act to exaggerate the deficit. It is thought that this amplification of the error forces the nervous system to correct it, which then leads to improved movement patterns when normal conditions are restored. To date, only transient improvements have been reported following a single session of upper or lower limb adaptation; however, it is likely that repeated training sessions are required to make the improvements more permanent.

Before we can apply these adaptive strategies to rehabilitation, it is essential to determine whether the learned pattern carries over to "real-world" activities, like walking over the ground, in the relevant clinical population. Recently, Reisman et al. (2009) investigated this issue and discovered that, although control subjects only transfer 30% of what they learned on the split-belt treadmill to walking over ground, people who have had a stroke transfer 60%. In other words, aftereffects observed overground are twice as large in stroke survivors as in age-matched controls. This may be because stroke survivors have difficulty changing movement patterns to accommodate different environmental demands (Lord and Rochester 2005; Dickstein 2008): once they learn a new walking pattern, these patients may lack the ability to quickly revert back to the old pattern when environmental conditions change. If so, it is interesting to note that a deficit in movement flexibility, which is considered to be disadvantageous for community ambulation, could be an advantage for rehabilitation by allowing subjects to transfer the benefits of treadmill training to activities of daily life. An alternative explanation is that, since the adapted walking pattern represents a gait improvement in stroke survivors, possibly resulting in benefits to balance or efficiency, it is more likely to be retained and applied to walking in a broader range of environmental contexts. It is not yet known whether there is increased transfer to other locomotor tasks (e.g., different speeds of walking) post-stroke but, if either of these explanations is true, we would expect greater generalization to occur here as well.

CONCLUSION

These recent studies demonstrate that there is enormous potential for the split-belt treadmill and other forms of adaptation in rehabilitation. However, questions remain regarding how to optimize learning. Using the split-belt paradigm, we have shown that adapted walking patterns are only temporarily stored following a single training session (Reisman et al. 2005; Reisman et al. 2007). Can we retrain a more permanent pattern over multiple training sessions? Moreover, split-belt adaptation is context- (Reisman et al. 2009) and task-specific (Choi and Bastian 2007; Vasudevan and Bastian 2010). How to structure training sessions to make more learning carry over to "real-world" walking is yet to be determined. It may be possible to adapt a more generalized pattern when errors made during movement are associated with one's own body, as opposed to an external device (e.g., Kluzik et al. 2008). Finally, although adaptive strategies have been successfully employed in people with cerebral damage (Reisman et al. 2007), they are not effective in people with cerebellar damage (Morton and Bastian, 2006). It is not clear whether alternative training strategies could be used to help retrain movements in this patient population. Future work in identifying the underlying principles and neural mechanisms of adaptation and generalization will shed light on these issues and allow us to transition the use of adaptive strategies from the laboratory to clinical practice.

REFERENCES

Arshavsky, Y.I., I.M. Gelfand, G.N. Orlovsky, and G.A. Pavlova. 1978. Messages conveyed by spinocerebellar pathways during scratching in the cat. II. Activity of neurons of the ventral spinocerebellar tract. *Brain Research* 151:493–506.

Berniker, M., and K. Kording. 2008. Estimating the sources of motor errors for adaptation and generalization. *Nature Neuroscience* 11:1454–61.

Bosco, G., J. Eian, and R.E. Poppele. 2005. Kinematic and non-kinematic signals transmitted to the cat cerebellum during passive treadmill stepping. *Experimental Brain Research* 167:394–403.

Bosco, G., J. Eian, and R.E. Poppele. 2006. Phase-specific sensory representations in spinocerebellar activity during stepping: evidence for a hybrid kinematic/kinetic framework. *Experimental Brain Research* 175:83–96.

Chambers, W.W., and J.M. Sprague. 1955a. Functional localization in the cerebellum. I. Organization in longitudinal cortico-nuclear zones and their contribution to the control of posture, both extrapyramidal and pyramidal. *Journal of Computational Neurology* 103:105–29.

Chambers, W.W., and J.M. Sprague. 1955b. Functional localization in the cerebellum. II. Somatotopic organization in cortex and nuclei. *AMA Archives of Neurology and Psychiatry* 74:653–80.

Choi, J.T., and A.J. Bastian. 2007. Adaptation reveals independent control networks for human walking. *Nature Neuroscience* 10:1055–62.

Choi, J.T., E.P. Vining, D.S. Reisman, and A.J. Bastian. 2009. Walking flexibility after hemispherectomy: split-belt treadmill adaptation and feedback control. *Brain* 132:722–33.

Conditt, M.A., F. Gandolfo, and F.A. Mussa-Ivaldi. 1997. The motor system does not learn the dynamics of the arm by rote memorization of past experience. *Journal of Neurophysiology* 78:554–60.

Cothros, N., J.D. Wong, and P.L. Gribble PL. 2006. Are there distinct neural representations of object and limb dynamics? *Experimental Brain Research* 173:689–97.

Dickstein, R. 2008. Rehabilitation of gait speed after stroke: a critical review of intervention approaches. *Neurorehabilitation and Neural Repair* 22:649–60.

Diedrichsen, J., Y. Hashambhoy, T. Rane, and R. Shadmehr. 2005. Neural correlates of reach errors. *Journal of Neuroscience* 25:9919–31.

Gandolfo, F., F.A. Mussa-Ivaldi, and E. Bizzi. 1996. Motor learning by field approximation. *Proceedings of the National Academy of Science U S A* 93:3843–46.

Gilbert, P.F., and W.T. Thach. 1977. Purkinje cell activity during motor learning. *Brain Research* 128:309–28.

Horak, F.B., and H.C. Diener. 1994. Cerebellar control of postural scaling and central set in stance. *Journal of Neurophysiology* 72:479–93.

Kluzik, J., J. Diedrichsen, R. Shadmehr, and A.J. Bastian. 2008. Reach adaptation: what determines whether we learn an internal model of the tool or adapt the model of our arm? *Journal of Neurophysiology* 100:1455–64.

Lam, T., and V. Dietz. 2004. Transfer of motor performance in an obstacle avoidance task to different walking conditions. *Journal of Neurophysiology* 92:2010–16.

Lang, C.E., and A.J. Bastian. 1999. Cerebellar subjects show impaired adaptation of anticipatory EMG during catching. *Journal of Neurophysiology* 82:2108–19.

Lord, S.E., and L. Rochester. 2005. Measurement of community ambulation after stroke: current status and future developments. *Stroke* 36:1457–61.

Malfait, N., D.M. Shiller, and D.J. Ostry. 2002. Transfer of motor learning across arm configurations. *Journal of Neuroscience* 22:9656–60.

Martin, T.A., J.G. Keating, H.P. Goodkin, A.J. Bastian, and W.T. Thach. 1996. Throwing while looking through prisms. I. Focal olivocerebellar lesions impair adaptation. *Brain* 119 (Pt 4): 1183–98.

Maschke, M., C.M. Gomez, T.J. Ebner, and J. Konczak. 2004. Hereditary cerebellar ataxia progressively impairs force adaptation during goal-directed arm movements. *Journal of Neurophysiology* 91:230–38.

McLean, D.L., and J.R. Fetcho. 2009. Spinal interneurons differentiate sequentially from those driving the fastest swimming movements in larval zebrafish to those driving the slowest ones. *Journal of Neuroscience* 29:13566–77.

McLean, D.L., M.A. Masino, I.Y. Koh, W.B. Lindquist, and J.R. Fetcho. 2008. Continuous shifts in the active set of spinal interneurons during changes in locomotor speed. *Nature Neuroscience* 11:1419–29.

Medina, J.F., and G.S. Lisberger. 2008. Links from complex spikes to local plasticity and motor learning in the cerebellum of awake-behaving monkeys. *Nature Neuroscience* 11:1185–92.

Morton, S.M., and A.J. Bastian. 2006. Cerebellar contributions to locomotor adaptations during splitbelt treadmill walking. *Journal of Neuroscience* 26:9107–16.

Orlovsky, G.N. 1972a. Activity of vestibulospinal neurons during locomotion. *Brain Research* 46:85–98.

Orlovsky, G.N. 1972b. The effect of different descending systems on flexor and extensor activity during locomotion. *Brain Research* 40:359–71.

Patton, J.L., M.E. Stoykov, M. Kovic, and F.A. Mussa-Ivaldi. 2006. Evaluation of robotic training forces that either enhance or reduce error in chronic hemiparetic stroke survivors. *Experimental Brain Research* 168:368–83.

Poppele, R.E., A. Rankin, and J. Eian. 2003. Dorsal spinocerebellar tract neurons respond to contralateral limb stepping. *Experimental Brain Research* 149: 361–70.

Reisman, D.S., H.J. Block, and A.J. Bastian. 2005. Interlimb coordination during locomotion: what can be adapted and stored? *Journal of Neurophysiology* 94:2403–15.

Reisman, D.S., R. Wityk, K. Silver, and A.J. Bastian. 2007. Locomotor adaptation on a split-belt treadmill can improve walking symmetry post-stroke. *Brain* 130:1861–72.

Reisman, D.S., R. Wityk, K. Silver, and A.J. Bastian. 2009. Split-belt treadmill adaptation transfers to overground walking in persons poststroke. *Neurorehabilitation and Neural Repair* 23:735–44.

Reynolds, R.F., and A.M. Bronstein. 2004. The moving platform aftereffect: Limited generalization of a locomotor adaptation. *Journal of Neurophysiology* 91:92–100.

Shadmehr, R., and F.A. Mussa-Ivaldi. 1994. Adaptive representation of dynamics during learning of a motor task. *Journal of Neuroscience* 14:3208–24.

Smith, M.A., and R. Shadmehr. 2005. Intact ability to learn internal models of arm dynamics in Huntington's disease but not cerebellar degeneration. *Journal of Neurophysiology* 93:2809–21.

Sprague, J.M., and W.W. Chambers. 1953. Regulation of posture in intact and decerebrate cat. I. Cerebellum, reticular formation, vestibular nuclei. *Journal of Neurophysiology* 16:451–63.

Thach, W.T., H.P. Goodkin, and J.G. Keating. 1992. The cerebellum and the adaptive coordination of movement. *Annual Reviews in Neuroscience* 15:403–42.

Vasudevan, E.V., and A.J. Bastian. 2010. Split-belt treadmill adaptation shows different functional networks for fast and slow human walking. *Journal of Neurophysiology* 103: 183–91.

Xu-Wilson, M., H. Chen-Harris, D.S. Zee, and R. Shadmehr. 2009. Cerebellar contributions to adaptive control of saccades in humans. *Journal of Neuroscience* 29:12930–39.

Yanagihara, D., and I. Kondo. 1996. Nitric oxide plays a key role in adaptive control of locomotion in cat. *Proceedings of the National Academy of Science U S A* 93:13292–97.

Yanagihara, D., and M. Udo. 1994. Climbing fiber responses in cerebellar vermal Purkinje cells during perturbed locomotion in decerebrate cats. *Neuroscience Research* 19:245–48.

Yanagihara, D., M. Udo, I. Kondo, and T. Yoshida. 1993. A new learning paradigm: Adaptive changes in interlimb coordination during perturbed locomotion in decerebrate cats. *Neuroscience Research* 18:241–44.

17

Aging and Movement Control

The Neural Basis of Age-related Compensatory Recruitment

Stephan P. Swinnen, Sofie Heuninckx, Annouchka Van Impe, Daniel J. Goble, James P. Coxon, and Nicole Wenderoth

Aging is characterized by a progressive decline of motor functioning with decreases in reaction time and movement speed as its most prominent features (Spirduso 1982; Welford 1984; Seidler and Stelmach 1995). Motor functioning is of primary concern to aging adults because it is intrinsic to many activities of daily living, such as walking, dressing, gardening, driving a car, and the like. Aging permeates all aspects of our life: physically, cognitively, psychologically, and socially. As a result of the demographic evolution in which older people occupy a gradually increasing cohort of the general population, it is of high socioeconomic importance to promote functional independence and comfort of living in this group. This requires a profound knowledge of the neural changes associated with aging and its sensorimotor consequences.

The underlying causes of senescence have been investigated at numerous levels of analysis, from the systems to the cellular level. A variety of factors have been identified at the microscopic level: changes in cellular metabolism, cell structure, cell–matrix interactions, neurotransmitter systems, and the rate and accuracy of DNA replication (Osiewacz and Hamann 1997; Ladislas 2000; Labat-Robert 2001; Campisi 2003; Troen 2003; Cabeza et al. 2005). With the increasing availability of brain imaging technologies, the systems level has come into the picture more prominently during the past decade. Blood oxygen level-dependent functional magnetic resonance imaging (BOLD fMRI) and positron emission tomography (PET) have been used most intensively to engender a breakthrough in the neuroscience of aging. Functional imaging has been complemented by structural imaging to assess age-related gray matter (voxel-based morphometry) and white matter changes (diffusion tensor imaging).

The majority of recent research on aging has focused on investigating the relationship between age-related changes in brain function and concomitant changes in cognitive/behavioral abilities (Grady et al. 1995; Gabrieli 1996; Madden et al. 1999; Della-Maggiore et al. 2000; Cabeza 2002; Craik and Grady 2002; Grady 2002a; Reuter-Lorenz 2002; Gazzaley and D'Esposito 2003; Buckner 2004; Park et al. 2004). It is, in fact, quite surprising that neuroimaging studies have so far mainly focused on cognitive aging, whereas knowledge about age-related changes in the underlying neural substrates of sensorimotor performance is rather scarce. In this chapter, we focus primarily on fMRI research identifying age-related changes in brain activation during the performance of simple and more complex motor tasks. Within this broader framework, we will devote special attention to recent work from our group on the neural basis of interlimb coordination, with a focus on coordinated hand–foot movements on the same side of the body (i.e., ipsilateral coordination). As will become evident, this type of task has served as a very powerful means for revealing sensorimotor-related aging processes, including the recruitment of cognitive resources to monitor movement.

We consider imaging research of critical importance for a better understanding of lifespan changes in neuromotor function. Not only has it provided refined information about the neurodegenerative changes that occur as a result of aging, but it has also generated encouraging evidence for overcoming these changes through mechanisms of neuroplasticity. Consequently, the traditional view of a static, rigid, and aging brain has gradually been replaced by a more optimistic dynamic view, emphasizing plastic changes into old age that allow continuous sculpturing of the brain. To this extent, a research program is now under way to determine the boundary conditions of such plasticity and the mechanisms that may allow its facilitation.

AGE-RELATED CHANGES IN BRAIN ACTIVATION DURING COGNITIVE TASK PERFORMANCE

During the past decade and a half, a considerable number of imaging studies have addressed age-related changes in brain activation during the performance of cognitive tasks. It is impossible to do justice to this work in a chapter focused on aging and sensorimotor function. However, due to the similarities in age-related neural changes across these task domains, it is meaningful to address some of the most prominent observations that have been made.

Whereas behavioral indices provide a general picture of slower and more error-prone performance in older than younger adults, neuroimaging studies have portrayed activation in older brains as being considerably different from that of the younger, rather than a mere reduced or depleted function. Across a wide range of cognitive task domains, four important trends are emerging. First, neuroimaging research has revealed localized regions of task-specific underactivation in older compared with younger adults, in the very brain regions that have been linked to proficient performance in young adults. This age-related underactivation often involves the prefrontal cortex (Moscovitch and Winocur 1995; West 1996). Second, even when behavioral performance is matched, younger and older adults show different activation patterns, suggesting that they engage distinctive brain areas to accomplish the same tasks (Grady et al. 1998). Third, older adults show conspicuous bilateral activation under conditions that produce highly lateralized activity in younger adults (Grossman et al. 2002; Hartley et al. 2001; Reuter-Lorenz et al. 2000). This phenomenon was coined the *H*emispheric *A*symmetry *R*eduction in *OLD* age (HAROLD) model by Cabeza (2002). Fourth, for some tasks, seniors exhibit increased brain activation that is correlated with task performance, suggesting compensatory potential in the aging brain (McIntosh et al. 1999; Rypma and D'Esposito 1999; Cabeza et al. 2002). This is also known as the compensation-related utilization of neural circuits or *CRUNCH* hypothesis (Grady 2000, 2008; Cabeza et al. 2002; Reuter-Lorenz and Lustig 2005).

In summary, it appears that older adults can show similar, lower, and/or higher brain activation as compared to the young adults. It remains to be investigated why and under what circumstances these different patterns are observed. The nature of the task, task performance instructions, and different ways to compare performance levels between age groups may all contribute to the brain activation patterns that are ultimately obtained. Further research is necessary to unravel these phenomena. However, it is striking to observe that the older brain is capable not only of showing decreased brain activation but also of displaying a surprising change and/or increase in brain activation that appears to be particularly evident in those elderly who preserve performance relative to their young counterparts, i.e., compensatory brain activation.

AGE-RELATED CHANGES IN BRAIN ACTIVATION DURING MOTOR TASK PERFORMANCE

As already mentioned, much less is known about age-related changes in brain activity during motor tasks. Only a handful of medical imaging experiments on aging and motor function have been conducted so far. These studies have revealed that elderly subjects exhibit altered brain activation patterns during simple isolated finger (Hutchinson et al. 2002; Mattay et al. 2002) or hand movements (Hutchinson et al. 2002; Ward and Frackowiak 2003). However, it remains largely unresolved which brain areas are recruited by elderly during the performance of more complex cyclical interlimb coordination tasks. In general, coordination is of primary concern to aging adults because it is intrinsic to many activities of daily living and shows up in many different forms or modes. Moreover, research has shown that different control principles emerge during the coordination of two or more limbs as compared to isolated limb movements. This is particularly evident from patient groups suffering from different types of brain disorders. Even though they can often produce isolated limb movements successfully, they encounter pronounced difficulties when limbs have to be coordinated (Debaere et al. 2001a; Serrien et al. 2000; Swinnen 2002; Swinnen et al. 1997). This provides sufficient justification to study cyclical interlimb coordination tasks.

Next, we will review fMRI studies in which age-related changes in cyclical hand and/or foot movements with different degrees of complexity were performed by younger and older adults. Brain activations were compared during the performance of isolated flexion-extension movements of the right hand and foot, as well as during their coordination, according to the "easy" isodirectional and "difficult" non-isodirectional mode. Before we elaborate on the observed brain activations, we first describe some behavioral findings from the perspective of the coordination principles they endorse. Subsequently, we will discuss the present work in relation to the broader field of imaging research on motor functions.

Task Paradigm for Studying Complex Coordination: Ipsilateral Hand–Foot Coordination

The study of interlimb coordination patterns has resulted in the identification of two elementary modes of movement coordination—the in-phase and anti-phase pattern (Kelso 1984; Swinnen 2002; Turvey 1990). With respect to bilateral finger, hand, or arm movements, in-phase coordination refers to the simultaneous timing of activation of homologous muscle groups (i.e., flexing or extending the arms, hands, or fingers simultaneously). Antiphase coordination refers to the simultaneous activation of nonhomologous muscle groups (i.e., flexing one limb segment while extending the other).

With respect to movements of the ipsilateral limbs (e.g., hand–foot coordination on the same side of the body), in-phase and anti-phase movements are defined with respect to movement direction in extrinsic space. In particular, in-phase refers to limb motions in the same direction (i.e., wrist flexion together with ankle plantarflexion, and vice versa—isodirectional, ISODIR), and anti-phase to motions in opposite directions (non-isodirectional, NONISODIR—i.e., wrist flexion combined with ankle dorsiflexion; see Fig. 17.1). To the best of our knowledge, this ipsilateral task was first introduced by Baldissera and coworkers (Baldissera et al. 1982). Later studies have adopted this paradigm, studying either hand–foot or forearm–lower leg coordination (Kelso and Jeka 1992; Serrien and Swinnen 1997; Serrien et al. 2000; Swinnen et al. 1995, 1997). Even though both the ISODIR and NONISODIR patterns are considered part of the intrinsic motor repertoire, studies have generally confirmed Baldissera's initial finding that they

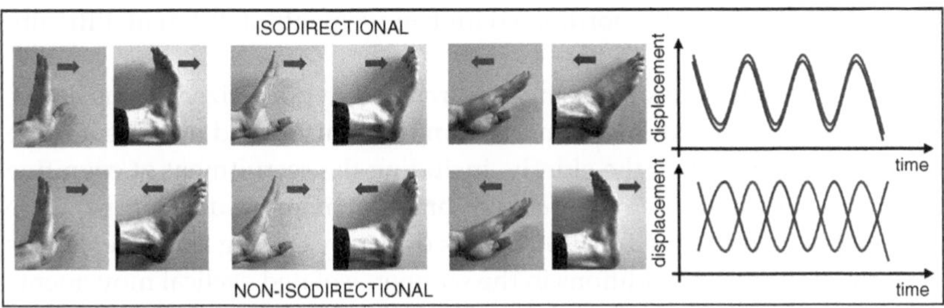

Figure 17.1 Isodirectional and non-isodirectional coordination of ipsilateral limb segments. The joint motions (*left side*) and angular displacements (*right side*) of the hand and foot are indicated during a partial movement cycle.

are not equally difficult, with ISODIR coordination preferentially coded by the central nervous system (CNS) (Baldissera et al. 2002; Byblow et al. 2007). Whereas isodirectional movements can be performed easily without much effort, the non-isodirectional coordination mode is more difficult and is produced with a lower degree of phase accuracy and stability (i.e., relative phase error and standard deviation, SD). This is particularly the case in elderly subjects (Serrien et al. 2000), as well as patients suffering from Parkinson's disease (Swinnen et al. 1997) or stroke (Debaere et al. 2001b). Furthermore, with increasing cycling frequency, participants often undergo an involuntary transition from the NONISODIR to the more stable ISODIR pattern if a critical frequency is reached (Baldissera et al. 1991; Carson et al. 1995, Kelso and Jeka 1992). More recently, research on the brain activation patterns associated with ipsilateral coordination has followed up on this behavioral work and has detailed the neural signature of the experienced differential difficulty between ISODIR and NONISODIR coordination (Debaere et al. 2001a; Caeyenberghs et al. 2009; Heuninckx et al. 2005, 2008; Rocca et al. 2007; Van Impe et al. 2009).

Age-related Brain Activation Changes During Ipsilateral Coordination

The study of motor tasks involving large effectors and/or displacements is particularly problematic in an fMRI context, not only because of artifacts induced by limb motion, but also because of the impact of effector displacement on head movements. Foot movements pose a specific problem in this respect because of the induced whole-body translation, which impacts on head movement. These effects can be minimized, however, through special precautions, such as inducing subject knee flexion and using a bite bar to stabilize the head. Aside from this, ipsilateral coordination is a meaningful task to study because it shares some similarities with locomotor patterns. Furthermore, the task affords different levels of coordinative complexity, ranging from isolated to coordinated limb movements of different difficulty levels.

We adopted this task for aging research and hypothesized that isolated, as well as coordinated, hand and foot movements would activate a more widespread network in the elderly, including the recruitment of cognitive resources. Furthermore, age-related brain activation differences were expected to increase as a function of task difficulty. Young and older adults performed different conditions in the scanner: isolated cyclical movements of the right hand (HAND) and foot (FOOT), and cyclical coordination of the hand and foot according to the isodirectional (ISODIR) and non-isodirectional (NONISODIR) mode. Angular displacements of the joints were registered using non-ferromagnetic encoders and, thus, did not interfere with image acquisition. Movements were paced by an electronic metronome. To equate difficulty level, we compared the older subjects' performance at 1 Hz to that of the younger subjects at 1.5 Hz. This was based on previous work demonstrating that these cycling frequencies represented a comparable ratio to the maximal frequency at which these patterns could be performed successfully by both groups (Heuninckx et al. 2004).

Our findings revealed that the overall movement characteristics were largely the same between young and elderly groups (cycling frequency and peak-to-peak amplitude). As expected, ISODIR coordination was performed with higher stability than NONISODIR coordination. With respect to relative phase, the absolute error did not reveal a group difference, but coordination variability was slightly more variable in the older adults than in the young.

With respect to brain activation, we will first report the results for the group differences pertaining to isolated hand and foot movements and then for the coordinated limb movements. Subsequently, we will specifically address the brain activation differences between ISODIR and NONISODIR coordination. A general picture of the activations obtained in younger (*gray*) and older adults (*white*) for each movement condition is provided in Figure 17.2.

Analysis of the group activations during both isolated limb movement conditions (Fig. 17.2A-B) revealed that the pattern of activation in the older group was more widespread and this effect was more prominent for foot than hand movements. A direct comparison of the groups revealed significantly higher activation in the older group in the left anterior insular cortex, left inferior frontal gyrus pars opercularis (IFGPO), left superior temporal gyrus, left inferior postcentral sulcus/secondary somatosensory cortex (S2), left supramarginal gyrus, and left fusiform gyrus (Fig. 17.2A-B, *white*). In addition, the older group exhibited significantly higher activation in a superior parietal cluster, with peak activation in right precuneus. No region was significantly more activated in the younger than in the older group. The increased activation surrounding the left frontal operculum is in agreement with earlier studies using auditory paced movements, yielding higher

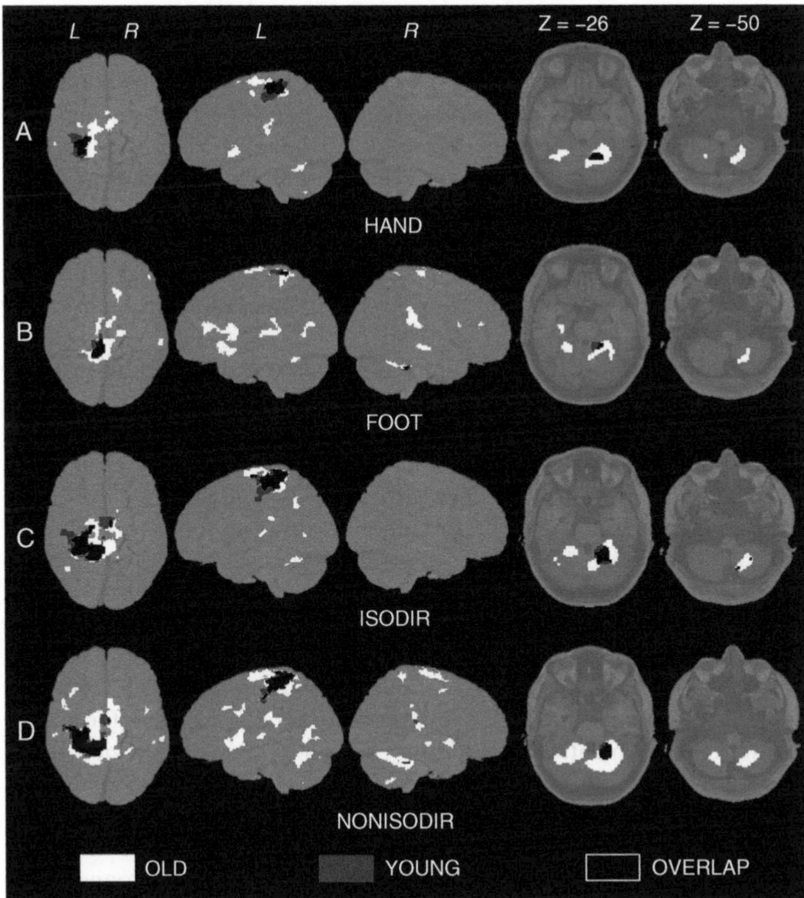

Figure 17.2 Group mean activations for each motor task (**A**: HAND; **B**: FOOT; **C**: ISODIR coordination; **D**: NONISODIR coordination) versus REST overlaid on standard MNI renders and templates. Significant voxels ($p < 0.001$; corrected for multiple comparisons) are indicated in white for the old group, in gray for the young group, and in black for overlap between activation of both groups; in each, the height threshold is $t = 6.98$. L, Left hemisphere; R, right hemisphere. Adapted from Heuninckx, S., N. Wenderoth, F. Debaere, R. Peeters, and S.P. Swinnen. 2005. Neural basis of aging: The penetration of cognition into action control. *Journal of Neuroscience* 25:6787–96, with permission of the publisher.

frontal operculum activation in old as compared to young subjects (Hutchinson et al. 2002). These areas are often involved in higher-order auditory processing (Platel et al. 1997; Bamiou et al. 2003; Thaut 2003), particularly in motor synchronization to an auditory rhythm (Lewis et al. 2004; Thaut 2003). This tentatively suggests that the older subjects relied more pervasively on external information sources (i.e., metronome pacing signal) for controlling their limb movements and complies with the broader view that the IFGPO is involved in interfacing external information about biological motion with internal representations of limb actions, as observed during movement observation, imitation, or imagery (Grezes et al. 1998; Iacoboni et al. 1999; Binkofski et al. 2000). Similarly, the fusiform gyrus, which was activated in the elderly but not in the young subjects, often emerges in relation to movement observation (Bonda et al. 1996; Grezes et al. 1998) and imagery (Jahn et al. 2004). Perhaps this reflects the use of some form of visualization strategy by elderly individuals to control their movements.

The older as compared to younger adults also exhibited additional activation in the left secondary somatosensory cortex (S2), left supramarginal gyrus, and right precuneus, consistent with earlier results obtained during various simple motor tasks (Hutchinson et al. 2002; Mattay et al. 2002; Ward and Frackowiak 2003). These areas are known to be involved in the integration of somatosensory information to guide motor actions (Cavada and Goldman-Rakic 1989; Kalaska et al. 1990; Ashe and Georgopoulos 1994; Ferraina and Bianchi 1994; Huttunen et al. 1996; Scott et al. 1997;Rizzolatti et al. 1998). Additionally, they are sometimes also related to the attentional effort required by a specific motor skill (Hari et al. 1990; Garcia-Larrea et al. 1991; Mima et al. 1998; Lam et al. 1999). These findings point to an increased focus on somatosensory processing to perform these rhythmical movements in the elderly. This is not surprising, in view of the decreased proprioceptive sensibility that occurs with aging (Goble et al. 2009).

Activation of the precuneus, located in the medial parietal cortex, is particularly noteworthy because it is highly and densely interconnected to many other brain areas, emphasizing its status as a central structural core with a prominent role in functional integration (Hagmann et al. 2008). The precuneus and superior parietal lobule are involved in top-down or goal-directed attention under the performer's control (Behrmann et al. 2004). Here, it is hypothesized to mediate increased attention to and spatial monitoring of the limb segments. Activation in the precuneus has also been documented in previous motor performance studies in the elderly (Zemke et al. 2003; Wu and Hallett 2005a), as well as in young and older patients suffering from motor-related disorders (Wu and Hallett, 2005b; Caeyenberghs et al. 2009). It appears to be a candidate area for compensatory recruitment in the suboptimal CNS (Serrien et al. 2007).

The general network for producing the ISODIR and NONISODIR coordination patterns was more extensive than for the isolated movements, and this effect was more pronounced in the older than young adults (Fig. 17.2C-D). Analysis of both coordination patterns combined revealed that the older adults exhibited significantly larger activation than the young group in the left anterior insular cortex, left IFGPO, left S2, left superior temporal gyrus, left supramarginal gyrus, left fusiform gyrus, and in the right precuneus. This is the same set of regions that was already discussed during the isolated hand and foot conditions. Additionally, the older group demonstrated significantly higher activation in the prefrontal cortex (PFC; i.e., in the left inferior frontal sulcus); in the ventral premotor cortex (PMv; i.e., in the left inferior precentral sulcus); in left and right pre-supplementary motor area (SMA); in the rostral part of the PMd, corresponding to the pre-PMd; in the right rostral anterior cingulate cortex (ACC); in the left angular gyrus; and in the left anterior and left and right posterior cerebellum. This latter set of brain areas differed from those observed during the isolated movements. Again, no region showed significantly higher activation in the younger than in the older group.

The increased brain activation observed in the older as compared to younger adults during coordination of both limb segments is noteworthy because it is supportive of a shift toward increased (pre)frontal involvement: pre-SMA, pre-PMd, RCC, and PFC. The latter two regions are not considered to represent classical "coordination areas." Pre-SMA and pre-PMd activation have previously emerged in age-related comparisons of hand-grip and visually paced button-press tasks (Mattay et al. 2002; Ward and Frackowiak 2003). There is increasing agreement that these areas are more closely related to cognitive than to motor processes, and their high connectivity with the PFC supports this (Keizer and Kuypers 1989; Lu et al. 1994; Geyer et al. 2000). These areas become typically activated with increasing cognitive demands of a motor task (for review, see Picard and Strick 2001). Interestingly, we have not observed activation of these areas in our previous coordination research on hand and/or foot movements in adolescents (Debaere et al. 2001a, 2003, 2004; Wenderoth et al. 2004a). In addition to these frontal areas, older adults also showed surplus activation in the anterior and posterior cerebellum (see Fig. 17.2C-D). The cerebellum is known to be involved in multilimb coordination (Debaere et al. 2001a, 2003, 2004; Ramnani et al. 2001; Tracy et al. 2001; Meyer-Lindenberg et al. 2002; Ullen et al. 2003), and it becomes increasingly activated when coordination complexity rises (Ullen et al. 2003; Debaere et al. 2004). This may refer to increasing demands on motor timing (Ivry 1997; Mima et al. 1999; Habas et al. 2004; Wenderoth et al. 2004b) and/or sensory processing (Jueptner et al. 1997; Bushara et al. 2001; Thickbroom et al. 2003). Overall, the picture that emerges from these findings is that hand–foot coordination strongly activated classical coordination areas, but, also several frontal regions interfacing motor control and cognition in older adults. This suggests that older subjects relied more on cognitive monitoring of the coordination tasks, consistent with recent behavioral results (Holtzer et al. 2005).

Our final analysis addressed old–young group differences during the NONISODIR versus the ISODIR coordination mode. We already mentioned that the NONISODIR mode is clearly perceived as being more difficult than the ISODIR coordination mode. Our results revealed that the

NONISODIR mode resulted in the recruitment of additional "coordination areas" in the older as compared to younger groups, such as the PMd, the posterior parietal cortex, and the cerebellum (Sadato et al. 1997; Stephan et al. 1999; Debaere et al. 2001a; Immisch et al. 2001; Ehrsson et al. 2002). Interestingly, a nonmotor network became also activated in the older adults, including the middle frontal gyrus (DLPFC), left superior frontal gyrus (pre-SMA), anterior rostral cingulate cortex (ACC), left insula, and left and right middle occipital gyrus (see Fig. 17.2 D). Remarkably, many of these regions (DLPFC, pre-SMA, aRCC) are involved in conflict monitoring and/or inhibitory control, as assessed by Stroop, Go/NoGo, Stop-signal, and Flanker tasks (e.g., Botvinick et al. 1999; Carter et al. 1999; Garavan et al. 1999; Casey et al. 2000; Kiehl et al. 2000; Menon et al. 2001; Watanabe et al. 2002; Aron et al. 2006; Coxon et al. 2009). Particularly, the aRCC is generally active in error detection and in suppression of conflicting response tendencies. Response inhibition has been shown to evoke a higher aRCC activity in old as compared to young subjects in cognitive tasks (Milham et al. 2002; Nielson et al. 2002). Here, it is reasonable to assume that aRCC activation in the elderly reflected larger efforts to suppress the regression from NONISODIR to ISODIR coordination. Overall, this suggests that the task may have been experienced as being quite difficult for our aged subjects. However, even if this task is performed at comfort pacing, increased activation is still evident in the elderly, albeit less pronounced (Van Impe et al. 2009).

In summary, our data suggest that the elderly exhibited higher and more extended brain activation than the young subjects across all motor tasks. The kinematic data suggested that task difficulty was reasonably matched between groups, such that the observed surplus activation in the elderly cannot be explained by differences in motor output between both age groups. The extended activation in the elderly became more pronounced with increasing task complexity. When overlooking the regions exhibiting an age-related increase in activation, it is possible to categorize the identified areas into distinct functional groups: increased activation in (a) the basic motor network, (b) areas responsible for sensory processing and (inter)sensory integration, (c) areas involved in imagery/visualization of movement, and (d) prefrontal areas reflecting increased cognitive control of movement and suppression of prepotent response tendencies (in the case of the more demanding NONISODIR pattern). This represents an interesting example of generic brain areas that span the motor and cognitive domains. Accordingly, our working hypothesis is that older, relative to young, adults show a shift from automatic to more controlled processing of movement, requiring recruitment of extra neural resources during complex interlimb coordination tasks. The important question that remains is why this overactivation occurs in the older as compared to younger adults, and what its functional meaning is. These issues are discussed next.

OVERACTIVATION IN THE AGING BRAIN: COMPENSATORY RECRUITMENT?

Seniors exhibit additional brain activation when compared with younger controls during the execution of various motor tasks (Mattay et al. 2002; Ward and Frackowiak 2003; Heuninckx et al. 2005). They either activate the same areas as their younger counterparts, but to a larger extent, and/or they activate additional areas that are not observed or do not reach significance in the young subjects. Even though this "overactivation" of the aging brain is now generally well documented for the motor system, the underlying neural mechanisms are still largely unknown. Unravelling these mechanisms is a complex and multidimensional problem because it may be a consequence of various age-related changes in the brain itself, but may also represent more peripheral changes, such as alterations in the musculoskeletal system, reflex control mechanisms, muscle (co)contraction properties, motor unit recruitment alterations, and the quality of sensory receptors providing input to the CNS. Here, we will attempt to undertake a first step toward answering this question by discussing some potential central mechanisms. Admittedly, this approach faces limitations and will most likely have to be amended in the longer term.

Inspired by cognitive aging studies, we formulate two major hypotheses regarding neural activation changes in the elderly. First, the *compensation hypothesis* predicts that age-related increases in activation, as well as the involvement of additional areas, counteracts age-related decline of brain function (Grady et al. 1998; Madden et al. 1999; Cabeza et al. 2000, 2002; Reuter-Lorenz et al. 2000; Grady 2002b; Reuter-Lorenz and Lustig 2005). Conversely, the *dedifferentiation hypothesis* assumes that age-related changes in functional activation reflect difficulties in recruiting specialized neural mechanisms (Li and Lindenberger 1999; Li et al. 2001). In the first case, overactivation is compensatory and meaningful to motor performance. It may reflect plasticity of the aging brain in the face of central and peripheral changes. In the second case, increased activation may reflect unwanted activation spreading or neural leakage, possibly as a consequence of reduced recruitment of inhibitory processes. Such increased activation does not support or may be indifferent to motor performance. It may result from the breakdown of inhibitory interactions between brain areas (Peinemann et al. 2001), in which case overactivation could reflect the nonselective recruitment of disinhibited regions (Li et al. 2001; Logan et al. 2002). Age-related changes in functional activation may also reflect deficits in neurotransmission, which in turn causes decreases in signal-to-noise ratio and less distinct neural representations (Li et al. 2001). Increases in activity then reflect spreading of activity due to reduced specialization of function. Time will tell whether this dissociation between compensation and dedifferentiation is as clear as proposed here, because it may not always be straightforward to demonstrate the (non-)functionality of surplus activation. Furthermore, age-related spontaneous unmasking of inhibitory connections within the brain may pave the road for exploiting these more widespread activation patterns to preserve or improve performance.

We tested these two hypotheses by correlating performance on ipsilateral hand–foot coordination tasks with brain activation. Functional MRI was conducted on 24 older adults and 11 young controls during the performance of the ISODIR and NONISODIR modes. The protocol was essentially the same as discussed previously. Subsequently, brain activation was correlated with motor performance. According to the *compensation hypothesis*, we predicted overactivation to be correlated with motor coordination performance; that is, activation was hypothesized to be larger in good than in poor elderly performers, and this effect should be more pronounced in more (NONISODIR) than less demanding (ISODIR) coordination tasks. Conversely, the *dedifferentiation hypothesis* assumed overactivation to be larger in poor than in successful motor performers due to nonfunctional neural irradiation.

Performance on the coordination task was quantified by means of the absolute phase error between the limbs, indicating coordination accuracy. To simplify interpretation, the relationship between error scores and performance was inverted (1/AE), such that high scores were indicative of good performance. Accordingly, positive correlations between brain activation and motor performance were considered to reflect *compensation* and negative correlations *dedifferentiation*. A distinction was made between (a) brain activation clusters that were equally activated in the young and elderly and (b) areas exhibiting overactivation in the elderly.

The results revealed activation levels in several areas to be correlated with performance. With respect to the *equally activated* regions during ISODIR coordination, a positive relationship was identified in the left pre- and postcentral gyrus (SM1) and in the right anterior cerebellar hemisphere. During NONISODIR coordination, a significant positive correlation between coordination performance and brain activation was observed in the left superior postcentral gyrus/sulcus, inferior post central gyrus, right SMA, and left CMA. Within the *overactivated* areas of the elderly, no significant relationships between activation and ISODIR coordination accuracy were identified. By contrast, for the more complex NONISODIR coordination mode, significant positive relationships were observed in the left inferior frontal gyrus pars opercularis (IFGPO) and pars triangularis (IFGPT) (Fig. 17.3B), anterior insular cortex (Fig. 17.3C), superior parietal gyrus (Fig. 17.3F), pre-PMd (Fig. 17.3E), DLPFC (Fig. 17.3A), and the right posterior cerebellum (Fig. 17.3H) ($p < 0.05$, cluster-wise FDR correction). Additionally, there was a trend toward a positive correlation in the left superior temporal gyrus (Fig. 17.3G) and left anterior cerebellar hemisphere (Fig. 17.3D) ($p < 0.001$, uncorrected). In Figure 17.3, the brain regions that were additionally activated by the elderly subjects while showing a positive relation between activation and coordination performance are encircled

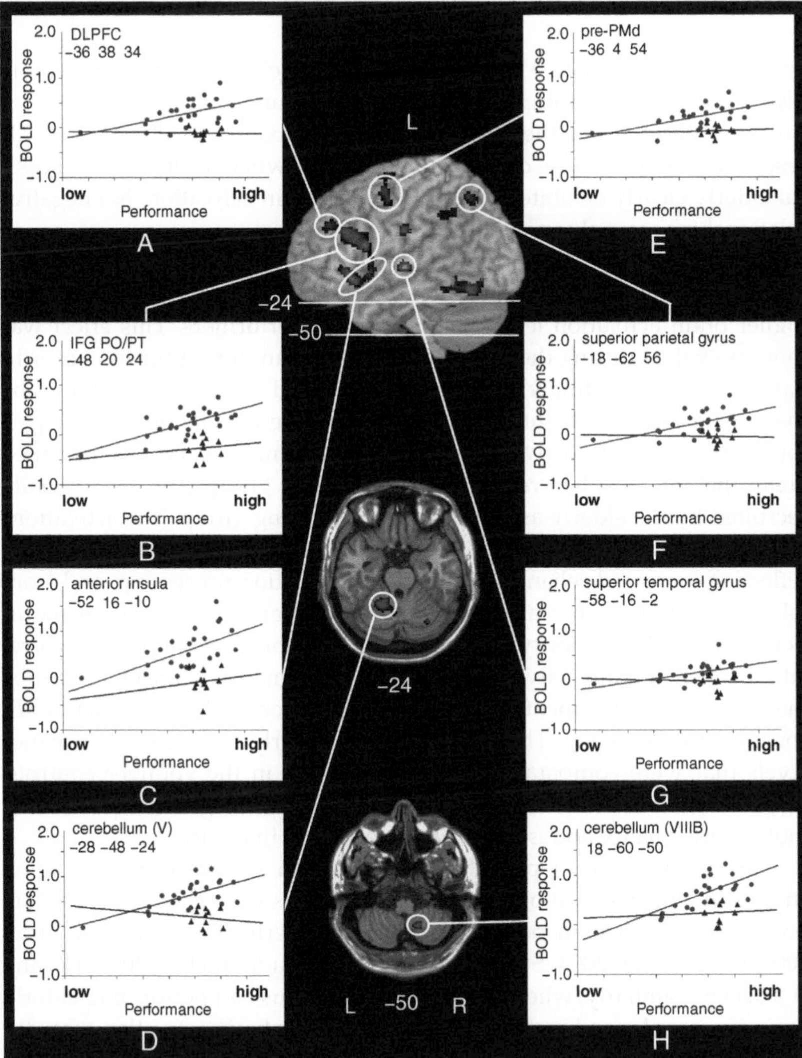

Figure 17.3 Statistical parametric mappings representing significantly larger activation in the older compared with the younger group during the NONISODIR coordination mode. Significant voxels ($p < 0.05$; corrected for multiple comparisons) are indicated in the gray spectrum, and the height threshold is $t = 4.00$. L, left hemisphere; R, right hemisphere. The brain regions that demonstrate a significant positive correlation between brain activity level and coordination performance are encircled. The graphics display each subject's BOLD response as a function of phase error, with the younger subjects in black triangles and the older subjects in gray circles. Note that low performance corresponds to a high phase error, and high performance to a low phase error. DLPFC, dorsolateral prefrontal cortex; pre-PMd, pre-dorsal premotor; IFG PO/PT, inferior frontal gyrus pars opercularis/triangularis. Adapted from Heuninckx S., N. Wenderoth, and S.P. Swinnen. 2008. Systems neuroplasticity in the aging brain: Recruiting additional neural resources for successful motor performance in elderly persons. *Journal of Neuroscience* 28:91–99, with permission of the publisher.

and the individual BOLD responses of the old (*light gray circles*) and young (*dark gray triangles*) subjects are displayed as a function of performance. It can be observed that the elderly performing poorly exhibited a BOLD response similar to those of the young controls, whereas the more successful elderly clearly exhibited higher levels of brain activation. No negative relationships were observed.

In summary, the older adults showed a significant positive correlation between activation and performance, such that good performers exhibited higher brain activation levels than did poor performers. This effect was more prevalent during the more demanding, than during the easy coordination task. Accordingly, our results provided strong support for the *compensation hypothesis*. Interestingly, this positive association between performance and brain activity was evident in some specific, well-defined areas that were either recruited by both age groups, or, additionally recruited by the elderly as compared to the young group. The activations refer to classical motor control areas, higher-level sensorimotor areas reflecting increased reliance on sensory information processing, and frontal areas reflecting increased cognitive control and monitoring of motor performance. The majority of these regions demonstrated a positive correlation between brain activation level and performance in the elderly, such that increased recruitment in these areas was associated with higher motor coordination accuracy. This enabled some elderly to reach performance levels that were comparable to those obtained in the younger controls, suggesting that the additional recruitment is meaningful for preserving motor performance and is largely compensatory in nature.

Our findings are in partial agreement with several cognitive aging studies in which activation levels in frontal areas were shown to correlate positively with overall performance in the elderly (Reuter-Lorenz et al. 2000; Grady et al. 2003; Scarmeas et al. 2003; Madden et al. 2004; Rosano et al. 2005). Similarly, when groups of good versus bad performing elderly were compared, good performers exhibited more brain activation than did bad performers (Cabeza et al. 2002; Rosen et al. 2002). However, it appears that, in motor control studies, the compensatory recruitment extends far beyond the prefrontal areas. Indeed, a more elaborate network involved in cognitive control and enhanced processing of sensory information for motor performance was correlated with motor performance.

The prefrontal recruitment is of particular interest here. For example, the DLPFC receives visual, somatosensory, and auditory information from the occipital, temporal, and parietal cortices (Goldman-Rakic and Schwartz 1982; Barbas and Pandya 1989; Seltzer and Pandya 1989; Pandya and Yeterian 1990; Petrides and Pandya 1999) and has preferential connections with the motor system structures (Miller and Cohen 2001). Accordingly, the DLPFC is likely to play a central role in the cognitive control of motor behavior (Miller and Cohen 2001). This penetration of cognition into motor performance appears to be a marker of successful aging and possibly reflects system-level neuroplasticity at higher age. Rehabilitation interventions that promote the exploitation of cognitive processing mechanisms for action control may find support through these observations.

Some additional points are noteworthy in the context of compensatory recruitment. First, the lack of positive correlations between brain activation and motor performance in younger adults does not imply that such correlations are or should be absent in this group. This is not the case, and part of the problem may be associated with the higher degree of performance homogeneity in the young group. Second, it may be a bit naïve to think that positive correlations will always be observed in older groups (Van Impe et al. 2009). There are a number of factors that may impact upon the size of the correlations, such as task features, task difficulty level, and other factors. In this context, we entertain the hypothesis that such correlations are more likely determined experimentally when task difficulty is sufficiently high, such that (a) reasonable neural recruitment levels can be obtained and (b) the performer is sufficiently probed to reveal CNS deficiencies more easily. Correlations provide only one potential piece of evidence in supporting the compensation hypothesis. In spite of these concerns, it is rather impressive that such positive correlations between brain and behavior are indeed observed.

CURRENT STATUS OF IMAGING RESEARCH ON AGING AND MOTOR CONTROL: AN EMERGING PICTURE

Compared to the wealth of imaging research on aging and cognition, few studies have addressed age-related changes in brain activation during motor performance. Even though commonalities emerge from the motor studies, a divergence in findings is also noted (for a review, see also Ward 2006). This is possibly a consequence of differing approaches to data analysis, statistics, experimental paradigms, task choice, and different ways to equate behavioral performance between young and old groups. Here, we will try to summarize some commonalities across the divergent motor task paradigms.

A few motor studies have reported only age-related decreases in extent or magnitude of primary and secondary motor area activation during a simple motor task (Hesselmann et al. 2001; Tekes et al. 2005). Both studies used fixed-effects analysis, which is currently considered a less optimal design when comparing two groups. This is a potential problem when looking for age-related changes because the error variance may be more dominated by *within-subject* variability. Random-effects analyses are more appropriate because the error variance is dominated by *between-subjects* variability (Ward 2006).

Hutchinson et al. (2002) also used a fixed-effects model to analyze age-related effects in brain activation during repetitive wrist flexion and extension, as well as index finger abduction and adduction. They demonstrated greater activation in contralateral sensorimotor and premotor cortices in the younger subjects, but greater activation in SMA in the older subjects for both tasks. Ipsilateral sensorimotor cortex activity was greater in the older subjects during finger movements only. Mattay et al. (2002) provided more convincing evidence of additional recruitment and compensatory reorganization in the elderly during performance of a visually paced button-press motor task with the dominant (right) hand. Recording of behavioral data enabled a distinction to be made between older subjects who performed at the same level as younger subjects, and those whose performance was in some way impaired. A random-effects model revealed that older subjects overactivated a number of regions in comparison to younger subjects, in particular the bilateral M1, SMA, premotor and parietal cortices, and cerebellum. Moreover, they observed a negative correlation in the older group between the magnitude of task-related activity and reaction time in bilateral M1, premotor cortex, SMA, contralateral parietal cortex, and ipsilateral cerebellum; that is, elderly subjects who showed greater activity in the aforementioned motor regions were able to react more quickly (Mattay et al. 2002). These results suggest functionally relevant reorganization of the cerebral motor network in some elderly subjects.

Both the increased age-related activations and the correlation between brain activation and performance are generally consistent with our ipsilateral coordination findings reported earlier. However, comparisons across studies also underscore that age-related changes are task specific. Using a simple motor task, Mattay et al. (2002) described age-related increases within known motor-related networks only, whereas our more complex motor task resulted in age-related increases in the motor network, as well as in areas related to higher-level sensorimotor processing and integration, and areas responsible for the cognitive surveillance of motor control.

Evidence for age-related additional activation in the motor network has also been provided by studies investigating, respectively, a thumb-to-index finger tapping task (Naccarato et al. 2006) and an index finger tapping task at increasing frequencies (2.0, 2.5, 3.0, 4.0, 5.0, and 6.0 Hz) (Riecker et al. 2006). In contrast to Hutchinson et al. (2002), Naccarato et al. (2006) observed age-related increased activation in the contralateral and ipsilateral M1.

At each single finger-tapping frequency, as well as across all finger-tapping frequencies, Riecker et al. (2006) found that the older subjects exhibited significantly greater activation than young subjects in the ipsilateral SM1 and premotor cortex. Assuming that incremental movement rates are associated with an increased functional demand on the motor system, the authors hypothesized that age-related areas of overactivation should either increase during higher movement rates or should show a close coupling between the movement rate and the hemodynamic response. However, they showed that the hemodynamic response magnitude in the overactivated regions remained constant across all frequencies. The authors concluded that age-related overactivation within the motor system was not related to the functional demand and did not necessarily reflect reorganization to compensate for the neurobiological changes of aging. In our study, however, we manipulated the functional demand on the motor system by using different degrees of movement complexity: isolated versus coordinated hand–foot movements under easy (ISODIR) and more difficult (NONISODIR) conditions. In addition to demonstrating age-related activation increases, the spatial distribution of brain activations also extended with increasing movement complexity in our study (see earlier discussion). Even though the tasks, as well as the experimental manipulations, differ from the frequency manipulation used in Riecker et al. (2006), our results show rather graded responses to increasing demands. Overall, it appears that simple single-effector versus complex multieffector tasks give rise to different results. Additional research is necessary to investigate the neural consequences of increasing task demands.

Wu and Hallett (2005) had younger and older subjects learn a button-pressing motor sequence until it became automatic. Subjects were scanned before and after learning, ensuring that any age-related differences in brain activation patterns more likely represented functionally relevant or compensatory reorganization. A random-effects analysis showed that brain activity was reduced at post-test as compared to pre-test in both groups, suggesting improved efficiency in task-relevant networks. The comparison of both groups after training revealed relative overactivations in the older group in the bilateral premotor and parietal cortices, bilateral cerebellum, and precuneus, as well as in the left prefrontal cortex, rostral SMA, anterior CMA, caudate nucleus, and thalamus. Given that task-related activity did not increase in any brain region after training in either group, this result is likely to indicate less training-related reduction in activity in the aforementioned brain regions for the older group. This is an intriguing result because the older subjects were able to perform at the same level in the post-training task even though their task-related network appeared less efficient (i.e., more elaborate). One possible explanation is that greater post-training activation was seen in the left sensorimotor cortex in the younger group compared to the old. Although speculative, this may refer to reduced capacity for change in M1 in older adults, and thus the more distributed network was possibly required for preserving performance levels.

Compared to the aforementioned studies looking for categorical differences between groups, Ward and Frackowiak (2003) examined the nature of the relationship between task-related signal changes across an age range of 21 to 80 years. A repetitive isometric hand-grip task was used with continuous visual feedback of the force produced. This task was performed by the dominant and nondominant hand and was found to activate a network of cortical and subcortical regions, typical for simple motor acts, as well as activation in a putative human "grasping circuit," involving the rostral PMv and intraparietal sulcus. Within this network, age-related increases were demonstrated in the left deep anterior central sulcus, caudal PMd, caudal cingulate sulcus, intraparietal sulcus, insula, frontal operculum, and cerebellar vermis. These results support again the view that an adaptable and plastic motor network is able to respond to or adjust for age-related changes in order to maintain performance levels on a visually paced hand-grip task.

Summarizing, it is difficult to make direct comparisons among studies because of differences in the experimental paradigms, subject selection features, analyses, and tasks used. These vary from button-pressing tasks (Mattay et al. 2002) to wrist or finger movement tasks (e.g. Hutchinson et al. 2002; Naccarato et al. 2006; Riecker et al. 2006), visuomotor tasks (e.g. Ward and Frackowiak 2003), interlimb coordination tasks (Heuninckx et al. 2005, 2008; Van Impe et al. 2009), and learned motor sequence tasks (Wu and Hallet 2005). The distributed networks for each task vary, resulting in differential age-related changes. Despite this, there appears to be mounting evidence for a wider recruitment of brain regions in older subjects during a variety of motor tasks. As tasks become more complex, the age-related increases expand from the known motor network to areas involved in higher-level sensorimotor processing/integration and cognitive monitoring of movement. Furthermore, results of Mattay et al. (2002) and those from our laboratory (Heuninckx et al. 2008) have additionally demonstrated positive relations between overactivation in the elderly and performance, suggestive of compensatory mechanisms in the aging brain. This is hypothesized to imply reorganization and redistribution of functional networks to compensate for presumed age-related structural and neurochemical changes. This hypothesis will have to be investigated in more detail in future studies. Even though evidence for age-related activation increases is prominent, decreases should also be taken into consideration, and will most likely be part of attempts to understand complex brain reorganization.

WHY DOES OVERACTIVATION OCCUR IN OLDER ADULTS?

Brain imaging research on aging has increasingly focused on an investigation of the relationship between age-related changes in brain function and concomitant changes in behavior. The largely unanticipated result from functional neuroimaging is overactivation. Age-related, region-specific overactivation is now well documented for a wide range of tasks referring to various cognitive (for reviews, see Grady 2000; Cabeza 2001; Reuter-Lorenz 2002; Hedden and Gabrieli 2004; Rajah and D'Esposito 2005; Reuter-Lorenz and Lustig 2005) and motor functions (Hutchinson et al. 2002; Mattay et al. 2002; Heuninckx et al. 2005, 2008; Naccarato et al. 2006; Riecker et al. 2006; Ward and Frackowiak 2003).

Compensatory changes in brain activation patterns are not unique to normally aging individuals. Consider Parkinson's disease (PD), in which hyperactivation in the ipsilateral cerebellum has been identified as a compensatory mechanism for the defective basal ganglia showing hypoactivity in the putamen, but also in the SMA and pre-SMA during performance of thumb-pressing movements (Yu et al. 2007). In addition, Helmich et al. (2009) have shown that, with increasing disease severity in PD, contributions of the basal ganglia to hand selection during a hand laterality judgment task and their effective connectivity with the medial frontal cortex (MFC) decreases, whereas involvement of the MFC increases (Helmich et al. 2009). Another example is found in patients with chronic subcortical hemiparetic stroke (Cramer et al. 1997; Cao et al. 1998; Newton et al. 2002; Ward et al. 2003a; Zemke et al. 2003). Overactivations in strokes are typically seen in secondary motor regions, such as the premotor cortex, SMA, and CMA, as well as in the parietal cortex. Moreover, these overactivations appear greater in patients with more motor impairment (Ward et al. 2003b) and greater damage to the corticospinal system (Ward et al. 2006).

At first sight, this pattern of reorganization in neurological populations appears similar to the shift from a focused to a more elaborate network in healthy older subjects under both cognitive and sensorimotor conditions. Whether this implies that overactivation in older adults also occurs directly in response to age-related deterioration remains to be seen. We are inclined to believe that the situation is more complex, but it does prompt questions about how compensation for functional and/or structural degeneration in the aging brain may trigger increased neural recruitment. This brings us back to the compensation–dedifferentiation hypotheses. As discussed previously, several lines of evidence support the compensatory viewpoint.

First, older adults show more activated regions for tasks that show minimal adverse performance effects due to age, such as autobiographical memory and verb generation (Maguire and Frith 2003; Persson et al. 2004), and when performance levels, effort exerted, or both, are matched (Ward and Frackowiak 2003). Second, activation levels have been shown to correlate positively with overall performance levels in motor and cognitive tasks (Mattay et al. 2002; Grady et al. 2003; Scarmeas et al. 2003; Madden et al. 2004; Heuninckx et al. 2008). In some cases, when subgroups of elderly individuals were examined, region-specific overactivations were characteristic for those groups that performed best (Cabeza et al. 2002; Rosen et al. 2002). These findings are consistent with our ipsilateral coordination results, in which additional recruitment of brain regions was especially observed in those older subjects who displayed performance levels comparable to those of the younger controls. Third, overactivations have been linked to trial outcome using event-related fMRI. Greater activity in prefrontal regions, especially lateral and inferior prefrontal sites, has been found in older adults in an encoding task when items were successfully remembered (Morcom et al. 2003; Gutchess et al. 2005). Thus, according to the functional compensation view, age-related decreases or absences in activation reflect deficits in brain function, and the concomitant increases in activation reflect successful compensation for these deficits, particularly when the increases are correlated with performance.

Overall, the aforementioned arguments support the compensatory view of overactivation in older adults. Even though this is an exciting and optimistic perspective, there may be some pitfalls: overactivation may have a hidden cost because it implies overall reduced economy in neural recruitment. More specifically, to the extent that older brains engage more neural circuitry at lower levels of task demand than younger adults do, seniors rely more on "cognitive reserve" (Scarmeas et al. 2003) and are thus more likely to reach a limit on the resources that can be brought to bear on task performance (DiGirolamo et al. 2001). As such, limitations in performance may emerge when task difficulty increases, or when multiple tasks have to be performed simultaneously. For example, the elderly's increased deployment of neural resources during motor performance, and particularly the recruitment of generic areas that span the motor and cognitive domains, may account for the extra difficulties they encounter when thinking or talking while walking (Lindenberger et al. 2000; Li et al. 2001). As such, the present findings have theoretical as well as clinical relevance for gerontology.

CONCLUSION

When summarizing current evidence on age-related brain function in the context of motor performance, the suggestion emerges that older adults utilize a partly different, more elaborate brain network during motor performance than do young adults, even when the same behavioral outcomes are produced. This suggests that preserved motor performance may be related to the ability of older adults to increase activation and/or to recruit new areas within sensorimotor and cognitive networks, and/or exhibit altered interactions among brain areas that constitute a specific network. This interpretation implies that an age-related compensatory mechanism is at work. The positive correlation between brain activation levels and behavioral performance seems to suggest that the compensatory recruitment is, at least under certain circumstances, beneficial to motor and cognitive performance. The observed brain activation increases during interlimb coordination are meaningful for older adults because they refer to enhanced recruitment in (a) the basic motor network, (b) areas responsible for sensory processing and (inter)sensory integration, (c) areas involved in imagery/visualization of movement, and (d) prefrontal areas reflecting increased cognitive control of movement. Accordingly, medical imaging research supports the view that aging is associated with a shift along the continuum from automatic to more controlled information processing for movement.

This field of study is still relatively young, and much more research is clearly needed. More specifically, for progress to be made, functional reorganization will need to be interpreted in connection with direct measures of structural/anatomical, as well as behavioral changes and age-related strategic changes in task performance. Diffusion tensor imaging has already been used to assess white matter tract integrity as a function of age (Madden et al. 2004, 2007; Sullivan and Pfefferbaum 2006). Voxel-based morphometry is instrumental in assessing age-related gray matter changes (Good et al. 2001; Alexander et al. 2006; Lehmbeck et al. 2006). Transcranial magnetic stimulation (TMS) has been used to assess age-related changes in intracortical inhibition (Peinemann et al. 2001). These measures could be used as more direct markers of age-related change with which to interpret age-related changes in motor-related organization (Ward 2006). A critical question is whether these complementary techniques will be able to demonstrate for what specific dysfunction or structural deterioration the brain compensates and whether there are boundaries in compensatory recruitment. Finally, investigations into age-related changes in functional and structural brain connectivity will hopefully reveal critical insights into modulation of the intensity and strength of interconnections among brain areas because these may also trigger alterations in functional brain activation. It is possible that compensatory recruitment is only part of the story and that decreased recruitment will have to be considered as part of a comprehensive model on aging. Our working hypothesis in this respect is that underactivation in one brain area may be compensated for by overactivation in other, more remote, areas in the ipsilateral or contralateral hemisphere. More specifically, it is possible that decreased integrity of subcortical structures will be compensated for by increased cortical recruitment to bypass the affected structures. This field of research is bound to become a very exciting yet highly complex endeavor at the interface between age-related structural, functional, and behavioral changes.

ACKNOWLEDGMENTS

This study was supported by grants from the Research Fund K.U. Leuven, Belgium (OT/07/073) and the Flanders Fund for Scientific Research (G.0593.08, G.0483.10). Post-doctoral funding from the above sources was also obtained by D. Goble (GP00408N & F/07/063) and J. Coxon (GP00608N & F/07/064). A. Van Impe was funded by a Ph.D. fellowship of the Research Foundation - Flanders (FWO).

REFERENCES

Alexander, G.E., K. Chen, T.L. Merkley, E.M. Reinman, R.J. Caselli, H. Aschenbrenner, et al. 2006. Regional network of magnetic resonance imaging gray matter volume in healthy aging. *Neuroreport* 17:951–56.

Aron, A.R., and R.A. Poldrack. 2006. Cortical and subcortical contributions to Stop signal response inhibition: role of the subthalamic nucleus. *Journal of Neuroscience* 26:2424–2433.

Ashe, J., and A.P. Georgopoulos. 1994. Movement parameters and neural activity in motor cortex and area 5. *Cerebral Cortex* 4:590–600.

Baldissera, F., P. Cavallari, and P. Civaschi. 1982. Preferential coupling between voluntary movements of ipsilateral limbs. *Neuroscience Letters* 34:95–100.

Baldissera, F., P. Cavallari, G. Marini, and G. Tassone. 1991. Differential control of in-phase and anti-phase coupling of rhythmic movements of ipsilateral hand and foot. *Experimental Brain Research* 83:375–80.

Baldissera, F., P. Borroni, P. Cavallari, G. Cerri. 2002. Excitability changes in human corticospinal projections to forearm muscles during voluntary movement of ipsilateral foot. *Journal of Physiology* 539:903–11.

Barbas, H., and D.N. Pandya. 1989. Architecture and intrinsic connections of the prefrontal cortex in the rhesus monkey. The *Journal of Comparative Neurology* 286:353–75.

Bamiou, D.E., F.E. Musiek, and L.M. Luxon. 2003. The insula Island of Reil and its role in auditory processing. Literature review. *Brain Research. Brain Research Reviews* 42:143–54.

Behrmann, M., J.J. Geng, and S. Shomstein. 2004. Parietal cortex and attention. *Current Opinion in Neurobiology* 14:212–17.

Binkofski, F., K. Amunts, K.M. Stephan, S. Posse, T. Schormann, H.J. Freund, et al. 2000. Broca's region subserves imagery of motion: A combined cytoarchitectonic and fMRI study. *Human Brain Mapping* 11:273–85.

Bonda, E., M. Petrides, D. Ostry, and A. Evans. 1996. Specific involvement of human parietal systems and the amygdala in the perception of biological motion. *Journal of Neuroscience* 16:3737–44.

Botvinick, M., L.E. Nystrom, K. Fissell, C.S. Carter, and J.D. Cohen. 1999. Conflict monitoring versus selection-for-action in anterior cingulate cortex. *Nature* 402:179–81.

Buckner, R.L. 2004. Memory and executive function in aging and AD: Multiple factors that cause decline and reserve factors that compensate. *Neuron* 44: 195–208.

Buckner, R.L., A.Z. Snyder, A.L. Sanders, M.E. Raichle, and J.C. Morris. 2000. Functional brain imaging of young, nondemented, and demented older adults. *Journal of Cognitive Neuroscience* 12 (Suppl 2): 24–34.

Bushara, K.O., J.M. Wheat, A. Khan, B.J. Mock, P.A. Turski, J. Sorenson, and B.R. Brooks. 2001. Multiple tactile maps in the human cerebellum. *Neuroreport* 12:2483–86.

Byblow, W.D., J.P. Coxon, C.M. Stinear, M.K. Fleming, G. Williams, J.F. Muller, and U. Ziemann. 2007. Functional connectivity between secondary and primary motor areas underlying hand–foot coordination. *Journal of Neurophysiology* 98: 414–22.

Cabeza, R. 2001. Cognitive neuroscience of aging: Contributions of functional neuroimaging. *Scandinavian Journal of Psychology* 42:277–86.

Cabeza, R. 2002. Hemispheric asymmetry reduction in older adults: The HAROLD model. *Psychology and Aging* 17:85–100.

Cabeza, R., N.D. Anderson, S. Houle, J.A. Mangels, and L. Nyberg. 2000. Age-related differences in neural activity during item and temporal-order memory retrieval: A positron emission tomography study. *Journal of Cognitive Neuroscience* 12:197–206.

Cabeza, R., N.D. Anderson, J.K. Locantore, and A.R. McIntosh. 2002. Aging gracefully: Compensatory brain activity in high-performing older adults. *NeuroImage* 17:1394–1402.

Cabeza, R., L. Nyberg, and D.C. Park. 2005. *Cognitive neuroscience of aging.* New York: Oxford University Press.

Cabeza, R., N.D. Anderson, J.K. Locantore, and A.R. McIntosh. 2002. Aging gracefully: Compensatory brain activity in high-performing older adults. *NeuroImage* 17:1394–1402.

Campisi, J. 2003. Cellular senescence and apoptosis: How cellular responses might influence aging phenotypes. *Experimental Gerontology* 38:5–11.

Cao, Y., L. D'Olhaberriague, E.M. Vikingstad, S.R. Levine, and K.M. Welch. 1998. Pilot study of functional MRI to assess cerebral activation of motor function after poststroke hemiparesis. *Stroke* 29:112–22.

Carter, C.S., M.M. Botvinick, and J.D. Cohen. 1999. The contribution of the anterior cingulate cortex to executive processes in cognition. *Reviews in the Neurosciences* 10:49–57.

Casey, B.J., K.M. Thomas, T.F. Welsh, R.D. Badgaiyan, C.H. Eccard, J.R. Jennings, and E.A. Crone. 2000. Dissociation of response conflict, attentional selection, and expectancy with functional magnetic resonance imaging. *Proceedings of the National Academy of Sciences of the USA* 97:8728–33.

Cavada, C., and P.S. Goldman-Rakic. 1989. Posterior parietal cortex in rhesus monkey: II. Evidence for segregated corticocortical networks linking sensory and limbic areas with the frontal lobe. *The Journal of Comparative Neurology* 287:422–45.

Caeyenberghs, K., N. Wenderoth, B.C. Smits-Engelsman, S. Sunaert, and S.P. Swinnen. 2009. Neural correlates of motor dysfunction in children with traumatic brain injury: Exploration of compensatory recruitment patterns. *Brain* 132:684–94.

Coxon, J.P., C.M. Stinear, and W.D. Byblow. 2009. Stop and go: The neural basis of selective movement prevention. *Journal of Cognitive Neuroscience* 21:1193–1203.

Cramer, S.C., G. Nelles, R.R. Benson, J.D. Kaplan, R.A. Parker, K.K. Kwong, et al. 1997. A functional MRI study of subjects recovered from hemiparetic stroke. *Stroke* 28:2581–27.

Carson, R.G., D. Goodman, J.A. Kelso, and D. Elliott. 1995. Phase transitions and critical fluctuations in rhythmic coordination of ipsilateral hand and foot. *Journal of Motor Behavior* 27:211–24.

Craik, F. I. M., C.L. Grady. 2002. Aging, memory and frontal lobe functioning. In *Principles of frontal lobe function* eds., D.T. Stuss and R.T. Knight, 528–41. New York: Oxford University Press.

Debaere, F., S.P. Swinnen, E. Beatse, S. Sunaert, P. Van Hecke, and J. Duysens. 2001a. Brain areas involved in interlimb coordination: A distributed network. *Neuroimage* 14:947–58.

Debaere, F., D. Van Assche, C. Kiekens, S.M. Verschueren, and S.P. Swinnen. 2001b. Coordination of upper and lower limb segments: Deficits on the ipsilesional side after unilateral stroke. *Experimental Brain Research* 141:519–29.

Debaere, F., N. Wenderoth, S. Sunaert, P. Van Hecke, and S.P. Swinnen. 2003. Internal vs. external generation of movements: Differential neural pathways involved in bimanual coordination performed in the presence or absence of augmented visual feedback. *NeuroImage* 19:764–76.

Debaere, F., N. Wenderoth, S. Sunaert, P. Van Hecke, and S.P. Swinnen. 2004. Changes in brain activation during the acquisition of a new bimanual coordination task. *Neuropsychologia* 42:855–67.

Della-Maggiore, V., A.B. Sekuler, C.L. Grady, P.J. Bennett, R. Sekuler, and A.R. McIntosh. 2000. Corticolimbic interactions associated with performance on a short-term memory task are modified by age. *Journal of Neuroscience* 20:8410–16.

DiGirolamo, G.J., A.F. Kramer, V. Barad, N.J. Cepeda, D.H. Weissman, M.P. Milham, et al. 2001. General and task-specific frontal lobe recruitment in older adults during executive processes: A fMRI investigation of task-switching. *Neuroreport* 12:2065–71.

Ehrsson, H.H., J.P. Kuhtz-Buschbeck, and H. Forssberg. 2002. Brain regions controlling nonsynergistic versus synergistic movement of the digits: A functional magnetic resonance imaging study. *Journal of Neuroscience* 22:5074–80.

Ehrsson, H.H., E. Naito, S. Geyer, K. Amunts, K. Zilles, H. Forssberg, and P.E. Roland. 2000. Simultaneous movements of upper and lower limbs are coordinated by motor representations that are shared by both limbs: A PET study. *European Journal of Neuroscience* 12:3385–98.

Ferraina, S., and L. Bianchi. 1994. Posterior parietal cortex: Functional properties of neurons in area 5 during an instructed-delay reaching task within different parts of space. *Experimental Brain Research* 99:175–78.

Gabrieli, J.D. 1996. Memory systems analyses of mnemonic disorders in aging and age-related diseases. *Proceedings of the National Academy of Sciences of the USA* 93:13534–40.

Gazzaley, A., and M. D'Esposito. 2003. The contribution of functional brain imaging to our understanding of cognitive aging. *Science of Aging Knowledge Environment* E2.

Garavan, H., T.J. Ross, and E.A. Stein. 1999. Right hemispheric dominance of inhibitory control: An event-related functional MRI study. *Proceedings of the National Academy of Sciences of the USA* 96:8301–06.

Garcia-Larrea, L., H. Bastuji, and F. Mauguiere. 1991. Mapping study of somatosensory evoked potentials during selective spatial attention. *Electroencephalography and Clinical Neurophysiology* 80:201–14.

Genovese, C.R., N.A. Lazar, and T. Nichols. 2002. Thresholding of statistical maps in functional neuroimaging using the false discovery rate. *NeuroImage* 15: 870–78.

Geyer, S., M. Matelli, G. Luppino, and K. Zilles. 2000. Functional neuroanatomy of the primate isocortical motor system. *Anatomy and Embryology Berl* 202: 443–74.

Goble, D.J., J.P. Coxon, N. Wenderoth, A. Van Impe, and S.P. Swinnen. 2009. Proprioceptive sensibility in the elderly: Degeneration, functional consequences and plastic-adaptive processes. *Neuroscience and Biobehavioral Reviews* 33:271–78.

Good, C.D., I.S. Johnsrude, J. Ashburner, R.N. Henson, K.J. Friston, and R.S. Frackowiak. 2001. A voxel-based morphometric study of ageing in 465 normal adult human brains. *NeuroImage* 14:21–36.

Goldman-Rakic, P.S., and M.L. Schwartz. 1982. Interdigitation of contralateral and ipsilateral columnar projections to frontal association cortex in primates. *Science* 216:755–57.

Grady, C.L., J.M. Maisog, B. Horwitzm, L.G. Ungerleider, M.J. Mentis, J.A. Salerno, et al. 1994. Age-related changes in cortical blood flow activation during visual processing of faces and location. *Journal of Neuroscience* 14:1450–62.

Grady, C.L. 2000. Functional brain imaging and age-related changes in cognition. *Biological Psychology* 54:259–81.

Grady, C.L. 2002a. Age-related differences in face processing: A meta-analysis of three functional neuroimaging experiments. *Canadian Journal of Experimental Psychology* 56:208–20.

Grady, C.L. 2002b. Introduction to the special section on aging, cognition, and neuroimaging. *Psychology and Aging* 17:3–6.

Grady, C.L. 2008. Cognitive neuroscience of aging. *Annals of the New York Academy of Sciences* 1124:127–44.

Grady, C.L., A.R. McIntosh, S. Beig, M.L. Keightley, H. Burian, and S.E. Black. 2003. Evidence from functional neuroimaging of a compensatory prefrontal network in Alzheimer's disease. *Journal of Neuroscience* 23:986–93.

Grady, C.L., A.R. McIntosh, F. Bookstein, B. Horwitz, S.I. Rapoport, and J.V. Haxby. 1998. Age-related changes in regional cerebral blood flow during working memory for faces. *NeuroImage* 8:409–25.

Grady, C.L., A.R. McIntosh, B. Horwitz, J.M. Maisog, L.G. Ungerleider, M.J. Mentis, et al. 1995. Age-related reductions in human recognition memory due to impaired encoding. *Science* 269:218–21.

Grezes, J., N. Costes, and J. Decety. 1998. Top-down effect of strategy on the perception of human biological motion: A PET investigation. *Cognitive Neuropsychology* 15:553–82.

Grossman, M., A. Cooke, C. DeVita, D. Alsop, J. Detre, W. Chen, and J. Gee. 2002. Age-related changes in working memory during sentence comprehension: An fMRI study. *NeuroImage* 15:302–17.

Gutchess, A.H., R.C. Welsh, T. Hedden, A. Bangert, M. Minear, L.L. Liu, and D.C. Park. 2005. Aging and the neural correlates of successful picture encoding: Frontal activations compensate for decreased medial-temporal activity. *Journal of Cognitive Neuroscience* 17:84–96.

Habas, C., H. Axelrad, T.H. Nguyen, and E.A. Cabanis. 2004. Specific neocerebellar activation during out-of-phase bimanual movements. *Neuroreport* 15: 595–99.

Hagmann P., L. Cammoun, X. Gigandet, R. Meuli, C.J. Honey, V.J. Wedeen, and O. Sporns. 2008. Mapping the structural core of human cerebral cortex. *PLoS Biology* 6:e159.

Hari, R., H. Hamalainen, M. Hamalainen, J. Kekoni, M. Sams, and J. Tiihonen. 1990. Separate finger representations at the human second somatosensory cortex. *Neuroscience* 37:245–49.

Hartley, A.A., N.K. Speer, J. Jonides, P.A. Reuter-Lorenz, and E.E. Smith. 2001. Is the dissociability of working memory systems for name identity, visual-object identity, and spatial location maintained in old age? *Neuropsychology* 15:3–17.

Hedden, T., and J.D. Gabrieli. 2004. Insights into the ageing mind: A view from cognitive neuroscience. *Nature Reviews. Neuroscience* 5:87–96.

Helmich, R.C., E. Aarts, F.P. de Lange, B.R. Bloem, and I. Toni. 2009. Increased dependence of action selection on recent motor history in Parkinson's disease. *Journal of Neuroscience* 29:6105–13.

Heuninckx, S., F. Debaere, N. Wenderoth, S. Verschueren, and S.P. Swinnen. 2004. Ipsilateral coordination deficits and central processing requirements associated with coordination as a function of aging. *Journal of Gerontology Series B: Psychological Sciences and Social Sciences* 59B:225–32.

Heuninckx, S., N. Wenderoth, F. Debaere, R. Peeters, and S.P. Swinnen. 2005. Neural basis of aging: The penetration of cognition into action control. *Journal of Neuroscience* 25:6787–96.

Heuninckx S., N. Wenderoth, and S.P. Swinnen. 2008. Systems neuroplasticity in the aging brain: Recruiting additional neural resources for successful motor performance in elderly persons. *Journal of Neuroscience* 28:91–99.

Hesselmann, V., O.Z. Weber, C. Wedekind, T. Krings, O. Schulte, H. Kugel, et al. 2001. Age related signal decrease in functional magnetic resonance imaging during motor stimulation in humans. *Neuroscience Letters* 308:141–44.

Hikosaka, O., K. Nakamura, K. Sakai, and H. Nakahara. 2002. Central mechanisms of motor skill learning. *Current Opinion in Neurobiology* 12:217–22.

Holtzer, R., Y. Stern, and B.C. Rakitin. 2005. Predicting age-related dual-task effects with individual differences on neuropsychological tests. *Neuropsychology* 19:18–27.

Hutchinson, S., M. Kobayashi, C.M. Horkan, A. Pascual-Leone, M.P. Alexander, and G. Schlaug. 2002. Age-related differences in movement representation. *NeuroImage* 17:1720–28.

Huttunen, J., H. Wikstrom, A. Korvenoja, A.M. Seppalainen, H. Aronen, and R.J. Ilmoniemi. 1996. Significance of the second somatosensory cortex in sensorimotor integration: Enhancement of sensory responses during finger movements. *Neuroreport* 7:1009–12.

Iacoboni, M., R.P. Woods, M. Brass, H. Bekkering, J.C. Mazziotta, and G. Rizzolatti. 1999. Cortical mechanisms of human imitation. *Science* 286:2526–28.

Immisch, I., D. Waldvogel, P. van Gelderen, and M. Hallett. 2001. The role of the medial wall and its anatomical variations for bimanual antiphase and in-phase movements. *NeuroImage* 14:674–84.

Ivry, R. 1997. Cerebellar timing systems. *International Review of Neurobiology* 41: 555–73.

Jahn, K., A. Deutschlander, T. Stephan, M. Strupp, M. Wiesmann, and T. Brandt. 2004. Brain activation patterns during imagined stance and locomotion in functional magnetic resonance imaging. *NeuroImage* 22:1722–31.

Jueptner, M., S. Ottinger, S.J. Fellows, J. Adamschewski, L. Flerich, S.P. Muller, et al. 1997. The relevance of sensory input for the cerebellar control of movements. *NeuroImage* 5:41–48.

Kalaska, J.F., D.A. Cohen, M. Prud'homme, and M.L. Hyde. 1990. Parietal area 5 neuronal activity encodes movement kinematics, not movement dynamics. *Experimental Brain Research* 80:351–64.

Keizer, K., and H.G. Kuypers. 1989. Distribution of corticospinal neurons with collaterals to the lower brain stem reticular formation in monkey *Macaca fascicularis*. *Experimental Brain Research* 74:311–18.

Kelso, J.A. 1984. Phase transitions and critical behavior in human bimanual coordination. *American Journal of Physiology* 246:R1000-R1004.

Kelso, J.A., and J.J. Jeka. 1992. Symmetry breaking dynamics of human multilimb coordination. *Journal of Experimental Psychology: Human Perception and Performance* 18:645–68.

Kiehl, K.A., P.F. Liddle, and J.B. Hopfinger. 2000. Error processing and the rostral anterior cingulate: An event-related fMRI study. *Psychophysiology* 37:216–23.

Lam, K., R. Kakigi, Y. Kaneoke, D. Naka, K. Maeda, and H. Suzuki. 1999. Effects of visual and auditory stimulation on somatosensory evoked magnetic fields. *Clinical Neurophysiology* 110:295–304.

Labat-Robert, J. 2001. Cell-matrix interactions, alteration with aging and age associated diseases. A review. *Pathologie-Biologie* 49:349–52.

Ladislas, R. 2000. Cellular and molecular mechanisms of aging and age related diseases. *Pathology Oncology Research* 6:3–9.

Lehmbeck, J.T., S. Brassens, W. Weber-Fahr, and D.F. Braus. 2006. Combining voxel-based morphometry and diffusion tensor imaging to detect age-related brain changes. *Neuroreport* 17:467–70.

Lewis, P.A., A.M. Wing, P.A. Pope, P. Praamstra, and R.C. Miall. 2004. Brain activity correlates differentially with increasing temporal complexity of rhythms during initialisation, synchronisation, and continuation phases of paced finger tapping. *Neuropsychologia* 42:1301–12.

Li, K.Z., U. Lindenberger, A.M. Freund, and P.B. Baltes. 2001. Walking while memorizing: Age-related differences in compensatory behavior. *Psychological Science* 12:230–37.

Lindenberger, U., M. Marsiske, and P.B. Baltes. 2000. Memorizing while walking: Increase in dual-task costs from young adulthood to old age. *Psychology and Aging* 15:417–36.

Li, S.C., and U. Lindenberger. 1999. Cross-level unification: A computational exploration of the link between deterioration of neurotransmitter systems dedifferentiation of cognitive abilities in old age. In *Cognitive Neuroscience of*

Memory eds., L.G. Nilsson and H.J. Markowitsch, 103–46. Seattle: Hogrefe & Huber.

Li, S.C., U. Lindenberger, and S. Sikstrom. 2001. Aging cognition: From neuromodulation to representation. *Trends in Cognitive Sciences* 5:479–86.

Li, S.C., and U. Lindenberger. 1999. Cross-level unification: A computational exploration of the link between deterioration of neurotransmitter systems dedifferentiation of cognitive abilities in old age. In *Cognitive Neuroscience of Memory* eds., L.G. Nilsson and H.J. Markowitsch, 103–46. Seattle: Hogrefe & Huber.

Li, S.C., U. Lindenberger, and S. Sikstrom. 2001. Aging cognition: From neuromodulation to representation. *Trends in Cognitive Sciences* 5:479–86.

Logan, J.M., A.L. Sanders, A.Z. Snyder, J.C. Morris, and R.L. Buckner. 2002. Underrecruitment and nonselective recruitment: Dissociable neural mechanisms associated with aging. *Neuron* 33:827–40.

Lu, M.T., J.B. Preston, and P.L. Strick. 1994. Interconnections between the prefrontal cortex and the premotor areas in the frontal lobe. *The Journal of Comparative Neurology* 341:375–92.

Madden, D.J., J. Spaniol, W.L. Whiting, B. Bucur, J.M. Provenzale, R. Cabeza, et al. 2007. Adult age differences in the functional neuroanatomy of visual attention: A combined fMRI and DTI study. *Neurobiology of Aging* 28:459–76.

Madden, D.J., T.G. Turkington, J.M. Provenzale, L.L. Denny, T.C. Hawk, L.R. Gottlob, and R.E. Coleman. 1999. Adult age differences in the functional neuroanatomy of verbal recognition memory. *Human Brain Mapping* 7:115–35.

Madden, D.J., W.L. Whiting, J.M. Provenzale, and S.A. Huettel. 2004. Age-related changes in neural activity during visual target detection measured by fMRI. *Cerebral Cortex* 14:143–55.

Maguire, E.A., and C.D. Frith. 2003. Aging affects the engagement of the hippocampus during autobiographical memory retrieval. *Brain* 126:1511–23.

Mattay, V.S., F. Fera, A. Tessitore, A.R. Hariri, S. Das, J.H. Callicott, and D.R. Weinberger. 2002. Neurophysiological correlates of age-related changes in human motor function. *Neurology* 58:630–35.

McIntosh, A.R., A.B. Sekuler, C. Penpeci, M.N. Rajah, C.L. Grady, R. Sekuler, and P.J. Bennett. 1999. Recruitment of unique neural systems to support visual memory in normal aging. *Current Biology* 9:1275–78.

Menon, V., N.E. Adleman, C.D. White, G.H. Glove, and A.L. Reiss. 2001. Error-related brain activation during a Go/NoGo response inhibition task. *Human Brain Mapping* 12:131–43.

Meyer-Lindenberg, A., U. Ziemann, G. Hajak, L. Cohen, and K.F. Berman. 2002. Transitions between dynamical states of differing stability in the human brain. *Proceedings of the National Academy of Sciences of the USA* 99:10948–53.

Miller, E.K., and J.D. Cohen. 2001. An integrative theory of prefrontal cortex function. *Annual Review of Neuroscience* 24:167–202.

Milham, M.P., K.I. Erickson, M.T. Banich, A.F. Kramer, A. Webb, T. Wszalek, and N.J. Cohen. 2002. Attentional control in the aging brain: Insights from an fMRI study of the Stroop task. *Brain and Cognition* 49:277–96.

Mima, T., T. Nagamine, K. Nakamura, and H. Shibasaki. 1998. Attention modulates both primary and second somatosensory cortical activities in humans: A magnetoencephalographic study. *Journal of Neurophysiology* 80:2215–21.

Mima T., N. Sadato, S. Yazawa, T. Hanakawa, H. Fukuyama, Y. Yonekura, and H. Shibasaki. 1999. Brain structures related to active and passive finger movements in man. *Brain* 122:1989–97.

Mima, T., N. Sadato, S. Yazawa, T. Hanakawa, H. Fukuyama, Y. Yonekura, and H. Shibasaki. 1999. Brain structures related to active and passive finger movements in man. *Brain* 122:1989–97.

Morcom, A.M., C.D. Good, R.S. Frackowiak, and M.D. Rugg. 2003. Age effects on the neural correlates of successful memory encoding. *Brain* 126:213–29.

Moscovitch, M., and G. Winocur. 1995. Frontal lobes, memory, and aging. *Annals of the New York Academy of Sciences* 769:119–50.

Naccarato, M., C. Calautti, P.S. Jones, D.J. Day, T.A. Carpenter, and J.C. Baron. 2006. Does healthy aging affect the hemispheric activation balance during paced index-to-thumb opposition task? An fMRI study. *NeuroImage* 32:1250–56.

Newton, J., A. Sunderland, S.E. Butterworth, A.M. Peter, K.K. Peck, and P.A. Gowland. 2002. A pilot study of event-related functional magnetic resonance imaging of monitored wrist movements in patients with partial recovery. *Stroke* 33:2881–87.

Nielson, K.A., S.A. Langenecker, and H. Garavan. 2002. Differences in the functional neuroanatomy of inhibitory control across the adult life span. *Psychology and Aging* 17:56–71.

Osiewacz, H.D., and A. Hamann. 1997. DNA reorganization and biological aging. A review. *Biochemistry* 62:1275–84.

Park, D.C., T.A. Polk, R. Park, M. Minear, A. Savage, and M.R. Smith. 2004. Aging reduces neural specialization in ventral visual cortex. *Proceedings of the National Academy of Sciences of the USA* 101:13091–95.

Pandya, D.N., and E.H. Yeterian. 1990. Prefrontal cortex in relation to other cortical areas in rhesus monkey: Architecture and connections. *Progress in Brain Research* 85:63–94.

Petrides, M., and D.N. Pandya. 1999. Dorsolateral prefrontal cortex: Comparative cytoarchitectonic analysis in the human and the macaque brain and corticocortical connection patterns. *The European Journal of Neuroscience* 11:1011–36.

Peinemann, A., C. Lehner, B. Conrad, and H.R. Siebner. 2001. Age-related decrease in paired-pulse intracortical inhibition in the human primary motor cortex. *Neuroscience Letters* 313:33–36.

Persson, J., C.Y. Sylvester, J.K. Nelson, K.M. Welsh, J. Jonides, and P.A. Reuter-Lorenz. 2004. Selection requirements during verb generation: Differential recruitment in older and younger adults. *NeuroImage* 23:1382–90.

Picard, N., and P.L. Strick. 2001. Imaging the premotor areas. *Current Opinion in Neurobiology* 11:663–72.

Platel, H., C. Price, J.C. Baron, R. Wise, J. Lambert, R.S. Frackowiak, et al. 1997. The structural components of music perception. A functional anatomical study. *Brain* 120:229–43.

Rajah, M.N., and M. D'Esposito. 2005. Region-specific changes in prefrontal function with age: A review of PET and fMRI studies on working and episodic memory. *Brain* 128:1964–83.

Ramnani, N., I. Toni, R.E. Passingham, and P. Haggard. 2001. The cerebellum and parietal cortex play a specific role in coordination: A PET study. *NeuroImage* 14:899–911.

Reuter-Lorenz, P. 2002. New visions of the aging mind and brain. *Trends in Cognitive Sciences* 6:394–400.

Reuter-Lorenz, P.A., J. Jonides, E.E. Smith, A. Hartley, A. Miller, C. Marshuetz, and R.A. Koeppe. 2000. Age differences in the frontal lateralization of verbal and spatial working memory revealed by PET. *Journal of Cognitive Neuroscience* 12:174–87.

Reuter-Lorenz, P.A., and C. Lustig. 2005. Brain aging: Reorganizing discoveries about the aging mind. *Current Opinion in Neurobiology* 15:245–51.

Riecker, A., K. Groschel, H. Ackermann, C. Steinbrink, O. Witte, and A. Kastrup. 2006. Functional significance of age-related differences in motor activation patterns. *NeuroImage* 32:1345–54.

Rizzolatti, G., G. Luppino, and M. Matelli. 1998. The organization of the cortical motor system: New concepts. *Electroencephalography and Clinical Neurophysiology* 106:283–96.

Rocca, M.A., R. Gatti, F. Agosta, P. Tortorella, E. Riboldi, P. Broglia, and M. Filippi. 2007. Influence of body segment position during inphase and antiphase hand and foot movements: A kinematic and functional MRI study. *Human Brain Mapping* 28: 218–27.

Rosano, C., H. Aizenstein, J. Cochran, J. Saxton, S. De Kosky, A.B. Newman, et al. 2005. Functional neuroimaging indicators of successful executive control in the oldest old. *NeuroImage* 28:881–89.

Rosen, A.C., M.W. Prull, R. O'Hara, E.A. Race, J.E. Desmond, G.H. Glover, et al. 2002. Variable effects of aging on frontal lobe contributions to memory. *Neuroreport* 13:2425–28.

Rypma, B.M., and M. D'Esposito. 1999. The roles of prefrontal brain regions in components of working memory: Effects of memory load and individual differences. *Proceedings of the National Academy of Sciences of the USA* 96:6558–63.

Sadato, N., Y. Yonekura, A. Waki, H. Yamada, and Y. Ishii. 1997. Role of the supplementary motor area and the right premotor cortex in the coordination of bimanual finger movements. *Journal of Neuroscience* 17:9667–74.

Scarmeas, N., E. Zarahn, K.E. Anderson, J. Hilton, J. Flynn, R.L. Van Heertum, et al. 2003. Cognitive reserve modulates functional brain responses during memory tasks: A PET study in healthy young and elderly subjects. *NeuroImage* 19:1215–27.

Scott, S.H., L.E. Sergio, and J.F. Kalaska. 1997. Reaching movements with similar hand paths but different arm orientations. II. Activity of individual cells in dorsal premotor cortex and parietal area 5. *Journal of Neurophysiology* 78:2413–26.

Seidler, R.D., and G.E. Stelmach. 1995. Reduction in sensorimotor control with age. *Quest* 47:386–94.

Seltzer, B., and D.N. Pandya. 1989. Intrinsic connections and architectonics of the superior temporal sulcus in the rhesus monkey. *The Journal of Comparative Neurology* 290:451–71.

Serrien, D.J., and S.P. Swinnen. 1997. Coordination constraints induced by effector combination under isofrequency and multifrequency conditions. *Journal of Experimental Psychology: Human Perception and Performance* 23:1–18.

Serrien, D.J., S.P. Swinnen, and G.E. Stelmach. 2000. Age-related deterioration of coordinated interlimb behavior. *Journal of Gerontology Series B: Psychological Sciences and Social Sciences* 55B:295–303.

Serrien, D.J., R.B. Ivry, and S.P. Swinnen. 2007. The missing link between action and cognition. *Progress in Neurobiology* 82: 95–107.

Spirduso, W.W. 1995. Issues of quantity and quality of life. In *Physical dimensions of aging*, ed., W.W. Spirduso, 5–30. Champaign, IL: Human Kinetics.

Spirduso, W.W. 1982. Physical fitness in relation to motor aging. In *The aging motor system*, eds., J.A. Mortimer and F.J.M.G.J. Pirozzolo, 120–51. New York: Prager.

Stephan, K.M., F. Binkofski, U. Halsband, C. Dohle, G. Wunderlich, A. Schnitzler, et al. 1999. The role of ventral medial wall motor areas in bimanual co-ordination. A combined lesion and activation study. *Brain* 122:351–68.

Sullivan, E.V., and A. Pfefferbaum. 2006. Diffusion tensor imaging and aging. *Neuroscience and Biobehavioral Reviews* 30:749–61.

Swinnen, S., K. Jardin, R. Meulenbroek, N. Dounskaia, and M. Hofkens-Van Den Brandt. 1997. Egocentric and allocentric constraints in the expression of patterns of interlimb coordination. *Journal of Cognitive Neuroscience* 9:348–77.

Swinnen, S.P. 2002. Intermanual coordination: From behavioral principles to neural-network interactions. *Nature Reviews. Neurosciences* 3:350–61.

Swinnen, S.P., N. Dounskaia, S. Verschueren, D.J. Serrien, and A. Daelman. 1995. Relative phase destabilization during interlimb coordination: The disruptive role of kinesthetic afferences induced by passive movement. *Experimental Brain Research* 105:439–54.

Swinnen, S.P., L. Van Langendonk, S. Verschueren, G. Peeters, R. Dom, and W. De Weerdt. 1997. Interlimb coordination deficits in patients with Parkinson's disease during the production of two-joint oscillations in the sagittal plane. *Movement Disorders* 12:958–68.

Tekes, A., M.A. Mohamed, N.M. Browner, V.D. Calhoun, and D.M. Yousem. 2005. Effect of age on visuomotor functional MR imaging. *Academic Radiology* 12:739–45.

Thaut, M.H. 2003. Neural basis of rhythmic timing networks in the human brain. *Annals of the New York Academy of Sciences* 999:364–73.

Thickbroom, G.W., M.L. Byrnes, and F.L. Mastaglia. 2003. Dual representation of the hand in the cerebellum: Activation with voluntary and passive finger movement. *NeuroImage* 18:670–74.

Tracy, J.I., S.S. Faro, F.B. Mohammed, A.B. Pinus, S.M. Madi, and J.W. Laskas. 2001. Cerebellar mediation of the complexity of bimanual compared to unimanual movements. *Neurology* 57:1862–69.

Troen, B.R. 2003. The biology of aging. *The Mount Sinai Journal of Medicine* 70:3–22.

Turvey, M.T. 1990. Coordination. *The American Psychologist* 45:938–53.

Ullen, F., H. Forssberg, and H.H. Ehrsson. 2003. Neural networks for the coordination of the hands in time. *Journal of Neurophysiology* 89:1126–35.

Van Impe, A., J.P. Coxon, D.J. Goble, N. Wenderoth, and S.P. Swinnen. 2009. Ipsilateral coordination at preferred rate: Effects of age, body side and task complexity. *Neuroimage* 47:1854–62.

Ward, N.S., and R.S. Frackowiak. 2003. Age-related changes in the neural correlates of motor performance. *Brain* 126:873–88.

Ward, N.S., M.M. Brown, A.J. Thompson, and R.S. Frackowiak. 2003a. Neural correlates of motor recovery after stroke: A longitudinal fMRI study. *Brain* 126:2476–96.

Ward, N.S. 2006. Compensatory mechanisms in the aging motor system. *Ageing Research Reviews* 5:239–54.

Ward, N.S., J.N. Newton, O.B. Swayne, L. Lee, A.J. Thompson, R.J. Greenwood, et al. 2006. Motor system activation after subcortical stroke depends on corticospinal system integrity. *Brain* 129:809–19.

Watanabe, J., M. Sugiura, K. Sato, Y. Sato, Y. Maeda, Y. Matsue, et al. 2002. The human prefrontal and parietal association cortices are involved in NO-GO performances: An event-related fMRI study. *NeuroImage* 17:1207–16.

Welford, A.T. 1984. Between bodily changes and performance: Some possible reasons for slowing with age. *Experimental Aging Research* 10:73–88.

Welford, A.T. 1988. Reaction time, speed of performance, and age. *Annals of the New York Academy of Sciences* 515:1–17.

Wenderoth, N., F. Debaere, and S.P. Swinnen. 2004. Neural networks involved in cyclical interlimb coordination as revealed by medical imaging techniques. In *Neuro-behavioral determinants of interlimb coordination: A multidisciplinary approach* eds., S.P. Swinnen and J. Duysens, 127–222. Boston/Dordrecht/London: Kluwer Academic Publishers.

Wenderoth, N., F. Debaere, S. Sunaert, P. Van Hecke, and S.P. Swinnen. 2004a. Parieto-premotor areas mediate directional interference during bimanual movements. *Cerebral Cortex* 14:1153–63.

Wenderoth, N., F. Debaere, and S.P. Swinnen. 2004b. Neural networks involved in cyclical interlimb coordination as revealed by medical imaging techniques. In *Neuro-behavioral determinants of interlimb coordination: A multidisciplinary approach* eds., S.P. Swinnen and J. Duysens, 127–222. Boston/Dordrecht/London: Kluwer Academic Publishers.

West, R.L. 1996. An application of prefrontal cortex function theory to cognitive aging. *Psychological Bulletin* 120:272–92.

Wu, T., and M. Hallett. 2005a. The influence of normal human ageing on automatic movements. *Journal of Physiology* 562:605–15.

Wu T., and M.A. Hallet. 2005b. functional MRI study of automatic movements in patients with Parkinsons's disease. *Brain* 128: 2250–59.

Yu, H., D. Sternad, D.M. Corcos, and D.E. Vaillancourt. 2007. Role of hyperactive cerebellum and motor cortex in Parkinson's disease. *Neuroimage* 5:222–33.

Zemke, A.C., P.J. Heagerty, C. Lee, and S.C. Cramer. 2003. Motor cortex organization after stroke is related to side of stroke and level of recovery. *Stroke* 34: 23–28.

Part 6

Lessons from Robotics

18

Decoding the Mechanisms of Gait Generation and Gait Transition in the Salamander Using Robots and Mathematical Models

Jeremie Knuesel, Jean-Marie Cabelguen, and Auke Ijspeert

An interesting aspect of animal locomotion is the ability to switch between different gaits; for instance, a horse or a cat can switch between a walk, a trot, and a gallop. The large number of degrees of freedom in the musculoskeletal system allows animals to use completely different gaits depending on the situation. This is a useful ability, as when optimizing the energetic cost for a desired speed (Hoyt and Taylor 1981; Srinivasan and Ruina 2006), adapting to different media (e.g., walking on ground and swimming in water), and improving postural stability.

Multiple studies have been made to characterize the gaits of vertebrates in terms of footfall patterns (Hildebrand 1966), kinematics, and electromyographic (EMG) activity. Although some animals tend to use a single gait for locomotion, many animals perform gait transition depending on speed and terrain. The same animal can, therefore, coordinate its limbs in drastically different ways; for instance, the interlimb coordination is very different between a quadruped trot and bound.

Whereas various gaits have been well characterized in various animals, the underlying principles are still not properly understood. Several experiments with decerebrated and spinalized animals, however, give an idea of the general organization of the locomotor system in vertebrates (Whelan 1996; Stein and Smith 1997; Bizzi et al. 2000; Tresch et al. 2002; Grillner 2006). These experiments have shown that many motor behaviors can be elicited without reference to the higher brain centers. Indeed, except for the corticospinal pathways that target specific motoneurons in primates (e.g., for hand muscles), higher-level control centers in the brain do not have direct control of motoneurons. The motor cortex, the cerebellum, and the basal ganglia instead appear to be mostly involved in the selection and modulation of motor patterns.

The brainstem plays a role in the transition between motor patterns: in decerebrated cats, salamanders, and birds, gait transitions can be induced with electrical stimulation of the mesencephalic locomotor region (MLR) (Shik et al. 1966; Steeves et al. 1987; Cabelguen et al. 2003). Such gait transitions induced by MLR stimulation have been observed in all classes of vertebrates and appear to be a common property of vertebrate locomotor control (Grillner et al. 1997). Gait transitions can also be triggered by sensory feedback (Rossignol 1996). For instance, intact, decerebrated, and spinalized cats on a motorized treadmill change gait depending on the treadmill speed.

The motor patterns themselves are in many cases implemented directly in the spinal cord. Rhythmic patterns in particular are produced by specialized networks called *central pattern generators* (CPGs). These neural networks, located in the spinal cord, are a key element of the locomotor system. They are capable of producing coordinated patterns of rhythmic activity without any rhythmic input from the periphery or from supraspinal centers (Delcomyn 1980; Grillner 1981).

Although the general design of the locomotor system is known, many points are still unclear about the exact organization of spinal circuits and descending pathways. These circuits and pathways represent the basic building blocks—the motor primitives—out of which movements are created. Properly understanding them is fundamental, since they represent the "vocabulary" of movement generation.

Several features of the salamander make it particularly useful for the investigation of the locomotor system of vertebrates. First, due to its amphibian nature, it is capable of both swimming and terrestrial walking. This makes the salamander a key element in the evolution of vertebrates, in particular for the transition from water to land. Second, its locomotor system has the same general organization as in mammals (and other vertebrates), but with much less complexity: It has orders of magnitude fewer neurons, which makes it more tractable for experimentation, analysis, and modeling. Third, its central nervous system is very close to that of the lamprey, which has arguably the best understood locomotor circuit among vertebrates. A large amount of experimental data on lampreys, and the numerous models derived from them, are therefore available to guide our investigations of the salamander locomotor circuitry. Fourth, salamanders have a mesencephalic locomotor region in which electrical stimulation can be used to trigger gait transitions (Cabelguen et al. 2003). This is very useful for the analysis of the mechanisms underlying gait transitions. Finally, salamanders are the only adult limbed vertebrates that can fully recover their locomotor functions following a transection at any level of the spinal cord (Piatt 1955; Davis et al. 1990; Chevallier et al. 2004). This regenerative capability is very useful, as it allows for the use of local lesions to study the connectivity and functionality of the spinal network.

In this chapter, we first overview the current knowledge of salamander locomotion and its underlying neural networks. We then present several models that have been developed of the salamander locomotor networks. Next, we discuss some questions that remain open concerning the mechanisms of gait generation and gait transition, and describe some preliminary modeling studies that explore how movement-related sensory feedback can shape the patterns produced by the CPG. The chapter concludes with a discussion of current and future work.

SALAMANDER LOCOMOTION AND THE UNDERLYING NEURAL CIRCUITS

Kinematics and Muscle Activity

The kinematics of salamander locomotion is well documented. There are several studies characterizing the axial movements during swimming and stepping (Frolich and Biewener 1992; Carrier 1993; Ashley-Ross 1994a; Delvolvé et al. 1997; Edwards 1977; Gillis 1997), the hindlimb kinematics (Ashley-Ross 1994b; Ashley-Ross 1994a) and backward walking (Ashley-Ross and Lauder 1997).

During swimming, the salamander uses an anguilliform gait very similar to the lamprey. A rostrocaudal wave of body undulation travels along the body, with the limbs folded backwards (Fig. 18.1, *left*). The wavelength is generally close to one body length, so that the body produces one complete wave (Frolich and Biewener 1992; Delvolvé et al. 1997).

During terrestrial stepping, salamanders usually use a walking trot, with diagonal limbs in phase, opposite limbs in antiphase, and a duty factor of more than 70% (Ashley-Ross 1994a; Ashley-Ross and Bechtel 2004; Ashley-Ross et al. 2009). A walking gait with only one limb at a time in swing phase has also been observed (Edwards 1977; Frolich and Biewener 1992), but is relatively rare. In the remainder of this chapter, "walking" will always refer to the walking trot.

In contrast to the traveling wave during swimming, walking is accompanied by an S-shaped *standing wave* of body curvature, with nodes (points of zero displacement) at the girdles (Fig. 18.1, *right*). The coordination between the standing wave in the trunk and the motion of the limbs is such that a forelimb is retracted during ipsilateral contraction of the trunk. With this coordination, the standing wave in the trunk has the positive effect of increasing the stride length (Roos 1964; Daan and Belterman 1968).

The traveling and standing waves of body curvature are reflected in EMG patterns that display similar waves of muscle activity (Frolich and Biewener 1992; Delvolvé et al. 1997), as illustrated in Figure 18.2. However, the kinematic and EMG waves travel at different speeds; the body dynamics thus contribute significantly to gait generation. This is discussed further in the section "Open Questions and Future Work." The EMG waves also

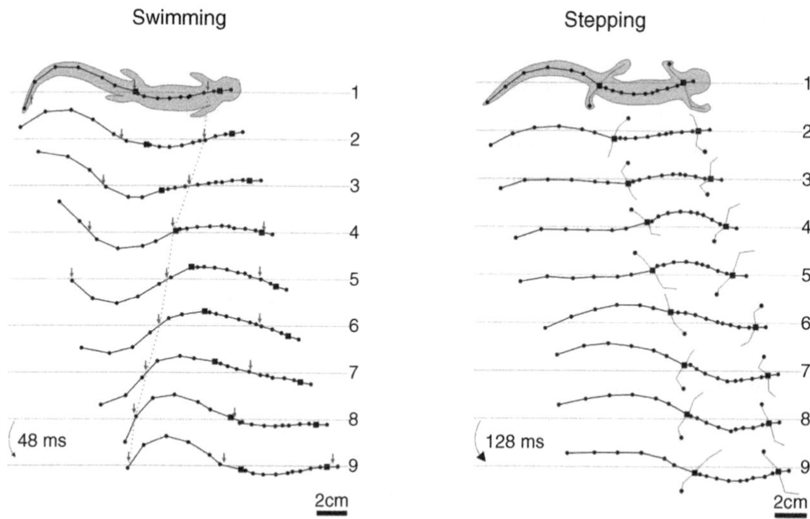

Figure 18.1 Kinematic recordings of a salamander (*Pleurodeles waltlii*), reconstructed from individual video frames. Squares indicate the girdles. Dots at the limb extremities indicate estimated foot contacts. Body configurations from successive frames are aligned according to the direction of overall forward motion. **Left**: Swimming gait. Arrows indicate the points of minimal displacement from the overall forward direction. A traveling wave of body curvature propagates down the body. **Right**: Walking gait. The body displays a standing wave of body curvature with nodes close to the girdles. Adapted from Ijspeert, A., A. Crespi, D. Ryczko, and J.M. Cabelguen. 2007. From swimming to walking with a salamander. *Science* 315(1):1416–20, with permission of the publisher.

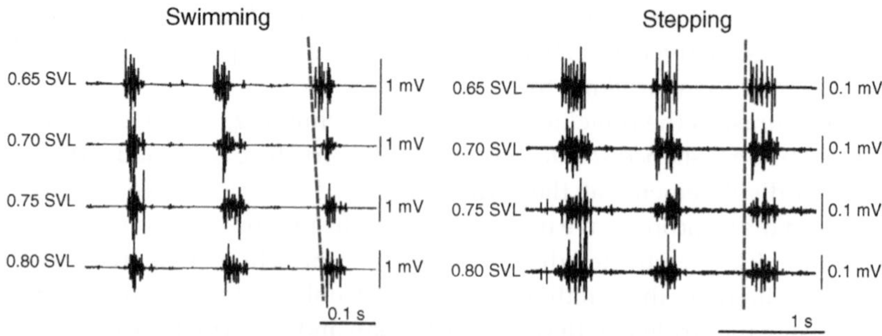

Figure 18.2 Electromyographic (EMG) recordings of epaxial muscle activity from four ipsilateral sites of the trunk of a salamander (*Pleurodeles waltlii*). Electrode positions are specified as fraction of the snout vent length (SVL), with 0.05 SVL corresponding to one spinal segment. Note the different calibrations for the left and right recordings. **Left**: A rostrocaudal phase lag of activities is observed during swimming, as indicated by the dashed line. **Right**: The muscle activity is synchronous in all sites during stepping. From S. Chevallier, unpublished data.

display some additional complexity compared to those of the lamprey. Whereas lampreys use smooth traveling waves of muscle activity during swimming (Wallén and Williams 1984; Williams et al. 1989), EMG recordings in salamanders show two discontinuities in the rostrocaudal phase lags at the girdles during swimming, and double-bursting in the neck and tail regions during walking (Delvolvé et al. 1997).

Central Generation of Locomotor Patterns

As in other vertebrates, salamander gaits are generated by central pattern generators located in the spinal cord (Wheatley et al. 1994; Delvolvé et al. 1997). This was demonstrated using in vitro preparations, in which the spinal cord was isolated from the body. Tonic excitation can be provided pharmacologically to the network by bath application of the excitatory amino acid N-methyl-D-aspartate (NMDA), resulting in periodic bursts of activity in the spinal cord. The CPG is composed of various oscillatory centers (groups of neurons that exhibit rhythmic activity). It is useful to distinguish a *body CPG*—the group of oscillatory centers that control the axial muscles—and a *limb CPG*—the oscillatory centers for the limb muscles.

As in the lamprey (Cohen and Wallen 1980; Grillner et al. 1995) and the *Xenopus* embryo (Tunstall and Roberts 1994; Combes et al. 2004), the generation of motor patterns for axial motion is distributed along the spinal cord (Ryczko et al. 2007). It has been shown recently that surgically isolated hemisegments are capable of rhythm generation (Ryczko et al. 2009). Simultaneous recordings from several ventral roots show that contralateral hemisegments are activated in antiphase, whereas consecutive segments are phase-locked, so as to create traveling waves of activity along the spinal cord. This pattern of ventral root activity is similar to the EMG pattern of muscle activity observed in intact animals during swimming. The coordinated patterns observed in vitro are thus referred to as *fictive swimming*. However, the traveling waves observed in vitro exhibit a large variability of wavelengths, which is not observed during swimming in vivo (Lamarque et al. 2009; Ryczko et al. 2009). Furthermore, standing waves of activity in vitro, which would correspond to fictive walking, are rarely observed (Delvolvé et al. 1999; Ryczko et al. 2009). These two points are discussed in the section "Current Issues with the Open-loop Model." Note that back-propagating (caudorostral) waves are observed in vitro and correspond to a struggling behavior in vivo (Lamarque et al. 2009; Ryczko et al. 2009).

The neural centers for the limb movements—forming the limb CPG—are located within the first to fifth segments for the forelimbs, and within the 14th to 18th segments for the hindlimbs (Székely and Czéh 1976; Wheatley et al. 1992; Cheng et al. 1998). Evidence from graft experiments (Brandle and Székely 1973) and spinal sections (Székely and Czéh 1976) show that these regions can be decomposed into left and right neural centers that independently control each limb. Furthermore, independent oscillatory centers for forelimb extensor and flexor motoneuron pools have been identified (Cheng et al. 1998; Cheng et al. 2002).

A mesencephalic locomotor region (MLR) has been identified in the salamander brainstem. Electrical microstimulation of the MLR can induce locomotion in semi-intact preparations (decerebrate animals with the forelimbs removed) (Cabelguen et al. 2003). The locomotor pattern can be modulated by adjusting the strength of the electrical stimulus (by varying either the stimulation current or its frequency). Walking is induced at low stimulation strengths. Increasing the stimulation strength successively leads to an increase of the walking frequency, a switch to the swimming gait, and a further increase of the swimming frequency.

The results obtained with electrical stimulations of the MLR are consistent with the general observation that swimming frequencies are always higher than walking frequencies in salamanders (Delvolvé et al. 1997) (see Table 18.1). Indeed, with a sprawling posture and short limbs, these animals are better adapted to swimming than to walking (Ashley-Ross 1994a; Ashley-Ross 1994b).

There is anatomical and electrophysiological evidence in different species that the MLR influences the activity of the CPG through reticulospinal (RS) neurons (Wannier 1994; Grillner et al. 1997). This is likely to be true also in the salamander (Bar-Gad et al. 1999). It remains to be seen whether the same RS neurons are recruited during MLR-induced swimming and walking, and whether the same cellular mechanisms are involved for both gaits.

MODELING

Understanding locomotion control is a problem that fundamentally requires a comprehensive and interdisciplinary modeling approach. Locomotion is a complex dynamic phenomenon that implies the interaction between the central and peripheral nervous systems, the musculoskeletal system, and

Table 18.1 Locomotor parameters in intact salamanders

	Overground stepping	Underwater stepping	Swimming
Intersegmental phase lag (% of cycle duration)	0.010 ± 0.050 N = 627	0.973 ± 0.087 N = 482	2.485 ± 0.162 N = 195
Cycle duration (ms)	752.9 ± 7.9 N = 626	1071.5 ± 15.1 N = 481	347.8 ± 4.2 N = 213

Data are recorded from six salamanders (*Pleurodeles waltlii*). They are expressed as means ± SEM. N is the total number of cycles. Differences between each of the gaits are statistically significant (ANOVA, $p < 0.001$). S. Lamarque, unpublished data.

the environment (see Prilutsky and Klishko, this volume). It is very unlikely that locomotion control will be properly understood by studying specific components in isolation. Focused studies on particular topics are clearly needed (e.g., on motoneuron properties, muscle properties, etc.), but comprehensive approaches are required to understand the whole picture—for example, to understand the feedback loops that are created through the physical interactions of the body with the environment, and through the different neural centers involved in locomotion control. Mathematical and numerical models are essential to understand these complex feedback loops. A (static) diagram of interactions between the different components will not be able to reflect the dynamic phenomena taking place.

Here, we overview past studies that are relevant to the modeling of gait generation and gait transitions in salamanders. We begin with a summary of the models of the lamprey swimming circuitry, which were often used as a source of inspiration for models of the salamander spinal network.

The lamprey spinal circuitry has been studied extensively (Buchanan and Grillner 1987; Grillner et al. 1988; Grillner et al. 1991; Grillner et al. 1995), which gave rise to numerous models of the swimming (axial) CPG. These models can be classified according to their level of abstraction. At the lowest level, biophysical models use relatively realistic (e.g., multicompartment Hodgkin-Huxley) neuron models. Such models can be used to validate our understanding of the physiological processes involved in rhythm generation (Ekeberg et al. 1991; Wallén et al. 1992). At an intermediate level, connectionist models use less realistic neuron models (e.g., leaky integrators), abstracting the complexity of internal neuron dynamics to focus on the interneuronal connectivity and how it can account in itself for the generation of different patterns of oscillations (Buchanan 1992; Williams 1992; Ekeberg 1993). At the most abstract level, the CPG is modeled as a chain of mathematical oscillators (e.g., phase oscillators), where each oscillator typically represents an oscillatory unit (i.e., a whole population of biological neurons). These models are used to investigate very general properties of the network without relying on the details of the biological implementation. Such network properties include the possible dominance of rostral coupling over caudal coupling (or vice versa), and the kind of network structure capable of producing a constant intersegmental phase lag independently of the frequency of oscillations (Kopell 1995; Williams and Sigvardt 1995). These models can also be used to investigate the global impact of feedback signals on the network dynamics.

We know of only five modeling studies concerning the neural circuits involved in the generation of the swimming and walking gaits of the salamander.

In Ermentrout and Kopell (1994), a chain of phase oscillators was used as an abstract model of a vertebrate's CPG. The ability of the chain to produce stable traveling waves and S-shaped standing waves was investigated analytically and numerically. Nearest-neighbor couplings, designed to induce synchrony, were supplemented by two kinds of long-range couplings: inward coupling from the extremities to the middle of the chain, and outward coupling from the middle to the extremities. Both inward and outward couplings were designed to induce antiphase between the parts that they connected. Their strengths determined the stable patterns of oscillations, which included synchrony, traveling waves, S-shaped standing waves, and antiwaves (two waves traveling in opposite directions). The ranges of strengths allowing for stable traveling waves and stable standing waves did not overlap. In other words, traveling and standing waves could be generated with the same network connectivity, but with different coupling strengths. The other models presented next explored other, more realistic possibilities to explain the transitions between traveling and standing waves, in particular without the need for the specific long-range couplings and without the need for changing coupling strengths between modes of locomotion.

In Ijspeert (2001), one of us developed a connectionist model of the salamander CPG based on leaky integrator neurons. The network was inspired by a model of the lamprey CPG (Ekeberg 1993), with the major addition of limb centers, represented by two additional segments: one for the forelimbs and one for the hindlimbs. The segmental network was modeled using six inhibitory interneurons. The range of intersegmental connections was limited to five segments. Forelimb and hindlimbs projected to all the trunk and tail segments, respectively. A genetic algorithm was used to adjust the synaptic weights of the intrasegmental, intersegmental, and limb–body connections. Standing waves were generated by the network when a tonic excitatory drive was applied to both body and limb oscillators. Traveling waves were released by suppressing the drive to the limb segments.[1] This work therefore served as a proof of concept that a lamprey-like network could be extended with limb CPGs to produce both swimming and walking gaits.

Another study by Bem et al. (2003) focused on reproducing the complexity of the salamander EMG patterns (see the section "Kinematics and Muscle Activity") in a model of the lamprey CPG (Ekeberg 1993). The generation of the walking pattern, with double-bursting in the neck and tail regions, required the reversal of the intersegmental inhibitory connections in the rostral part of the network, as well as an increase of the tonic drive at the girdles and a phasic drive outside the girdle regions. Generation of the swimming pattern also required drive adjustments. Because of its modified connectivity, the rostral part of the network generated a caudorostral wave under uniform tonic excitation. This was compensated for by increasing the tonic drive in the rostral part of the network. Additional increases in

[1] An inhibitory drive to the limb segments was actually used to prevent slow oscillation in the limb networks.

regions slightly caudal to the girdles were able to reproduce the discontinuities in the salamander swimming pattern. The same effect could be achieved by suppressing the sensory feedback in the girdle regions. In this chapter, we will present new modeling results that similarly explore the possible role of sensory feedback in shaping the swimming and walking pattern. Special focus will be given to new data showing the large variability of traveling waves during fictive locomotion, and to the question of how these various traveling waves can be transformed into the specific traveling and standing waves observed in EMG recordings during swimming and walking.

In Ijspeert et al. (2005), we used a neuromechanical simulation to explore more systematically different potential body-limb CPGs configurations underlying salamander locomotion. In particular, we compared local and global connectivity patterns between the limb and body CPGs. In configurations with local connectivity, the limb oscillators are connected only to the nearest segments of the body; see Figure 18.3 (*left*) for an example. With the global connectivity, forelimb oscillators are connected to all trunk oscillators, and hindlimb oscillators to all tail oscillators. This is also illustrated in Figure 18.3 (*right*). Inhibitory connections were used between limb oscillators, and between the left and right oscillator of the same segment, in order to induce antiphase behavior. Excitatory connections were used between limb and body oscillators to induce in-phase behavior. Ascending and descending connections were both excitatory and inhibitory, which allowed for arbitrary phase relationships. The simulation results showed that, in the absence of sensory feedback, only the configurations with global coupling can produce standing waves as observed during walking. Local coupling configurations always resulted in traveling waves in the CPG output. However, using these traveling waves as the control signal for the mechanical simulation on the ground still resulted in quasi-standing waves of body undulation. This was attributed to the environment interaction forces on the ground, which differ from interaction forces in water. The addition of sensory feedback then entrained the CPG itself to standing wave–like patterns of oscillations. The role of sensory feedback will be discussed further in this chapter, in the section "Closing the Loop." The discontinuities observed in the rostrocaudal phase lags during swimming could also be reproduced by making the intersegmental coupling stronger in the rostral direction and setting the girdle segments to slightly lower intrinsic frequencies.

In our most recently published study (Ijspeert et al. 2007), we investigated the mechanisms of automatic transitions between swimming and walking. We used a network of amplitude-controlled phase oscillators with global connections from limb to body oscillators, and bidirectional connections between nondiagonal limbs (Fig. 18.3, *right*).

We sought to reproduce the MLR stimulation experiments (see earlier discussion) where a switch from low-frequency stepping to high-frequency

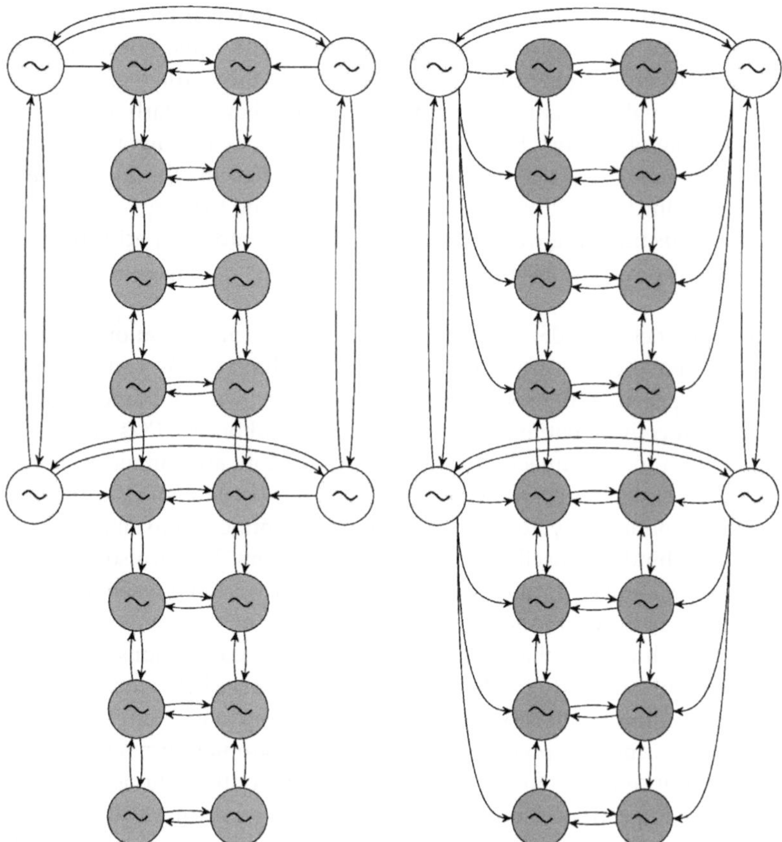

Figure 18.3 Two models of the salamander spinal cord. The axial network is composed of two columns of eight oscillators (*gray*) with nearest-neighbor couplings. Each limb oscillator (*white*) connects to the axis, as well as to all other nondiagonal limb oscillators. **Left**: Local coupling from limb oscillators to axial oscillators. **Right**: Global coupling from limb to body oscillators. In this configuration, the forelimb oscillators connect to all ipsilateral oscillators from the trunk, and the hind limb oscillators to all ipsilateral oscillators from the tail. Adapted from Ijspeert, A., A. Crespi, D. Ryczko, and J.M. Cabelguen. 2007. From swimming to walking with a salamander. *Science* 315(1):1416–20, with permission of the publisher.

swimming could be induced by increasing the intensity of the electrical stimulation in the MLR. This was achieved through the introduction of two hypotheses. First, that limb oscillators saturate at high frequencies: They stop oscillating at high levels of stimulation. Second, that for the same level of stimulation, limb oscillators have lower intrinsic frequencies than do the body oscillators. Numerical simulations showed that the first hypothesis provides a mechanism for the automatic transition between walking and swimming similar to that observed in MLR stimulation experiments. It also explains why walking frequencies are always lower than swimming frequencies, as shown by kinematic recordings (Frolich and Biewener 1992). The second hypothesis explains the rapid increase of frequencies observed when the salamander switches from walking to swimming: During walking, the lower frequency of the limb oscillators slows down the rhythm of the body CPG. When the limb oscillators saturate, the body oscillators suddenly become free to oscillate at their higher intrinsic frequency. This mechanism also explains a gap observed between the walking and swimming frequencies. We were able to verify the second hypothesis in vitro: The midtrunk and limb segments were isolated by transections of the spinal cord, and an identical tonic drive applied pharmacologically to all parts resulted in slower rhythms in the limb segments than in the midtrunk (see supplementary material in Ijspeert et al. 2007). In this chapter, we will present ongoing work on the extension of this model to account for new biological observations, in particular through the incorporation of sensory feedback.

We also tested the CPG model on an amphibious salamander robot capable of swimming and walking (Fig. 18.4). The robot was used to demonstrate that the CPG model can generate forward locomotion with variable speed and heading, as this requires a mechanical body and cannot be studied at the neuronal level alone. The robot also allowed us to compare quantitatively the gaits generated by our model to the gaits of the animal.

CLOSING THE LOOP

Our current model of the salamander spinal cord (Ijspeert et al. 2007) was described in the preceding section. The motor commands generated by this

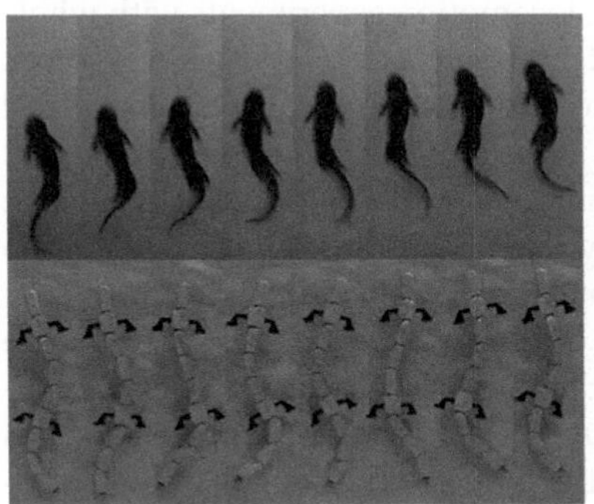

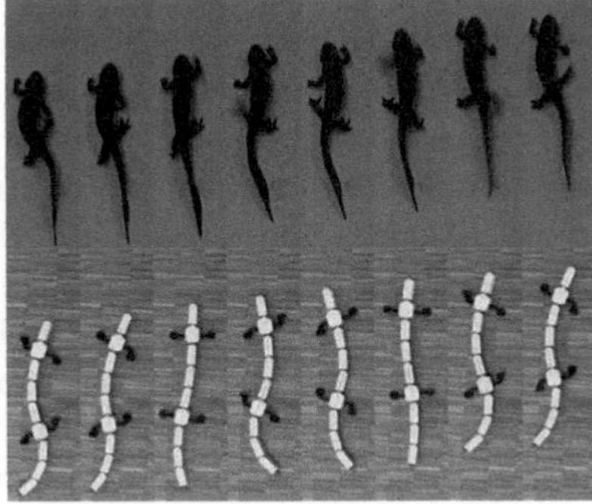

Figure 18.4 Swimming gait (*left*) and walking gait (*right*) in the salamander (*Pleurodeles waltlii*) and the robot Salamandra Robotica. From Ijspeert, A., A. Crespi, D. Ryczko, and J.M. Cabelguen. 2007. From swimming to walking with a salamander. *Science* 315(1):1416–20, with permission of the publisher (supplementary material).

model are not affected by the interactions of the body with its environment. It is thus an *open-loop* model. We will now expose two issues with this model, as revealed by recent experimental results, and discuss how sensory feedback can address them. We will then present some preliminary work toward a *closed-loop* model of the salamander spinal cord; that is, a model that includes some kind of sensory feedback.

Current Issues with the Open-loop Model

The model of the salamander spinal cord published in Ijspeert et al. (2007) is an open-loop model. The output of the CPG does not depend on sensory feedback, such as the proprioceptive signals due to the actual movements of the body. This model was successful in reproducing important features of salamander locomotion, including the generation of traveling waves for swimming and standing waves for stepping, and a mechanism of transition between these gaits similar to that observed in MLR stimulation experiments. However, the model needs to be adapted to account for recent experimental data regarding the formation of standing waves in the trunk, and the variability of intersegmental phase lags observed in vitro, as we will explain next.

Generation of Standing Waves in the Trunk

In the open-loop model, the formation of standing waves and the gap of frequencies between swimming and stepping are due to the influence of the limb centers on the axial (trunk and tail) centers. In particular, the extensive connections from limb to axial centers, where each forelimb oscillator connects to all the ipsilateral trunk oscillators, mean that limb activity is inseparable from standing waves in the trunk. However, standing wave patterns are rarely observed in fictive locomotion experiments with whole spinal cords that include the limb centers (Delvolvé et al. 1999; Ryczko et al. 2009). When active, the limb centers do slow down the axial centers, but fail to impose a standing wave of activity in the trunk (Ryczko et al. 2009). And recently, EMG recordings during underwater stepping have shown that traveling waves in the trunk and rhythmic limb muscle activity can also occur together in vivo (Lamarque et al. 2009; see also Table 18.1). This suggests that connections from the limb centers to the axial centers affect the frequency but not the phase of trunk and tail oscillators. In terms of couplings, this suggests a strong local coupling of the limbs to a few oscillators of the trunk and the tail, resulting in the frequency locking of axial oscillators at the girdles, which would entrain other oscillators in the trunk and the tail without restricting the formation of traveling waves. The model therefore needs to be updated to reflect this local coupling pattern, as opposed to the current global coupling from limb to axial centers.

If limb oscillators project only locally to the axial oscillators, they cannot account alone for the formation of the standing waves in the trunk. The network would then generate traveling waves even during walking on land, which is in contradiction with the EMG recordings during terrestrial stepping. We propose that additional mechanisms are at play, such as a phase regulator and/or modulation by sensory feedback.

Reduction of the Variability of In-Vitro Phase Lags

Fictive locomotion experiments (see the section "Central Generation of Locomotor Patterns") have shown that isolated spinal cords of salamanders activated by bath application of an NMDA receptor agonist can produce coordinated traveling waves, as in the lamprey. An important feature of the pattern of oscillations is the intersegmental phase lag: the delay between the activation of two consecutive segments, expressed as a fraction of the complete cycle.

EMG experiments show that intact salamanders swim with an intersegmental phase lag of about 2.5% (see Table 18.1).[2] Since the salamander has about 40 segments, this corresponds roughly to the body making one complete traveling wave. By contrast, recent in vitro preparations show a great variability of phase lags between individuals, with values distributed between –12.61% and 12.44% per spinal segment (Ryczko et al. 2009).

In the model, the phase lag is specified explicitly for each ascending and descending coupling. In the absence of limb activity, this intrinsic phase lag is directly reflected in the output of the CPG, and thus in the motor patterns. Generating a regular motor pattern from diverse intrinsic phase lags requires the addition of a mechanism to reduce this variability (i.e., to explain how a large variety of open-loop patterns are transformed into more stereotyped closed-loop patterns).

Adapting the Spinal Cord Model

We present here two principles that could account for the formation of standing waves in the trunk and the reduction of the variability of the intersegmental phase lag: (a) a strong proprioceptive feedback, and (b) a phase regulator. The first principle will be presented next and explored in more depth in the following section, using an extension of our model.

[2] An intersegmental phase lag of 2.5% is consistently observed during steady swimming; however, other behaviors are characterized by different phase lags, such as 0% during terrestrial stepping, 1% during underwater stepping (Table 18.1) and negative phase lags during pelvis-induced struggling (Lamarque et al. 2009).

The Role of Proprioceptive Feedback

Both of the issues presented in at the beginning of the chapter relate to differences between in vitro and in vivo experiments. One of the main differences between these two conditions is the presence of movement-related (phasic) sensory feedback during the in vivo recordings. From a control theory perspective, the in vitro preparation is an open-loop system, whereas the in vivo preparations used for EMG recordings, which include phasic sensory feedback, constitute a closed-loop system. In particular, the CPG of the in vitro preparation does not elicit actual movements and thus receives no phasic mechanical feedback signals, for instance from stretch receptors within the muscles and spinal cord itself.[3]

Proprioceptive feedback[4] offers a likely explanation for the formation of standing waves of EMG patterns recorded in vivo during walking. In the intact animal, different interaction forces with the ground and the water could result in feedback patterns that favor the production of standing waves versus traveling waves. This is supported by our previous modeling work (Ijspeert et al. 2005). As described in a preceding section, a neuromechanical simulation controlled by traveling waves of muscle activity exhibited quasi-standing waves of body undulation These standing waves were reflected in the proprioceptive feedback signals, which were used to entrain the CPG toward a standing wave pattern of oscillations. Similar results were obtained in experiments with lampreys trying to swim on a wet bench: The actual motion of the animal resembles a standing wave (Bowtell and Williams 1991).

In addition to imposing a standing wave during locomotion on ground, proprioceptive feedback could also contribute to the reduction of the variability of intersegmental phase lags during both swimming and walking. In the lamprey, such feedback is known to be strong enough to allow for mechanical entrainment of the CPG from half to almost the double of its rest frequency (Williams et al. 1990). Mechanical entrainment has been shown to affect phase lags and stabilize irregular rhythms during in vitro experiments (McClellan and Sigvardt 1988).

In the next section (Exploring the Role of Phasic Sensory Feedback: Preliminary Modeling), a preliminary modeling study will confirm the plausibility of the role of sensory feedback in modulating the locomotor patterns.

---

[3] The lamprey spinal cord is known to include stretch receptor neurons that project locally to CPG interneurons (McClellan and Sigvardt 1988; Viana Di Prisco et al. 1990). Similar cells have been found in the salamander spinal cord, although their stretch-sensitive function has not been confirmed (Schroeder and Egar 1990).

[4] The role of tonic sensory feedback, which is also present in vitro, will not be considered here. The term "proprioceptive feedback" will be used to refer to phasic movement-related feedback only.

A Phase Regulator

Another possibility for the reduction of phase lag variability is the presence of a phase regulator in the brainstem–spinal cord network. Deviations from the phase lag observed in vivo could, in principle, be corrected by differential activation of the oscillatory centers distributed along the spinal cord, in contrast to the homogeneous activation of the in vitro preparation by the amino acid bath. Differential activation has been shown to have the ability to change phase lags in the lamprey. For instance, bath application of NMDA with different concentrations for the rostral and caudal parts of the spinal cord can modulate the intersegmental phase lag (Matsushima and Grillner 1992). Similar results were obtained in a modeling study of the lamprey spinal cord using a chain of phase oscillators with nearest-neighbor coupling. In that study, the activation of spinal cord segments in the animal can be related to the intrinsic frequencies of the oscillators in the model. It was shown that the model's intersegmental phase lag could be controlled by changing the intrinsic frequencies of the oscillators along the chain (Cohen et al. 1982). This approach of phase lag modulation will be explored in future models.

Exploring the Role of Phasic Sensory Feedback: Preliminary Modeling

We present here some preliminary modeling that was done to test the viability of two hypotheses related to the role of sensory feedback:

- That proprioceptive feedback can reduce the variability of phase lags observed during fictive locomotion experiments by entraining the axial oscillators to phase patterns as found in EMG recordings from intact animals
- That proprioceptive feedback can entrain the axial oscillators from a traveling wave pattern to the standing wave pattern during walking

To evaluate the feedback strengths necessary for these two types of entrainment, and the contributions of ipsilateral and contralateral feedback, we subjected a model of the axial network to artificial feedback patterns (external signals designed to approximate the feedback signals of a closed-loop system). This was done as a first step before the development of a closed-loop system (a similar approach has been used in Bem et al. 2003).

The Network Model

The spinal cord model presented here builds on a previous model (Ijspeert et al. 2007) based on dynamical systems. Each oscillator represents the activity of an oscillatory pool of neurons corresponding to a hemisegment of the animal's spinal cord. This high level of abstraction allows us to focus on the interactions between the oscillatory centers and their mechanism of activation and modulation through descending drive signals and sensory feedback. We thus take for granted the generation of rhythm in each oscillatory center, and look at the general principles governing the modulation of these rhythms. Such principles include the strength of couplings between oscillatory centers and the strength of sensory feedback.

The axial salamander CPG was modeled as a chain of 40 identical segments, to match the number of segments in the animal (Fig. 18.5).

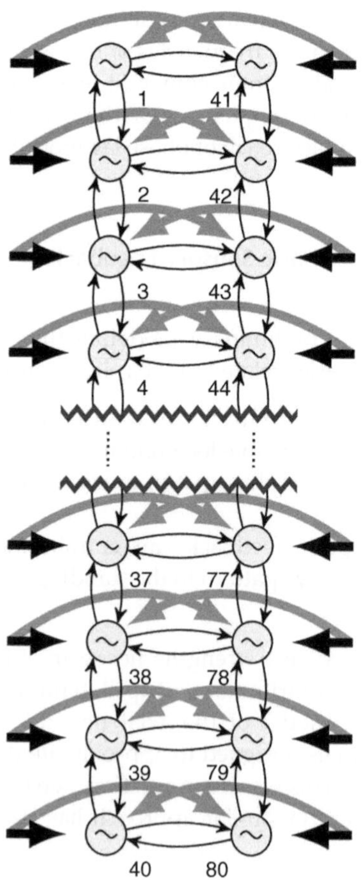

Figure 18.5 Model of the axial network of the salamander spinal cord. The network is made of 80 oscillators organized in two columns, with nearest-neighbor coupling. The two columns represent the two hemicords of the animal. Wide black and wide gray arrows represent ipsilateral and contralateral feedback signals, respectively.

Each segment was made of two Hopf oscillators, and a diffusive nearest-neighbor coupling was used to set the global oscillation pattern to a traveling wave. By comparison, the model in Ijspeert et al. (2007) was made of eight segments for the axis, each composed of two amplitude-controlled phase oscillators, with the addition of four limb oscillators with extensive couplings to the body.

The Hopf oscillator was chosen because of its limit cycle behavior and the fact that it can easily be expressed in polar and Cartesian coordinates. The latter are useful for the integration of signals without explicit phase information, as is the case with sensory feedback (see below).

We first wrote the oscillator equations in polar coordinates, in which phase relations can be expressed easily:

$$\begin{aligned} \dot{r}_i &= \gamma(R^2 - r_i^2)r_i \\ \dot{\theta}_i &= 2\pi\nu + \sum_{j=1}^{N} w_{ij} r_j \sin(\theta_j - \theta_i - \phi_{ij}) \end{aligned} \qquad \text{(Eq. 1)}$$

with N the number of segments, i the segment index, r the amplitude, R the intrinsic amplitude, θ the phase, ν the intrinsic frequency, γ a convergence factor, w_{ij} a coupling weight different from zero when oscillators i and j are nearest neighbors, and ϕ_{ij} the intrinsic phase lag $\theta_j - \theta_i$ between the two oscillators. The parameter values are given in Table 18.2.

Ascending and descending coupling weights were set to 200, which allowed the network to converge to the desired amplitudes, frequencies, and phase lags from random initial values (between –1 and 1) in just one or two cycles. Similar speeds of convergence have been observed in animals in vivo (Ashley-Ross and Bechtel 2004) (transitions between swimming and walking) and in vitro (Delvolvé et al. 1999) (transitions between two fictive rhythmic motor patterns). For lateral coupling weights, a value of 1 was found to be sufficient. We set ϕ_{ij} to π for lateral couplings, in order to keep the left and right oscillators in antiphase. The phase lags of all ascending couplings were set to the same value ϕ; the opposite value was used for descending couplings. With oscillators 1 and 41 (Fig. 18.5) representing the rostral end of the spinal cord, a positive ϕ corresponds to a rostrocaudal traveling wave of oscillations. The number of wave cycles between the rostral and caudal extremities is directly related to the intersegmental phase lag ϕ:

$$k = \frac{N\phi}{2\pi} \qquad \text{(Eq. 2)}$$

A wave number $k = 1$ corresponds to the natural swimming gait (intersegmental phase lag of 2.5%, or $\varphi = \frac{2\pi}{40}$).

Table 18.2 Network parameters

Name	Symbol	Value
Number of segments	N	40
Coupling weights	w_{ij}	200 (axial), 1 (lateral)
Convergence factor	γ	1
Intrinsic amplitude	R	1
Intrinsic frequency	ν	varied $\in$ [0.9, 3.8] Hz
Intrinsic phase lag	ϕ_{ij}	ϕ (ascending), $-\phi$ (descending), π (lateral)
Intrinsic axial phase lag	ϕ	Varied $\in$ [-5, 5]
Intrinsic wave number	k	$\frac{N\phi}{2\pi}$
Ipsilateral signal strength	α	varied $\in$ [0, 1000]
Contralateral signal strength	β	0 or -α
Feedback pattern wave number	k_f	1
Feedback pattern frequency	ν_f	2 Hz

To introduce the feedback pattern, the oscillator equations were rewritten in the Cartesian space (van den Kieboom 2009):

$$\begin{aligned}
\dot{x}_i &= \gamma(R^2 - r_i^2)x_i - 2\pi\bar{\nu}x_i + \alpha\cos^+[\varphi_i(t)] + \beta\cos^+[\varphi_i(t) + \pi] \\
\dot{y}_i &= \gamma(R^2 - r_i^2)y_i + 2\pi\bar{\nu}y_i \\
\bar{\nu} &= \nu + \sum_{j=1}^{N} \frac{w_{ij}}{r_i}[(x_i y_j - x_j y_i)\cos\phi_{ij} - (x_i x_j + y_i y_j)\sin\phi_{ij}]
\end{aligned} \quad \text{(Eq. 3)}$$

with $\varphi_i(t) = 2\pi\nu_f + \varphi_i(0)$ the artificial feedback pattern of frequency $2\pi\nu_f$, and $\cos^+[\varphi] = \max(0, \cos\varphi)$. The initial values $\varphi_i(0)$, $i = 1,\ldots,$ N encode the shape of the pattern, which was either a traveling wave or a standing wave with nodes at the extremities and a third node at the middle segment (oscillators 20 and 60, representing the lower girdle of the salamander).

The α term in Equation 3 corresponds to the ipsilateral feedback, shown with wide black arrows in Figure 18.5, and the β term corresponds to contralateral feedback (*wide gray arrows*). With $\alpha > 0$ and $\beta < 0$, the ipsilateral term is the positive half of a sine wave and the contralateral term a negative half. This was chosen as an approximation of the signals received from stretch receptors, which can be either excitatory or inhibitory. When $\beta = -\alpha$ the sum of both terms is a full sine wave.

Entrainment Simulations

Networks of different intrinsic wave number k and frequency ν were entrained to a feedback pattern of wave number $k_f = 1$ and frequency $\nu_f = 2$ Hz, using different ipsilateral and contralateral signal strengths (α and β respectively). The network was given 5 seconds to synchronize to its intrinsic pattern before artificial feedback signals were activated.

We used network wave numbers (k) between –5 and 5, which corresponds to an intersegmental phase lag between –12.5% and 12.5% (Equation 2). These wave numbers were selected to reproduce the variability of phase lags observed in vitro (phase lags between –12.61% and 12.44%, cf. "Current Issues with the Open-loop Model").

Intrinsic or "rest" frequencies (ν) were varied between 1 Hz and 4 Hz, in order to have a range of frequency ratios ν / ν_f between 0.5 and 2. This range was selected to include the range of entrainment observed in lampreys (from 0.5 to 1.8 times the rest frequency) (Williams et al. 1990).

To judge whether entrainment was successful, errors in frequency and axial coordination were estimated separately. The axial coordination error was measured on the left column of oscillators as the average per-segment deviation between the expected and actual phase lags, expressed in percentage of the whole cycle. The frequency error was taken as the deviation between actual and expected frequencies, in percentage of the expected frequency. The actual frequency was calculated as the average frequency over all oscillators, over all periods in the time range considered. The network was said to be properly entrained if both error measures were below 2%.

Results

Figure 18.6 shows contour plots of the minimal signal strength necessary to entrain the networks toward the frequency and phase lags of the feedback patterns, using either ipsilateral signals only ($\beta = 0$, left plot) or both ipsilateral and contralateral signals (of equal strength: $\beta = -\alpha$, right plot).

At constant phase lag (k=1), the whole range of frequencies (from 50% to 200% of the target frequency) could be entrained with ipsilateral and contralateral signals of strength 30, which corresponds to 15% of the axial coupling strength (Fig. 18.5, *right*). Using only ipsilateral signals, a strength of 30 cannot entrain frequencies beyond 150% of the target frequency; entrainment of the whole range of frequencies requires an ipsilateral signal strength of 350. It appears that, in the absence of contralateral signals, slowing down a network of high intrinsic frequency is more difficult than entraining a "slow" network to higher frequencies. Interestingly, similar observations were made on the lamprey: although extreme slow-down by entrainment has been observed (down to 50% of the rest frequency, Williams et al. 1990), it is generally easier to entrain the lamprey CPG to faster rhythms (Williams et al. 1990; Tytell and Cohen 2008).

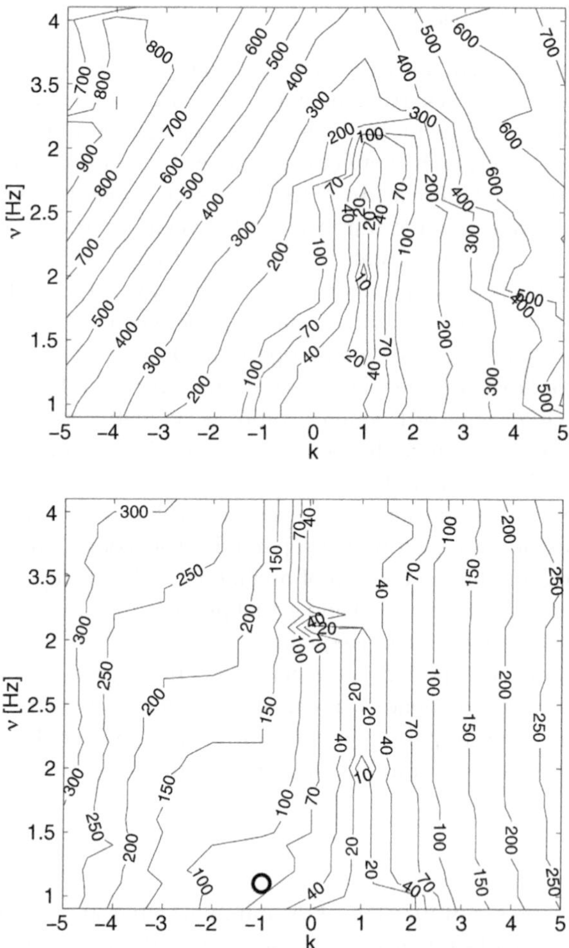

Figure 18.6 Contour plot of the minimal artificial feedback strength α necessary for entraining a network of frequency ν and wave number k to a pattern $\nu_f = 2\text{Hz}$, $k_f = 1$. The range of wave numbers k corresponds to the variability of intersegmental phase lags observed in vitro. The range of frequency ratios ν/ν_f was selected to match the range of entrainment observed in lampreys. **Top**: Using only ipsilateral signals ($\beta = 0$). **Bottom**: Using ipsilateral and contralateral signals of the same strength ($\beta = -\alpha$). The process of synchronization for network parameters indicated by the black ring is shown in Figure 18.7 (*bottom*).

At constant frequency ($\nu = 2$ Hz) and with ipsilateral signals only, entrainment of phase lags over the whole range of variability observed in vitro requires artificial feedback strengths of 710, or 355% of the axial coupling strength. Using both ipsilateral and contralateral feedback patterns (of equal strength), the phase lags can be entrained with feedback patterns of strength 330, or 165% of the axial coupling strength.

To illustrate the process of convergence to the intrinsic and entrained patterns, a time series plot is shown in Figure 18.7 (*bottom*), using the network indicated by a black circle. Each dot marks the completion of one cycle for the corresponding segment, and the gray line shows the expected pattern. The left part of the plot shows the convergence to the intrinsic pattern. After activation of the artificial feedback signal (indicated by a vertical black bar on the plots), the network quickly converged to the entrained pattern.

An ipsilateral signal about as strong as the axial couplings was found to be sufficient for the entrainment of a swimming pattern to a walking pattern of identical frequency and wave number (Fig. 18.7, *top*). The addition of a contralateral signal did not affect the required signal strength significantly (not shown).

It should be noted that, in our simulations, the mechanisms of integration of the feedback signal in the CPG were the same for all segments. This might not be the case in the salamander. Entrainment experiments with lampreys have shown that the phase relationship between CPG bursts and the bending stimulus depends on the location of the stimulus along the body (Tytell and Cohen 2008).

It should also be noted that the addition of artificial feedback patterns to an open-loop system does not constitute a closed-loop system. The results presented here are only a first step in ongoing investigations on the role of sensory feedback in the generation of locomotor patterns in the salamander. They do show, however, that relatively strong feedback is required in our model, if it must account alone for the reduction of variability in intersegmental phase lags and the formation of standing waves in the body. They also show that phase lags can be entrained over a much wider range using ipsilateral and contralateral feedback, which are both known to exist in the lamprey (Viana Di Prisco et al. 1990), compared to ipsilateral feedback only. Finally, our results suggest that contralateral feedback has a dramatic effect on the range of frequencies over which the network can be entrained, with a ten-fold drop in the strength required to entrain a network to the half of its rest frequency.

DISCUSSION

In our latest model (Ijspeert et al. 2007), the generation of S-shaped standing waves of muscle contractions along the body was hypothesized to be a purely central mechanism: It was produced by the CPG without any

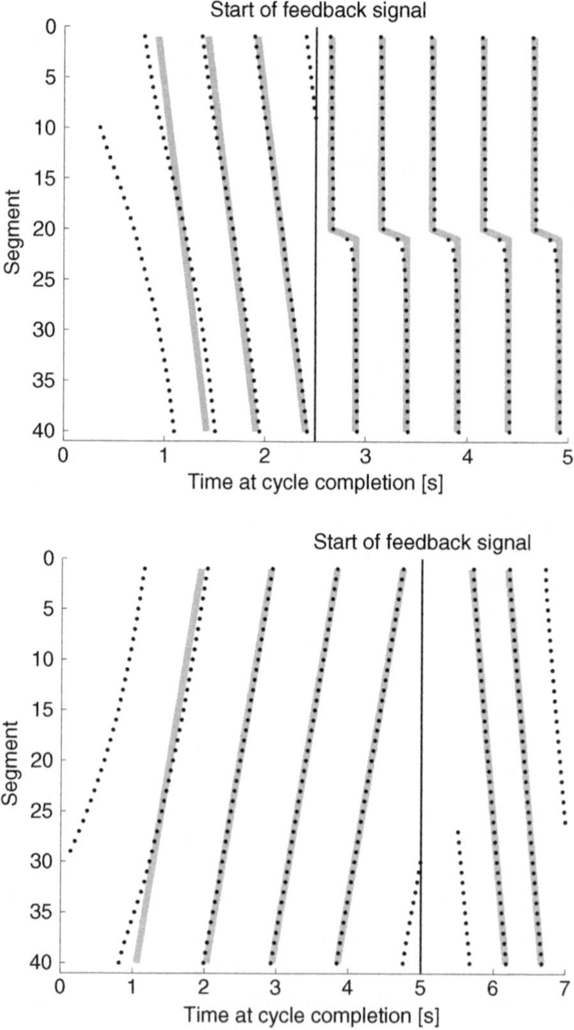

Figure 18.7 Process of convergence of the network to intrinsic patterns, followed by the convergence to the feedback pattern after activation of the artificial feedback signals. The vertical black line indicates the time of activation of the artificial feedback. Each dot marks the completion of one cycle for the corresponding segment. The gray line shows either the intrinsic pattern (before activation of the artificial feedback signals) or the feedback pattern (after activation of the signals). **Top**: A network of intrinsic wave number $k=1$, frequency $\nu=2$ Hz is entrained to a walking pattern (standing wave) using ipsilateral signals of strength $\alpha=200$. Signals were normally started after 5 seconds, but this was adapted here for legibility and compactness. **Bottom**: A network of wave number $k=-1$, frequency $\nu=1.1$ Hz is entrained to a swimming pattern $k_f=1$, $\nu_f=2$ Hz using both ipsilateral and contralateral signals of strength $\alpha=80$, $\beta=-80$.

sensory feedback. Indeed, the traveling wave output of the axial CPG became a standing wave because of the strong couplings from the limb oscillators to the various axial oscillators. The model also assumed that, in the absence of limb activity, intrinsic network properties tend to the production of a traveling wave with an appropriate wavelength of about one body length. Earlier, we mentioned new biological evidence from in vitro experiments that seem to contradict both of these assumptions: Activity in the limb CPGs does not generally result in standing waves of activity in the trunk, and a wide range of wavelengths are observed for traveling waves in the trunk. We have also mentioned that traveling waves are present in the trunk during underwater stepping, which provides in vivo evidence against the first hypothesis (see "Current Issues with the Open-loop Model"). The same biological experiments strengthen the support for other assumptions of the model. One such assumption is that the salamander's CPG can be decomposed into axial and limb components, and that the axial component is very similar to the lamprey CPG and can be modeled as a double chain of oscillators (Ryczko et al. 2007). The lower intrinsic frequency of the limb CPG, and its slow-down effect on the axial CPG, were also confirmed (Ryczko et al. 2009). We are thus seeking to extend the current model to account for the latest experimental data and at the same time, retain features that are supported by biological observations.

In this chapter, we suggested that sensory feedback could play a significant role in reducing the variability of wavelengths and in forcing the travelling wave to become a standing wave during walking. The section "Exploring the Role of Phasic Sensory Feedback: Preliminary Modeling" presented the first steps in our ongoing modeling work to test these hypotheses. We used artificial feedback patterns to entrain networks of various intersegmental phase lags to natural swimming and walking patterns. We found that, in our model, ipsilateral and contralateral signals slightly stronger than the intersegmental coupling can entrain the whole range of phase lags observed in the animal in vitro. Using only ipsilateral feedback patterns required signals 3.5 times stronger than the intersegmental coupling.

The simulations also support our hypothesis that proprioceptive feedback contributes to the formation of standing waves in the trunk: Results suggest that feedback signals of strength similar to the intersegmental coupling can account for the formation of a standing wave with a node at the lower girdle. Interestingly, EMG recordings of salamanders walking underwater display a small intersegmental phase lag, which lies between the traveling wave of swimming and the standing wave of terrestrial walking (see Table 18.1). This intermediate phase lag might reflect sensory feedback signals halfway between terrestrial walking feedback and swimming feedback. Due to the buoyant support of the water, contacts with the ground are much reduced during underwater stepping. For example, in the *Taricha torosa*, underwater stepping is characterized by a duty factor of 41%, compared with 77% for terrestrial stepping (Ashley-Ross et al. 2009). The "reduced gravity" during underwater stepping also affects the cycle durations, which are significantly longer than during overground stepping (see Table 18.1).

In principle, it would also be possible that descending signals from the brainstem contribute directly to the formation of standing waves in the CPG, without the need for sensory feedback. For instance, the spinal network could receive a (rostrocaudally) negative gradient of excitation from the brainstem. Electrical stimulation of the MLR can induce both swimming and walking gaits in a semi-intact in vitro preparation, depending on the intensity of the stimulation (Cabelguen et al. 2003; see "Central Generation of Locomotor Patterns"). In these experiments, the salamander was placed in a chamber filled with amphibian Ringer's solution. The front limbs were removed and the cranium and first two vertebrae were pinned down to the chamber for stabilization. There was no other contact between the salamander body and the border of the chamber; nevertheless, standing waves of activity were observed in the trunk. However, this preparation, with the front limbs removed, the hindlimbs not in contact with the bottom of the chamber, and the rostral end attached to the chamber, is not representative of the sensory feedback conditions in an intact animal. Also, during fictive locomotion experiments (i.e., without movement-related sensory feedback) with preparations that included the brainstem, standing waves were almost never observed (Delvolvé et al. 1999; Ryczko et al. 2009). It thus appears that, although the brainstem can elicit stepping, the shaping of standing waves on the trunk could require sensory feedback.

Regarding the variability of phase lags observed during in vitro experiments, we should note that the nature of the excitation could contribute to the variability of the fictive locomotor patterns. Most of the data collected with salamander in vitro preparations use NMDA to excite the spinal network. In the lamprey spinal cord, NMDA-induced rhythms show a variability of phase lags (Matsushima and Grillner 1992), whereas D-glutamate-induced patterns are very close to EMG patterns recorded on intact lampreys (Wallén and Williams 1984). Unfortunately, there is no published evidence of a successful use of D-glutamate to induce fictive swimming in the salamander spinal cord (see Lavrov and Cheng 2004, for D-glutamate-induced limb activity). The extreme phase lags observed in vitro might thus be an artifact of NMDA excitation; it would be interesting to see if they can be reproduced using other sources of excitation (e.g., D-glutamate or MLR stimulation). In conclusion, the strengths of the feedback connections relative to the body intersegmental couplings that we found likely constitute upper bounds for the strength needed to impose the closed-loop patterns.

Future work will seek to validate the results from the preliminary modeling experiments in a closed-loop model of the salamander in simulation, as well as in a robot. Biological experiments would also be needed to confirm the conclusions of the modeling study.

Validation of the model could be achieved through hybrid experiments in which the central nervous system of the salamander is interfaced with the robot. Previous experiments of this type include interfacing an isolated lamprey brain with a wheeled robot (Karniel et al. 2005), and interfacing a rat brain (Chapin et al. 1999) or a monkey brain (Carmena et al. 2003; Velliste et al. 2008) with a robot arm. In our case, as a first step, recordings from descending pathways in the animal could be used to drive the robot in open-loop. In a subsequent experiment, a closed-loop system could be implemented in which live recordings from the animals are used to drive the robot, and sensors are used to feed, for example, visual or tactile stimuli back to the animal. Successful experiments with this setup would provide an outstanding validation of the spinal cord model.

Open Questions and Future Work

Many aspects of salamander locomotion are still not properly understood; the role of proprioceptive feedback is only one of them. We give here an overview of additional open questions and some suggestions for future biological experiments.

The Nature of the Feedback Signals

Many sensory modalities can potentially affect the generation of locomotor patterns. Examples include the position and velocity of elongation in muscles, tendons, and intraspinal cells, as well as cutaneous feedback. In our open-loop simulations with artificial feedback patterns, the nature of the sensory information is not very significant as long as the signals can be assumed to be periodic (the case of cutaneous feedback as a discrete stimulus is considered below). The results of our work in preliminary modeling can thus be applied to some extent to various sensory modalities. In a closed-loop model, however, the origin of the signal is fundamental, as it determines the phase relationship between the motor command and the feedback signal. It is an important consideration for our ongoing work on a closed-loop model of the salamander locomotor system. We will have to determine the most appropriate phase relationships for the feedback signals in the closed-loop model. This might prove useful for our understanding of salamander locomotion, as it could lead to interesting hypotheses regarding the contribution of different sensory modalities to the modulation of the salamander CPG.

Tactile Feedback and Gait Transitions

It would be interesting to investigate the role of tactile feedback in motor pattern generation, particularly for gait transitions. Manipulations with salamanders suggest that simple contacts with the head or abdomen can trigger a transition from swimming to aquatic walking (J.-M. Cabelguen, unpublished observations). It is also known that tactile stimuli can elicit locomotion in lampreys (Wallén and Williams 1984; McClellan 1988; Viana Di Prisco et al. 1997). This information seems to be integrated in reticulospinal neurons, which then send descending commands to the CPG and motoneurons (Viana Di Prisco et al. 1997; Viana Di Prisco et al. 2000). It would be interesting to investigate whether salamanders use a similar process to translate cutaneous stimuli into gait transitions, and whether higher centers are involved or not. A possible experiment would be to try to elicit gait transitions by tactile stimulation in a semi-intact preparation.

Speed and Efficiency of Locomotion

Swimming experiments with our lamprey robots have shown that the intersegmental phase lag strongly influences the speed of locomotion and that it must be adjusted depending on the frequency of motion to obtain the highest speeds (Crespi and Ijspeert 2006). At low frequencies, the highest speed is obtained with a wave number $k = 0.5$. At frequencies above 0.8 Hz, the highest speeds are obtained with $k = 1$. In the lamprey however, the intersegmental phase is almost constant (k close to 1) and thus independent of the frequency (Wallén and Williams 1984; Williams et al. 1989). This is also true for the salamander, at least in the tail (Frolich and Biewener 1992; D'Août and Aerts 1997; Delvolvé et al. 1997). We naturally do not expect animals to optimize their locomotion patterns on speed only. At the least, a tradeoff between speed and energy must be involved. Robots could be very useful in investigating the importance of different factors in such a tradeoff: Their energy consumption can be readily measured and could be related to kinematic parameters, such as the intersegmental phase lag and the amplitude of undulations, for both swimming and walking gaits. Because of the modularity of our robots, different trunk and tail lengths can be explored by the simple addition or removal of segments. Limbs can also be easily replaced. The robots could thus be a very useful platform for a comparative study of the body morphology and ecological niche of various species of lizards and salamanders in relation to their speed and efficiency of locomotion. Robots and simulations could also help to better understand the role of the tail during terrestrial walking; recent modeling work suggests that the tail might play a role in stability as well as propulsion (Karakasiliotis and Ijspeert 2009).

Also related to the efficiency of locomotion is the relative timing between muscle activation and body undulation. In lampreys and other fishes, waves of muscle activity travel faster than waves of body undulation (Williams et al. 1989). The phase delay between muscle activation and body curvature depends on the species. A comparative study has shown how the phase delay is affected by the fish morphology and how it relates to muscle function (Wardle and Videler 1994). The muscle performs positive work when it is activated during its shortening phase. Conversely, it performs negative work when activated during the lengthening phase. In that case, the muscle is stiffening the body to facilitate the caudal transmission of mechanical power. In carangiform swimmers, there is a strong increase of the phase delay from the head to the tail. Rostral muscles generate positive work, and muscles along the body are mostly used to transmit this power to the caudal fin. Anguilliform swimmers, such as the lamprey, display a smaller increase of the phase delay down the body. These fishes have no tail blade and use most of their body to generate positive work. Experiments with swimming salamanders gave similar results, with positive work generated in muscles located at up to 80% of the body length (D'Août et al. 1996). We intend to measure the phase delay in our swimming robot, to evaluate how it is affected by the frequency and intersegmental activation phase lag, and how it relates to swimming speed and power consumption.

Rich Motor Skills

Models of the locomotor system of lower vertebrates generally focus on the reproduction of stereotypic gaits, such as steady-state walking (a walking trot in the case of the salamander) and swimming along a straight line. However, these animals can also exhibit more complex behaviors. The lamprey, for instance, is capable of backward swimming and C-start escape responses (Grillner and Wallén 1984). The C-start is a C-like shape of body curvature used by many fishes to initiate an escape response when startled (Domenici and Blake 1997); it is also observed in salamanders (Azizi and Landberg 2002). We are now in the process of documenting the diversity of behaviors in the salamander *Pleurodeles waltlii*. Observed behaviors include an underwater pace gait, rhythmic movements of two of the four limbs only, and backward stepping[5] (unpublished observations).

Our current models fail to exhibit the richness of salamander motor skills. Questions remain on how other motor behaviors are implemented. It is well known that the spinal cord contains circuits that generate coordinated movements of single limbs, both for discrete and rhythmic movements (Bizzi et al. 2000; Tresch et al. 2002). In particular, questions remain whether subparts of our CPG model (i.e., a small set of oscillatory centers) can be activated independently of each other, for instance, just the oscillators for one limb. From a theoretical point of view, selective activation of a part of the spinal network can be obtained in different ways, including multiple descending pathways, finely tuned time-varying descending signals, additional spinal circuits, or time-varying connection topologies

[5] Backward stepping has been previously observed in the Pacific giant salamander *Dicamptodon tenebrosus* (Ashley-Ross 1997).

(for instance, under the influence of neuromodulators—see the next section—or by activating or inactivating relay centers).

Mechanisms of Gait Transition

The mechanisms that underlie the suppression of periodic limb activity during swimming are still not clear. Are the mechanisms implemented in the MLR, the reticular formation (RF), or the spinal cord? Electric stimulation of the MLR shows that walking is induced at low levels of stimulation, and swimming at higher levels (Cabelguen et al. 2003). The MLR-RF-spinal cord ensemble contains, therefore, a mechanism such that limb oscillatory centers stop oscillating when the descending drive is too high. In Ijspeert et al. (2007), we showed that a CPG architecture based on this idea could explain several features of gait transition, but it is not clear how and where this mechanism is implemented. In particular, it is not clear whether it is implemented by some gating mechanisms in the MLR or reticular formation (i.e., high drive signals are not transmitted to limb oscillatory centers), or whether it is a spinal mechanism (limb oscillatory centers saturate and become tonic when receiving too much stimulation). Interestingly, it has been shown in the lamprey that high-frequency swimming involves populations of reticulospinal neurons different from those used in the initiation and maintenance of slow swimming (Brocard and Dubuc 2003).

A more detailed knowledge of the activity of descending pathways during locomotor behaviors would contribute greatly to the understanding of both the generation of rich motor skills and gait transitions. A possible experiment would be to use a technique, such as calcium imaging, to characterize the activity of reticulospinal neurons during walking, swimming, and during the expression of rich motor skills.[6] This could reveal the selective activity of reticulospinal subgroups involved in specific motor behaviors.

We have assumed that global connections from the limb centers to the trunk and the tail are incompatible with the diversity of synchronization patterns observed in salamanders. We concluded that limb centers must connect only locally to the axial centers. However, the functional coupling between limb and axial centers could also be altered dynamically by neuromodulators, allowing the network to switch between different connectivity patterns for swimming and walking. Extensive connections from limb to axial oscillators could be enabled during walking for frequency locking and the generation of standing waves, and reduced or totally suppressed during swimming to release the traveling waves. Modulations of functional coupling in the spinal network by neuromodulators were recently identified

[6] Calcium imaging has been used to record reticulospinal neuron activity in the lamprey (Di Prisco 1997, 2000).

in the *Xenopus* (Rauscent et al. 2009). It would be interesting to try to reproduce these results in salamanders and to measure how modifications of the functional coupling by neuromodulators affect the frequencies of the limb and body CPGs.

CONCLUSION

We have presented our current knowledge of the salamander locomotor system and shown that the salamander shares many similarities with the lamprey, while also presenting features that are observed in frog and other limbed vertebrates including reptiles and mammals. We also discussed the state of modeling of this system in light of recent biological data from in vivo and in vitro experiments. These new data raise two questions in particular: How can the same spinal network generate a variety of synchronization patterns in vitro, and more stereotyped patterns in vivo? And, what mechanisms allow for both traveling and standing waves in the trunk concurrently with rhythmic limb activity? We looked at the possible role of proprioceptive feedback in answering these questions. Open-loop simulations showed that signals as strong as, or stronger than, the intersegmental coupling are required in the current model to account for the observed behaviors, whereas much weaker signals can account for the entrainment of frequency observed in lampreys. Closed-loop simulations and robotic experiments will be used to validate these results. New biological experiments will also be required, in particular to elucidate the role of the MLR in pattern generation and gait transitions.

Finally, we should note that, while we address these questions in the salamander, most of them are of great importance for all vertebrates. For instance, gait transitions by MLR stimulation have been observed in all classes of vertebrates and appear to be a common but yet poorly understood property of vertebrate locomotor control (Grillner et al. 1997). Also, the problem of properly coordinating trunk and limb movements is relevant to all limbed vertebrates.

ACKNOWLEDGMENTS

This work was funded by the European Commission's seventh EU framework programme (FP7) under the theme "BIO-ICT convergence," project LAMPETRA. We would like to acknowledge Alessandro Crespi, André Guignard, and André Badertscher for their help in designing and constructing the salamander robot, as well as Stéphanie Chevallier, Stéphanie Lamarque, Dimitri Ryczko, Konstantinos Karakasiliotis, and Andrej Bicanski, for useful discussions.

REFERENCES

Ashley-Ross, M. 1994a. Hindlimb kinematics during terrestrial locomotion in a salamander *(Dicamptodon tenebrosus)*. *Journal of Experimental Biology* 193:255–83.

Ashley-Ross, M. 1994b. Metamorphic and speed effects on hindlimb kinematics during terrestrial locomotion in the salamander *(Dicamptodon tenebrosus)*. *Journal of Experimental Biology* 193:285–305.

Ashley-Ross, M., and B. Bechtel. 2004. Kinematics of the transition between aquatic and terrestrial locomotion in the newt *Taricha torosa*. *Journal of Experimental Biology* 207(3):461–74.

Ashley-Ross, M., and G. Lauder. 1997. Motor patterns and kinematics during backward walking in the pacific giant salamander: Evidence for novel motor output. *Journal of Neurophysiology* 78:3047–60.

Ashley-Ross, M., R. Lundin, and K. Johnson. 2009. Kinematics of level terrestrial and underwater walking in the California newt *(Taricha torosa)*. *Journal of Experimental Zoology Part A: Ecological Genetics and Physiology* 311(4):240–57.

Azizi, E., and T. Landberg. 2002. Effects of metamorphosis on the aquatic escape response of the two-lined salamander *(Eurycea bislineata)*. *Journal of Experimental Biology* 205(6):841–49.

Bar-Gad, I., I. Kagan, and M.L. Shik. 1999. Behavior of hindbrain neurons during the transition from rest to evoked locomotion in a newt. *Progress in Brain Research* 123:285–94.

Bem, T., J.M. Cabelguen, O. Ekeberg, and S. Grillner. 2003. From swimming to walking: A single basic network for two different behaviors. *Biological Cybernetics* 88:79–90.

Bizzi, E., M. Tresch, P. Saltiel, and A. d'Avella. 2000. New perspectives on spinal motor systems. *Nature Review of Neuroscience* 1:101–08.

Bowtell, G., and T. Williams. 1991. Anguilliform body dynamics: Modelling the interaction between muscle activation and body curvature. *Philosophical Transactions of the Royal Society of London. Series B Biological Sciences* 334: 385–90.

Brandle, K., and G. Székely. 1973. The control of alternating coordination of limb pairs in the newt *(Triturus vulgaris)*. *Brain Behavior and Evolution* 8:366–85.

Brocard, F., and R. Dubuc. 2003. Differential contribution of reticulospinal cells to the control of locomotion induced by the mesencephalic locomotor region. *Journal of Neurophysiology* 90(3):1714–27.

Buchanan, J. 1992. Neural network simulations of coupled locomotor oscillators in the lamprey spinal cord. *Biological Cybernetics* 66:367–74.

Buchanan, J., and S. Grillner. 1987. Newly identified 'glutamate interneurons' and their role in locomotion in the lamprey spinal cord. *Science* 236:312–14.

Cabelguen, J.M., C. Bourcier-Lucas, and R. Dubuc. 2003. Bimodal locomotion elicited by electrical stimulation of the midbrain in the salamander *(Notophthalmus viridescens)*. *Journal of Neuroscience* 23(6):2434–39.

Carmena, J.M., M.A. Lebedev, R.E. Crist, J.E. O'Doherty, D.M. Santucci, D.F. Dimitrov, et al. 2003. Learning to control a brain-machine interface for reaching and grasping by primates. *PLoS Biology* 1(2):e42.

Carrier, D. 1993. Action of the hypaxial muscles during walking and swimming in the salamander *(Dicamptodon ensatus)*. *Journal of Experimental Biology* 180: 75–63.

Chapin, J., K. Moxon, R. Markowitz, and M. Nicolelis. 1999. Real-time control of a robot arm using simultaneously recorded neurons in the motor cortex. *Nature Neuroscience* 2:664–70.

Cheng, J., K. Jovanovic, Y. Aoyagi, D. Bennett, Y. Han, and R. Stein. 2002. Differential distribution of interneurons in the neural networks that control walking in the mudpuppy *(Necturus maculatus)* spinal cord. *Experimental Brain Research* 145(2):190–98.

Cheng, J., R. Stein, K. Jovanovic, K. Yoshida, D. Bennett, and Y. Han. 1998. Identification, localization, and modulation of neural networks for walking in the mudpuppy *(Necturus maculatus)* spinal cord. *Journal of Neuroscience* 18(11):4295–304.

Chevallier, S., M. Landry, F. Nagy, and J.M. Cabelguen. 2004. Recovery of bimodal locomotion in the spinal-transected salamander *(Pleurodeles waltlii). European Journal of Neuroscience* 20(8):1995–2007.

Cohen, A., P. Holmes, and R. Rand. 1982. The nature of coupling between segmented oscillations and the lamprey spinal generator for locomotion: A mathematical model. *Journal of Mathematics and Biology* 13:345–69.

Cohen, A., and P. Wallen. 1980. The neural correlate of locomotion in fish. "Fictive swimming" induced in a in vitro preparation of the lamprey spinal cord. *Experimental Brain Research* 41:11–18.

Combes, D., S.D. Merrywest, J. Simmers, and K.T. Sillar. 2004. Developmental segregation of spinal networks driving axial- and hindlimb-based locomotion in metamorphosing xenopus laevis. *Journal of Physiology* 559(1):17–24.

Crespi, A., and A. Ijspeert. 2006. AmphiBot II: An amphibious snake robot that crawls and swims using a central pattern generator. Proceedings of the 9th International Conference on Climbing and Walking Robots. CLAWAR 2006, pp. 19–27.

Daan, S., and T. Belterman. 1968. Lateral bending in locomotion of some lower tetrapods. *Proceedings of the Koninklijke Nederlandse Akademie van Wetenschappen*, 71:245–66.

D'Août, K., and P. Aerts. 1997. Kinematics and efficiency of steady swimming in adult axolotls *(Ambystoma mexicanum). Journal of Experimental Biology* 200(13):1863–71.

D'Août, K., P. Aerts, and F. de Vree. 1996. The timing of muscle strain and activation during steady swimming in a salamander *(Ambystoma mexicanum). Netherlands Journal of Zoology* 46:263–71.

Davis, B., J. Ayers, L. Koran, J. Carlson, M. Anderson, and S. Simpson. 1990. Time course of the salamander spinal cord regeneration and recovery of swimming: HRP retrograde pathway tracing and kinematic analysis. *Experimental Neurology* 108:198–213.

Delcomyn, F. 1980. Neural basis for rhythmic behaviour in animals. *Science* 210: 492–98.

Delvolvé, I., T. Bem, and J.M. Cabelguen. 1997. Epaxial and limb muscle activity during swimming and terrestrial stepping in the adult newt *(Pleurodeles waltl). Journal of Neurophysiology* 78:638–50.

Delvolvé, I., P. Branchereau, R. Dubuc, and J.M. Cabelguen. 1999. Fictive rhythmic motor patterns induced by NMDA in an in vitro brain stem-spinal cord preparation from an adult urodele. *Journal of Neurophysiology* 82:1074–77.

Domenici, P., and R. Blake. 1997. The kinematics and performance of fish fast-start swimming. *Journal of Experimental Biology* 200(8):1165–78.

Edwards, J. 1977. The evolution of terrestrial locomotion. In *Major patterns in vertebrate evolution*, eds., M.K. Hecht, P.C. Goody and B.M. Hecht, 553–77. New York: Plenum Press.

Ekeberg, Ö. 1993. A combined neuronal and mechanical model of fish swimming. *Biological Cybernetics* 69:363–74.

Ekeberg, Ö., P. Wallén, A. Lansner, H. Traven, L. Brodin, and S. Grillner. 1991. A computer-based model for realistic simulations of neural networks I: The single neuron and synaptic interaction. *Biological Cybernetics* 65:81–90.

Ermentrout, B., and N. Kopell. 1994. Inhibition-produced patterning in chains of coupled nonlinear oscillators. *Siam Journal of Applied Mathematics* 54(2): 478–507.

Frolich, L., and A. Biewener. 1992. Kinematic and electromyographic analysis of the functional role of the body axis during terrestrial and aquatic locomotion in the salamander *(Ambystoma tigrinum). Journal of Experimental Biology* 62:107–30.

Gillis, G. 1997. Anguilliform locomotion in an elongate salamander *(Siren intermedia)*: Effects of speed on axial undulatory movements. *Journal of Experimental Biology* 200:767–84.

Grillner, S. 1981. Control of locomotion in bipeds, tetrapods and fish. In *Handbook of physiology the nervous system 2 motor control*, ed., V. Brooks, 1179–1236. Bethesda, MD: American Physiology Society.

Grillner, S. 2006. Biological pattern generation: The cellular and computational logic of networks in motion. *Neuron* 52(5):751–66.

Grillner, S., J. Buchanan, P. Wallén, L. Brodin. 1988. Neural control of locomotion in lower vertebrates. In *Neural control of rhythmic movements in vertebrates*, eds., A.H. Cohen, S. Rossignol and S. Grillner, 1–40. New York: John Wiley and Sons.

Grillner, S., T. Degliana, Ö Ekeberg, A. El Marina, A. Lansner, G. Orlovsky, and P. Wallén. 1995. Neural networks that co-ordinate locomotion and body orientation in lamprey. *Trends in Neuroscience* 18(6):270–79.

Grillner, S., A.P. Georgopoulos, L.M. Jordan. 1997. Selection and initiation of motor behavior. In *Neurons networks and motor behavior*, eds., P.S.G. Stein, S. Grillner, A. Selverston and D.G. Stuart. Cambridge, MA: MIT press.

Grillner, S., and P. Wallén. 1984. How does the lamprey central nervous system make the lamprey swim? *Journal of Experimental Biology* 112(1):337–57.

Grillner, S., P. Wallén, and L. Brodin. 1991. Neuronal network generating locomotor behavior in lamprey: Circuitry, transmitters, membrane properties, and simulation. *Annual Review of Neuroscience* 14:169–99.

Hildebrand, M. 1966. Analysis of the symmetrical gaits of tetrapods. *Folia Biotheoretica* 6:9–22.

Hoyt, D., and R. Taylor. 1981. Gait and the energetics of locomotion in horses. *Nature* 292:239–40.

Ijspeert, A. 2001. A connectionist central pattern generator for the aquatic and terrestrial gaits of a simulated salamander. *Biological Cybernetics* 84(5):331–48.

Ijspeert, A., A. Crespi, and J. Cabelguen. 2005. Simulation and robotics studies of salamander locomotion. Applying neurobiological principles to the control of locomotion in robots. *Neuroinformatics* 3(3):171–96.

Ijspeert, A., A. Crespi, D. Ryczko, and J.M. Cabelguen. 2007. From swimming to walking with a salamander. *Science* 315(1):1416–20.

Karakasiliotis, K., and A. Ijspeert. 2009. Analysis of the terrestrial locomotion of a salamander robot. *Proceedings of IROS*.

Karniel, A., M. Kositsky, K. Fleming, M. Chiappalone, V. Sanguineti, S. Alford, and F. Mussa-Ivaldi. 2005. Computational analysis in vitro: Dynamics and plasticity of a neuro-robotic system. *Journal of Neural Engineering* 2(3):250–65.

Kopell, N. 1995. Chains of coupled oscillators. In *The handbook of brain theory and neural networks*, ed., M. Arbib, 178–83. Cambridge, MA: MIT Press.

Lamarque, S., D. Ryczko, H. Didier, and J.M. Cabelguen. 2009. Dynamics of the axial locomotor network in intact, freely moving salamanders. 31st International Symposium of the GRSNC, Montréal. Canada.

Lavrov, I., and J. Cheng. 2004. Activation of NMDA receptors is required for the initiation and maintenance of walking-like activity in the mudpuppy

(*Necturus maculatus*). *Canadian Journal of Physiology & Pharmacology* 82(8-9): 637–44.

Matsushima, T., and S. Grillner. 1992. Neural mechanisms of intersegmental coordination in lamprey: Local excitability changes modify the phase coupling along the spinal cord. *Journal of Neurophysiology* 67:373–88.

McClellan, A. 1988. Brainstem command systems for locomotion in the lamprey: Localization of descending pathways in the spinal cord. *Brain Research* 457(2):338–49.

McClellan, A., and K. Sigvardt. 1988. Features of entrainment of spinal pattern generators for locomotor activity in the lamprey spinal cord. *Journal of Neuroscience* 8:133–45.

Piatt, J. 1955. Regeneration of the spinal cord in the salamander. *Journal of Experimental Zoology* 129(1):177–207.

Rauscent, A., J. Einum, D.L. Ray, J. Simmers, and D. Combes. 2009. Opposing aminergic modulation of distinct spinal locomotor circuits and their functional coupling during amphibian metamorphosis. *Journal of Neuroscience* 29(4): 1163–74.

Roos, P. 1964. Lateral bending in newt locomotion. *Proc Ned Akad Wetten Ser C* 67:223–32.

Rossignol, S. 1996. Neural control of stereotypic limb movements. In *Handbook of physiology Section 12 exercise: Regulation and integration of multiple systems,* eds., L. Rowell and J. Sheperd. Bethesda, MD: American Physiology Society.

Ryczko, D., A. Ijspeert, F. Nagy, and J.M. Cabelguen. 2007. Mechanisms of rhythm generation in spinal cord segments of the salamander. Society for Neuroscience, 37th Annual Meeting, San Diego.

Ryczko, D., S. Lamarque, H. Didier, and J.M. Cabelguen. 2009. Dynamics of the axial locomotor network in the isolated spinal cord of the salamander. Society for Neuroscience, 39th Annual Meeting, Chicago.

Schroeder, D., and M. Egar. 1990. Marginal neurons in the urodele spinal cord and the associated denticulate ligaments. *The Journal of Comparative Neurology* 301:93–103.

Shik, M., F. Severin, and G. Orlovsky. 1966. Control of walking and running by means of electrical stimulation of the mid-brain. *Biophysics* 11:756–65.

Srinivasan, M., and A. Ruina. 2006. Computer optimization of a minimal biped model discovers walking and running. *Nature*, 439(5):72–75.

Steeves, J., G. Sholomenko, and D. Webster. 1987. Stimulation of the pontomedullary reticular formation initiates locomotion in decerebrate birds. *Brain Research* 401(2):205–12.

Stein, P.S.G., J.L. Smith. 1997. Neural and biomechanical control strategies for different forms of vertebrate hindlimb motor tasks. In *Neurons networks and motor behavior*, eds., P.S.G. Stein, S. Grillner, A. Selverston and D.G. Stuart, 61–73. Cambridge, MA: MIT Press.

Székely, G., G. Czéh. 1976. Organization of locomotion. In *Frog neurobiology a handbook*, 765–92. Berlin: Springer Verlag.

Tresch, M., P. Saltiel, A. d'Avella, and E. Bizzi. 2002. Coordination and localization in spinal motor systems. *Brain Research Reviews* 40(1-3):66–79.

Tunstall, M., and A. Roberts. 1994. A longitudinal gradient of synaptic drive in the spinal cord of xenopus embryos and its role in co-ordination of swimming. *Journal of Physiology* 474(3):393–405.

Tytell, E.D., and A.H. Cohen. 2008. Rostral versus caudal differences in mechanical entrainment of the lamprey central pattern generator for locomotion. *Journal of Neurophysiology* 99(5):2408–19.

van den Kieboom, J. 2009. Biped locomotion and stability: A practical approach. Master's thesis, University of Groningen. Netherlands, Dept. of Artificial Intelligence.

Velliste, M., S. Perel, M.C. Spalding, A. Whitford, and A. Schwartz. 2008. Cortical control of a prosthetic arm for self-feeding. *Nature* 453(7198):1098–101.

Viana Di Prisco, G., E. Pearlstein, D.L. Ray, R. Robitaille, and R. Dubuc. 2000. A cellular mechanism for the transformation of a sensory input into a motor command. *Journal of Neuroscience* 20(21):8169–76.

Viana Di Prisco, G., E. Pearlstein, R. Robitaille, and R. Dubuc. 1997. Role of sensory-evoked NMDA plateau potentials in the initiation of locomotion. *Science* 278(5340):1122–25.

Viana Di Prisco, G., P. Wallén, and S. Grillner. 1990. Synaptic effects of intraspinal stretch receptor neurons mediating movement-related feedback during locomotion. *Brain Research* 530:161–66.

Wallén, P., Ö Ekeberg, A. Lansner, L. Brodin, H. Traven, and S. Grillner. 1992. A computer-based model for realistic simulations of neural networks II: The segmental network generating locomotor rhythmicity in the lamprey. *Journal of Neurophysiology* 68:1939–50.

Wallén, P., and T. Williams. 1984. Fictive locomotion in the lamprey spinal cord in vitro compared with swimming in the intact and spinal animal. *Journal of Physiology* 347(1):225–39.

Wannier, T. 1994. Rostro-caudal distribution of reticulospinal projections from different brainstem nuclei in the lamprey. *Brain Research* 666:275–78.

Wardle, C.S., J.J. Videler. 1994. The timing of lateral muscle strain and EMG activity in different species of steadily swimming fish. In *Mechanics and physiology of animal swimming*, eds., L. Maddock, Q. Bone and J.M.V. Rayner, 111–18. Cambridge: Cambridge University Press.

Wheatley, M., M. Edamura, and R. Stein. 1992. A comparison of intact and in-vitro locomotion in an adult amphibian. *Experimental Brain Research* 88:609–14.

Wheatley, M., K. Jovanovic, R. Stein, and V. Lawson. 1994. The activity of interneurons during locomotion in the in vitro necturus spinal cord. *Journal of Neurophysiology* 71(6):2025–32.

Whelan, P. 1996. Control of locomotion in the decerebrate cat. *Progress in Neurobiology* 49:481–515.

Williams, L., S. Grillner, V. Smoljaninov, P. Allen, S. Kashin, and S. Rossignol. 1989. Locomotion in lamprey and trout: The relative timing of activation and movement. *Journal of Experimental Biology* 143:559–66.

Williams, T. 1992. Phase coupling by synaptic spread in chains of coupled neuronal oscillators. *Science* 258:662–65.

Williams, T., K. Sigvardt. 1995. Spinal cord of lamprey: Generation of locomotor patterns. In *The handbook of brain theory and neural networks*, ed., M. Arbib, 918–21. Cambridge, MA: MIT Press.

Williams, T., K. Sigvardt, N. Kopell, G. Ermentrout, and M. Rempler. 1990. Forcing of coupled nonlinear oscillators: Studies of intersegmental coordination in the lamprey locomotor central pattern generator. *Journal of Neurophysiology* 64:862–71.

19

Aerial Navigation and Optic Flow Sensing

A Biorobotic Approach

NICOLAS FRANCESCHINI, FRANCK RUFFIER, AND JULIEN SERRES

Insects are no longer the dumb creatures they used to be called. Some insects have well-developed learning and memory capacities whose essential mechanisms do not differ drastically from those of vertebrates (Giurfa and Menzel 1997, Giurfa 2003). Flying insects have been in the business of sensory–motor integration for more than a hundred millions years. These star pilots navigate swiftly through the most unpredictable environments, often attaining a level of agility that greatly outperforms that of both vertebrate animals and present-day aerial robots. Insects are capable of dynamic stabilization, three-dimensional autonomous navigation, ground avoidance, collision avoidance with stationary and nonstationary obstacles, tracking, docking, decking on movable substrates, autonomous takeoff, hovering, landing, and more. They also behave in a predictive manner, making the appropriate anticipatory postural adjustments that will allow them to take off in the right direction when they notice an approaching threat (Card and Dickinson 2008).

No wonder that insects' neural circuits are highly complex—commensurate with the sophisticated behavior they mediate. However, these circuits can be investigated at the level of single, *uniquely identifiable neurons*, i.e., neurons that can be reliably identified in all the individuals of the species on the basis of their location in the ganglion, their exact shape, and their consistent electrical responses. This great advantage of insect versus vertebrate neuroscience enables insect neuroscientists to accumulate knowledge during anything from a few days to several decades about a given individual neuron or a well-defined neural circuit (Strausfeld 1976; Hausen and Egelhaaf 1989; Frye and Dickinson 2001).

This chapter deals with the autopilot systems that may allow insects to fly safely without bumping into things. The chapter summarizes our recent attempts to formulate explicit control schemes explaining how insects may navigate *without requiring any distance or speed measurements.* The aim of these studies was not to produce a detailed neural circuit but rather to obtain a picture that abstracts some basic control laws. We attempted to determine the variables the insect needs to measure, the variables it needs to control, and the causal and dynamic relationships between the sensory and motor variables involved.

The last decades have provided evidence that flying insects guide themselves visually by processing the *optic flow* (OF) that is generated on their eyes as a consequence of their locomotion. In the animal's reference frame, the translational OF is the *angular speed* ω at which contrasting objects in the environment move past the animal as a consequence of locomotion (Kennedy 1939, 1951; Gibson 1950; Lee 1980; Koenderink 1986).

Our progress was achieved not only by performing simulation experiments but also by testing our control schemes onboard miniature aerial robots. Constructing a bio-inspired robot first requires exactly formulating the signal-processing principles at work in the animal. It gives us, in return, a unique opportunity of checking the soundness and robustness of those principles by bringing them face to face with the real physical world (see also Webb 2001).

Like the early terrestrial Robot-Fly (the "robot-mouche": Pichon et al. 1989; Franceschini et al. 1992), our aerial robots are based on the use of electronic *OF sensors* (Blanès 1986; Franceschini et al. 1986) inspired by the housefly *elementary motion detectors* (EMDs), which we previously studied in our laboratory (see: Riehle and Franceschini, 1984; Franceschini 1985, 1992; Franceschini et al. 1989).

After recalling some aspects of the fly visual system and its motion sensitive neurons, we focus on the realization of fly-inspired OF sensors. We then examine the problem of ground avoidance by flying creatures and introduce the principle of *OF regulation.* The micro-helicopter demonstrator we built is then described, equipped with an electronic OF sensor and an *OF regulator.* The extent to which the OF regulator concept accounts for the actual behavioral patterns observed in insects is discussed. The results of recent behavioral experiments on honeybees trained to enter a corridor led us to introduce the *dual OF regulator,* an OF-based autopilot that is able to control both speed and clearance from the walls. This autopilot's performance was tested in simulation on a micro-hovercraft. We conclude by discussing the potential applications of these insect-derived principles to the navigation of aerial vehicles, in particular Micro Aerial Vehicles (MAVs) and Micro Space Vehicles (MSVs), which, like insects, are not supposed to carry the prohibitively large and power-hungry sensors and control systems present on conventional aircraft.

THE FLY VISUAL SYSTEM AND ITS MOTION-SENSITIVE NEURONS

Each compound eye consists of an array of small eyes, the *ommatidia*. The frontend of each *ommatidium* is a facet lens that focusses light on a small set of photoreceptor cells (Fig. 19.1, *right*). The fly retina is among the most complex and best organized retinal mosaic in the animal kingdom. It has been described in great detail, with its different spectral types of photoreceptor cells, polarization sensitive cells, and sexually dimorphic cells. There exists a typical division of labor within the retina (see Franceschini 1984, 1985; Hardie 1985):

- The two central photoreceptor cells, R7–8, display various spectral sensitivities that are randomly scattered across the retinal mosaic, as attested by the characteristic R7 autofluorescence colors (Fig. 19.1). R7 and R8 are thought to participate in color vision.

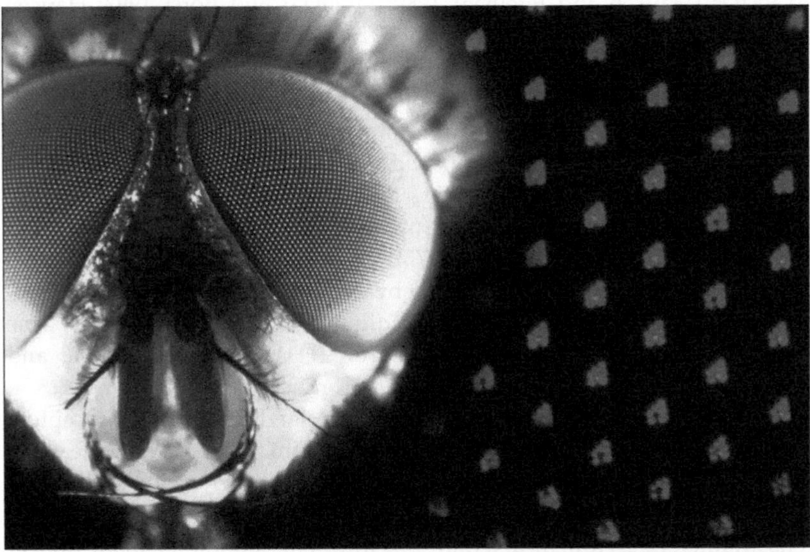

Figure 19.1 Head of the blowfly *Calliphora erythrocephala* with its panoramic compound eyes (*left*). The right part shows about 2% of the housefly retinal mosaic. A cluster of micrometer-sized photoreceptors is located in the focal plane of each facet lens: six outer receptors (R1–6) surround a central cell R7 (prolonged by an R8, not seen here). These are the natural *autofluorescence* colors of the receptors observed *in vivo* under blue excitation (Franceschini et al., 1981a,b), after "optical neutralization of the cornea." From Franceschini, N. 2007. Sa majesté des mouches. In: *Voir l'Invisible* eds., J.P. Gex, and E. Fox-Keller, 28–29. *Voir l'Invisible,* Paris: Omniscience, with permission of the publisher.

- The outer six photoreceptor cells (R1–6) all have the same, dual-peak spectral sensitivity (blue-green + UV). Within each R1-6 cell, signal-to-noise ratio is improved by the presence of an ultraviolet sensitizing pigment that enhances the quantum catch while making the cell panchromatic (Kirschfeld et al. 1977). Sensitivity of the R1-6 visual pathway is also improved by an exquisite opto-neural projection called *neural superposition* (Trujillo-Cenoz and Melamed, 1966; Braitenberg 1967; Kirschfeld 1967; Kirschfeld and Franceschini 1968). The R1–6 photoreceptors therefore make for a high-sensitivity ("scotopic") system (Kirschfeld and Franceschini 1968) that is devoted, in particular, to motion perception (Buchner 1984; Heisenberg and Wolf 1984; Riehle and Franceschini 1984).

To estimate the OF, insects use *motion-sensitive neurons*. Flies analyze the OF locally, pixel-by-pixel, via a neural circuit, the EMD. Further down the neural pathways, more precisely in that part of the third optic ganglion called the *lobula plate* (LP), about 60 large-field collator neurons called lobula plate tangential cells (LPTCs) integrate the outputs of large numbers of EMDs (Hausen and Egelhaaf 1989; Egelhaaf and Borst 1993; Hausen 1993). The LPTC neurons analyze the OF field generated by the animal's movements (Krapp et al. 1998; Borst and Haag 2002; Taylor and Krapp 2008). Some of these neurons transmit electrical signals via the neck to the thoracic interneurons directly or indirectly responsible for driving the wing, leg, or head muscles (Strausfeld and Bassemir, 1985). Other LPTCs (in particular, the H1 neuron, Fig. 19.2B) send relevant signals to the contralateral eye. Taking advantage of the micro-optical techniques we had developed earlier (Franceschini 1975), we were able to activate a single EMD in the eye of the living housefly by stimulating single identified photoreceptor cells within a single ommatidium, while recording the response of an identified motion sensitive neuron (H1) in the LP (Riehle and Franceschini 1984; Franceschini 1985, 1992; Franceschini et al. 1989).

We applied pinpoint stimulation to two neighboring photoreceptors (diameter ≅ 1μm) within the selected ommatidium (Fig. 19.2A) by means of a high-precision instrument (a hybrid between a microscope and a telescope: Figure 19.2D), in which the main objective lens was a single facet lens (diameter ≅ 25 μm, focal length ≅ 50 μm). This laboratory-made optical instrument served to: (a) select the facet lens (Fig. 19.2A), (b) select two out of the seven receptors visible *in vivo* in the back focal plane of the facet lenslet, and (c) stimulate these two photoreceptors (R1 and R6) *successively* with 1 μm light spots. Sequential stimulation produced an "apparent motion" that would simulate a real motion within the small visual field of the selected ommatidium. The H1 neuron responded with a vigorous spike discharge only when the motion was mimicked in the preferred direction (see Fig. 19.2C, *top trace*). The null response observed for the reverse sequence (Fig. 19.2C, *bottom trace*) attests to the remarkable sequence-discriminating ability of an EMD, which is indeed *directionally selective* (Franceschini 1992).

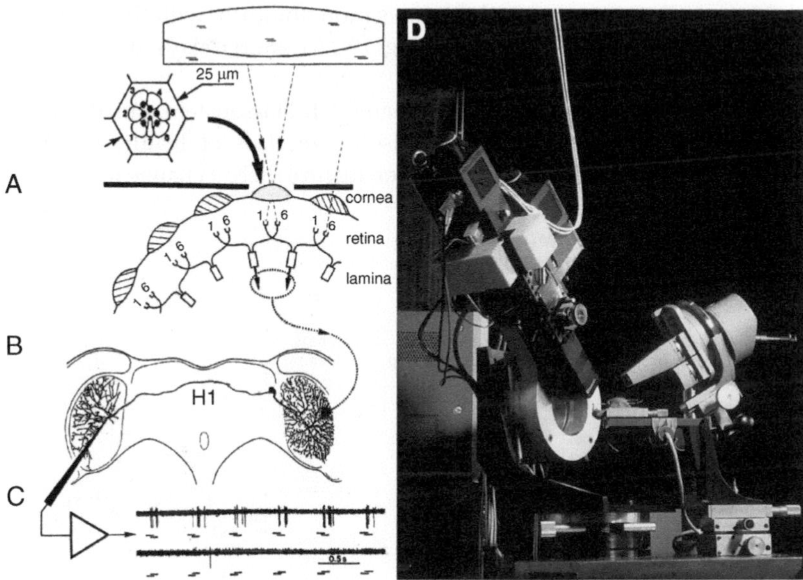

Figure 19.2 **A–C**: Principle of the experiment aimed at deciphering the principle of motion vision in flies, using optical stimulation of single photoreceptors. **D**: Triple-beam incident light "microscope-telescope" that delivers a 1μm light spot to two neighboring photoreceptor cells, R1 and R6, *successively* (see A). A microelectrode (C) records the unit response (nerve impulses) of the motion sensitive neuron H1 to this "apparent motion." From Franceschini, N., A. Riehle, A. Le Nestour. 1989. Directionally selective motion detection by insect neurons. In: *Facets of vision*, eds., D.G. Stavenga and R.C. Hardie, 360–90. Berlin: Springer, with permission of the publisher.

From many experiments of this kind, in which various sequences of light steps and/or pulses were applied to selected receptor pairs, an EMD block diagram was obtained, and the dynamics and nonlinearity of each block were characterized (Franceschini 1985, 1992; Franceschini et al. 1989). Although not unveiling the EMD cellular details—still elusive in both vertebrates and invertebrates—our analysis at least allowed the EMD principle to be understood functionally, paving the way for some transcription into another, man-made technology, such as electronics.

NEUROMIMETIC OPTIC FLOW SENSORS

In the mid 1980s, we designed a neuromorphic optic flow sensor (Blanès 1986; Franceschini et al. 1986), the signal processing scheme of which was inspired by what we had learned from the fly EMD. The OF is an angular speed ω [rad.s^{-1}] that corresponds to the inverse of the time Δt taken by a contrasting feature to travel between the visual axes of two adjacent photoreceptors, separated by an angle $\Delta\varphi$. Our OF sensor processes this delay Δt

so as to generate a response that grows monotonically with the inverse of Δt, and hence with the optic flow ω (Fig. 19.3A). Short delays Δt give higher voltage outputs and vice versa.

Our scheme is not a correlator scheme (cf. Hassenstein and Reichardt 1956; Reichardt 1969). It corresponds to the class of feature-matching schemes (Ullman 1981), in which a given feature (here a change in intensity

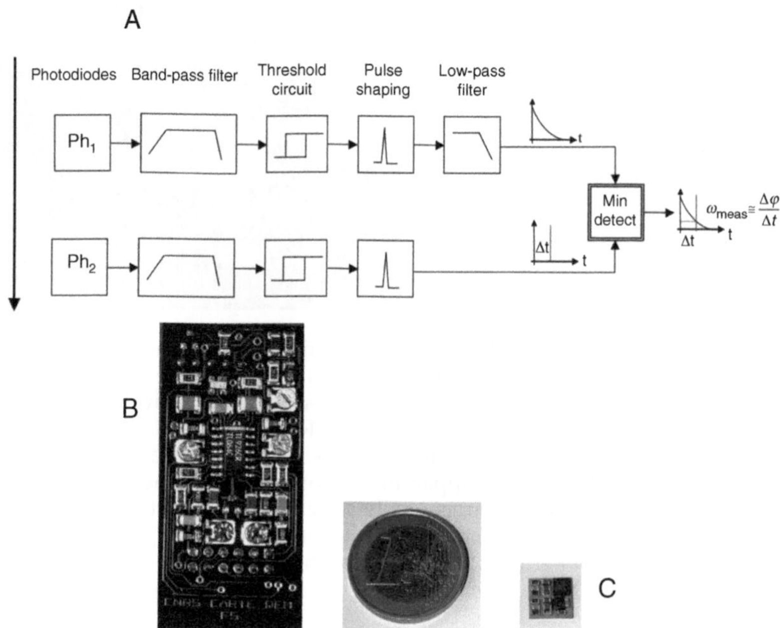

Figure 19.3 **A**: Principle of the electro-optic flow sensor derived from our electrophysiological analyses of the housefly's EMD (Blanes, 1986, Franceschini et al., 1986). **B**: Purely analogue version (weight 5 grams) built in 1989 for Robot-Fly, whose compound eye housed a ring of 114 EMDs of this type (Pichon et al., 1989; Franceschini et al., 1992). **C**: Hybrid (analog + digital) version (size: 7×7 mm, mass 0.2 grams) based on a microcontroller and built using low-temperature co-fired ceramics technology (LTCC) (Pudas et al., 2007). From Blanès, C. 1986. Appareil visuel élémentaire pour la navigation à vue d'un robot mobile autonome. MS thesis in Neuroscience, University of Aix-Marseille II, Marseille, France; Franceschini, N., C. Blanès, and L. Oufar. 1986. Passive, noncontact optical velocity sensor *Technical Report ANVAR/DVAR*, No. 51549, Paris (in French); Pichon, J.M., C. Blanès, N., and Franceschini. 1989. Visual guidance of a mobile robot equipped with a network of self-motion sensors. In *Mobile robots IV*, eds., W.J. Wolfe and W.H. Chun, 44–53. Bellingham, U.S.A: SPIE, Vol. 1195; Franceschini, N., J.M. Pichon, and C. Blanès. 1992. From insect vision to robot vision. *Philosophical Transactions of the Royal Society London B* 337: 283–294; and Pudas, M., S. Viollet, F. Ruffier, A. Kruusing, S. Amic, S. Leppävuori, and N. Franceschini. 2007. A miniature bio-inspired optic flow sensor based on low temperature co-fired ceramics (LTCC) technology. *Sensors and Actuators A* 133: 88–95, with permission of the respective publishers.

that may represent an edge) is extracted and tracked in time. Once bandpass filtered, the photodiode signal of each channel (Fig. 19.3A) actually resembles the analog signal measured in the large monopolar neurons postsynaptic to the photoreceptors in the fly lamina (Zettler and Weiler 1974; Laughlin 1984). The next processing step consists of hysteresis thresholding and generation of a unit pulse. In the EMD version built in 1989 for Robot-Fly (Fig. 19.3B), the unit pulse from one channel was sampling a long-lived decaying exponential function generated by the other channel, via a nonlinear circuit called a *minimum detector*, to give an output $\omega_{measured}$ that grows as a monotonic function of the angular velocity $\omega = \Delta\varphi/\Delta t$ (Fig. 19.3) (Blanès 1986; Franceschini et al. 1986). The thresholding operation makes the voltage output largely independent of texture and contrast—unlike the Reichardt correlator—and the circuit responds as well to natural scenes (Portelli et al. 2008). A very similar EMD principle has been conceived, independently, a decade later by C. Koch's group at CALTECH, where it became known as the "facilitate-and-sample" velocity sensor (Kramer et al. 1995). Another variant of our original "time-of-travel" principle was proposed yet another decade later (Moeckel and Liu 2007).

Since our original analog implementation, we have built various versions of OF sensors based on the same principle. In the EMD currently used onboard our aerial robotic demonstrators, the signals are processed using a mixed (analog + digital) approach (Ruffier et al. 2003). Such OF sensors can be small and lightweight (the smallest one weighs only 0.2 grams: Fig. 19.3C) and an array of sensors can be integrated on a miniature field programmable gate array (FPGA) (Aubépart et al. 2004; Aubépart and Franceschini 2007).

THE PROBLEM OF GROUND AVOIDANCE

To control an aircraft, it has been deemed essential to measure state variables such as ground height, ground speed, descent speed, etc. The sensors developed for this purpose (usually emissive sensors such as radio-altimeters, laser rangefinders, Doppler radars, GPS receivers, forward-looking infrared sensors, etc.) are far too cumbersome for insects or even birds to carry and to power. The OF sensors evolved by natural flyers over the last few hundred million years are at odds with these avionic sensors. OF sensors are *nonemissive* sensors.

The ventral OF experienced in the vertical plane by flying creatures—including aircraft pilots—is the relative angular velocity ω generated by a point directly below on the flight track (Gibson et al. 1955; Whiteside and Samuel 1970). As shown in Figure 19.4A, the *translational OF* perceived vertically downward depends on both the ground speed V_x and the ground height h and is equal to the ratio between these two variables:

$$\omega = V_x / h [\text{rad.s}^{-1}] \qquad \text{(Eq. 1)}$$

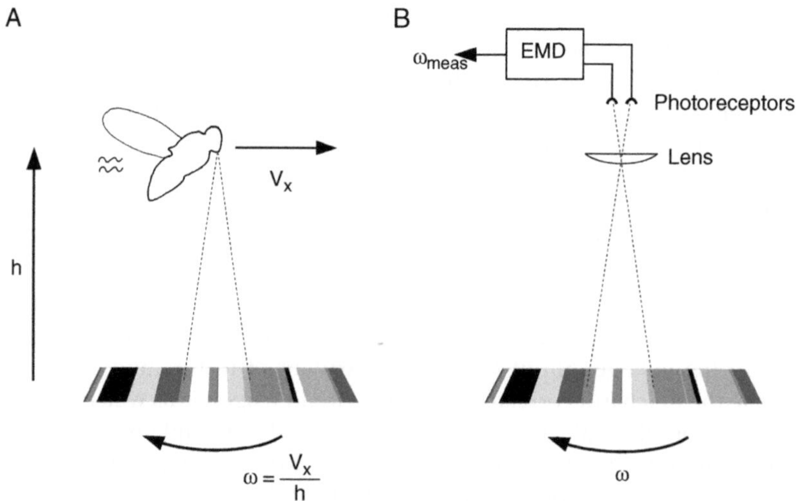

Figure 19.4 **A**: Definition and measurement of the ventral optic flow ω experienced by an insect (or a robot) flying in translation in the vertical plane. **B**: An EMD of the type shown in Figure 19.3, like the EMDs driving the honeybees' VT neurons (Ibbotson, 2001), is able to measure the ventral OF (i.e., the angular speed ω at which any contrasting feature moves under the flying agent). From Franceschini, N., F. Ruffier, and J. Serres. 2007. A bio-inspired flying robot sheds light on insect piloting abilities. *Current Biology* 17: 329–335.

We know that flies and bees are able to react to the *translational OF*, ω independently of the spatial texture and contrast (David 1982; Kirchner and Srinivasan 1989; Srinivasan et al. 1991, 1993; Baird et al. 2005). We also know that some of their visual neurons may be involved in this reaction because they respond monotonically to ω with little dependence on texture and contrast (Ibbotson 2001; Shoemaker et al. 2005; Straw et al. 2008). Neurons facing downward can therefore act as ventral OF sensors, and thus assess the V_x / h ratio (Fig. 19.4).

Based on laboratory experiments on mosquitoes and field experiments on locusts, Kennedy put forward an hypothesis, according to which flying insects maintain a "preferred retinal velocity" with respect to the ground below (Kennedy 1939, 1951). In response to wind, for example, insects may adjust their ground speed or ground height to restore the apparent velocity of the ground features. Kennedy's hypothesis has been repeatedly confirmed during the last 30 years: both flies and bees were found to maintain a constant OF with respect to the ground while cruising or landing (David 1978; Preiss 1992; Srinivasan et al. 1996, 2000; Baird et al. 2006).

The problem is *how* insects may achieve this feat, since maintaining a given OF is a kind of chicken-and-egg problem, as illustrated by Equation 1: An insect may hold its ventral OF, ω constant by adjusting either its ground speed (if it knows its ground height) or its ground height (if it knows its ground speed). In addition, the insect could maintain an OF of 1 rad/s (i.e., 57 degrees/s), for instance, by flying at a speed of 1 m/s at a height of 1 meter or by flying at a speed of 2 m/s at a height of 2m: An infinitely large number of possible combinations of ground speed and ground height will give rise to the same "preferred OF."

Drawing on the experience we had with OF-based visual navigation of a terrestrial robot (Pichon et al. 1989; Franceschini et al. 1992), we attempted early to develop an explicit flight-control scheme for aerial navigation in the vertical plane. Our first tentative step on these lines was not particularly successful, because we were cornered in the general notion that prevailed in those days that insect navigation relies on *gauging range* (Kirchner and Srinivasan 1989; Srinivasan et al. 1991; Franceschini et al. 1992; Srinivasan 1993). In the experimental simulations we performed in 1994, for example (Mura and Franceschini 1994), we assumed that the insect (or the robot) would know its ground speed V_x (by whatever means), so that by measuring ω it would be able to gauge the distance h from the ground (Eq. 1) and react accordingly to avoid it. Although this procedure is still used in robotics (see, e.g., Barber et al. 2005; Srinivasan et al. 2006; Garratt and Chahl 2008), where ground speed can be determined (e.g., via GPS), this makes the way insects operate all the more elusive.

In 1999, we established (in simulation) how a rotorcraft (or an insect) might be able follow a terrain (Fig. 19.5A) and land (Fig. 19.5B) on the sole basis of OF cues, *without measuring its ground speed and ground height* (Netter and Franceschini 1999).

The landing manoeuvre was achieved under permanent visual feedback from a 20-pixel forward-looking eye driving 19 EMDs. The progressive loss in altitude was *caused* by the decrease in the horizontal flight speed that occurred when the rotorcraft (or the insect) decreased its speed to land, either voluntarily or in the presence of a headwind. The landing trajectory obtained in this simulation (Fig. 19.5B) already resembles the final approach of bees landing on a smooth surface (Srinivasan et al. 1996). The principle was first validated onboard FANIA, a miniature tethered helicopter having a single (variable-pitch) rotor, an accelerometer, and a forward-looking eye with 20 pixels (and, therefore, 19 EMDs) arranged in the frontal meridian (Netter and Franceschini 2002). This 0.8 kg rotorcraft had three degrees of freedom (surge, heave, and pitch). Mounted at the tip of a flight mill, the robot lifted itself by increasing its rotor collective pitch. Upon remotely inclining the servo-vane located in the propeller wake, the operator made the helicopter pitch forward by a few degrees so that it gained speed and, therefore, climbed to maintain a reference OF with respect to the terrain below. FANIA was able to jump over a rising terrain by increasing its collective pitch as a function of the fused signals from its 19 EMDs (Fig. 19.5C).

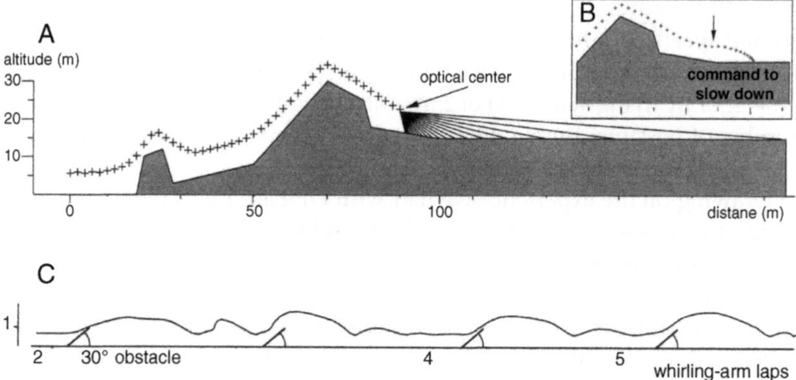

Figure 19.5 Optic flow-based terrain following and landing of a miniature helicopter whose eye (20 pixels, 19 EMDs) covers a frontal FOV of 75 degrees in the vertical plane, centered at 40 degrees below the horizon. **A**: Simulation of nap-of-the-earth flight (initial conditions: height: 5m, speed 2m.s $^{-1}$; iteration step 1s). **B**: Landing initiated by simply decreasing the rotorcraft horizontal speed at every iteration while retaining the same request to maintain a reference OF value (Netter and Franceschini, 1999). **C**: Actual flight path of the tethered FANIA rotorcraft, which repeatedly jumped over a 30-degree rising terrain (Netter and Franceschini, 2002). From Netter, T., and N. Franceschini. 1999. Neuromorphic optical flow sensing for nap-of-the-Earth flight. In *Mobile Robots XIV*, eds., D. Gage and H. Choset, 208–16. Bellingham, U.S.A.: SPIE, Vol. 3838; and Netter, T., and N. Franceschini. 2002. A robotic aircraft that follows terrain using a neuromorphic eye. In *Proceedings of the IEEE International Conference on Intelligent Robots and Systems* (IROS) Lausanne, Switzerland, pp. 129–34, with permission of the publishers.

THE OPTIC FLOW REGULATION PRINCIPLE

In spite of this early success to explain how an insect could navigate on an OF basis, we considered that Kennedy's insightful hypothesis was calling for a clear formalization that would bring to light:

- The flight variables really involved
- The sensors really required
- The dynamics of the various system components
- The causal and dynamic links existing between the sensory output(s) and the variable(s) to be controlled
- The point of application of the various disturbances that an insect will experience in flight and the variables it will have to control to compensate for these disturbances

We came up with an autopilot called OCTAVE (Optical altitude Control sysTem for Autonomous VEhicles) that is little demanding in terms of neural (or electronic) implementation and could be just as appropriate for insects as it would be for aircraft (Ruffier and Franceschini 2003). A ventral

OF sensor was integrated into a feedback loop that would drive the robot's lift, and thus the ground height, so as to compensate for any deviations of the OF sensor's output from a given set point (Ruffier and Franceschini 2003, 2004a,b, 2005; Franceschini et al. 2007). As we will see, this simple autopilot (Fig. 19.6A) enabled a micro-helicopter to perform challenging tasks such as take-off, terrain following, reacting suitably to wind, and landing.

The OCTAVE autopilot can be said to be an *OF regulator*. The word "regulator" is used here as in control theory to denote a *feedback control system* designed to maintain an output signal constantly equal to a given set point. The Watt flyball governor from the 18th century, for instance, was not only one of the first servomechanisms ever built: it was also the very first angular speed regulator. It served to maintain the rotational speed of a steam engine shaft at a given set point, whatever interferences occurred as the result of unpredictable load disturbances. The Watt regulator was based on a rotational speed sensor (meshed to the output shaft), whereas the OF regulator is based on a noncontact rotational speed sensor—an *OF sensor*—that measures the ventral OF (again in rad/s).

Specifically, the OF signal ω_{meas} delivered by the OF sensor (see Fig. 19.6A) is compared with the OF set point, ω_{set}. The comparator produces an error signal: $\varepsilon = \omega_{meas} - \omega_{set}$ which drives a controller adjusting the lift L, and thus the ground height h, so as to minimize ε. All the operator does is set the pitch angle Θ and therefore the airspeed (see Figure 19.6A): The OF regulator does the rest; that is, it attempts to keep ω constant by adjusting the ground height h proportionally to the current ground speed V_x. In the

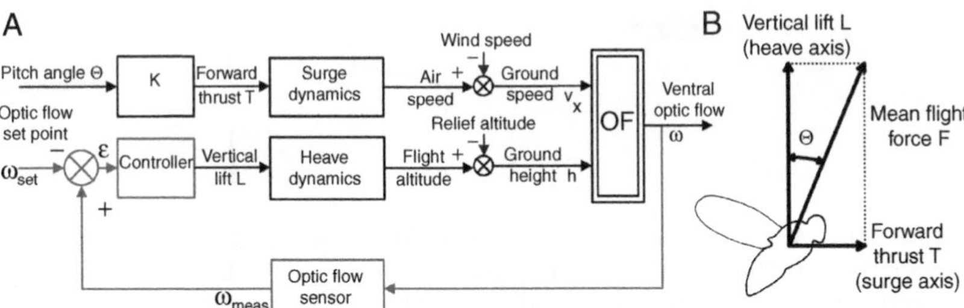

Figure 19.6 A: The OCTAVE optic flow regulator (bottom feedback loop) controls the mean flight force vector and hence the lift, and hence the ground height, so as to maintain the ventral optic flow ω constant and equal to the set-point ω_{set}. **B**: Flies, like helicopters, pitch forward slightly to increase their forward thrust, and hence their airspeed. As long as they pitch forward by $\Theta<10°$, the lift component L does not incur any major loss. From Franceschini, N., F. Ruffier, and J. Serres. 2007. A bio-inspired flying robot sheds light on insect piloting abilities. *Current Biology* 17: 329–35, with permission of the publisher.

steady state ($t = \infty$), $\omega_{meas} \cong \omega_{set}$, and the ground height becomes proportional to the ground speed.

$$h = KV_x(\text{with } K = 1/\omega_{SET} = constant) \qquad \text{(Eq. 2)}$$

The controller includes proportional and derivative (PD) functions, which ensure closed-loop stability in the ground speed range of 0–3m.s^{-1}. Controlling F (via the rotor speed) actually affects not only L but also T. This coupling is negligible, however, because Θ is always ≤10 degrees for the highest speed attained (3m.s^{-1}), so that the ensuing change in L is at least six times (cotan 10°) greater than the change in T.

A MICRO-HELICOPTER EQUIPPED WITH AN OF SENSOR AND AN OF REGULATOR

We tested the idea that insects may be equipped with a similar OF regulator by comparing the behavior of insects with that of a "seeing helicopter" placed in similar situations. The robot we built (Fig. 19.7A) is a micro-helicopter (MH) equipped with a simple, two-pixel ventral eye driving an EMD acting as an OF sensor (Fig. 19.7A). The 100-gram robot is tethered to an instrumented flight mill consisting of a light pantographic arm driven in

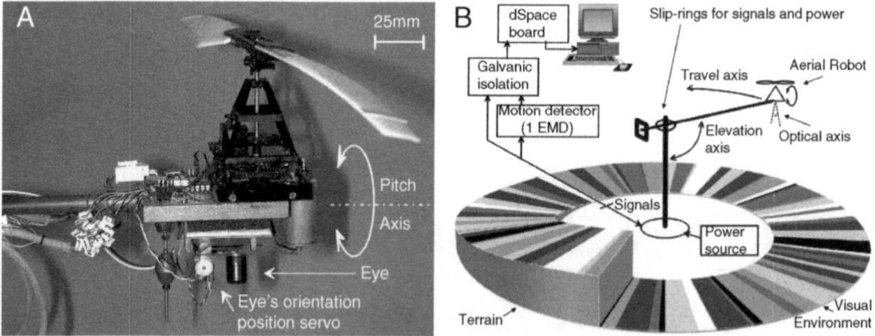

Figure 19.7 **A**: 100-gram micro-helicopter (MH) equipped with a ventral OF sensor (Figure 19.3E) and the OF regulator shown in A. **B**: The MH can be remotely pitched forward by a small angle Θ while keeping its roll attitude. It lifts itself and circles counterclockwise at speeds up to 3m/s and heights up to 3 m over a large arena (outside diameter: 4.5 m), giving rise to the flight patterns given in Figures 19.8 and 19.9 The flight mill is equipped with ground-truth azimuthal and elevation sensors with which the position and speed of the MH can be monitored accurately in real time. From Ruffier, F., and N. Franceschini. 2003. OCTAVE, a bioinspired visuo-motor control system for the guidance of Micro-Air Vehicles. In *Bioengineered and bioinspired systems*, ed., A. Rodriguez-Vazquez, et al., 1–12. Bellingham, U.S.A: SPIE, Vol. 5119, with permission of the publisher.

terms of its elevation and azimuth by the MH's lift and forward thrust, respectively (Fig.19.7B).

Any increase in the rotor speed causes the MH to rise, and the slightest (operator-mediated) forward ("nose-down") tilting by a few degrees produces a forward thrust component that causes the MH to gain forward speed. The flight mill is equipped with ground-truth azimuthal and elevation sensors that allow the position and speed of the MH to be monitored at high accuracy and in real time. Since the MH's purpose was to demonstrate a basic principle, it was equipped with an elementary ventral eye composed of only two photoreceptors driving a single EMD built according to the principle shown in Fig. 19.3A (Ruffier and Franceschini 2003; Ruffier et al. 2003).

MICRO-HELICOPTER'S VERSUS INSECTS' BEHAVIORAL PATTERNS

OCTAVE's OF regulator scheme results in the behavioral patterns shown in Figure 19.8. Between arrowheads 1 and 2, the operator simply pitched the MH forward rampwise by an angle $\Delta\Theta = +10°$. The ensuing increase in ground speed V_x (up to 3m.s^{-1}, see Fig. 19.8B) automatically made the MH take off, since the feedback loop consistently increased h proportionally to V_x to comply with Equation 2.

Once reaching a constant speed, the MH flew level at a ground height of approximately 1 m, the value imposed by the OF set point ω_{set} = 3 rad.s^{-1} = 172°.s^{-1} (Fig. 19.8C). After covering 42 m, the MH was pitched backward rampwise by an opposite angle $\Delta\Theta = -10°$ (between arrowheads 3 and 4), and the ensuing deceleration (see Fig. 19.8B) effectively produced an automatic descent and landing—a safe landing maneuver, since it is performed "under visual control." The actual OF (Fig. 19.8D) is seen to have been held relatively—but not perfectly—constant throughout the journey, even during the take-off and landing maneuvers, where the ground speed can be seen to vary considerably (Fig. 19.8B).

Figure 19.9 shows that the various robot's flight patterns are extremely robust and reproducible, including those over a rising terrain and in the presence of wind.

The OF regulator concept was found to account for a series of puzzling, seemingly unconnected flying abilities observed in various insect species, as summarized below (details in Franceschini et al. 2007):

- *Automatic terrain following*. A gradual increase in relief constitutes a "disturbance" that impinges on the system at a particular point (see Fig. 19.6A). The closed feedback loop overcomes this disturbance by increasing the flight altitude, resulting in a constant ground height over the rising terrain (Fig. 19.9B). This may account for the well-documented terrain- and canopy-following abilities of migrating insects (e.g., Srygley and Oliveira 2001).

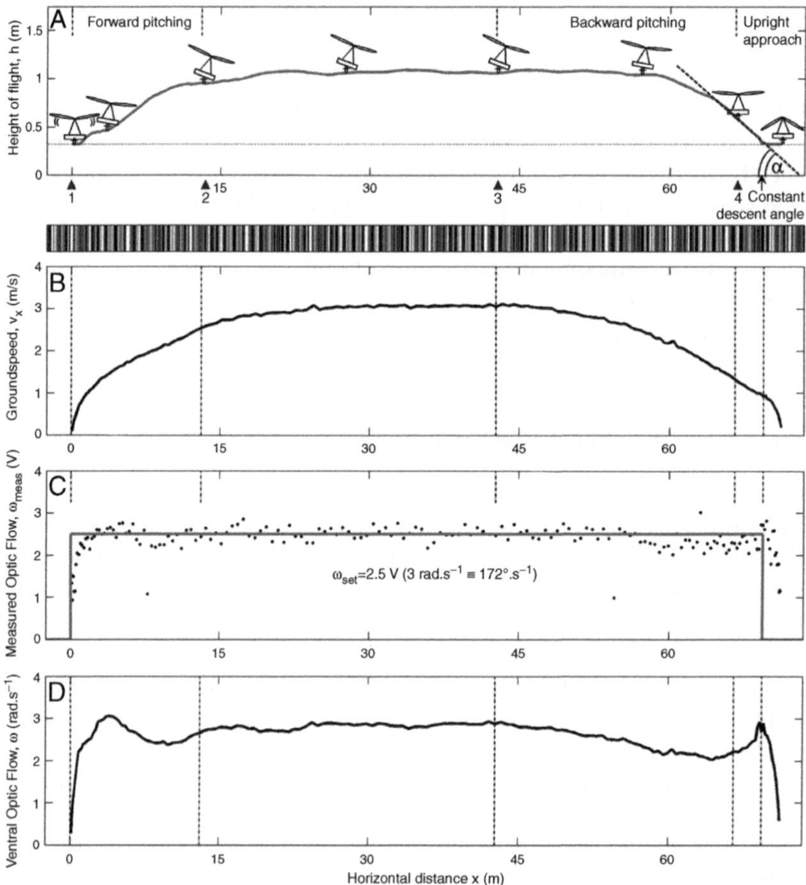

Figure 19.8 Flight variables monitored during a 70-meter flight of the micro-helicopter over a flat, randomly textured pattern (shown at the bottom of A), including take-off, level flight, and landing at a constant descent angle. **A**: Flight path consisting of about six laps on the circular test arena. **B**: Groundspeed V_x. **C**: Output ω_{meas} of the OF sensor. **D**: Actual OF, ω (calculated as V_x / h) resulting from the behavioral reaction. From Franceschini, N., F. Ruffier, and J. Serres. 2007. A bio-inspired flying robot sheds light on insect piloting abilities. *Current Biology* 17: 329–35, with permission of the publisher.

- *Suitable reactions to headwind.* Wind speed is a disturbance that impinges on the system at a different point (see Fig. 19.6A) and reduces the ground speed. The feedback loop overcomes this disturbance by forcing the robot to descend (and even to land smoothly by strong wind) (Fig. 19.9D). A similar reaction was observed in locusts, honeybees and dung beetles.

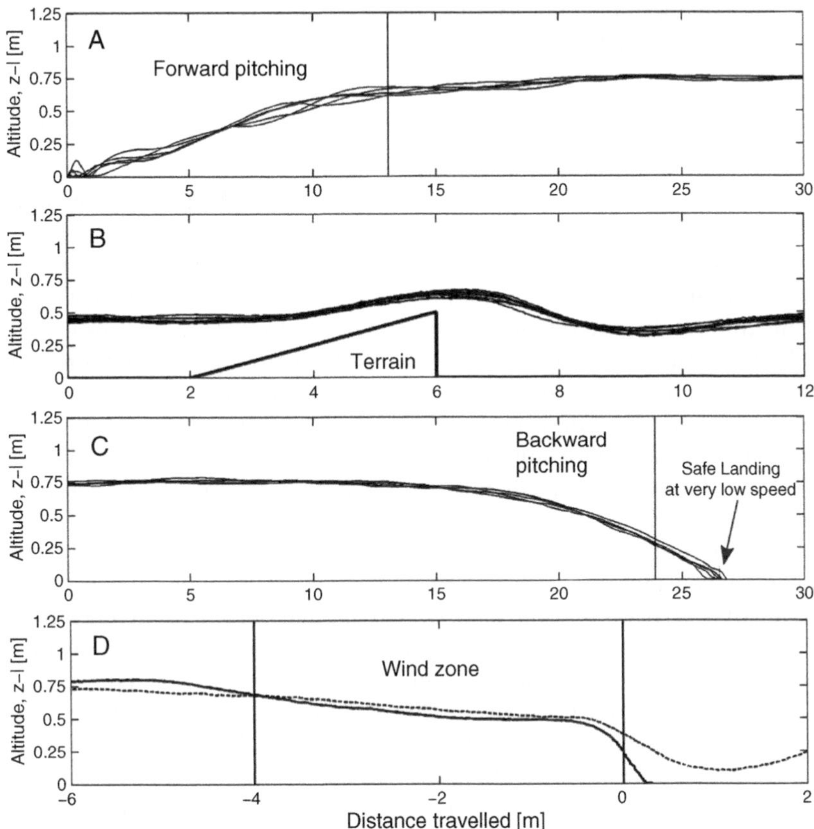

Figure 19.9 Performance and reproducibility of the micro-helicopter's flight path in the longitudinal plane. **A**: Automatic take-off obtained by gradually pitching the rotorcraft forward (nose-down) by 10 degrees from the vertical. **B**: Automatic terrain following over the rising terrain shown in Figure 19.7B. **C**: automatic approach and landing upon gradually raising the rotor axis vertically (nose-up). **D**: A light headwind made the rotorcraft descend (*dotted trajectory*). A strong headwind forced the MH to land (*continuous curve*) at negligible vertical and forward speeds. From (Ruffier and Franceschini, © 2004a IEEE).

- *Flying over a no-contrast zone.* Here the OF sensor fails to respond (see Figure 19.6A), which irremediably causes the robot to crash, just as honeybees crash into mirror-smooth water (Heran and Lindauer 1963).
- *Landing on a flat surface.* During the *final approach,* which starts when the MH has regained its completely upright position (arrowhead 4 in Fig. 19.8A and right vertical line in Fig. 19.9C), the OF

regulator forces the MH to land smoothly at a *constant descent angle*, α which can be calculated as follows:

$$\alpha = -\arctan\left(\frac{1}{\omega_{set}\tau}\right) \qquad \text{(Eq. 3)}$$

where ω_{set} [rad.s^{-1}] is the OF set-point, and τ [s] is the MH's *surge time constant* (τ_{MH} = 2.15s).

Interestingly, honeybees were also observed to land with a constant slope on flat surfaces, but how they may achieve this feat has been explained quite differently. According to Srinivasan et al. (2000), landing bees would follow two rules: "(a) adjusting the speed of forward flight to hold constant the angular velocity of the image of the surface as seen by the eye, and (b) making the speed of descent proportional to the forward speed." By contrast, the OF regulator automatically generates smooth landing with a constant slope while adjusting neither the forward speed nor the speed of descent.

The OF set-point ω_{set} is the reference signal that the feedback loop must maintain constant under all circumstances. ω_{set} would thus correspond to Kennedy's early ideas about a "preferred angular velocity of image movement" (Kennedy 1939, 1951). By increasing its ω_{set} (see Fig. 19.6A), the flier will follow the terrain at a lower height, as typically observed in the case of the MH (Ruffier and Franceschini 2003). Conversely, by setting ω_{set} near zero, the animal will rise farther from the ground, as also typically observed on the MH. This OF set point ω_{set} may well be under the control of other (e.g., visual or olfactory) sensors, but it may also depend on other external and/or internal factors such as a "drive for migration" (in the case of locusts: see Preiss 1992).

Taken together, these data show that an aerial vehicle equipped with an OF regulator will be able to take off, navigate over flat or rising terrain, react sensibly to headwind and land without ever measuring and holding any ground heights, ground speeds, or descent speeds. A similar principle was recently applied to a 0.4 kg flying wing, which, by flying at a constant cruise speed (imposed by an extra airspeed regulator) was able to maintain its altitude from its ventral OF measurement (Beyeler et al. 2009).

MICRO-HOVERCRAFT AGAINST HONEYBEES' BEHAVIORAL PATTERNS

Behavioral experiments on several insect species have long shown that motion perceived by the *lateral* part of their compound eyes affects the forward thrust, and hence the forward speed (for review, see Franceschini et al. 2007). First, when flying through a *tapered corridor*, honeybees slowed down as they approached the narrowest section and speeded up when the corridor widened beyond this point (Srinivasan et al. 1996). The authors concluded that bees tended to adjust their speed proportionally to the local corridor width by regulating the image velocity. Second, when flying through a *straight corridor*, honeybees tended to fly along the midline (Srinivasan et al. 1991). To explain this "centering behavior," the authors hypothesized that bees were balancing the speeds of the retinal images (i.e., the lateral OFs) of the two walls, a hypothesis that subsequently gave rise to many wheeled and aerial robots capable of centering in a corridor (e.g., Coombs and Roberts 1993; Duchon and Warren 1994 Santos-Victor et al. 1995).

We recently found, however, that honeybees trained to fly along a *larger* corridor do not systematically center on the corridor midline (Fig. 19.10B,C). They keep remarkably close to one wall, even when part of the opposite wall is missing (Fig. 19.10D). Distance from that wall (D_R or D_L) and forward speed V_x were, on average, such that the speed-to-distance ratio (i.e., the lateral OF) was maintained practically constant, at about 230°/s in our 95 cm wide corridor (Serres et al. 2008a).

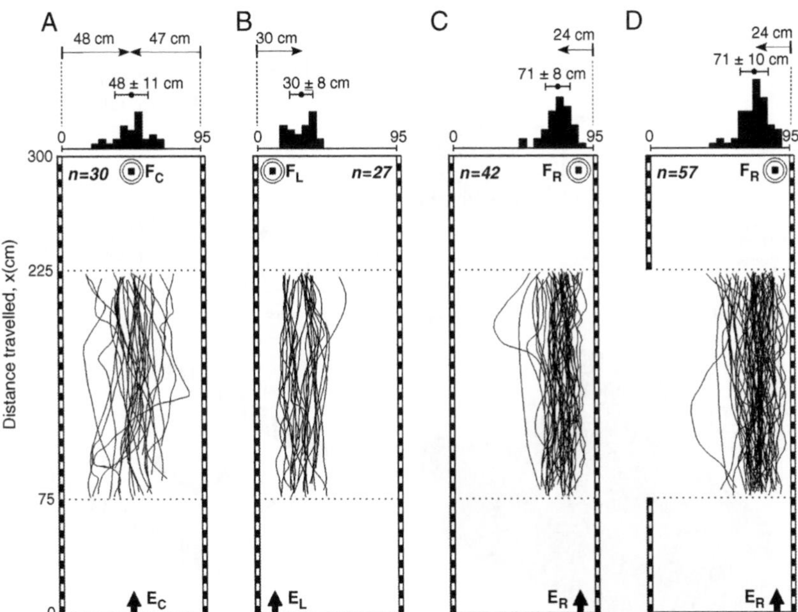

Figure 19.10 Honeybees' *centering* and *wall-following* behaviors. Bees were trained to enter a wide (width 0.95 m) 3-meter long corridor, formed by two 0.25-m high walls lined with vertical white-and-gray stripes (period 0.1 m; contrast m = 0.41). The bee's entrance (E_C) and the feeder (F_C) were placed either on the corridor midline (a) or on one side (b, c, d). In (d), part of the left wall was removed during the trials. Mean distances distribution as shown on top. From Serres, J., G. Masson, F. Ruffier, and N. Franceschini. 2008. A bee in the corridor: Centring and wall following. *Naturwissenschaften* 95: 1181–87, with permission of the publisher.

With a view to explaining the various honeybee behaviors observed in the various corridors, we came up with the design of the LORA III autopilot (LORA III stands for Lateral Optic flow Regulator Autopilot, mark III), which is able to control both the forward speed V_x of an aerial vehicle and its lateral distances D_R and D_L from the two corridor walls jointly, *without ever measuring any speeds or distances* (Fig. 19.11A) (Serres et al. 2008b). A micro-hovercraft (HO) was used, which can produce insect-like forward and sideward slips independently, because the two added lateral thrusters *LT1* and *LT2* (Fig. 19.11B,C) make it *fully actuated.* It travels at a constant altitude (~2 mm) and senses the environment with two laterally oriented eyes measuring the right and left OFs. The HO's heading is maintained along the X-axis of the corridor (Fig. 19.11C) by a heading lock system that

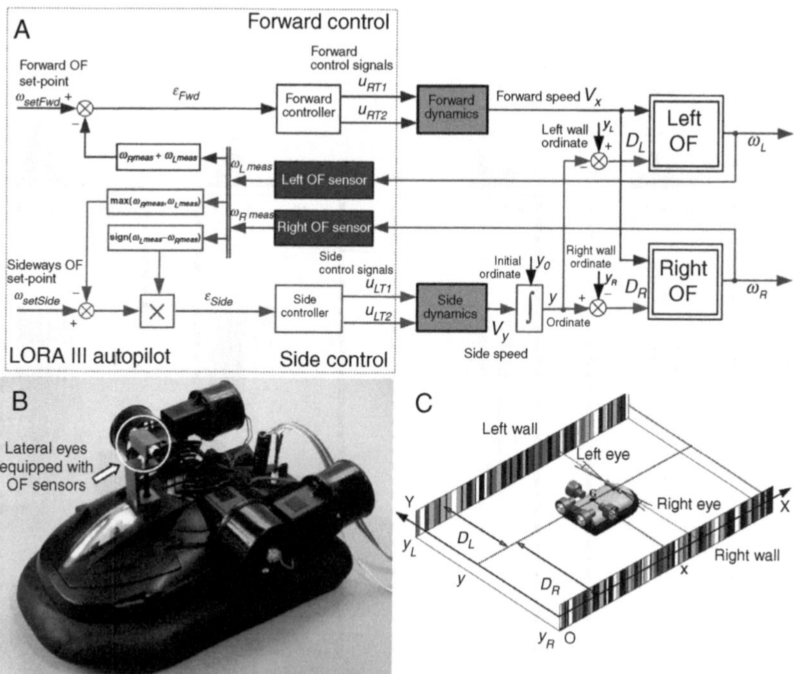

Figure 19.11 **A**: LORA III autopilot enabling a hovercraft to navigate in a corridor by controlling its forward speed and its distance to the walls *jointly, without measuring any speeds or distances.* **B,C**: *Fully actuated* hovercraft (HO) equipped with two OF sensors looking sidewards at an angle of +90/–90 degrees The corridor walls are randomly textured. From Serres, J., D. Dray, F. Ruffier, and N. Franceschini. 2008. A vision-based autopilot for a miniature air vehicle: Joint speed control and lateral obstacle avoidance. *Autonomous Robots* 25: 103–22, with permission of the publisher.

compensates for any yaw disturbances by controlling the two rear thrusters differentially. This system mimics the honeybee's heading lock system, which is based on a polarized light compass (Rossel and Wehner 1984) and gives the insect an impressively straight course, even in the presence of wind (Riley and Osborne 2001).

The LORA III autopilot is based on only two OF sensors (one looking to the right, one to the left). The forward speed V_x is controlled (via a proportional-integral controller) by the error signal ε_{Fwd} between the *sum* of the two OFs (right and left) and the forward OF set-point ω_{setFwd}. The side slip speed V_y, and hence the lateral distances D_L and D_R to the walls, is controlled (via a proportional derivative controller) by the error signal ε_{Side} between the *larger* of the two OFs and the sideways OF set-point $\omega_{setSide}$. The HO's behavior is entirely determined by these two OF set points: $\omega_{setFwd} = 300°/s$ and $\omega_{setSide} = 230°/s$.

Simulation experiments in which the HO navigated in a straight or tapered corridor accounted for all the honeybee behaviors reported earlier (Serres et al. 2008b). Figure 19.12 illustrates, for example, the HO's behavior in a tapered corridor. Whatever the position of its initial ordinate y_0, the HO automatically decelerated on approaching the narrowest section of the corridor and accelerated when the corridor widened (Fig. 19.12B). It can be seen that the *forward control system* succeeded in keeping the sum of the two lateral OFs measured nearly constant and equal to the forward OF set-point $\omega_{setFwd} = 300°/s$ (Fig. 19.12C). Likewise, the *side control system* succeeded in keeping the *larger* of the two lateral OFs measured practically constant and equal to the sideways OF set-point $\omega_{setSide} = 230°/s$ (Fig.19.12E). The result is that the HO automatically tuned both its ground speed and its distance to the walls jointly, without any knowledge about the current corridor width, the ground speed, or the clearance from the walls.

The field of view (FOV) of the eyes and the provocatively small numbers of pixels (four) and EMDs (two) will obviously need to be increased for dealing with navigation in more sparsely textured environments. It will also be necessary to control the heading direction (e.g., Zufferey 2008) to enable the HO to successfully negotiate more challenging corridors, including L-junctions and T-junctions (cf. Humbert and Hyslop 2010).

CONCLUSION

In studying the types of operations that insects may perform to guide their flight on the basis of optic flow (OF) cues, we came up with several bio-inspired autopilot principles that harness the power of the *translatory OF* parsimoniously and therefore offer interesting prospects for MAV autonomous guidance. The micro-helicopter's outstanding visuomotor performance (Figs. 19.8 and 19.9) suggests how insects and MAVs may take off, follow terrain, and land if they are equipped with OF sensors facing the ground and an OF regulator that servos the measured OF to a

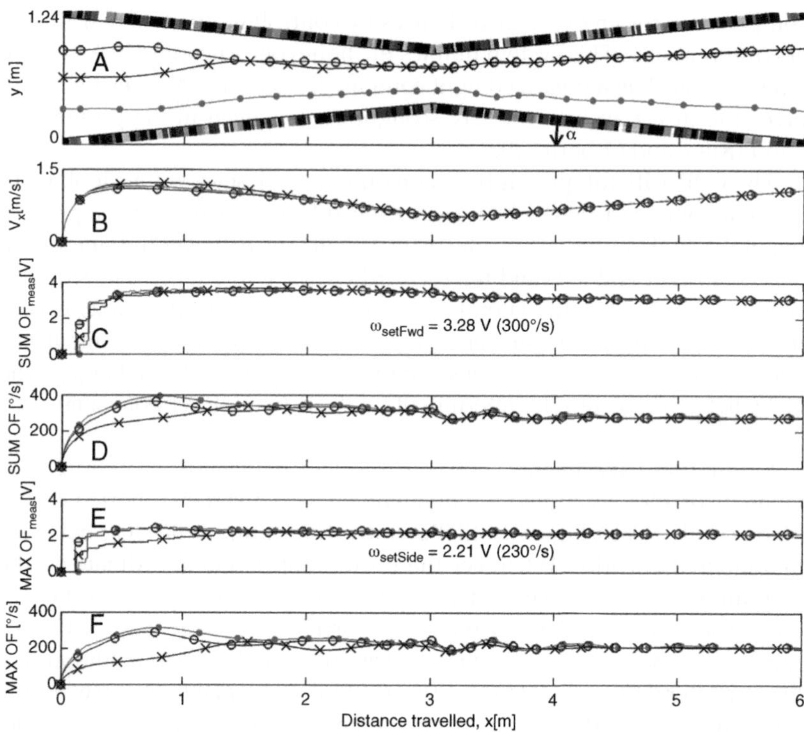

Figure 19.12 Simulated navigation of the hovercraft (HO) along a tapered corridor, requiring no data on the corridor width, tapering angle α, nor any measurements of groundspeed and distance to the walls. **A**: Simulated trajectories of the HO moving to the right along the corridor (tapering angle α = 7°) with three initial ordinates y_0 (*open dots*: y_0 = 0.90 m; *crosses*: y_0 = 0.60 m; *full dots*: y_0 = 0.30 m). **B**: Forward speed profile. **C,D**: Sum and maximum of the two lateral OFs *measured*, respectively. **E,F**: Sum and maximum of the two *actual* OFs, respectively. From Serres, J., D. Dray, F. Ruffier, and N. Franceschini. 2008. A vision-based autopilot for a miniature air vehicle: Joint speed control and lateral obstacle avoidance. *Autonomous Robots* 25: 103–22, with permission of the publisher.

given set-point (Fig. 19.6). The great advantage of this autopilot is that it requires neither to measure nor to compute nor to regulate (i.e., hold constant) any ground speeds or ground heights. The only variable it needs to measure and regulate is the OF—a variable that can be accessed straightforwardly by dedicated sensors called OF sensors (Fig. 19.3). The recent finding that bees gradually descend when they fly in a corridor the floor of which is moved in the same direction as their flight, is fully consistent with the OCTAVE autopilot model (Portelli et al. 2010a). The OCTAVE principle differs markedly from another OF-based navigation strategy that requires measuring not only the ventral OF, ω but also the ground speed V_x (e.g., from GPS), with an aim to estimate the ground height (see Eq. 1) (Barber et al. 2005; Srinivasan et al. 2006; Garratt and Chahl 2008).

OCTAVE and LORA III autopilots consist of *interdependent OF regulators*, which control the lift, lateral thrust, and forward thrust, on which the ground height, lateral position, and ground speed, respectively, depend. The block diagrams (Figs. 19.6A and 19.10A) show which variables need to be measured, which are controlled, and which are regulated, as well as the point of application of the various disturbances.

In contrast with the control schemes presented by Conroy et al. (2009) for a quadrotor navigating a straight corridor, OCTAVE's task is not to hold a "desired height" and LORA III's task is not to hold a "desired forward speed" and a "desired lateral position" in the corridor. Before entering the corridor, our hovercraft does not know how fast it will eventually fly and whether or not it will center or rather follow one wall: it is the environment itself that constrains both its speed and its distance to the walls, depending on the OF set-points (Fig. 19.12). These explicit control schemes account for a series of flying abilities observed in numerous insect species, including honeybees' habit of landing at a constant slope and their flight pattern along a straight or tapered corridor. Our recent finding that bees do not center systematically in a corridor but may follow a wall unilaterally (Fig. 19.10D) cannot be accounted for by the optic flow balance hypothesis (Srinivasan et al. 1991) but is convincingly accounted for by the LORA III model, in which centering behavior arises as a particular case of wall-following behavior (Serres et al. 2008b). OCTAVE and LORA III interdependent OF regulators were recently combined in a comprehensive model, called ALIS (AutopiLot using an Insect-based vision System), which allows a simulated bee to travel safely along (horizontally or vertically) tapered tunnels, by automatically controlling both its speed and its clearance from the right wall, left wall, ground, and roof, without ever estimating any ground speeds or distances (Portelli et al. 2010b). The simulated bee navigates on the basis of two parameters alone: the forward OF set-point and the positioning OF set-point. Although it is conceivable that on board insects, the OF set-points may depend on either innate, internal or external factors, MAVs could receive their OF set-points from the control station via a radio link.

Once engineered further, the OF feedback control systems we have described here could serve to improve navigation aids and automatic maneuvers. When measured on a commercial aircraft, a ventral OF greater than the set-point would mean that the current altitude is "too low for the current ground speed" (Franceschini et al. 2003). Installed on board a MAV, the OCTAVE autopilot would enable it to automatically take off, fly level at a ground height proportional to the ground speed, follow shallow terrains, make it react automatically to unpredictable headwind or tailwind disturbances (by descending or climbing, respectively), and land safely

(Franceschini et al. 2003; Ruffier and Franceschini 2004a,b, 2005b). Both OCTAVE and LORA III could potentially guide MAVs indoors or through complex terrains such as mountain or urban canyons, without using any computationally intensive visuomotor algorithms. Since these autopilots do not rely on GPS and ILS, and do not require any bulky (and power-hungry) emissive sensors such as RADARs, SONARs, FLIRs, or laser rangefinders, they can be of very small size, lightweight, and power-lean, and therefore meet the challenge of future insect-scale MAVs. For the same reasons, these simple autopilots could potentially be adapted to micro- or nano-space vehicles (MSVs) landing on command on other celestial bodies or performing rendezvous and docking missions in space. A recent paper presented the first simulation experiment conducted in our laboratory, showing an OCTAVE-based descent to the Moon (Valette et al. 2010). Over the last 2.6 km, the lander actuated its thrusters as a function of its current pitch and braked from 1800 km/h down to only 15 km/h. This descent (from 500 m down to 10 m above the Moon surface) occurred steadily under visual control, thanks to the ventral OF sensor and the OF regulator, without using any altimeters or speedometers. Throughout descent, the lunar lander maintained an approximately constant OF of about 0.3 rad.s^{-1} (i.e., 17.2° s^{-1}).

An aerial Martian rover equipped with more elaborate OCTAVE and LORA III autopilots could take off autonomously and explore an area, skimming the ground and hugging the walls of a canyon, and adapting its ground speed and clearance from the walls automatically to the width of the canyon. With ground and obstacle avoidance at a premium, the rover could perform its mission successfully in uncharted environments, despite being unaware of its own ground speed and altitude at all times (Franceschini 2009). The orbiter (or the Earth-based control station) would simply be required to send the rover a set of low bandwidth signals: the values of the OF set-points.

ACKNOWLEDGMENTS

We are grateful to S. Viollet, F. Aubépart, G.P., Masson, D. Dray, L. Kerhuel, and G. Portelli for their help and fruitful suggestions during this research. We are also thankful to M. Boyron, and F. Paganucci for their expert technical assistance, and J. Blanc for revising the English manuscript. The work presented here was supported by CNRS (Life Science and Engineering Science), EU contracts (IST/FET 1999-29043 and IST/FET 2009-237940), DGA contracts (05-34022 and 0451037), and an ESA contract (08-6303b).

REFERENCES

Aubépart, F., and N. Franceschini. 2007. Bio-inspired optic flow sensors based on FPGA: Application to micro-air vehicles. *Journal Microprocessors and Microsystems* 31:408–19.

Aubépart, F., M. El Farji, and N. Franceschini. 2004. FPGA implementation of elementary motion detectors for the visual guidance of micro-air vehicles. *Proceedings of IEEE International Symposium on Industrial Electronics (ISIE'2004)*, Ajaccio, France, 71–76.

Baird, E., M.V. Srinivasan, S.W. Zhang, and A. Cowling. 2005. Visual control of flight speed in honeybees. *Journal of Experimental Biology* 208:3895–905.

Baird, E., M.V. Srinivasan, S.W. Zhang, R. Lamont, A. Cowling. 2006. Visual control of flight speed and height in the honeybee. In S. Nolfi et al. (eds.), *From Animals to Animats* 9, 4095, 40–51.

Barber, D.B., S.R. Griffiths, T.W. McLain, and R.W. Beard. 2005. Autonomous landing of miniature aerial vehicles. *Proceedings of American Institute of Aeronautics and Astronautics Conference.*

Beyeler, A., J.C. Zufferey, and D. Floreano. 2009. Vision-based control of near-obstacle flight. *Autonomous Robots* 27:201–19.

Blanès, C. 1986. Appareil visuel élémentaire pour la navigation à vue d'un robot mobile autonome. *MS thesis in Neuroscience*, University of Aix-Marseille II, Marseille, France.

Borst, A., and J. Haag. 2002. Neural networks in the cockpit of the fly. *Journal of Comparative Physiology A* 188:419–37.

Braitenberg, V. 1967. Patterns of projection in the visual system of the fly, I/Retina-Lamina projections. *Experimental Brain Research* 3:271–98.

Buchner, E. 1984. Behavioral analysis of spatial vision in insects. In *Photoreception and Vision in Invertebrates*, ed., M Ali, 561–621. New York: Plenum.

Card, G., and M. Dickinson. 2008. Visually mediated motor planning in the escape response of drosophila. *Current Biology* 18:1300–07.

Conroy, J., G. Grémillon, B. Ranganathan, and J.S. Humbert. 2009. Implementation of wide-field integration of optic flow for autonomous quadrotor navigation. *Autonomous Robots* 27:189–98.

Coombs, D., and K. Roberts. 1993. Centering behavior using peripheral vision. *Proceedings IEEE Conference on Computer Vision and Pattern Recognition New York.*

David, C. 1978. The relationship between body angle and flight speed in free-flying Drosophila. *Physiological Entomology* 3:191–95.

David, C. 1982. Compensation for height in the control of groundspeed by *Drosophila* in a new 'barber's pole' wind tunnel. *Journal of Comparative Physiology* A147: 485–493.

Duchon, A.P., and W.H. Warren. 1994. Robot navigation from a Gibsonian viewpoint. *Proceedings IEEE International Conference on Systems Man and Cybernetics* (SMC), Piscataway, USA, 2272–2277.

Egelhaaf, M., A. Borst. 1993. Movement detection in arthropods. In *Visual motion an its role in the stabilization of gaze* eds., F. Miles and J. Wallman, 53–77. Amsterdam: Elsevier.

Franceschini, N. 1975. Sampling of the visual environment by the compound eye of the fly: Fundamentals and applications. In *Photoreceptor optics*, eds., A. Snyder and R. Menzel, 98–125. Berlin: Springer.

Franceschini, N. 1984. Chromatic organisation and sexual dimorphism of the fly retinal mosaic. In *Photoreceptors*, eds., A. Borsellino and L. Cervetto, 319–350. New-York: Plenum Press.

Franceschini, N. 1985. Early processing of colour and motion in a mosaic visual system. *Neuroscience Research* (Suppl 2):517–49.

Franceschini, N. 1992. Sequence-discriminating neural network in the eye of the fly. In *Analysis and modeling of neural systems*, ed., F.H.K. Eeckman, 142–150. Norwell: Kluwer Academy Publications.

Franceschini, N. 2007. Sa majesté des mouches. In *Voir l'Invisible,* eds., J.P. Gex and E. Fox-Keller, 28–29. Paris: Omniscience.

Franceschini, N. 2009. Towards automatic visual guidance of aerospace vehicles: From insects to robots. *Acta Futura* 3:15–34.

Franceschini, N., C. Blanès, and L. Oufar. 1986. Passive, noncontact optical velocity sensor *Technical Report ANVAR/DVAR,* No. 51549, Paris (in French).

Franceschini, N., J.M. Pichon, and C. Blanès. 1992. From insect vision to robot vision. *Philosophical Transactions of the Royal Society London B* 337:283–94.

Franceschini, N., K. Kirschfeld, and B. Minke. 1981a. Fluorescence of photoreceptor cells observed *in vivo. Science* 213:1264–67.

Franceschini, N., R.C. Hardie, W. Ribi, and K. Kirschfeld. 1981b. Sexual dimorphism in a photoreceptor. *Nature* 291:241–44.

Franceschini, N., A. Riehle, A. Le Nestour. 1989. Directionally selective motion detection by insect neurons. In *Facets of vision,* eds., D.G. Stavenga and R.C. Hardie, 360–90. Berlin: Springer.

Franceschini, N., F. Ruffier, and J. Serres. 2007. A bio-inspired flying robot sheds light on insect piloting abilities. *Current Biology* 17:329–35.

Franceschini, N., F. Ruffier, S. Viollet, and M. Boyron. 2003. Steering aid system for altitude and horizontal speed, perpendicular to the vertical, of an aircraft, and aircraft equipped therewith. *International Patent* PCT/FR2003/002611.

Frye, M., and M. Dickinson. 2001. Fly flight: A model for the neural control of complex behavior. *Neuron* 32:385–88.

Garratt, M.A., and J.S. Chahl. 2008. Vision-based terrain following for an unmanned rotorcraft. *Journal of Field Robotics* 25:284–301.

Gibson, J.J. 1950. *The perception of the visual world.* Boston: Houghton Mifflin.

Gibson, J.J., P. Olum, and F. Rosenblatt. 1955. Parallax and perspective during aircraft landings. *American Journal of Psychology* 68:372–95.

Giurfa, M. 2003. The amazing mini-brain: Lessons from a honeybee. *Beeworld* 84:5–18.

Giurfa, M., and R. Menzel. 1997. Insect visual perception: Complex ability of simple nervous systems. *Current Opinion in Neurobiology* 7:505–13.

Hardie, R.C. 1985. Functional organization of the fly retina. In *Progress in sensory physiology* 5 ed., D. Ottosson, 2–79. Berlin: Springer.

Hassenstein, B., and W. Reichardt. 1956. Systemtheoretische Analyse der Zeitreihenfolgen und Vorzeichenauswertung bei der Bewegungsperzeption des Rüsselkäfers Chlorophanus. *Zeitschrift für Naturforschung* 11b:513–24.

Hausen, K. 1993. Decoding of retinal image flow in insects. In *Visual motion and its role in the stabilization of gaze,* eds., F.A. Miles and J. Wallman, 203–35. Amsterdam: Elsevier.

Hausen, K., M. Egelhaaf. 1989. Neural mechanisms of course control in insects. In *Facets of vision* eds., D.G. Stavenga and R.C. Hardie, 391–424. Berlin: Springer.

Heran, P., and M. Lindauer. 1963. Windkompensation und Seitenwindkorrektur der Bienen Flug über Wasser. *Zeitschrift für vergleichende Physiologie* 47:39–55.

Heisenberg, M., R. Wolf. 1984. *Vision in Drosophila.* Berlin: Springer.

Humbert, J.S., and A.M. Hyslop. 2010. Bioinspired visuomotor convergence. *IEEE Transactions on Robotics* 26:121–30.

Ibbotson, M.R. 2001. Evidence for velocity-tuned motion-sensitive descending neurons in the honeybee. *Proceedings of the Royal Society London B* 268:2195–201.

Kennedy, J.S. 1939. Visual responses of flying mosquitoes. *Proceedings of the Zoogical Society of London* 109:221–42.

Kennedy, J.S. 1951. The migration of the desert locust (Schistocerca gregaria Forsk.) I. The behaviour of swarms. *Philosophical transactions of the Royal Society of London. Series B* 235:163–290.

Kirchner, W.H., and M.V. Srinivasan. 1989. Freely moving honeybees use image motion to estimate distance. *Naturwissenchaften* 76:281–82.

Kirschfeld, K. 1967. Die Projektion der optischen Umwelt auf das Raster der Rhabdomere im Komplexauge von Musca. *Experimental Brain Research* 3:248–70.

Kirschfeld, K., and N. Franceschini. 1968. Optische Eigenschaften der Ommatidien im Komplexauge von Musca. *Kybernetik* 5:47–52.

Kirschfeld, K., N. Franceschini, and B. Minke. 1977. Evidence for a sensitizing pigment in fly photoreceptors. *Nature* 269:386–90.

Koenderink, J.J. 1986. Optic flow. *Vision Research* 26:161–79.

Kramer, J., R. Sarpeshkar, and C. Koch. 1995. An analog VLSI velocity sensor. *Proceedings of IEEE International Symposium on Circuits and Systems,* Seattle, USA, 413–16.

Krapp, H., B. Hengstenberg, and R. Hengstenberg. 1998. Dendritic structure and receptive-field organisation of optic flow processing interneurons in the fly. *Journal of Neurophysiology* 79:1902–17.

Laughlin, S. 1984. The role of parallel channels in early visual processing by the arthropod compound eye. In *Photoreception and vision in invertebrates* ed., M.A. Ali, 457–481. New York: Plenum.

Lee, D.N. 1980. The optic flow field: The foundation of vision. *Philosophical Transactions of the Royal Society London B* 290:169–79.

Moeckel, R., and S.C. Liu. 2007. Motion detection circuits for a time-to-travel algorithm. *Proceedings IEEE International Symposium Circuits and Systems* (ISCAS07): 3079–3082.

Mura, F., N. Franceschini. 1994. Visual control of altitude and speed in a flying agent. In *From Animals to Animats III,* ed., D. Cliff, 91–99. Cambridge: MIT Press.

Netter, T., N. Franceschini. 1999. Neuromorphic optical flow sensing for nap-of-the-Earth flight. In *Mobile Robots XIV,* eds., D.V. Gage and H.M. Choset, 208–216. Bellingham, U.S.A.: SPIE, Vol. 3838.

Netter, T., and N. Franceschini. 2002. A robotic aircraft that follows terrain using a neuromorphic eye. *Proceedings of the IEEE International Conference on Intelligent Robots and Systems* (IROS) Lausanne, Switzerland: 129–34.

Pichon, J.M., C. Blanès, N. Franceschini. 1989. Visual guidance of a mobile robot equipped with a network of self-motion sensors. In *Mobile Robots IV,* eds., W.J. Wolfe and W.H. Chun, 44–53. Bellingham, U.S.A: SPIE, Vol. 1195.

Portelli, G., J. Serres, F. Ruffier, and N. Franceschini. 2008. An insect-inspired visual autopilot for corridor-following. *Proceedings of the 2nd Biennial IEEE International Conference on Biomedical Robotics and Biomechatronics,* BioRob 08, Scottsdale, USA, 19–26.

Portelli, G., F. Ruffier, and N. Franceschini. 2010a. Honeybees change their height to restore their optic flow. *Journal of Comparative Physiology A* 196:307–313.

Portelli, G., J. Serres, F. Ruffier, and N. Franceschini. 2010b. Modelling honeybee visual guidance in a 3-D environment. *Journal de Physiologie* 104:27–39.

Preiss, R. 1992. Set point of retinal velocity of ground images in the control of swarming flight of desert locusts. *Journal Comparative Physiology A* 171:251–56.

Pudas, M., S. Viollet, F. Ruffier, A. Kruusing, S. Amic, S. Leppävuori, and N. Franceschini. 2007. A miniature bio-inspired optic flow sensor based on low temperature co-fired ceramics (LTCC) technology. *Sensors and Actuators A* 133:88–95.

Reichardt, W. 1969. Movement perception in insects. In *Processing of Optical Data by Organisms and by Machines,* ed., W. Reichardt, 465–93. New York: Academic Press.

Riehle, A., and N. Franceschini. 1984. Motion detection in flies: Parametric control over ON-OFF pathways. *Experimental Brain Research* 54:390–94.

Riley, J.R., J.L. Osborne. 2001. Flight trajectories of foraging insects: Observations using harmonic radar. In *Insect movement: Mechanisms and consequences*, eds., T.P. Woiwod, D.R. Reynolds and C.D. Thomas, 129–57. Wallingford, UK: CABI Publishing, CAB International.

Rossel, S., and R. Wehner. 1984. How bees analyze the polarization pattern in the sky. Experiments and model. *Journal of Comparative Physiology A* 154:607–15.

Ruffier, F., N. Franceschini. 2003. OCTAVE, a bioinspired visuo-motor control system for the guidance of micro-air vehicles. In *Bioengineered and Bioinspired Systems* ed., A. Rodriguez-Vazquez, 1–12. Bellingham, U.S.A: SPIE, Vol. 5119

Ruffier, F., and N. Franceschini. 2004a. Visually guided micro-aerial vehicle: Automatic take-off, terrain following, landing and wind reaction. *Proceedings IEEE International Conference on Robotics and Automation* (ICRA04), New Orleans: 2339–46.

Ruffier, F., and N. Franceschini. 2004b. Optic flow based AFCS for rotorcraft automatic maneuvring (terrain following, takeoff and landing). *Proceedings of the 30th European Rotorcraft Forum* AAF/CEAS, Marseille, 71.1–71.9.

Ruffier, F., and N. Franceschini. 2005. Optic flow regulation: The key to aircraft automatic guidance. *Robotics and Automomous Systems* 50:177–94.

Ruffier, F., S. Viollet, S. Amic, and N. Franceschini. 2003. Bio-inspired optical flow circuits for the visual guidance of micro-air vehicles. *Proceedings the IEEE International Symposium on Circuits and Systems* (ISCAS), Bangkok, Thaïland, Vol. III, 846–49.

Santos-Victor, J., G. Sandini, F. Curotto, and S. Garibaldi. 1995. Divergent stereo in autonomous navigation: From bees to robots. *International Journal of Computer Vision* 14:159–77.

Serres, J., G. Masson, F. Ruffier, and N. Franceschini. 2008a. A bee in the corridor: Centring and wall following. *Naturwissenschaften* 95:1181–87.

Serres, J., D. Dray, F. Ruffier, and N. Franceschini. 2008b. A vision-based autopilot for a miniature air vehicle: Joint speed control and lateral obstacle avoidance. *Autonomous Robots* 25:103–22.

Shoemaker, P.A., D.C. O'Caroll, and A.D. Straw. 2005. Velocity constancy and models for wide-field visual motion detection in insects. *Biological Cybernetics* 93:275–87.

Srinivasan, M.V. 1993. How insects infer range from visual motion. In *Visual motion and its role in the stabilization of gaze* eds., F.A. Miles and J. Wallman, 139–56. Amsterdam: Elsevier.

Srinivasan, M., S. Thurrowgood, and D. Soccol. 2006. An optical system for guidance of terrain following in UAVs. *Proceedings of the IEEE International Conference on Video and Signal Based Surveillance* AVSS06.

Srinivasan, M.V., M. Lehrer, W.H. Kirchner, and S.W. Zhang. 1991. Range perception through apparent image speed in freely flying honeybees. *Visual Neuroscience* 6:519–535.

Srinivasan, M.V., S.W. Zhang, and K. Chandrashekara. 1993. Evidence for two distinct movement-detecting mechanisms in insect vision. *Naturwissenchaften* 80:38–41.

Srinivasan, M.V., S.W. Zhang, M. Lehrer, and T. Collett. 1996. Honeybee navigation en route to the goal: Visual flight control and odometry. *Journal of Experimental Biology* 199: 237–44.

Srinivasan, M.V., S.W. Zhang, J.S. Chahl, E. Barth, and S. Venkatesh. 2000. How honeybees make grazing landings on flat surface. *Biological Cybernetics* 83:171–83.

Srygley, R.B., E.G. Oliveira. 2001. Orientation mechanisms and migration strategies within the flight boundary layer. In *Insect movements: Mechanisms and consequences*, eds., T.P. Woiwod, D.R. Reynolds and C.D. Thomas, 183–206. Wallingford, UK: CABI Publishing, CAB International.

Strausfeld, N.J. 1976. *Atlas of an insect brain*. Berlin: Springer.

Strausfeld N.J. and U.K. Bassemir. 1985. Lobula plate and ocellar interneurons converge onto a cluster of descending neurons leading to leg and neck motor neuropil in *Calliphora erythrocephala*. *Cell and Tissue Research* 240:617–640.

Straw, A.D., T. Rainsford, and D.C. O'Carroll. 2008. Contrast sensitivity of insect motion detectors to natural images. *Journal of Vision* 8:1–9.

Taylor, G.K., H.G. Krapp. 2008. Sensory systems and flight stability: What do insects measure and why? In *Advances in Insect Physiology 34: Insect mechanisms and control*, eds., J. Casas and S.J. Simpson, 231–316. Amsterdam: Elsevier.

Trujillo-Cenoz O. and J. Melamed. 1966. Compound eye of Dipterans: anatomical basis for integration, An electron microscopy study. *Journal of ultrastructure Research* 16:395–398.

Ullman, S. 1981. Analysis of visual motion by biological and computer systems. *Computer* 14:57–69.

Valette, F., F. Ruffier, S. Viollet, and T. Seidl. 2010. Biomimetic optic flow sensing applied to a lunar landing scenario. *Proceedings IEEE International Conference of Robotics and Automation*, Anchorage, USA, 2253–2260.

Webb, B. 2001. Can robots make good models of biological behavior? *Behavioral and Brain Sciences* 24:6.

Whiteside, T.C., and G.D. Samuel. 1970. Blur zone. *Nature* 225:94–95.

Zettler, F., R. Weiler. 1974. Neuronal processing in the first optic neuropile of the compound eye of the fly. In *Neural principles in vision*, eds., F. Zettler and R. Weiler, 226–37. Berlin: Springer.

Zufferey, J.C. 2008. *Bio-inspired flying robots*. Boca Raton, FL: EPFL Press/CRC Press.

20

Models and Architectures for Motor Control

Simple or Complex?

Emmanuel Guigon

Motor control is a fantastic challenge for the central nervous system. In fact, efficient motor coordination theoretically requires the mastering of the laws of Newtonian mechanics, and it is well known, from any textbook, that the equations of motion for systems with many degrees of freedom (DOFs), as it is the case for the human body, are nonlinear and complex (Bernstein 1967). Furthermore, ongoing actions can be unexpectedly disrupted by deterministic (e.g., obstacles) or stochastic (e.g., noise) perturbations. Yet, we know that humans are capable of highly skillful motor behaviors (e.g., dancing, riding a bicycle, etc.). From the point of view that the brain should face unconquerable difficulties and incredible computational burdens to faithfully represent the laws of movement, it is tempting to suggest that some "simplifying" strategies have been discovered (e.g., through phylogenetic processes) to alleviate the "cost" of motor control (Lee 1984; Macpherson 1991; Mussa-Ivaldi and Bizzi 2000; Latash et al. 2007). We have identified at least four (more or less formalized) approaches to motor control that concur with the idea of simplification. Following a thorough analysis and discussion, we conclude that the proposed strategies do not actually tackle the overall problem of motor coordination. Then, we present a principled approach that provides an overarching account to motor control.

The scope of this chapter is restricted to the case of discrete movements (as defined in Hogan and Sternad 2007). We consider, following recent theoretical and experimental works (e.g., Schaal et al. 2004, 2007; Huys et al. 2008), that discrete and rhythmic movements are subserved by distinct control mechanisms. Thus, conclusions drawn for one type of movement are likely to be irrelevant or even wrong for the other type.

MOTOR CONTROL: WHAT NEEDS TO BE SOLVED

We start with a brief description of some well-known problems in the framework of motor control.

Bernstein's Problem

Despite multiple levels of redundancy, noisy sensors and actuators, and the complexity of biomechanical elements to be controlled, the nervous system elaborates well-coordinated movements with disconcerting ease (Bernstein 1967). In fact, Bernstein (1967) observed that a motor goal can be successfully reached, even though each attempt to reach this goal has unique, nonrepetitive characteristics. To succeed in this daunting control task, powerful mechanisms should be at work in brain circuits. Their properties should encompass the capacity: (a) to reach a goal with little error and small energy expenditure (i.e., to choose an appropriate set of motor commands among an infinite number of solutions; a degrees-of-freedom problem); and (b) to face deterministic (e.g., change in goal, force applied on the moving limb) and stochastic (e.g., noise in motor commands) perturbations (variability problem). Bernstein's problem, which encompasses both the degrees-of-freedom and variability problems, is illustrated in Figure 20.1 for a reaching movement. In this example, the moving arm has three degrees of freedom (Fig. 20.1A; shoulder, elbow, wrist), and moves in a two-dimensional space to reach a target (Fig. 20.1B). Thus, there exists an infinite number of articular displacements that are appropriate to capturing the target (Fig. 20.1C). In the presence of noise, the reaching movements are successful, but have different characteristics (Fig. 20.1D).

Posture/Movement

The apparent ease of motor control hides the paradoxical problem of interference between posture and movement (Ostry and Feldman 2003). The central issue is why processes that are responsible for postural control do not appear to overtly interfere with movement control. Consider the following example: A mass which can move along a line and which is attached to two muscle-like actuators (Fig. 20.2A). Each actuator is represented by a muscle unit (Zajac 1989): a force generator and a parallel elastic element. The purpose is to capture two main features of muscular functioning: The muscle generates force in response to a stimulation; and the muscle generates a restoring force when lengthened. Thus, a more detailed model is not necessary here. The mass is initially in equilibrium due to the equal and opposite actions of the actuators' forces. The goal is to displace the mass to a new position (e.g., to the right), and maintain it in equilibrium at this position.

We observe that activation of the rightward muscle displaces the mass to the right, but that the final position requires maintained activation of this

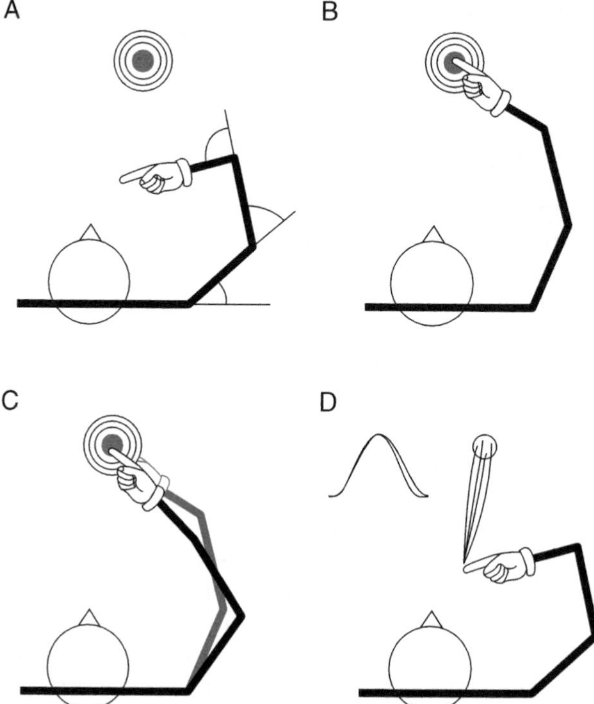

Figure 20.1 Illustration of Bernstein's problem. **A**: Planar reaching movement with a redundant arm (three degrees of freedom [DOF]). **B**: A successful movement reaches the target region (*central gray circle*). **C**: Two successful movements with different final postures. **D**: Several successful movements with different spatiotemporal characteristics. **Inset**: Velocity profiles. Reproduced from Figure 1 of Guigon, E., P. Baraduc, and M. Desmurget. 2008b. Optimality, stochasticity, and variability in motor behavior. *Journal of Computational Neuroscience* 24(1):57–68, with permission of the publisher.

muscle to compensate for the leftward restoring force induced by the displacement (Fig. 20.2B). In this case, posture interferes with displacement, and initial and final postures are not equivalent. This example shows that the specification of a displacement by a force is not appropriate to managing the conflict between postural maintenance and the initiation/termination of movement (Ostry and Feldman 2003). An alternative approach is to create a force through a change in the origin of the muscles (Fig. 20.2C). In this case, one and the same mechanism is used for posture and movement, and the initial and final postures are of the same nature.

These two examples raise the fundamental issue of the integration between posture and movement that should be addressed by any model of motor control.

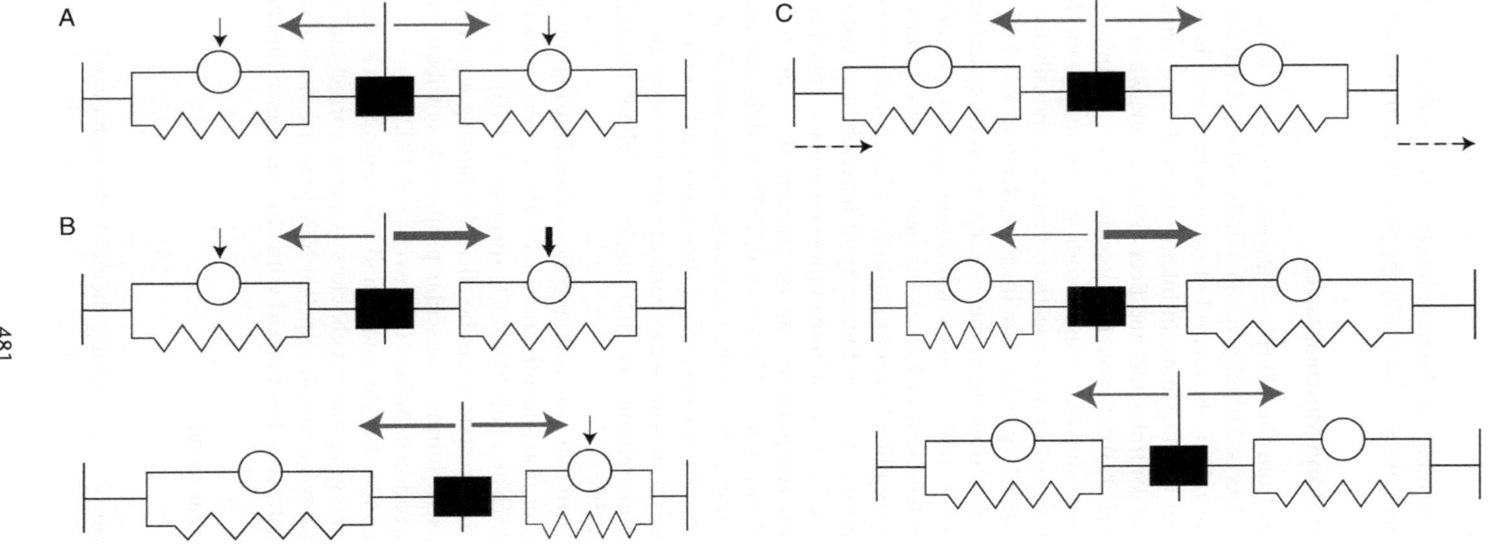

Figure 20.2 Illustration of the posture/movement problem. **A**: A mass is at equilibrium due to the equal and opposite forces of two muscles (*gray horizontal arrows*: actual forces exerted on the mass; *black vertical arrows*: control forces). **B**: To displace the mass, the equilibrium is modified by changing the control forces (more force to the right). **C**: To displace the mass, the equilibrium is modified by changing the origin of the muscles (displacement to the right).

SIMPLIFICATIONS

Here, we describe strategies at different levels in the brain–body system that could provide simplified solutions to the problem of motor control.

At the Biomechanical and Muscular Levels

Motor control arises from the interplay between processes at the neural and musculoskeletal levels. Although it is generally believed that the neural level has a dominant role in the control of movements, there is evidence that the mechanics of moving limbs in interaction with the environment can also contribute to control (Chiel and Beer 1997; Nishikawa et al. 2007). Raibert and Hodgins (1993) defended the view that "the mechanical system has a mind on its own," and that "the nervous system and the mechanical system should be designed to work together, sharing responsibility for the behaviour that emerges" (p. 350). For instance, Kubow and Full (1999) showed in a model that running in the cockroach can be generated by a feedforward controller with a self-stabilization against perturbations through mechanical feedback that alters leg moment arms. In this sense, mechanics can act to simplify the control task. The idea of *intelligent mechanics* has been developed mainly in the study of invertebrates, but related ideas can be found in the study of human movements (van Ingen Schenau 1989). Morphological computation can be performed by the tendinous network of human hand (Valero-Cuevas et al. 2007), and the mechanics of the ocular plant (Demer 2006). In the latter case, mobile soft-tissue sheets (pulleys) in the orbit influence the pulling direction of extraocular muscle. This organization could provide a mechanical basis for simplified oculomotor control by constraining eye movements to follow Listing's law (Quaia and Optican 1998).

It is also well known that muscles can play a self-stabilizing role during movement due to their force-length and force-velocity properties (Brown and Loeb 2000; Jindrich and Full 2002; Richardson et al. 2005). For instance, an immediate restoring response can be elicited following a perturbation that stretches a muscle. Intrinsic muscular properties contribute to compensation for perturbation in human (Rothwell et al. 1982).

Although the premise that the neural and mechanical levels share the responsibility for emerging motor behaviors is surely correct and makes sense for reactive control, it remains unclear how proper coordination and predictive motor control can be obtained with "two drivers in the car."

At the Neuromuscular Level

Synergies

The concept of synergy is a recurring theme in the framework of motor control (Bernstein 1967; Lee 1984; Macpherson 1991; Tresch and Jarc 2009;

see also Chapter 5, and Chapter 1, this volume). Historically, a synergy has been broadly defined as a set of anatomical or functional elements acting together. Such a "lumping" was thought to simplify the coordination task of the CNS in the face of multiple levels of redundancy (motor units, muscles, degrees of freedom, etc.). Macpherson (1991) addressed the issue of muscular synergies and concluded that, if they exist, these synergies are not hard-wired, but highly flexible, versatile, and task-dependent (see also Soechting and Lacquaniti 1989; Maier and Hepp-Reymond 1995; Mercer and Sahrmann 1999). In her view, a description of motor behavior in terms of muscular synergies is a way of saying that there exists an underlying efficient, but inaccessible process of coordination.

In recent years, the concept has been redefined in more functional terms, but in at least three qualitatively different ways. One definition is derived from microstimulation experiments in the spinal cord that have identified a motor map of convergent force fields—that is, neural synergies that generate movements toward an equilibrium position (Bizzi et al. 2000; Mussa-Ivaldi and Bizzi 2000). These spinal modules that produce specific pattern of muscle activation, would form a set of *motor primitives*—the "building blocks," and basis functions that could be combined to construct complex motor behaviors (Mussa-Ivaldi and Bizzi 2000). The feasibility of this idea has been assessed in a computational model (Mussa-Ivaldi 1997).

The second definition can be considered as an extension of the first. It is based on the hypothesis that a small set of time-varying patterns is sufficient to generate, through appropriate scaling and time-shifting, the entire set of muscle patterns across a range of motor behaviors (d'Avella et al. 2003). This view has been widely used to describe dimensionality reduction in the motor system for different species (frog, cat, monkey, human, etc. tasks (posture, locomotion, grasping, etc.), and conditions (perturbations, motor disorders, etc.) (Krouchev et al. 2006; Klein Breteler et al. 2007; Torres-Oviedo and Ting 2007; Overduin et al. 2008). In these cases, as the natural behavior of freely moving animals was considered, it was not possible to directly ascertain the actual biomechanical effects of synergies. Yet, in some studies, the muscle synergies were shown to be correlated to the control of task-related variables (e.g., endpoint kinematics or kinetics, displacement of the center of pressure) (Ivanenko et al. 2003; Krishnamoorthy et al. 2003; Ting and Macpherson 2005; Torres-Oviedo et al. 2006). Furthermore, a modular organization of movement control at the task level is consistent with observation of neural population recordings (Georgopoulos et al. 1993) and microstimulation experiments (Graziano et al. 2002; Lemay and Grill 2004). A central premise of this approach is to equate a synergy to an open-loop process that unfolds independently of feedback signals (i.e., a *motor program*; d'Avella et al. 2003). This hypothesis on the nature of synergies has been challenged by Kargo and Giszter (2008). They showed that distortion of sensory feedback through muscle vibration modified the timing of burst signals that control wiping movements in the frog. More generally, control cast in terms of motor programs fails to reflect the flexible nature of motor behaviors (see below; Desmurget and Grafton 2000; Todorov and Jordan 2002).

The third definition is based on the uncontrolled manifold (UCM) approach, a technical procedure that identifies stable performance variables from trial-to-trial variability (Schöner 1995). This method makes a partition of the variance of a set of measured variables (e.g., joint angles of a redundant limb) into two components: a component that modifies the value of a performance variable (e.g., the endpoint position of the limb) and one (the uncontrolled manifold) that does not affect it. The structure of the variability revealed by the UCM defines synergies characterized by stability against perturbations and flexibility to solve concurrent tasks (Latash et al. 2007; Chapter 1, this volume).

Overall, the identification of synergies is a meaningful step toward understanding which performance variables are controlled by the CNS, and how the CNS translates task goals into appropriate spatio-temporal patterns of muscle activation. Yet, it remains that synergies are obtained as the outcome of a data processing/statistical analysis process. The point raised by Macpherson (1991) of the actual coordination process that produces synergies remains an open issue: What computational mechanism could solve the problem of motor control by a reduction of dimensionality compatible with the characteristics of synergies? One mechanism could be the minimum intervention principle—the fact that variability in task-irrelevant directions remains uncorrected (Todorov and Jordan 2002; Valero-Cuevas et al. 2009; see below).

It is interesting that even some of the most ardent supporters of the notion of synergy recognize the difficulties and ambiguities raised by this notion (Tresch and Jarc 2009).

Elimination

It has been proposed that a strategy to solve a redundant task is the freezing of supernumerary DOFs (Bernstein 1967; Newell 1991; Vereijken et al. 1992). This strategy would entail a radical simplification by drastically restricting the space of possible mechanical solutions. Yet, as mechanical coupling induces interaction forces between segments of a moving limb, freezing a DOF necessarily involves an active control. Gribble and Ostry (1999) showed that a pure forearm movement evokes electromyographic (EMG) activity in shoulder muscles that stabilizes the upper arm and is proportional to elbow velocity.

A related strategy has been observed in the control of eye movements. According to Donders' law, possible gaze positions in three-dimensional space are restricted to a plane (Wong 2004); that is, eye torsion is automatically defined by the choice of horizontal and vertical displacements. We can make two remarks. First, Donders' law does not apply in general to arm movements (Gielen et al. 1997). Second, the mechanical origin of this law is debated (Angelaki and Hess 2004; Demer 2006; Tweed 2007). For instance, frequent violations of Donders' law are observed during the vestibulo-ocular reflex and sleep.

At the Control Level

The control level encompasses processes that convert task goals into muscle activations.

Equilibrium Point Theory

The equilibrium point theory (EPT) proposes that movement results from imbalance between the spring forces generated by a shift of the origin of the springs (Fig. 20.2C) (Feldman and Levin 1995). In this framework, movement is a series of continuous transitions between postures along an *equilibrium trajectory*, defined by time-varying changes in the origin of the muscles. Postural maintenance is a natural product of the control scheme. A central tenet of the theory is that realistic movements can be generated without knowledge of the dynamics of the object to be controlled; the equilibrium trajectory is derived from kinematic characteristics of the planned movement. The validity of this tenet is highly debated, as the arguments for or against the theory are based on the nature of muscle models and level of stiffness considered (Gomi and Kawato 1996; Gribble et al. 1998; Kistemaker et al. 2006, 2007). Paradoxically, the debate over EPT has focused on the problem of movement generation, whereas its main weakness is probably on the postural side of the problem. In fact, according to the EPT, posture is a passive stiffness-based process, which raises at least two remarks. We first note that the geometry of muscular insertion can threaten postural stability (Shadmehr and Arbib 1992; Dornay et al. 1993). Second, the issue of the magnitude of stiffness is crucial: Is stiffness sufficient to oppose the destabilizing effect of gravity (Winter et al. 1998; Morasso and Schieppati 1999)? Although agreement is still lacking on this point, converging evidence from recent studies on postural control indicates that ankle stiffness is too low for passive postural maintenance (Loram and Lakie 2002; Morasso and Sanguineti 2002; Casadio et al. 2005; van Soest and Rozendaal 2008).

We can also ask whether EPT really entails a simplification of motor control, since compensation for loads applied during arm movement requires information about the loads and arm dynamics (Gribble and Ostry 2000). In the same way, it is unclear how anticipation of the effects of interjoint coupling can occur without knowledge of limb inertia (Shapiro et al. 1995; Gribble and Ostry 1999).

Dynamical Systems Theory

The dynamical system approach to motor control attributes emergent behaviors to regularities of nonlinear dynamical systems (Schöner and Kelso 1988). In this framework, spatiotemporal patterns can emerge spontaneously from interactions between coupled subsystems. If applicable, this approach entails a clear-cut simplification in control, as computation is merely replaced by a natural evolution in space and time. This could be the case for rhythmic movement patterns that are observed in a wide variety of coordinated behaviors (e.g., finger tapping, locomotion, etc.). Application to discrete movements is more controversial, as it is widely held that discrete and rhythmic movements are subserved by distinct control mechanisms (Schaal et al. 2004, 2007; Huys et al. 2008). Schöner (1990) proposed a model for discrete movement generation in which movement kinematics emerged from the alternation of a fixed-point regime and a limit-cycle regime in the same dynamical system. The model was able to produce the timing properties of discrete movements of a mass point in a single dimension (spatial coordination was not described). This model was extended to a nonlinear redundant biomechanical system by Martin (2006), yet with a glaring loss in the expected simplification. We note that an important limitation of the dynamical system approach to discrete movements is to define posture as a fixed-point attractor (i.e., posture is an asymptotically stable behavior, unlike what has been observed experimentally; Kiemel et al. 2002; Bottaro et al. 2005).

Muscular Strategies

Discrete movements are characterized by typical and reproducible EMG patterns. For instance, fast arm movements are accompanied by a triphasic agonist–antagonist EMG (Hallett et al. 1975). Analysis of the relationship between EMG characteristics (intensity, timing) and movement kinematics (amplitude, duration, velocity) and dynamics (load) has led to propose descriptive rules for EMG; that is, how to build the proper EMG, given movement characteristics, such as the speed control hypothesis (Freund and Büdingen 1978), the pulse-step control theory (Ghez 1979), the impulse timing theory (Wallace 1981), the dual strategy (Gottlieb et al. 1989), and more. We will not enter into the details of these strategies, but simply note that they only apply to single-joint movements. Extension to multijoint movements would require complex rules to deal with interaction forces and directional anisotropy of inertia and velocity-dependent forces. A simple scaling rule is not sufficient in the case of two-joint arm movements, as the fine details of motor coordination and timing can hardly be embedded in a rule (Buneo et al.1995).

At the Functional Level

Separation of Planning/Execution and Kinematics/Dynamics

The observed invariance of trajectories and velocity profiles has led to the proposal that movements are represented at a geometric (Torres and

Zipser 2002; Biess et al. 2007) or a kinematic (Flash and Hogan 1985) level. The planned spatiotemporal path would then serve as a reference input for a trajectory tracking system (Flash 1987; Flanagan et al. 1993). In the framework of a strict separation between planning and execution, a planned movement is executed irrespective of possible changes in task requirements (e.g., unexpected target displacement). A strategy for movement correction is a simple linear superposition of the trajectories planned for the initial target position and for the perturbed position (Flash and Henis 1991). A notable aspect of this model is that no information about actual hand position is necessary to generate online corrections. This greatly simplifies the problem of motor control by suppressing the need for forward modeling. Kinematic planning can also be considered as an online process that makes no distinction between planning and execution (Torres and Zipser 2002). The main limiting factor of these approaches is the necessity for a trajectory tracking system that should faithfully translate kinematics into dynamics. This "motor implementation stage" (Torres and Zipser 2002) is frequently associated to the equilibrium point theory, with its known limitations (see earlier discussion).

Separation of Posture and Movement

Various experimental data point to a necessary dissociation between posture and movement control (Frank and Earl 1990; Massion 1992). The timing of anticipatory postural adjustments can vary independently from the onset of focal movement (Brown and Frank 1987; Schepens and Drew 2003). The timing also varies with the importance of the destabilizing effect of the focal movement on balance (Zattara and Bouisset 1986). These results suggest that the postural and movement components may be controlled and planned separately. A possible scenario could involve a canonical, predefined postural synergy that would guarantee the maintenance of upright stance during performance of the focal movement (Nashner and McCollum 1985; Frank and Earl 1990).

It should be noted that authors arguing for specialized posture and movement processes basically argue against a single process, and they fail to propose a clear computational scheme that would illustrate the duality of posture and movement. In particular, it is unclear how proper coordination can be guaranteed in a separation scheme (Latash et al. 1995).

Is It Possible to Simplify?

If we try to find what is common to the preceding proposals, we see that simplification is frequently discussed in relation to *simplified* motor control problems. For instance, discrete hard-wired synergies have been described for postural control in the sagittal plane (Rushmer et al. 1983; Nashner and McCollum 1985), but such a description is not valid for the general case of postural sway in the horizontal plane (Macpherson 1988; Moore et al. 1988). The EPT has addressed the control of single- (St-Onge et al. 1997; Gribble et al. 1998; Kistemaker et al. 2006) and two-joint (Flash 1987; Flanagan et al. 1993) arms, but not kinematically redundant systems (although it has been claimed to be feasible; Balasubramaniam and Feldman 2004). These remarks lead to the following conclusion: If simplification is a solution to motor control, it remains to be proven in a case that encompasses the main and difficult issues of motor control.

CONTROL WITH INTERNAL MODELS

Although simplification should remain an objective, it should also be in keeping with a general solution to motor control. A general solution should not be a mere description of all the complex problems that the CNS faces in generating motor actions and a catalogue of mechanisms that could solve these problems, but a principled approach that captures the spirit of motor coordination and provides computational processes that create it. The EPT and the dynamical systems theory could be candidate solutions, but they fail to be comprehensive enough.

In fact, from a design perspective, it would seem necessary that motor control processes should incorporate detailed knowledge on the functioning of the object to be controlled (see Chapter 11, this volume). This view has led to the notion of internal models; that is, structures that define the relationship between commands and outcomes (*forward models*), or desired outcomes and commands (*inverse models*). Two kinds of architecture have been proposed that exploit internal models.

Inverse Dynamics and Impedance Control

This architecture involves (a) a feedforward controller that translates a *desired trajectory* into appropriate control signals, and (b) a feedback controller that can correct deviations between the actual and the desired trajectory (Kawato 1999; Fig. 20.3). The feedforward controller is an inverse model of the dynamics of the object to be controlled that guarantees an efficient guidance of the object toward its goal. The feedback controller exploits the viscoelastic properties of the neuromuscular system to compensate for unexpected perturbations exerted on the controlled object (Shadmehr and Mussa-Ivaldi 1994; Franklin et al. 2003; Berniker and Körding 2008).

We can make two remarks on this architecture. First, it is unclear how one and the same neuromuscular unit can produce the appropriate combination of feedforward and feedback commands. On the one hand, the feedforward command is a direct specification of the force (or torque) to be produced by the neuromuscular system. On the other hand, the feedback command, which is a viscoelastic term that depends on the actual and

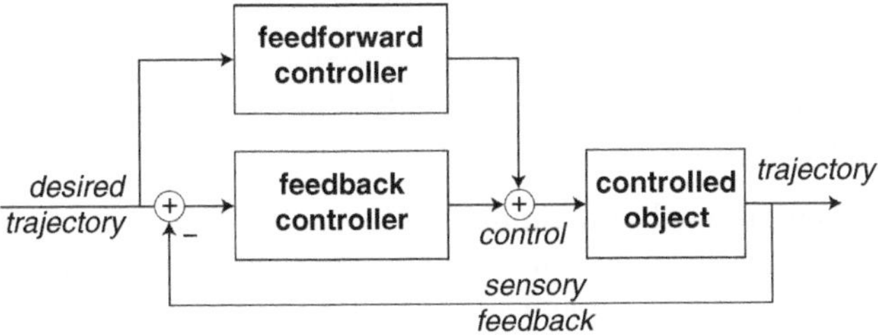

Figure 20.3 Architecture for inverse dynamics and impedance control.

desired state of the controlled object, must be produced by force-length and force-velocity mechanisms at the neuromuscular level, independently of and without interference with the feedforward command. Thus, control requires a combination of force- and position-based commands (Ostry and Feldman 2003) that has never been precisely described. Second, the notion of desired trajectory, which is central to the robustness of this approach, has been strongly criticized, as it fails to account for the flexibility of motor behavior (Bernstein 1967; Sporns and Edelman 1993; Todorov and Jordan 2002).

Control and Estimation

This architecture involves (a) a controller that elaborates appropriate control signals to reach a *desired goal* for a given state of the system, and (b) a state estimator that constructs an estimated state of the system based on commands and sensory feedback (Fig. 20.4).

A rationale for a control/estimation architecture in the framework of motor control has been developed recently by (Todorov and Jordan 2002).

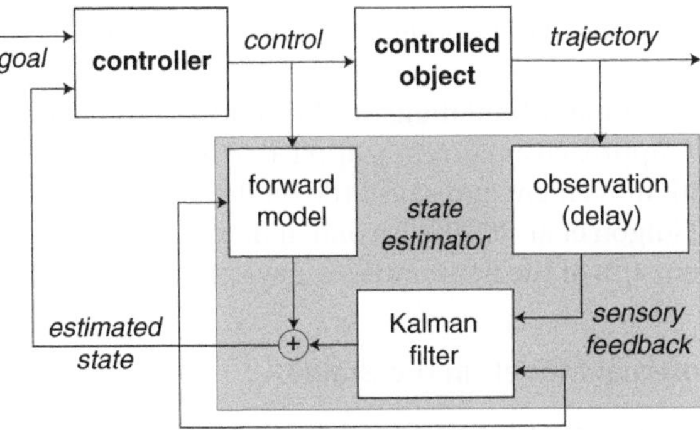

Figure 20.4 Architecture for control and estimation.

Central to their analysis is the observation that, for reaching a behavioral goal, the CNS is directly pursuing it rather than trying to reproduce a predetermined pattern that would fulfill it. This fact was already noticed by Bernstein (1967), and formalized by Abbs et al. (1984):

> Program is more likely the representation of the dynamic processes whereby the appropriate sensorimotor contingencies are set up to ensure cooperative complementary contribution of the multiple actions to a common, predetermined goal.

To capture this notion, Todorov and Jordan (2002) proposed a computational mechanism (stochastic optimal feedback control, SOFC; see also Bryson and Ho 1975; Stengel 1986; Todorov 2004, 2005) that precisely accounts for the goal-directed nature of motor actions. The recipe has three components. First, it is based on feedback control. This component is a ubiquitous feature in the field of motor control (Houk and Rymer 1981), but is generally used in the sense defined in classical control theory (e.g., PID control), with its well-known limitations (e.g., necessity of high gains, oscillatory behavior for long feedback delays). In the framework of SOFC, the feedback control is defined by time-varying gains elaborated from a full knowledge of the properties of the object to be controlled, and does not suffer the same limitations as classical feedback. The second component is an optimality principle, which is also frequently encountered in computational motor control to solve redundancy problems (reviewed in Todorov 2004). Interestingly, optimality not only solves redundancy, but also implements a "minimum intervention principle": The controller does not compensate for a deviation that does not interfere with the success of the task not to incur an unjustifiable cost. The third component is stochastic control, the capacity to control a system in the presence of uncertainty (e.g., noise).

The control/estimation architecture can account for kinematics, kinetics, muscular and neural characteristics of arm movements (Todorov and Jordan 2002; Guigon et al. 2007a,b), online movement corrections (Saunders and Knill 2004; Liu and Todorov 2007), structure of motor variability (Todorov and Jordan 2002; Guigon et al. 2008a,b), formation of synergies (Todorov and Jordan 2002), and Fitts' law and control of precision (Guigon et al. 2008a).

There are two main limitations to the control/estimation architecture and the SOFC approach as currently applied to motor control. First, it deals generally with movement and says little on the integration of posture and movement (Guigon et al. 2007b). Second, it does not take into account low-level characteristics of the neuromuscular system (reflex, stiffness).

Are There Internal Models in the Brain?

Although the concept of internal models is a widely used theoretical construct in the framework of motor control (Kawato 1999), its cogency has been questioned (see Chapter 1, this volume). Early on, Turvey et al. (1978) were concerned with the possibility of performing movement coordination through a detailed central specification of muscular operations. They raised the issue of the coordination of multiple degrees of freedom (Bernstein's problem), and the problem of context-conditioned variability (i.e., the fact that muscles can have context-dependent mechanical actions). Incidentally, they noted that the presence of sensory feedback information can alleviate the issue of context-conditioned variability, an observation that anticipated the necessary role of online feedback control (Desmurget and Grafton 2000). More recently, Ostry and Feldman (2003) discussed the failure of control based on internal models to properly address the posture–movement problem (see Fig. 20.2B). This issue is fundamental, all the more so because it is generally ignored in the field of computational motor control (Hoff and Arbib 1993; Wolpert and Ghahramani 2000; Todorov and Jordan 2002; Todorov 2004). We will return to this point in the following section.

PRINCIPLES FOR MOTOR CONTROL

On the basis of the preceding observations, here, we describe several principles that provide a unified basis for motor control.

Optimality

Optimality as an overarching principle for motor control is a well-substantiated idea (reviewed in Todorov 2004). From a theoretical point of view, it provides an efficient solution to Bernstein's problem as it generates realistic movements in the face of spatial, temporal, kinematic, and muscular redundancy (Todorov and Jordan 2002; Guigon et al. 2007b). The idea applies equally well to different motor tasks involving the hand, arm, eye, or whole body (Harris and Wolpert 1998; Tweed 2007). There is also empirical evidence that humans behave according to optimal laws (Arechavaleta et al. 2008), or can learn to discover near-optimal solutions to real-world tasks (Inooka and Koitabashi 1990; Engelbrecht et al. 2003; Chhabra and Jacobs 2006; Izawa et al. 2008; Sherback and D'Andrea 2008).

Efficiency

Optimality entails the choice of a cost function, which indicates a quantity to minimize. The nature of the cost function is a highly debated issue. Part of the confusion arises from the fact that all the proposed cost functions (jerk, energy, torque change, etc.) make similar predictions on basic qualitative characteristics of movement; for example, trajectories and velocity profiles (Flash and Hogan 1985; Uno et al. 1989; Alexander 1997; Harris and Wolpert 1998; Todorov and Jordan 2002; Guigon et al. 2007b). Yet, a thorough quantitative analysis is generally lacking and could provide more contrasted results. For instance, the minimum torque change model fails to produce the observed quantitative characteristics of velocity profile (Engelbrecht and Fernandez 1997) and the appropriate curvature of two-dimensional movements (Soechting and Flanders 1998).

With the minimum variance model, Harris and Wolpert (1998) have drastically changed the viewpoint on the cost functions. Their proposal is to use a behaviorally relevant measure (variance) rather than an arbitrary and behaviorally meaningless quantity (e.g., acceleration derivative) as a cost. This is a radical departure from the previous optimal control models in the sense that characteristics of motor behavior emerge from a general principle rather than from a level-specific (e.g., kinematic, dynamic, muscular), effector-specific (e.g., arm, eye) or task-specific (e.g., posture, locomotion, etc.) criterion (see Todorov 2004, for a review). This analysis was further refined by Todorov and Jordan (2002), leading to an error/effort cost function, in which the effort is the size of central signals that eventually generate the movement. The rationale for this choice is discussed in Kawato (1996). In a series of studies, Guigon et al. (2007a,b, 2008a,b) have used a cost function with a single effort term, error being considered as a constraint to be fulfilled. The two types of cost function have been able to explain a wide range of observations on motor control (Todorov and Jordan 2002; Saunders and Knill 2004; Todorov and Li 2005; Li 2006; Guigon et al. 2007a,b; Liu and Todorov 2007; Guigon et al. 2008a). Yet, the two approaches differ on what is considered a cost and what is considered a constraint (Guigon et al. 2008b). This point raises subtle and interesting issues, if one is to identify the actual cost function that governs motor behaviors (Liu and Todorov 2007; O'Sullivan et al. 2009). The mixed error/effort function would predict that subjects can make a trade-off between error and effort (e.g., sustain a larger error in order to minimize their effort). This issue could likely be tested in an experiment (see, e.g., Liu and Todorov 2007).

Feedback

Feedback is probably one of the oldest notions used for the formal description of motor control. Yet, there is some confusion on the nature and role of feedback. The nature of feedback is clearly illustrated in the stretch reflex (e.g., Houk and Rymer 1981). Muscle lengthening leads to increased afferent discharge through Ia and II fibers on the one hand, and increased motoneuronal discharge and muscle force on the other hand. One component of feedback has a sensory dimension and can carry information on the state of the muscle. This information is transmitted through ascending tracts to the cortex and the cerebellum, and it can contribute to central representations of posture and movement. The other component has a motor dimension that can be exploited to compensate for perturbations, but also to produce movements (Houk and Rymer 1981; Feldman and Levin 1995).

On this basis, the possible role of feedback can be addressed. On the motor side, feedback can contribute directly to movement production, as in the EPT (Feldman and Levin 1995), or indirectly by correcting deviations from a desired trajectory (Shadmehr and Mussa-Ivaldi 1994). This view is not backed up by observations in deafferentated patients, showing that they move somewhat normally under visual feedback (Ghez et al. 1990). Although the general motor behavior of deafferentated patients is strongly affected, the basic capacity to move appears to be preserved (Forget and Lamarre 1987). On the sensory side, feedback provides information on the state of the body, and is the basis for the widely acknowledged role of state estimation (Wolpert et al. 1995; Shadmehr and Krakauer 2008). The tight link between estimation and control has led to the idea that motor commands are continuously updated by internal feedback loops (Desmurget and Grafton 2000), and to the notion of optimal feedback control (Hoff and Arbib 1993; Todorov and Jordan 2002; Guigon et al. 2008b).

Effort

In motor control models, a movement is generally specified by its amplitude and duration. Yet, although humans can performed timed actions, for instance rhythmic movements, not all their actions are actually timed—for example, ambulatory locomotion movements, movements around postural states, or reaching movements are not in general specified to have a particular duration (Schöner 2002). Psychophysical studies have shown that movement duration depends on movement parameters: for example, amplitude/duration scaling (Fitts 1954; Wadman et al. 1979; Gordon et al. 1994b), load/duration scaling (Bock 1990; Hatzitaki and McKinley 2001), and systematic direction/duration variations (Gordon et al. 1994b; Pellegrini and Flanders 1996). Furthermore, subjects fail to adapt to time-dependent perturbations (e.g., force fields that explicitly depend on time [Conditt and Mussa-Ivaldi 1999]), and they do consider time-dependent force fields as state-dependent force fields.

If duration is not specified for a given movement (defined as its initial position and its amplitude), it should arise from a computational process. The constant effort principle proposes to calculate actual duration from a desired level of effort using the relationship between amplitude, duration, and effort prescribed by the optimality principle (Guigon et al. 2007b, 2008b); that is, for a given amplitude and effort, there exists a unique duration such that the optimal movement for this amplitude and duration is associated with this (minimum) effort. This principle provides a quantitative account of amplitude/duration and load/duration scaling, and direction-dependent changes in movement duration (Guigon et al. 2007b). A related idea is time minimization to match a given level of terminal variability (Meyer et al. 1988; Harris and Wolpert 1998). However, this solution predicts that scaling is associated with constant terminal variability. Experimental observations show that variability can increase with movement amplitude for series of movements obeying an amplitude/duration scaling law (Gordon et al. 1994a; van Beers et al. 2004). A competing proposal to explain direction-dependent changes in movement duration is that the nervous system fails to compensate for the inertial anisotropy of the arm (Gordon et al. 1994b; see Todorov 1998 for a model). Yet, this view is not backed up by experimental observations (e.g., Flanagan and Lolley 2001).

CONCLUSION

The idea that the nervous system could solve problems of motor control through simplifications was thoroughly reviewed. No appropriate strategy was persuasively and unambiguously identified that could actually address the complex issue of movement coordination. Putting simplification aside, a set of principles was presented based on the idea that the nervous system should possess detailed knowledge on the functioning of the objects to be controlled. Although these principles appeared highly successful for a computational description of motor control, it should not lead us to forget the good reasons that have driven the search for simplifications (Turvey et al. 1978; Ostry and Feldman 2003). First, finding a solution to optimal control problems is a highly demanding issue in computer science (Bryson 1999), and it is unclear how it could be discovered and realized by neural hardware. More generally, the neural substrate for the proposed principles remains elusive. Second, the problem of posture/movement integration is only partially and unpersuasively addressed. In particular, the lack of consideration for low-level characteristics of the neuromuscular system (reflex, stiffness) is problematic, and prevents the study of perturbation-induced changes in motor behavior. These limitations provide directions for future developments in the framework of computational motor control.

Two perspectives are interesting. First, the principles were applied to the control of the humanoid robot HRP2 (Tran et al. 2008). Interesting preliminary results were obtained on the coordination of seven- and nine-DOF configurations involving the trunk and the arm. On the one hand, the application of biologically inspired principles to robotics can offer an alternative to classical control techniques that are robust, but less flexible than the solutions discovered by the nervous system. On the other hand, the study of robotic systems could help validate the principles on more realistic kinematic chains (using larger numbers of DOFs). Second, the principles could apply to understanding the neuroanatomy of motor control and associated motor disorders (e.g., Shadmehr and Krakauer 2008). For instance, the concept of effort could play a central role in inferring the functions of basal ganglia (Shadmehr and Krakauer 2008) and explaining behavioral disorders in Parkinson disease (Mazzoni et al. 2007).

REFERENCES

Abbs, J.H., V.L. Gracco, and K.J. Cole. 1984. Control of multimovement coordination: Sensorimotor mechanisms in speech motor programming. *Journal of Motor Behavior* 16(2):195–231.

Alexander, R.M. 1997. A minimum energy cost hypothesis for human arm trajectories. *Biological Cybernetics* 76(2):97–105.

Angelaki, D.E., and B.J.M. Hess. 2004. Control of eye orientation: Where does the brain's role end and the muscle's begin? *European Journal of Neuroscience* 19(1):1–10.

Arechavaleta, G., J.-P. Laumond, H. Hicheur, and A. Berthoz. 2008. An optimality principle governing human walking. *IEEE Transactions on Robotics* 24(1): 5–14.

Balasubramaniam, R., A.G. Feldman. 2004. Guiding movements without redundancy problems. In *Coordination dynamics*, eds., V.K. Jirsa and J.A.S. Kelso, 155–76. New York: Springer.

Berniker, M., and K. Körding. 2008. Estimating the sources of motor errors for adaptation and generalization. *Nature Neuroscience* 11(12):1454–61.

Bernstein, N. 1967. *The co-ordination and regulation of movements*. Oxford, UK: Pergamon Press.

Biess, A., D.G. Liebermann, and T. Flash. 2007. A computational model for redundant human three-dimensional pointing movements: Integration of independent spatial and temporal motor plans simplifies movement dynamics. *Journal of Neuroscience* 27(48):13045–64.

Bizzi, E., M.C. Tresch, P. Saltiel, and A. d'Avella. 2000. New perspectives on spinal motor systems. *Nature Reviews. Neuroscience* 1(2):101–08.

Bock, O. 1990. Load compensation in human goal-directed arm movements. *Behavioral Brain Research* 41(3):167–77.

Bottaro, A., M. Casadio, P.G. Morasso, and V. Sanguineti. 2005. Body sway during quiet standing: Is it the residual chattering of an intermittent stabilization process? *Human Movement Science* 24(4):588–615.

Brown, I.E., G.E. Loeb. 2000. A reductionist approach to creating and using neuromusculoskeletal models. In *Biomechanics and neural control of posture and movement*, eds., J.M. Winters and P.E. Crago, 148–63. New York: Springer.

Brown, J.E., and J.S. Frank. 1987. Influence of event anticipation on postural actions accompanying voluntary movement. *Experimental Brain Research* 67(3):645–50.

Bryson, A.E. 1999. *Dynamic optimization*. Englewood Cliffs, NJ: Prentice-Hall.

Bryson, A.E., Y.-C. Ho. 1975. *Applied optimal control - optimization, estimation, and control*. New York: Hemisphere Publishing Corp.

Buneo, C.A., J. Boline, J.F. Soechting, and R.E. Poppele. 1995. On the form of the internal model for reaching. *Experimental Brain Research* 104(3):467–79.

Casadio, M., P.G. Morasso, and V. Sanguineti V. 2005. Direct measurement of ankle stiffness during quiet standing: Implications for control modelling and clinical application. *Gait & Posture* 21(4):410–24.

Chhabra, M., and R.A. Jacobs. 2006. Near-optimal human adaptive control across different noise environments. *Journal of Neuroscience* 26(42):10883–87.

Chiel, H., and R.D. Beer. 1997. The brain has a body: Adaptive behavior emerges from interactions of nervous system, body, and environment. *Trends in Neuroscience* 20(12):553–57.

Conditt, M.A., and F.A. Mussa-Ivaldi. 1999. Central representation of time during motor learning. *Proceedings of the National Academy of Sciences of the USA* 96(20):11625–30.

d'Avella, A., P. Saltiel, and E. Bizzi. 2003. Combinations of muscle synergies in the construction of a natural motor behavior. *Nature Neuroscience* 6(3):300–08.

Demer, J.L. 2006. Current concepts of mechanical and neural factors in ocular motility. *Current Opinion in Neurology* 19(1):4–13.

Desmurget, M., and S. Grafton. 2000. Forward modeling allows feedback control for fast reaching movements. *Trends in Cognitive Science* 4(11):423–31.

Dornay, M., F.A. Mussa-Ivaldi, J. McIntyre, and E. Bizzi. 1993. Stability constraints for the distributed control of motor behavior. *Neural Network*, 6(9):1045–59.

Engelbrecht, S.E., N.E. Berthier, and L.P. O'Sullivan. 2003. The undershoot bias: Learning to act optimally under uncertainty. *Psychological Science* 14(3):257–61.

Engelbrecht, S.E., and J.P. Fernandez. 1997. Invariant characteristics of horizontal-plane minimum-torque-change movements with one mechanical degree of freedom. *Biological Cybernetics* 76(5):321–29.

Feldman, A.G., and M.F. Levin. 1995. The origin and use of positional frames of reference in motor control. *Behavioral Brain Science* 18(4):723–44.

Fitts, P.M. 1954. The information capacity of the human motor system in controlling the amplitude of movement. *Journal of Experimental Psychology* 47(6):381–91.

Flanagan, J.R., and S. Lolley. 2001. The inertial anisotropy of the arm is accurately predicted during movement planning. *Journal of Neuroscience* 21(4):1361–69.

Flanagan, J.R., D.J. Ostry, and A.G. Feldman. 1993. Control of trajectory modifications in target-directed reaching. *Journal of Motor Behavior* 25(3):140–52.

Flash, T. 1987. The control of hand equilibrium trajectories in multi-joint arm movements. *Biological Cybernetics* 57(4–5):257–74.

Flash, T., and E. Henis. 1991. Arm trajectory modifications during reaching towards visual targets. *Journal of Cognitive Neuroscience*, 3(3):220–30.

Flash, T., and N. Hogan. 1985. The coordination of arm movements: An experimentally confirmed mathematical model. *Journal of Neuroscience* 5(7):1688–703.

Forget, R., and Y. Lamarre. 1987. Rapid elbow flexion in the absence of proprioceptive and cutaneous feedback. *Human Neurobiology* 6(1):27–37.

Frank, J.S., and M. Earl. 1990. Coordination of posture and movement. *Physical Therapy*, 70(12):855–63.

Franklin, D.W., R. Osu, E. Burdet, M. Kawato, and T.E. Milner. 2003. Adaptation to stable and unstable dynamics achieved by combined impedance control and inverse dynamics model. *Journal of Neurophysiology* 90(5):3270–82.

Freund, H.-J., and H.J. Büdingen. 1978. The relationship between speed and amplitude of the fastest voluntary contractions of human arm muscles. *Experimental Brain Research* 31(1):1–12.

Georgopoulos, A.P., M. Taira, and A. Lukashin. 1993. Cognitive neurophysiology of the motor cortex. *Science* 260:47–52.

Ghez, C. 1979. Contributions of central programs to rapid limb movement in the cat. In *Integration in the nervous system*, eds., H. Asanuma and V.J. Wilson, 305–20. Tokyo: Igaku-Shoin.

Ghez, C., J. Gordon, M.F. Ghilardi, C.N. Christakos, and C.E. Cooper. 1990. Roles of proprioceptive input in the programming of arm trajectories. *Cold Spring Harbor Symposia on Quantitative Biology* 55:837–47.

Gielen, C.C.A.M., E.J. Vrijenhoek, T. Flash, and S.F.W. Neggers. 1997. Arm position constraints during pointing and reaching in 3-D space. *Journal of Neurophysiology* 78(2):660–73.

Gomi, H., and M. Kawato. 1996. Equilibrium-point control hypothesis examined by measured arm stiffness during multijoint movement. *Science* 272(5258):117–20.

Gordon, J., M.F. Ghilardi, and C. Ghez. 1994a. Accuracy of planar reaching movements. I. Independence of direction and extent variability. *Experimental Brain Research* 99(1):97–111.

Gordon, J., M.F. Ghilardi, S.E. Cooper, and C. Ghez. 1994b. Accuracy of planar reaching movements. II. Systematic extent errors resulting from inertial anisotropy. *Experimental Brain Research* 99(1):112–30.

Gottlieb, G.L., D.M. Corcos, and G.C. Agarwal. 1989. Strategies for the control of voluntary movements with one mechanical degree of freedom. *Behavioral Brain Science* 12(2):189–250.

Graziano, M.S.A., C.S. Taylor, and T. Moore. 2002. Complex movements evoked by microstimulation of precentral cortex. *Neuron* 34(5):841–51.

Gribble, P.L., and D.J. Ostry. 1999. Compensation for interaction torques during single- and multijoint limb movement. *Journal of Neurophysiolog,* 82(5): 2310–26.

Gribble, P.L., and D.J. Ostry. 2000. Compensation for loads during arm movements using equilibrium-point control. *Experimental Brain Research* 135(4):474–82.

Gribble, P.L., D.J. Ostry, V. Sanguineti, and R. Laboissière. 1998. Are complex control signals required for human arm movement? *Journal of Neurophysiology* 79(3):1409–24.

Guigon, E., P. Baraduc, and M. Desmurget. 2007a. Coding of movement- and force-related information in primate primary motor cortex: A computational approach. *European Journal of Neuroscience* 26(1):250–60.

Guigon, E., P. Baraduc, and M. Desmurget. 2007b. Computational motor control: Redundancy and invariance. *Journal of Neurophysiology* 97(1):331–47.

Guigon, E., P. Baraduc, and M. Desmurget. 2008a. Computational motor control: Feedback and accuracy. *European Journal of Neuroscience,* 27(4):1003–16.

Guigon, E., P. Baraduc, and M. Desmurget. 2008b. Optimality, stochasticity, and variability in motor behavior. *Journal of Computational Neuroscience* 24(1): 57–68.

Hallett, M., B.T. Shahani, and R.R. Young. 1975. EMG analysis of stereotyped voluntary movements in man. *Journal of Neurology, Neurosurgery, and Psychiatry* 38(12):1154–62.

Harris, C.M., and D.M. Wolpert. 1998. Signal-dependent noise determines motor planning. *Nature* 394(6695):780–84.

Hatzitaki, V., and P. McKinley. 2001. Effect of single-limb inertial loading on bilateral reaching: Interlimb interactions. *Experimental Brain Research* 140(1): 34–45.

Hoff, B., and M.A. Arbib. 1993. Models of trajectory formation and temporal interaction of reach and grasp. *Journal of Motor Behavior* 25(3):175–92.

Hogan, N., and D. Sternad. 2007. On rhythmic and discrete movements: Reflections, definitions and implications for motor control. *Experimental Brain Research* 181(1):13–30.

Houk, J.C., W.Z. Rymer. 1981. Neural control of muscle length and tension. In *Handbook of physiology, sect. 1: The nervous system, vol. II: Motor control, Part 1,* ed., V.B. Brooks, 257–323. Bethesda, MD: American Physiological Society.

Huys, R., B.E. Studenka, N.L. Rheaume, H.N. Zelaznik, and V.K. Jirsa. 2008. Distinct timing mechanisms produce discrete and continuous movements. *PLoS Comput Biology* 4(4):e1000061.

Inooka, H., and T. Koitabashi. 1990. Experimental studies of manual optimization in control tasks. *IEEE Control Systems Magazine* 10(5):20–23.

Ivanenko, Y.P., R. Grasso, M. Zago, M. Molinari, G. Scivoletto, V. Castellano, et al. 2003. Temporal components of the motor patterns expressed by the human spinal cord reflect foot kinematics. *Journal of Neurophysiology* 90(5):3555–65.

Izawa, J., T. Rane, O. Donchin, and R. Shadmehr. 2008. Motor adaptation as a process of reoptimization. *Journal of Neuroscience* 28(11):2883–91.

Jindrich, D.L., and R.J. Full. 2002. Dynamic stabilization of rapid hexapedal locomotion. *Journal of Experimental Biology* 205(18):2803–23.

Kargo, W.J., and S.F. Giszter. 2008. Individual premotor drive pulses, not time-varying synergies, are the units of adjustment for limb trajectories constructed in spinal cord. *Journal of Neuroscience* 28(10):2409–25.

Kawato, M. 1996. Bi-directional theory approach to integration. In *Attention and performance, vol. XVI: Information integration in perception and communication*, eds., T. Inui and J.M. McClelland, 335–67. Cambridge, MA: MIT Press.

Kawato, M. 1999. Internal models for motor control and trajectory planning. *Current Opinion in Neurobiology* 9(6):718–27.

Kiemel, T., K.S. Oie, and J.J. Jeka. 2002. Multisensory fusion and the stochastic structure of postural sway. *Biological Cybernetics* 87(4):262–77.

Kistemaker, D.A., A.J. van Soest, and M.F. Bobbert. 2006. Is equilibrium point control feasible for fast goal-directed single-joint movements? *Journal of Neurophysiology* 95(5):2898–912.

Kistemaker, D.A., A.K. van Soest, and M.F. Bobbert. 2007. Equilibrium point control cannot be refuted by experimental reconstruction of equilibrium point trajectories. *Journal of Neurophysiology* 98(3):1075–082.

Klein Breteler, M.D., K.J. Simura, and M. Flanders. 2007. Timing of muscle activation in a hand movement sequence. *Cerebral Cortex* 17(4):803–15.

Krishnamoorthy, V., M.L. Latash, J.P. Scholz, and V. Zatsiorsky. 2003. Muscle synergies during shifts of the center of pressure by standing persons. *Experimental Brain Research* 152(3):281–92.

Krouchev, N., J.F. Kalaska, and T. Drew. 2006. Sequential activation of muscle synergies during locomotion in the intact cat as revealed by cluster analysis and direct decomposition. *Journal of Neurophysiology* 96(4):1991–2010.

Kubow, T.M., and R.J. Full. 1999. The role of the mechanical system in control: A hypothesis of self-stabilization in hexapedal runners. *Philosophical Transactions of the Royal Society of London. Series B, Biological Sciences* 354(1385):849–61.

Latash, M.L., A.S. Aruin, and M.B. Shapiro. 1995. The relation between posture and movement: A study of a simple synergy in a two-joint task. *Human Movement Science* 14(1):79–107.

Latash, M.L., J.P. Scholz, and G. Schöner. 2007. Toward a new theory of motor synergies. *Motor Control* 11(3):276–308.

Lee, W.A. 1984. Neuromotor synergies as a basis for coordinated intentional action. *Journal of Motor Behavior* 16(2):135–70.

Lemay, M.A., and W.M. Grill. 2004. Modularity of motor output evoked by intraspinal microstimulation in cats. *Journal of Neurophysiology* 91(1):502–14.

Li, W. 2006. Optimal control for biological movement systems. Ph.D. thesis, University of California, San Diego.

Liu, D., and E. Todorov. 2007. Evidence for the flexible sensorimotor strategies predicted by optimal feedback control. *Journal of Neuroscience* 27(35):9354–68.

Loram, I.D., and M. Lakie. 2002. Direct measurement of human ankle stiffness during quiet standing: The intrinsic mechanical stiffness is insufficient for stability. *Journal of Physiology* 545(3):1041–53.

Macpherson, J.M. 1988. Strategies that simplify the control of quadrupedal stance. II. Electromyographic activity. *Journal of Neurophysiology* 60(1):218–31.

Macpherson, J.M. 1991. How flexible are muscle synergies? In *Motor control: Concepts and issues*, eds., D.R. Humphrey and H.J. Freund, 33–48. Chichester, UK: Wiley.

Maier, M.A., and M.C. Hepp-Reymond. 1995. EMG activation patterns during force production in precision grip. 2. Muscular synergies in the spatial and temporal domain. *Experimental Brain Research* 103(1):123–36.

Martin, V. 2006. A dynamical systems account of the uncontrolled manifold and motor equivalence in human pointing movements. Ph.D. thesis, Institut fur Neuroinformatik, Ruhr Universitat Bochum.

Massion, J. 1992. Movement, posture and equilibrium: Interaction and coordination. *Progress in Neurobiology* 38(1):35–56.

Mazzoni, P., A. Hristova, and J.W. Krakauer. 2007. Why don't we move faster? Parkinson's disease, movement vigor, and implicit motivation. *Journal of Neuroscience* 27(27):7105–16.

Mercer, V.S., and S.A. Sahrmann. 1999. Postural synergies associated with a stepping task. *Physical Therapy* 79(12):1142–52.

Meyer, D.E., R.A. Abrams, S. Kornblum, C.E. Wright, and J.E.K. Smith. 1988. Optimality in human motor performance: Ideal control of rapid aimed movement. *Psychological Review* 95(3):340–70.

Moore, S.P., D.S. Rushmer, S.L. Windus, and L.M. Nashner. 1988. Human automatic postural responses: Responses to horizontal perturbations of stance in multiple directions. *Experimental Brain Research* 73(3):648–58.

Morasso, P.G., and V. Sanguineti. 2002. Ankle muscle stiffness alone cannot stabilize balance during quiet standing. *Journal of Neurophysiology* 88(4):2157–62.

Morasso, P.G., and M. Schieppati. 1999. Can muscle stiffness alone stabilize upright standing? *Journal of Neurophysiology* 82(3):1622–26.

Mussa-Ivaldi, F.A. 1997. Nonlinear force fields: A distributed system of control primitives for representing and learning movements. *Proceedings of the IEEE International Symposium on Computational Intelligence in Robotics and Automation*, 84–90.

Mussa-Ivaldi, F.A., and E. Bizzi. 2000. Motor learning through the combination of primitives. *Philosophical Transactions of the Royal Society of London. Series B, Biological Sciences* 355(1404):1755–69.

Nashner, L.M., and G. McCollum. 1985. The organization of human postural movements: A formal basis and experimental synthesis. *Behavioral Brain Science* 8(1):135–72.

Newell, K.M. 1991. Motor skill acquisition. *Annual Review of Psychology* 42:213–37.

Nishikawa, K., A.A. Biewener, P. Aert, A.N. Ahn, H.J. Chiel, M.A. Daley, et al. 2007. Neuromechanics: An integrative approach for understanding motor control. *Integrative and Comparative Biology* 47(1):16–54.

Ostry, D.J., and A.G. Feldman. 2003. A critical evaluation of the force control hypothesis in motor control. *Experimental Brain Research* 153(3):275–88.

O'Sullivan, I., E. Burdet, and J. Diedrichsen. 2009. Dissociating variability and effort as determinants of coordination. *PLoS Computative Biology* 5(4):e1000345.

Overduin, S.A., A. d'Avella, J. Roh, and E. Bizzi. 2008. Modulation of muscle synergy recruitment in primate grasping. *Journal of Neuroscience*, 28(4):880–92.

Pellegrini, J.J., and M. Flanders. 1996. Force path curvature and conserved features of muscle activation. *Experimental Brain Research* 110(1):80–90.

Quaia, C., and L.M. Optican. 1998. Commutative saccadic generator is sufficient to control a 3-D ocular plant with pulleys. *Journal of Neurophysiology* 79(6): 3197–215.

Raibert, M.H., J.A. Hodgins. 1993. Legged robots. In *Biological neural networks in invertebrate neuroethology and robotics*, eds., R. Beer, R. Ritzmann and T. McKenna, 319–54. Boston, MA: Academic Press.

Richardson, A.G., J.J. Slotine, E. Bizzi, and M.C. Tresch. 2005. Intrinsic musculoskeletal properties stabilize wiping movements in the spinalized frog. *Journal of Neuroscience* 25(12):3181–91.

Rothwell, J.C., M.M. Traub, B.L. Day, J.A. Obeso, P.K. Thomas, and C.D. Marsden. 1982. Manual motor performance in a deafferented man. *Brain* 105(3):515–42.

Rushmer, D.S., C.J. Russell, J.M. Macpherson, J.O. Phillips, and D.C. Dunbar. 1983. Automatic postural responses in the cat: Responses to headward and tailward translation. *Experimental Brain Research* 50(1):45–61.

Saunders, J.A., and D.C. Knill. 2004. Visual feedback control of hand movements. *Journal of Neuroscience* 24(13):3223–34.

Schaal, S., P. Mohajerian, and A. Ijspeert. 2007. Dynamics systems vs. optimal control: A unifying view. *Progress in Brain Research,* 165:425–45.

Schaal, S., D. Sternad, R. Osu, and M. Kawato. 2004. Rhythmic arm movement is not discrete. *Nature Neuroscience* 7(10):1136–43.

Schepens, B., and T. Drew. 2003. Strategies for the integration of posture and movement during reaching in the cat. *Journal of Neurophysiology* 90(5):3066–86.

Schöner, G. 1990. A dynamic theory of coordination of discrete movement. *Biological Cybernetics* 63(4):257–70.

Schöner, G. 1995. Recent developments and problems in human movement science and their conceptual implications. *Ecological Psychology* 7(4):291–314.

Schöner, G. 2002. Timing, clocks, and dynamical systems. *Brain Cognition* 48(1):31–51.

Schöner, G., and J.A.S. Kelso. 1988. Dynamic pattern generation in behavioral and neural systems. *Science* 239(4847):1513–20.

Shadmehr, R., and M.A. Arbib. 1992. A mathematical analysis of the force-stiffness characteristics of muscles in control of a single joint system. *Biological Cybernetics* 66(6):463–77.

Shadmehr, R., and J.W. Krakauer. 2008. A computational neuroanatomy for motor control. *Experimental Brain Research* 185(3):359–81.

Shadmehr, R., and F.A. Mussa-IvaldiA. 1994. Adaptive representation of dynamics during learning a motor task. *Journal of Neuroscience* 14(5Pt2):3208–24.

Shapiro, M.B., A.S. Aruin, and M.L. Latash. 1995. Velocity-dependent activation of postural muscles in a simple two-joint synergy. *Human Movement Science* 14(3):351–69.

Sherback, M., and R. D'Andrea. 2008. Visuomotor optimality and its utility in parametrization of response. *IEEE Transactions on Bio-medical Engineering* 55(7):1783–91.

Soechting, J.F., M. Flanders. 1998. Movement planning: Kinematics, dynamics, both or neither? In *Vision and action*, eds., L.R. Harris and M. Jenkin, 332–49. Cambridge, UK: Cambridge University Press.

Soechting, J.F., and F. Lacquaniti. 1989. An assessment of the existence of muscles synergies during load perturbations and intentional movements of the human arm. *Experimental Brain Research* 74(3):535–48.

Sporns, O., and G.M. Edelman. 1993. Solving Bernstein's problem: A proposal for the development of coordinated movement by selection. *Child Development* 64(4):960–81.

St-Onge, N., S.V. Adamovich, and A.G. Feldman. 1997. Control processes underlying elbow flexion movements may be independent of kinematic and electromyographic patterns: Experimental study and modelling. *Neuroscience* 79(1):295–316.

Stengel, R.F. 1986. *Stochastic optimal control: Theory and application*. New York: Wiley.

Ting, L.H., and J.M. Macpherson. 2005. A limited set of muscle synergies for force control during a postural task. *Journal of Neurophysiology* 93(1):609–13.

Todorov, E. 1998. Studies of goal-directed movements. Ph. D. thesis, Department of Brain and Cognitive Sciences, Massachusetts Institut of Technology, Cambridge, MA.

Todorov, E. 2004. Optimality principles in sensorimotor control. *Nature Neuroscience* 7(9):907–15.

Todorov, E. 2005. Stochastic optimal control and estimation methods adapted to the noise characteristics of the sensorimotor system. *Neural Computations* 17(5):1084–108.

Todorov, E., and M.I. Jordan. 2002. Optimal feedback control as a theory of motor coordination. *Nature Neuroscience* 5(11):1226–35.

Todorov, E., and W. Li. 2005. A generalized iterative LQG method for locally-optimal feedback control of constrained nonlinear stochastic systems. *Proceedings of the American Control Conference* 1:300–06.

Torres, E.B., and D. Zipser. 2002. Reaching to grasp with a multi-jointed arm. I. Computational model. *Journal of Neurophysiology* 88(5):2355–67.

Torres-Oviedo, G., J.M. Macpherson, and L.H. Ting. 2006. Muscle synergy organization is robust across a variety of postural perturbations. *Journal of Neurophysiology* 96(3):1530–46.

Torres-Oviedo, G., and L.H. Ting. 2007. Muscle synergies characterizing human postural responses. *Journal of Neurophysiology* 98(4):2144–56.

Tran, M.T., P. Souères, M. Taïx, and E. Guigon. 2008. A principled approach to biological motor control for generating humanoid robot reaching movements. *Proceedings of the 2nd IEEE RAS & EMBS International Conference on Biomedical Robotics and Biomechatronics*, 783–88.

Tresch, M., and A. Jarc. 2009. The case for and against muscle synergies. *Current Opinion in Neurobiology* 19(6):601–07.

Turvey, M.T., R.E. Shaw, W. Mace. 1978. Issues in the theory of action: Degrees of freedom, coordinative structures and coalitions. In *Attention and performance, vol. VII*, ed., J. Requin, 557–98. Hillsdale, NJ: Erlbaum.

Tweed, D. 2007. Sensorimotor optimization in higher dimensions. *Progress in Brain Research* 165:181–91.

Uno, Y., M. Kawato, and R. Suzuki. 1989. Formation and control of optimal trajectory in human multijoint arm movement: Minimum torque change model. *Biological Cybernetics* 61(2):89–101.

Valero-Cuevas, F.J., M. Venkadesan, and E. Todorov. 2009. Structured variability of muscle activations supports the minimal intervention principle of motor control. *Journal of Neurophysiology* 102(1):59–68.

Valero-Cuevas, F.J., J.W. Yi, D. Brown, R.V. McNamara, C. Paul, and H. Lipson. 2007. The tendon network of the fingers performs anatomical computation at a macroscopic scale. *IEEE Transactions on Bio-medical Engineering* 54(6Pt2): 1161–66.

van Beers, R.J., P. Haggard, and D.M. Wolpert. 2004. The role of execution noise in movement variability. *Journal of Neurophysiology* 91(2):1050–63.

van Ingen Schenau, G.J. 1989. From rotation to translation: Constraints in multi-joint movements and the unique role of biarticular muscles. *Human Movement Science* 8(4):301–37.

van Soest, A.J., and L.A. Rozendaal. 2008. The inverted pendulum model of bipedal standing cannot be stabilized through direct feedback of force and contractile element length and velocity at realistic series elastic element stiffness. *Biological Cybernetics* 99(1):29–41.

Vereijken, B., R.E.A. van Emmerik, H.T.A. Whiting, and K.M. Newell. 1992. Free(z) ing degrees of freedom in skill acquisition. *Journal of Motor Behavior* 24(1): 133–42.

Wadman, W.J., J.J. Denier van der Gon, R.H. Geuze, and C.R. Mol. 1979. Control of fast goal-directed arm movements. *Journal of Human Movement Studies* 5:3–17.

Wallace, S.A. 1981. An impulse-timing theory for reciprocal control of muscular activity in rapid, discrete movement. *Journal of Motor Behavior* 13(3):1144–60.

Winter, D.A., A.E. Patla, F. Prince, M. Ishac, and K. Gielo-Perczak. 1998. Stiffness control of balance in quiet standing. *Journal of Neurophysiology* 80(3):1211–21.

Wolpert, D.W., and Z. Ghahramani. 2000. Computational principles of movement neuroscience. *Nature Neuroscience* 3(Suppl):1212–17.

Wolpert, D.M., Z. Ghahramani, and M.I. Jordan. 1995. An internal model for sensorimotor integration. *Science* 269:1880–82.

Wong, A.M.F. 2004. Listing's law: Clinical significance and implications for neural control. *Survey of Ophthalmology* 49(6):563–75.

Zajac, F.E. 1989. Muscle and tendon: Models, scaling, and application to biomechanics and motor control. *Critical Reviews in Biomedical Engineering* 17(4): 359–415.

Zattara, M., and S. Bouisset. 1986. Chronometric analysis of the posturo-kinetic programming of voluntary movement. *Journal of Motor Behavior* 18(2):215–23.

Index

Note: Page numbers followed by "*f*" and "*t*" denote figures and tables, respectively.